CRITICAL
THINKING
IN
RESPIRATORY
CARE

A Problem-Based Learning Approach

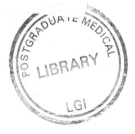

NOTICE

CRITICAL THINKING IN RESPIRATORY CARE

A Problem-Based Learning Approach

Shelley C. Mishoe, PhD, RRT, FAARC

Professor, Respiratory Therapy and Graduate Studies
Associate Dean, School of Allied Health Sciences
Medical College of Georgia
Augusta, Georgia

Melvin A. Welch, Jr., MPH, RRT, RCP

Professor
Health Science Department
Santa Monica College
Santa Monica, California

McGraw-Hill
MEDICAL PUBLISHING DIVISION

New York   Chicago   San Francisco   Lisbon   London
Madrid   Mexico City   Milan   New Delhi   San Juan
Seoul   Singapore   Sydney   Toronto

McGraw-Hill

*A Division of The **McGraw·Hill** Companies*

1234567890 DOC DOC 01234567890

ISBN 0-07-134474-8

This book was set in Times by V&M Graphics / Joanna V. Pomeranz.
The editors were Sally J. Barhydt and Karen Davis.
The production supervisor was Lisa T. Mendez.
The cover designer was Mary McKeon.
The text was designed by Marsha Cohen / Parallelogram.
The index was prepared by Editorial Services / Maria Coughlin.
R.R. Donnelley/Crawfordsville was printer and binder.

This book is printed on acid-free paper.

Library of Congress Cataloging-in-Publication Data
Clinical thinking in respiratory care : a problem-based learning approach / [edited by]
Shelley C. Mishoe, Melvin A Welch, Jr.
     p. ; cm.
  ISBN 0-07-134474-8
   1. Respiratory therapy. 2. Respiratory therapy — Decision making. I. Mishoe, Shelley
C., 1955-II. Welch, Melvin A.
  [DNLM: 1. Respiratory Tract Diseases—therapy. 2. Problem-based Learning. 3.
Respiratory Therapy. WF 145 C934 2001]
  RC735.I5 C75 2001
  616.2'0046—dc21   00-065390

Dedication

This book would not be possible without the love and support of my husband, Ken Mishoe, and our sons, Wesley and Jeffrey. I spent many weekends and evenings working first on my dissertation, which is the basis for the critical thinking framework for this textbook, and then over these past three years working on this project. My family's support has been profound throughout these times. I dedicate this book to my family with love, admiration, and appreciation for their genuine interest in my work and my life. I also pay tribute with this book to all who strive to improve their critical thinking through their reflective skepticism, self-discipline, lifelong learning, and openness to new ideas, strategies, and possibilities.

S.C.M.

I am indebted to the hundreds of students I have worked with over the past 25 plus years in respiratory care education. Their endless desire to learn, to understand, and to grasp for success has provided me the inspiration and motivation to continue to strive to improve my ability to motivate and teach those who desire to learn. I am hopeful that this text will aid those who wish to develop their knowledge and skills beyond that of simple "knowing of facts." I also owe my wife of 28 years, Cheryl, daughter, Michelle, and son, Michael, for their continuing support and understanding as "Dad" once again buried himself in his "other" lifelong love . . . his profession.

M.A.W.

Acknowledgments

There are many people we would like to acknowledge that made this work possible. We thank Sally Barhydt, our editor, for her guidance, dedication, expertise and encouragement throughout all phases of the project. There are insufficient words to adequately thank our editor Karen Davis, for her attention to detail, responsiveness to our suggestions, and kind ways of dealing with unforeseen problems and delays. We also thank Steven Zollo for seeing the potential of our idea and providing valuable insight and work with the concept development, proposal, and approval in the early phases of this project. We thank Mike Shelton, who we affectionately refer to as "OUR" copyeditor, for his sense of how to improve our original chapters with corrections, questions, and suggestions. We acknowledge all contributors to this textbook, not only for their chapters, but also for their feedback throughout the project. We thank our faculty and students for the invaluable ways they facilitated our understanding and experience with problem-based learning to facilitate critical thinking. Finally, we acknowledge the respiratory therapists who participated in the research study of critical thinking, who are the unsung heroes of respiratory care. There are many others we acknowledge, too numerous to mention, in our classes, at our universities, at the hospitals and other clinical rotations, and in our professional organizations who we have helped shape our careers, ideas, and this textbook.

CONTENTS

PART II
PATIENT PROBLEMS IN RESPIRATORY CARE / 313

CONTRIBUTORS

R. Randall Baker, PhD, RRT, RCPT
Associate Professor and Interim Chair
Department of Respiratory Therapy
School of Allied Health Sciences
Medical College of Georgia
Augusta, Georgia

Paul Bellamy, MD
Professor of Medicine
University of California, Los Angeles Medical Center
Los Angeles, California

J. M. Cairo, PhD, RRT
Professor of Cardiopulmonary Science and Physiology
Department Head of Cardiopulmonary Science
School of Allied Health Professions
Louisiana State University Health Sciences Center
New Orleans, Louisiana

Bruce A Feistner, MSS, RRT
Associate Professor and Director
Respiratory Care Program
Dakota State University
Madison, South Dakota

Sheena Mari Ferguson, MSN, RN, CCRN
Pulmonary Clinical Nurse Specialist
Adult Cystic Fibrosis Center
University of New Mexico
  Health Sciences Center
Albuquerque, New Mexico

James B. Fink, MS, RRT, FAARC
Director, Respiratory Programs
AeroGen, Inc.
Sunnyvale, CA
Research Associate, Pulmonary and Critical Care
Loyola Chicago Stritch School of Medicine
Maywood, Illinois

Brian H. Foresman, DO, FCCP, FACSM
Medical Director, Indiana University Center for
  Sleep Disorders
Medical Director, MidWest Regional Sleep
  Disorders Center
Clinical Assistant Professor of Medicine
Indiana University Schoo of Medicine
Indianapolis, Indiana

Linda Thomas Goodfellow, EdD, MBA, RRT
Director of Clinical Education
Department of Cardiopulmonary Care Services
Georgia State University
Atlanta, Georgia

Charles R. Hall, Sr., MS, RRT, RPFT
Assistant Professor, School of Allied Health Sciences
Department of Respiratory Therapy
Medical College of Georgia
Augusta, Georgia

Kathleen M. Hernlen, MBA, RRT
Instructor, School of Allied Health Sciences
Department of Respiratory Therapy
Medical Colleges of Georgia
Augusta, Georgia

Timothy B. Op't Holt, EdD, RRT
Professor, Cardiorespiratory Care
University of South Alabama
Mobile, Alabama

Tara Orfanello Jones, BS, RRT
Instructor, Department of Cardiopulmonary Science
School of Allied Health Professions
Louisiana State University Health Sciences Center
New Orleans, Louisiana

Robert Wayne Lawson, MS, RRT
Assistant Professor, School of Allied Health Sciences
Department of Respiratory Care
University of Texas Health Science Center
    at San Antonio
San Antonio, Texas

Terry S. LeGrand, PhD, RRT
Assistant Professor, School of Allied Health Sciences
Director of Clinical Education
Department of Respiratory Care
The University of Texas Health Science Center
    at San Antonio
San Antonio, Texas

Terry P. Lyle, MA, RRT
Respiratory Care Program Director
Modesto Junior College
Modesto, California

Stephen P. Mikles, EdS, RRT
Professor and Program Director
Saint Petersburg Junior College
Pinellas Park, Florida

Pamela Minkley, RPSGT, RRT
Supervisor, Ingham Regional Sleep / Wake Center
Ingham Regional Medical Center
Lansing, Michigan

Shelley C. Mishoe, PhD, RRT, FAARC
Professor, Respiratory Therapy and Graduate Studies
Associate Dean, School of Allied Health Sciences
Medical College of Georgia
Augusta, Georgia

Orna Molayeme, MA, RRT
Respiratory Therapy Department
University of California, Los Angeles Medical Center
Los Angeles, California

Joseph A. Morelos, BS, RRT
Clinical Instructor
Respiratory Therapy Program
Albuquerque Technical-Vocational Institute
Albuquerque, New Mexico

Leslie C. Patzwahl, BS, RRT
Clinical Specialist
Department of Pulmonary and Critical Care Medicine
The Cleveland Clinic Foundation
Cleveland, Ohio

Mary L. Reinesch, BA, RRT
Director of Clinical Education,
Respiratory Care Program
Dakota State University
Madison, South Dakota

Salvatore A. Sanders, MS, RRT, CPFT
Instructional Technology Specialist
Center for Teaching and Learning Technology
Youngstown State University
Youngstown, Ohio

David C. Shelledy, PhD, RRT
Chair, Department of Respiratory Care
University of Texas Health Sciences Center
    at San Antonio
San Antonio, Texas

Robert Tanaka, MD, FCCP
Gould Medical
Modesto, California

J. Michael Thompson, BS, RRT, RPFT
Associate Professor and Director of Clinical Education
Respiratory Therapy Program, East Los Angeles College
Monterey Park, California

Amy Travis, BS, RRT
Staff Respiratory Therapist
Charleston Pulmonary Associates
Charleston, South Carolina

Melvin A. Welch, Jr., MPH, RRT, RCP
Professor, Health Science Department
Santa Monica College
Santa Monica, California

John Wright, MBA, BS, RRT
Assistant Director
Respiratory Therapy Department
University of California, Los Angeles Medical Center
Los Angeles, California

PREFACE

Why This Textbook?

A major trend which influences *Critical Thinking in Respiratory Care* is the interest in preparing and developing a new kind of respiratory care practitioner who can function effectively in current and future health care delivery systems. It is a tremendous challenge to prepare graduates to have the clinical assessment and decision-making skills that they need to become competent practitioners. Traditionally, we have trained respiratory therapists and other health professionals to work primarily in acute care to treat disease using clinical knowledge. Today, we are challenged further to prepare graduates who can work in a variety of health care settings with an emphasis on health promotion and disease management.

Graduates must also have additional skills beyond their clinical and technical expertise. Additional professional skills required in respiratory care and health care include teamwork, communications, collaborative problem solving, and development of care plans. Health care professionals must also have an appreciation of patient education needs, ethics, quality of life issues, and economic factors. Consequently, there is growing interest in problem-based learning. *Critical Thinking in Respiratory Care: A Problem-Based Learning Approach* is the first book to address these issues and learning needs. This book appears at a crucial time in the development of the respiratory therapy profession and fills a need as an authoritative source for the preparation of a new kind of health care professional.

The major goal of this book is to provide information and learning experiences for students to develop a deep and broad understanding of respiratory care content based on sound clinical decision making. This book provides strategies to enhance cognitive and practical critical thinking skills and traits by incorporating numerous individual and group exercises. This book requires students to solve practical problems in health care and respiratory care using a case-based approach. In addition, faculty will find several options with instructions on how to use the textbook to incorporate problem-based learning (PBL) in their curricula. Critical thinking is essential for effective respiratory care practice across the continuum of health care, which is greatly influenced today by managed care. Educators want to enhance students' critical thinking, but they may lack the resources to design and evaluate effective learning experiences. This book includes actual clinical cases for critical analysis, patient assessment, clinical application, discussion, and decision making.

Why Problem-Based Learning?

PBL is a process by which learners work their way through situations, often solving "problems" that arise while working through "cases." This method of learning is believed to be particularly useful in developing an understanding of the material beyond the simple learning of "facts." The PBL process is student directed, allowing for trial and error and learning through mistakes, research, discussion, and reflection. The role of faculty is to facilitate the process while giving the learner much control over the direction of their learning (the discussions, research, pace, sequencing). Consequently, PBL assists in developing the learners' problem-solving and critical thinking abilities and traits.

PBL is a process; however, a textbook is a product. Consequently, a major challenge to creation of this textbook was to take this "process of PBL" and to provide enough structure and direction in the chapters, while still leaving room for students to provide direction in resolving the problems presented. The "Critical Thinking Exercises" accomplish this, with expert responses to the various exercises available only in the Instructor Guide. The "expert responses" often identify multiple responses, each potentially appropriate to the various exercises posed during the cases. Furthermore, the cases and exercises are designed in such a way to allow for continual incorporation of the newest and best evidence as the most appropriate suggestions and solutions for the particular problem. Often there is not one correct solution or response being advocated.

In addition, the Instructor Guide provides advice for faculty on several variations of a PBL approach that may be used to incorporate the textbook into their curricula across a variety of courses. This book is ideal for incorporation into traditional pathophysiology courses, providing a fresh, new approach. This book is unique in that it focuses on biopsychosocial aspects of cardiorespiratory disease and does not provide "answers" with the text. We decided early in this project that potential responses and expert opinions would be available to faculty, but not students. The success of this book will partly depend on the ability of educators to provide students with timely, consistent, and detailed feedback without undermining the intent of the book through wide circulation of the instructor-intended supporting materials.

There are two major sections to this book. Part I consists of the first ten chapters that are background material to provide students with a foundation that will give them a better understanding of PBL, critical thinking, problem solving, and selected topics. The selected topics are those that we feel are particularly important to understand prior to attempting to solve the problems brought forth in the case chapters. Part II consists of thirteen chapters that focus on developing the student's critical thinking skills through

cases that deal with various common respiratory illnesses. With our contributors, we made a definitive choice to include cases that are most likely to appear on credentialing examinations, including the Written Registry Examinations and the Clinical Simulation Examinations offered by the National Board for Respiratory Care.

The book is different in that it accepts the reality that health care and respiratory care practice are complex, and that critical thinking dictates that there are often multiple solutions to the problems we encounter. Students must be aware that in "real life" there is often not just one perspective or one answer.

Why "Critical Thinking" for Respiratory Therapists?

The days of "task orientation" are numbered. The respiratory therapists who want to just "follow physician orders and perform procedures" are rapidly becoming a disappearing species. The changing health care delivery systems demand practitioners who can be "resource managers" to ensure the focus of care is on quality and cost-effectiveness with an emphasis on outcomes. To maximize our professional potential and contribute to quality patient care, critical thinking skills and traits must become the "norm" not the exception.

A famous person once said something like this when referring to problems of poverty and hunger, "it is better to teach a person to fish and farm, than to give them food." After many years of teaching respiratory care we have come to the conclusion that it is far better to teach the student how to think and learn than to give them lots of facts to memorize about respiratory care. We hope our efforts provide students, educators, and practitioners with insight, knowledge, and experiences to help them think and learn throughout life.

Shelley C. Mishoe
Melvin A. Welch, Jr.

PART

I

PROFESSIONAL SKILLS IN RESPIRATORY CARE

1

INTRODUCTION TO PROBLEM-BASED LEARNING

Shelley C. Mishoe

Learning without thought is labor lost.
CONFUCIUS

LEARNING OBJECTIVES

1. Describe problem-based learning (PBL).
2. Compare traditional teaching methods and PBL to enhance learners' critical thinking.
3. Compare and contrast the similarities and differences between covering the material (lecture) and learning the material (PBL).
4. Discuss the goals of PBL and the various roles of students and facilitators.
5. Differentiate the teacher as lecturer and the teacher as facilitator.
6. Describe the importance of student participation in PBL discussions and ways students can overcome reluctance or hesitancy to speak.
7. Elaborate the various ways that students are graded for PBL curricula and courses.
8. Discuss how PBL and evidenced-based medicine (EBM) should be incorporated together to develop an evidence-based approach to respiratory care practice.
9. Explain why self-directed and lifelong learning is essential for respiratory therapists.
10. Utilize the exercises and cases in this textbook to develop the skills and traits for critical thinking and an evidence-based approach to practice.

KEY WORDS

Critical Thinking Exercises
Evidence-Based Medicine (EBM)
Facilitator
Group Exercises
Learning Guide
Learning Issues
Levels of Evidence
Patient Problem
Peer Evaluation
Problem-Based Learning (PBL)
Reader
Scribe
Strength of the Evidence
Traditional Teaching
Tutor

ESSENTIALS OF PROBLEM-BASED LEARNING (PBL)

What is PBL?

Problem-based learning (PBL) is a student-centered rather than a teacher-centered approach to learning. With PBL, students actively learn their discipline while solving problems like the ones they will encounter in the real world when they graduate. PBL is a teaching-learning strategy that places more emphasis on learning and less emphasis on teaching.

Unlike the lecture method of teaching, the PBL approach assumes that students are self-directed learners who can work together to solve practice-related problems. With PBL, the role of faculty shifts from that of lecturer to one of coach, facilitator, mentor, and tutor. PBL permits students to have some influence over the direction, speed, and depth of their instruction. Most importantly, PBL focuses on development of cognitive strategies and professional skills including teamwork, communication, and clinical decision making. Later sections dealing with implementation and evaluation will further explain PBL.

CRITICAL CONTENT

PROBLEM-BASED LEARNING (PBL)

A teaching-learning strategy whereby students direct their learning by working in small groups to solve problems like the ones they will encounter in the real world in their professional practice.

How is PBL Different from Lecture-Based Courses?

PBL requires students to direct their learning by working through problems, asking questions, doing research, working in groups, using current evidence to make informed decisions, and discussing pertinent aspects of health care. With the traditional lecture method, the teacher decides what is important and how a course will proceed. In addition, some teachers rely heavily on textbooks and lecture notes as primary resources, even though the information may be out-of-date or unnecessarily biased. PBL requires learners to research current topics and controversial aspects of practice to enhance their professional development.

In practice, the health care professional must be able to seek information and answers to patient problems using a variety of resources. Respiratory therapists need the experience and skills to identify alternatives to solve work-related problems in the real world. Passively listening to lectures does not contribute to the abilities to critically read, write, speak, or think. Therefore the traditional lecture does not adequately prepare health care professionals to acquire skills that can be applied to clinical practice. Generally, students taught by the lecture method cannot apply their knowledge to solve problems or make decisions. There is little transfer of learning to the clinical setting. Unlike PBL, traditional teaching does not challenge students to research topics of interest or to independently review areas of weakness. Furthermore, students are rarely able to bring up topics for discussion such as related clinical cases or something relevant they learned in previous semesters.

In actual practice, there are usually multiple approaches to patient care and numerous possibilities to choose from when deciding what is best for each patient. PBL shifts the responsibility for ascertaining the answers from the teacher to the learner. Today it is rare that any single person or resource has all the answers to the clinical problems that arise. Lecture-based courses perpetuate the idea that there is only ONE correct answer and that the teacher is the expert who has all the answers! During lectures, some instructors discourage questions from students or even refuse to answer questions because they find it distracting to their presentation. In some cases, instructors may not like being put on the spot and having to come up with responses to questions because they have the erroneous idea that they should be able to answer all questions! PBL promotes and develops students' questioning and analytical skills. Furthermore, PBL provides opportunities for students to find and use medical information to solve practical, clinical problems.

PBL encourages group problem solving through interactive discussion of complex and controversial topics. This type of experience helps novices to understand the complexities of solving clinical problems. In health care today, the team approach is emphasized and required so that patients can benefit from the collective expertise of specialists in medicine and the other health care disciplines. PBL shifts the traditional role of the faculty member from one of expert to that of role model, colleague, and team member.

The instructional setting for PBL is usually a small group (6 to 7 students) with a faculty tutor who facilitates the group learning process. The faculty member functions as an equal member of the group, relinquishing ownership of the group learning process to the students. A skilled facilitator may be able to handle a larger group discussion. However, as the number of people in a group increases, the increased size can jeopardize the opportunity for equal participation by all students. Equal participation of all students promotes self-directed learning and enhances student opportunities to develop their reasoning and communication skills.

Is PBL New?

PBL is not a new teaching-learning strategy, but it is being utilized more than ever before. The problem-based curriculum originates in medicine and is built upon research into the problem-solving skills of physicians and principles of educational psychology.[1] More recently, PBL has been advocated as a useful way to educate allied health care practitioners for the future. PBL is utilized in many professional programs, including architecture, engineering, aviation, medicine, psychology, nursing, occupational therapy, physical therapy, physician assistant, and respiratory therapy programs.[2–7]

The term *problem-based learning* must be considered a genus for which there are many species and subspecies, with each addressing different objectives to varying degrees.[1] The essential components of PBL include an integrated curriculum rather than one separated into clinical and theoretical components; curriculum organized around problems versus disciplines; and an emphasis on cognitive skills as well as knowledge.[8] There are various approaches to incorporating PBL into professional preparation curricula. There are also numerous approaches to implementation of PBL itself.

CRITICAL CONTENT

COMPARISON OF PBL WITH TRADITIONAL TEACHING

PBL

- Student-directed
- Active learning
- Centered on patient cases
- Emphasis on cognitive skills
- Curriculum organized around problems
- Retrieval and use of medical information
- Centers on group discussion, communication skills, and problem solving
- Addresses biological, clinical, and psychosocial issues

LECTURE

- Teacher-directed
- Passive listening
- Centered on lecture notes
- Emphasis on knowledge acquisition
- Curriculum organized around disciplines
- Relies on textbooks and notes
- Centers on listening, independent reading, testing to assess knowledge
- Primarily focuses on treatment of pathophysiology

What Are the Goals of PBL?

PBL enables students to direct their own learning by using a variety of resources to manage and solve work-related problems that are similar to the actual problems they will encounter in professional practice. Students are encouraged to discuss and evaluate the **biological**, **clinical**, and **psychosocial** issues related to the clinical problem. Biological issues include application of knowledge from the basic sciences, including physiology and pathophysiology. Clinical issues include the various aspects of the prevention, diagnosis, treatment, and long-term management of disease. Psychosocial issues include patient understanding, education, compliance, and self-management, as well as societal factors such as ethics, cost, and access, which influence health care. PBL also gives students experience discussing and evaluating the numerous issues involved in the diagnosis and management of acute and chronic cardiopulmonary disease.

The PBL approach requires students to draw upon their abilities to work collaboratively with others; to manage time and resources; and to develop the skills and characteristics of a critical thinker. Most importantly, students have the opportunity to interact with faculty mentors who role model critical thinking skills. Role modeling is perhaps the best strategy for developing the skills and traits needed by critical thinkers.[8,9]

How is PBL Implemented?

PBL utilizes progressive disclosure of an actual patient case to allow students the opportunity to solve problems similar to the ones they will encounter in clinical practice. During PBL courses faculty members assign students various clinical cases (the problems), which gradually unfold over multiple group sessions. **Part II of this textbook provides numerous clinical cases that allow students and faculty members to implement PBL.**

Scheduling PBL

Each group session may last anywhere from 2 to 4 hours depending on the clinical problem, learning issues, size of the group, students' abilities, and facilitator's skills. Faculty can determine along with the students the scheduling of patient problems (the cases), group sessions, and length of time of each session. For example, some programs may choose to meet for 3 hours once a week for 6 weeks to discuss each patient case (6 sessions). Another program may decide that groups will meet 2 times per week for 2 hours per session, requiring about 4 weeks (8 sessions). These decisions will determine the schedule for PBL during each semester of

a curriculum. There is no single best way for faculty to schedule PBL courses and patient cases. Faculty members of each program will need to experiment to find the best schedule for their students. Faculty must also determine the amount and types of program content to be incorporated into PBL courses versus those studied in lectures, labs, or clinical situations. The amount of PBL incorporated into any program is often determined by the size of the faculty and the number of students.

Group Learning Sessions

Each patient problem begins with a brief case scenario. During each group session, someone from the group acts as the "reader" who reads aloud the clinical problem given to the group by the facilitator. The group may decide to read **one line at a time**, one paragraph at a time, or one page at a time. We highly encourage students to read one line at a time, based on our experience facilitating PBL with both medical students and respiratory therapy students. Someone else from the group acts as the "scribe." The scribe records the discussions of the group using a blackboard, overhead projector, newsprint, or computer with projector, in such a way that everyone can see the group's notes. The scribe makes five columns to record information from the group discussions on what they know, what they need to know, what they hypothesize, what they recommend, and what topics they will research, as shown in Table 1-1. As one person reads the case line by line, the scribe records the group's discussions.

The students prepare the column entitled "What do we know," with the scribe writing down the information provided with the case (the patient problem). From this information, students determine what they need to know, which is equivalent to information-gathering on the clinical simulation examination (CSE). Students form hypotheses regarding what is happening with the patient, what might happen next, and what the health professionals should do as the case evolves.

During each session, the group decides their learning issues based on what information the group needs to solve the patient problem. The learning

TABLE 1-1   FORMAT TO RECORD A GROUP'S PBL DISCUSSIONS

Biological			Clinical		Psychosocial
What do we know?	What do we need to know?	What do we hypothesize?	What do we recommend?	What topics will we research?	

issues become the group's research project to be done prior to the next group meeting. Learning issues are formulated by the group when they realize they need to find information previously learned on a particular topic in order to apply it to this problem. Learning issues are also determined when the group realizes it is confronted by a new topic that no one knows much about, one that is important to understanding and solving the patient problem. Learning issues can be highly diverse, from the simple to the complex. The facilitator should help the group achieve an equitable and reasonable distribution of work to accomplish the required research. The facilitator should continually encourage students to apply the learning issue to the patient problem, reminding students why it became a topic for research and how the research facilitates understanding and management of the patient case.

The medical model for PBL utilizes three or four columns to record group discussions. However, we suggest adding a column to include respiratory therapy recommendations as shown in Table 1-1. The recommendation column can help respiratory therapy students to prepare for the NBRC examinations, especially the CSEs. Persons who take the advanced practice examinations must evaluate respiratory care recommendations throughout each CSE. Furthermore, the professional role of respiratory therapists requires clinicians who are prepared to make recommendations and provide input and feedback for the acute and chronic management of cardiopulmonary disease.[4] It is useful to give students access to the NBRC exam matrices so they will have a better understanding of the types of recommendations expected on the CSE and in practice.

Students evaluate what they know from the problem, what they need to know, and what they hypothesize. Based on the group discussions, students determine their recommendations for respiratory care. The group also collectively determines their learning issues. The scribe uses the last column to record students' learning issues. Students decide their learning issues when the group realizes they need to review or investigate a topic further to understand the clinical problem within each part of every case. The learning issues are essentially the subject areas and questions that require further research because the group is lacking information or the knowledge base to make further clinical decisions.

Research of Learning Issues

Students should be encouraged to incorporate an evidence-based approach to their research of learning issues and their problem solving, using evidence-based medicine (EBM) as described later in this chapter. Before PBL, students should have instruction on how to use MEDLINE to incorporate EBM and other resources into their research of learning issues. Faculty should also inform students that other resources for their research include clinical practice guidelines (CPGs), journal articles, indexes, dictionaries, textbooks, the Internet, and medical experts on and off campus. The faculty can provide a list of resources, including persons and agencies to contact for each particular case. Alternatively, the faculty can require students to identify their own resources as part of the PBL process. The faculty should work with experts in the community to build a rich, supportive resource pool of mentors who are willing to answer student questions, be interviewed, and provide materials such as patient data forms, patient surveys, and patient educational materials.

Students can use a variety of strategies within their PBL groups to tackle their leaning issues. Ideally, every student should research every learning issue so each member comes to the next meeting prepared with the knowledge necessary to discuss the case. Purists would argue that this approach is fundamental to true PBL because critical thinking can only occur with an informed understanding of the problem. However, it is possible to implement variations regarding how each group deals with their learning issues.

One alternative is to have selected students be responsible for researching specific learning issues, with each one assigned to report to the group at the next session. For example, at the end of each PBL session the group would finalize their learning issues and members of the group could negotiate who will research each learning issue. Each group member assumes responsibility to research the assigned learning issue(s) and report to the group at the next session. Another alternative would be to have random selection of the learning issues, leaving the individual assignments to chance. A third alternative would be some type of rotating order that would allow each student to take their turn at selecting first from the list of the learning issues that the group will research. Faculty and students should determine together which strategy would best meet the learning needs based on the resources, schedules, and patient problems.

After the students and faculty determine the group method for researching the learning issues, students self-direct their research efforts. Students gather information and data to resolve their assigned problem (either individually or in smaller groups).

When the entire group reconvenes, each member presents learning issues and provides handouts and information to present solutions to the group. Students must indicate the sources of their information so that the group can evaluate the accuracy, validity, and relevance of the information for solving the clinical problem. In addition, this part of the experience will encourage an evidence-based approach to clinical practice.

Group Process

After the initial session, students reconvene and discuss their learning issues. Every member of the group should have the scribed notes from previous sessions as well as all parts of the patient case as known to date. At the beginning of each session, the group identifies their reader and scribe. It is best for students to rotate these responsibilities. The students decide with assistance from their facilitator the amount of time dedicated to discussion of the learning issues. Following this part of the discussion (which generally takes about 60 to 90 minutes), the group continues with the patient problem through further disclosure of the patient case.

It is important to the group process that no one from the group reads ahead into the patient case because this can interfere with the discussion. Problem solving, communication, active listening, and assessment of the group's learning are best

CRITICAL CONTENT

GROUP PROCESS FOR PBL

- Everyone comes prepared for learning sessions.
- No one should read ahead because active listening is essential.
- Everyone should remain focused on discrete, specific pieces of information.
- The group works together to enhance one another's problem solving, communication, thinking, and decision making skills.

achieved if everyone remains focused on a discrete, limited amount of information. Since all of us can read and hear much faster than someone can speak, you can understand why this process is critically important. Later in the chapter, we describe how the groups should utilize the cases in Part II for PBL.

What Is the Role of the Facilitator?

PBL facilitators are guides and coaches, not lecturers or resources. I like to use the common expression that "The PBL facilitator is the coach on the side, not the sage on the stage!" This may sound simple, but the majority of faculty members will need training in facilitation to become effective facilitators. Since most of us were taught by lecture, it is difficult for faculty members to shift from the teaching role to the facilitating role. Although each facilitator has a personal style, his or her principal role is to promote student-centered learning and critical thinking within the group. Facilitators do this by posing nondirective questions at appropriate times to encourage analytical thought and aid the group process. The facilitator also helps to handle conflict within a group, promotes professional debate of controversial issues, provides feedback on individual and group performance, and provides direction to facilitate group learning.

The faculty facilitator should promote interaction, guide and focus discussion, help students integrate new and prior knowledge, and promote immediate feedback. During group sessions the facilitator should:

- Organize the group and establish a comfortable atmosphere
- Maintain a log of attendance, punctuality, and participation
- Assure the group has a reader, a scribe, and possibly a patient
- Distribute case materials
- Keep the group focused

Additionally, throughout a PBL course and curriculum the facilitator will:

- Monitor the discussion and keep records
- Stimulate group questions

- Assure self-evaluation at the end of each session (to assess process and performance)
- Evaluate student performance and participation
- Evaluate PBL learning modules
- Coordinate peer evaluations
- Obtain anonymous evaluations of the course and facilitator
- Assign grades

The facilitator should role model the desirable PBL behaviors by demonstrating **R**isk, **O**peness, **P**articipation, **E**xperience, and **S**ensitivity (ROPES). See the critical content box for specific examples of facilitating comments to role model. Gradually, students in the group will assume greater responsibility for facilitation and will be posing these types of questions to the group.

CRITICAL CONTENT

FACILITATING QUESTIONS

- Does everyone know what that means?
- What are you thinking? Feeling? Wondering? Anticipating? Prioritizing?
- What do you hypothesize?
- What does the group want to do next?
- Who has questions or comments on this?
- How will you proceed? What next?
- What do you conclude?
- Is that a learning issue? Why?
- How does the group wish to deal with this? (or Who agrees and who disagrees with this? Why?)

An effective facilitator does not provide direct answers, but instead helps achieve student interaction with each other, not with the facilitator! In addition, he or she facilitates student control of the discussions, activities, time management, learning, and evaluation. The successful facilitator holds students accountable via peer feedback and assessments, allowing student problem solving. Effective facilitators foster honest dialogue and critical thinking. Facilitating PBL is such an important component that a **faculty web site** is available to support the entire PBL process.

What Are the PBL Challenges for Students?

The student's major challenge with PBL is to learn to rely on their own abilities to understand, discover, and apply knowledge and skills that they can transfer to the real world. A major obstacle from the student's perspective is the degree to which they have been taught to rely on the "expert." Students are naturally curious and eager to solve problems. However, traditional learning methods have stifled the natural tendencies for learners to ask questions and to seek more information about a subject. PBL shifts the role from passive student to active learner. All of us have come to rely on the instructor's role as the expert who will tell us what we need to know. We have been lulled into a false assumption that our learning is complete when a teacher "covers" a topic.

Unfortunately, the traditional approach has placed too much emphasis on knowing facts versus problem solving. Thus, PBL works best when faculty members shift from teachers to mentors and when students shift to their primary role as active learners. Students may initially be reluctant to assume so much responsibility for their learning, including doing the research and coming prepared for class discussions. However, every student has a responsibility to come prepared to participate fully because this is how students will develop the needed skills and traits of critical thinking. In addition, fulfilling this responsibility is how they will prepare themselves for entry into professional clinical practice.

Some students are naturally reserved or quiet and are hesitant to join group discussions, which is counterproductive in PBL. It is the different experiences, knowledge, perceptions, and ways of thinking shared by the group and applied in active discussions that makes PBL such a powerful learning method![10] Furthermore, it is by speaking out in a group that you can test your ideas, which is a hallmark of critical thinking. If you do not express

your own thoughts and solutions, you miss the opportunity to test the accuracy and validity of your ideas. Group participation provides the opportunity to learn how to communicate, negotiate, and reflect on your ideas, beliefs, and actions. Quietness in a group discussion can also be misinterpreted as apathy or ignorance. Each student must participate so the faculty facilitator and group members can assess how well you understand the group discussions and how much you have learned.

CRITICAL CONTENT

ACTIVE PARTICIPATION

Students must actively participate in group discussions because it provides opportunities to develop thinking, communicating, negotiating, and reflecting abilities that will be needed in their professional practice. Speaking up in a group discussion is the major way to test the validity and accuracy of your ideas, which is the hallmark of critical thinking.

STRATEGIES FOR USING THIS TEXT FOR PBL

This textbook is a radical departure from most textbooks because there are no answers with the questions and cases! In addition, there is no glossary or definition of key words in this textbook. At first, faculty and students may feel uneasy about these aspects of the text. However, rest assured that the editors and authors made painstaking efforts to facilitate PBL. Providing answers or definitions with the text would interfere with problem solving, self-directed learning, student pacing, sequencing of the learning issues, and most other aspects of PBL. Furthermore, in the real world there is seldom only one right answer to a professional or clinical problem. Therefore, we feel strongly that faculty should have the opportunity to provide feedback and expert opinions about the cases and questions, only **AFTER** the students have done so using PBL. Program faculties have an instructor's guide and a supportive web site to facilitate providing feedback to students regarding the patient problems and exercises within this textbook, without interfering with the PBL process.

This textbook is also a radical departure from most student workbooks because the emphasis is on development of cognitive strategies and professional skills. This is **NOT** a lab book or workbook to help students develop psychomotor skills or to correctly answer fact-based questions. This textbook is designed to stimulate thought, dialogue, controversy, application, and analysis within the framework of respiratory care cases and problems. This textbook is designed to help professionals understand and appreciate the numerous ethical, legal, political, economic, and practical aspects of their practice. Consequently, many of the cases in Part II also incorporate several group exercises such as debates to foster professional development. Most importantly, this textbook is designed to enhance professional communications and team building, which are essential to effective health care practice. Faculty and students are encouraged to take the time to incorporate this textbook into their curricula to facilitate their professional development.

Part I

We recommend that students and faculty begin their PBL process with Part I in order to form the foundation for students' development of the needed professional skills. Part I deals specifically with the numerous aspects of professional practice, including patient assessment, critical thinking, problem solving, communication, negotiation, health care delivery systems, ethical and cost considerations, and several others. If necessary, Chapters 5 and 8 through 10 could be delayed until later in the curriculum or PBL process. Chapter 7, "Patient Assessment and Respiratory Care Plan Development," is a foundational chapter that should be covered before discussion of the respiratory care problems outlined in Part II. Each chapter in Part I is designed

to facilitate acquisition of the necessary skills to actively participate in PBL and professional practice. Part I primarily utilizes individual and group exercises to help students form the foundation for both PBL and professional practice, and it could be incorporated into existing foundational courses or seminars.

Part I of the text includes coverage of PBL and critical thinking. Faculty will want to assign these chapters and their exercises to assist student understanding of why critical thinking skills and traits are important to their professional development. Part I also provides coverage of topics that will broaden student knowledge in areas that are most important for the expanding professional roles of respiratory therapists. Part I of the text is designed to give students the foundation for developing the professional skills and traits important to respiratory care.

Part II

Part II contains sample patient problems in respiratory care. Faculty should assign Chapter 11 as the initial patient problem in respiratory care because there are more details to assist students and faculty in using the textbook to implement PBL. Each chapter includes a brief synopsis of various aspects of cardiopulmonary pathophysiology, including acute and chronic diseases. In addition, various aspects of disease management are incorporated, including age-specific factors, economic issues, ethical problems, and patient adherence. Part II includes cases designed to give students the opportunity to further apply their critical thinking skills and traits within the context of respiratory care cases. Part II is designed to assist students in grasping the content of respiratory care by solving problems presented in clinical cases that are similar to the problems they will encounter in the workplace.

Variations of PBL

We believe that this textbook could be incorporated in several ways with at least three variations of PBL: 1) student-directed (full PBL); 2) modified

PBL (partial PBL); or 3) introduction to PBL (minimal PBL). We describe each of these approaches to assist faculty and students in the implementation of PBL within their curricula using this textbook.

Student-Directed PBL (Full PBL). A student-directed approach allows students to set the pace and the direction of their learning in the context of solving the patient problems presented with each case. No specific exercises or questions are presented or assigned to the students when using full PBL, a purist's approach. Student-directed PBL presents the students with clinical problems within patient cases and the students determine their own learning issues. The students determine their learning issues after discussions of what they know, what they need to know, what they hypothesize, and what they recommend for each portion of a clinical problem or case. Students proceed from one part of the problem to the next over several group sessions.

The faculty and students determine the pace of moving through each case, depending on their course schedules. After deciding the group's learning issues during each small group discussion of the patient problem, the group collectively determines which issues each student will research. Students utilize a variety of resources, including journal articles, discussions with experts, consensus statements, textbooks, the Internet, and others to research their learning issues. Students report back on their learning issues at the beginning of the next small group session as a means to review and present the information needed to discuss all aspects of the case. The faculty serves as group facilitators who gently guide students to a predetermined core of learning issues. The faculty does not lecture or present learning issues. Rather, the faculty guides students in the learning necessary to resolve each case.

The faculty may also choose to utilize a full PBL approach in place of the chapter exercises. If the purist's approach to PBL is adopted, students should be directed to consider choosing any of the exercises incorporated into each case as part of the group's learning issues. Implementation of PBL that is truly student-directed will require a realistic

schedule that allows regular meeting times for small group interaction with a faculty facilitator. Small groups and individual students will also need to meet outside of the scheduled time to research and prepare learning issues. Programs must identify those faculty members who have training in group facilitation and are familiar with the patient problem or case and learning issues to effectively guide group discussions.

Modified PBL. Each patient case includes a suggested list of learning issues provided in the instructor's guide to assist faculty members in their facilitation of each patient problem. However, a modified PBL process can also be used, whereby the instructor uses these learning issues and the exercises in the book as the basis for student research and learning. Using the learning issues and/or the exercises in the textbook can guide the PBL process, providing direction to faculty facilitators and students. A modified approach will also allow students to direct their learning through the performance of the exercises. However, the instructor rather than the students determines the pace and direction of the learning with this modified approach. We recommend the modified approach for those programs whose faculty may not have had training in facilitation because the textbook exercises with the instructor materials will help guide the process.

The chapter exercises are designed to facilitate development of the critical thinking skills and characteristics that are essential in respiratory care practice. The modified approach is another form of PBL because students will assume greater responsibility for their learning than with a traditional lecture technique. The modified PBL approach can also facilitate students' development of professional skills while acquiring a knowledge base.

Faculty should review all the exercises and questions when assigning a specific case from the textbook. Faculty can then determine which are most appropriate to meet the goals of their program. Faculty who have the desire and make the time for PBL will likely decide to incorporate as many exercises as possible within their programs. Faculty should allow students to work on exercises in small groups with considerable lead time for student-directed research and learning on the topic. This would then be followed by faculty-facilitated discussions.

Introduction to PBL.   Some programs may not have the time, faculty, flexibility, schedule and/or other resources to implement specific PBL courses and curricula. However, most faculties want to introduce their students to PBL and encourage lifelong learning. We recommend that faculty members choose a variety of exercises to be used throughout the course of study, including in labs and clinical experiences, to enhance student learning. Faculty members may opt to assign selected cases and/or exercises within their programs as a means to expose their students to PBL and to facilitate critical thinking within program constraints. The assigned exercises can be performed in small groups, followed by group discussion with a facilitator. If necessary, faculty members may choose to facilitate a larger group discussion following small group research and discussion. However, whenever possible, groups of 6 to 8 students are recommended to maximize learning and development of professional skills. Students may be required to develop written responses to chapter exercises as a means to facilitate critical reading and writing. However, we recommend collaborative activities and group discussion to enhance critical thinking whenever possible. Our ideas, decisions, and actions must be validated through discourse with others to enhance critical thinking skills and traits.

When time and other resources are limited, we recommend that faculty members pick and choose from the available exercises to facilitate learning a specific skill or trait. Utilizing a variety of the exercises from the textbook on a limited basis will provide a mechanism to encourage problem solving, clinical decision making, and lifelong learning, even though a full or modified PBL approach may not be possible.

CRITICAL CONTENT

**USING THE TEXTBOOK CASES
FOR VARIATIONS OF PBL**

Full PBL: Students use the cases to fully self-direct their learning, deciding their own learning issues and group activities without any faculty assignments.

Modified PBL: Students self-direct their learning by working through the cases with more faculty direction of the learning issues, critical thinking exercises, and group exercises.

Introduction to PBL: Faculty members direct more of the student learning by providing the learning issues for each case in addition to assignment of individual and group exercises.

Assignment of Cases and Learning Issues

We strongly advise students **NOT** to read the cases in this textbook until directed to do so by their faculty. The cases are designed in such a way that they can be used in a variety of ways to incorporate PBL into the curriculum. If the purist's approach is adopted, students work through each case, line by line, generating their learning issues as previously described. However, faculty members can provide students with the learning issues developed for each case if a modified or introductory approach to PBL is being used. To promote a self-directed approach to learning, which is a hallmark of PBL, students will have to access additional resources in addition to the information provided in the details of the case studies in the text. Many of the chapter questions were designed with the assumption that students would be referring to additional resources as a means to develop their abilities to access medical information. As with the exercises, if there are time constraints, faculty may choose to assign only selected learning issues or exercises.

At the completion of each case, faculty members should provide students with feedback from their instructors' guide, including a list of the expected learning issues with possible answers, as well as expert opinions about the chapter exercises chosen for the course.

Individual and Group Critical Thinking Exercises

Each chapter has a variety of critical thinking exercises and group critical thinking exercises in addition to the list of learning issues provided to the faculty. Not all chapters utilize all potential exercises; each chapter utilizes those exercises most pertinent to their particular case(s).

The critical thinking exercises (not specified as group exercises) can be assigned to individual students **OR** may be done in small groups. The activities allow students to apply strategies that promote critical thinking and stress specific skill development (eg, prioritizing, anticipating, reflecting, etc). The research time required of the students to respond to these exercises varies from minimal to moderate, thus facilitating their implementation in most programs.

The group critical thinking exercises are specifically designed to be group activities that allow students to practice specific critical thinking skills. The exercises assume students will present their responses in a group setting with the benefit of a facilitator to assist the group during the discussions. The faculty-support web site provides tips and information useful to the facilitator during these student discussions. It is expected that the amount of student research and preparation time would be greater for these group exercises. Therefore, adequate lead time and time for debate and discussion should be planned. It will not be feasible to attempt to do all of the exercises in a single course because of time constraints. If PBL is implemented throughout the curriculum in several courses, then the majority of exercises in this textbook could be accomplished.

Student Feedback

It is critical that students receive regular, specific feedback regarding their individual performance,

the group's performance, and the expected learning to be accomplished for each case. Students could receive a text-based learner's guide at the completion of each patient case, that would include the expected learning issues, possible responses, and expert opinions for the critical thinking exercises. Or, students could participate in a feedback session in which the faculty or peers could present an overview of the case that would provide this same information. Peer and facilitator evaluations should determine a percentage of the grade for each PBL course. In addition, each PBL session should provide opportunities at the end for the facilitator and each group member to comment on group and individual performance during the session.

EVALUATION OF PBL

How Are Students Evaluated with PBL?

The evaluation methods for PBL should include an assessment of student learning and an assessment of student performance. PBL assessment should include peer evaluation and the facilitator's evaluation of the abilities to summarize issues clearly, offer information from diverse sources, utilize information from previous cases (including clinical experiences), and reconsider hypotheses and decisions. Course grading should reflect these goals and priorities. Student performance during group discussion, preparation of the learning issues, research of problems, and self-directed learning should be evaluated as the major components of the overall course grade.

Written examinations should comprise a smaller portion of the total course grade. Furthermore, written examinations should be case-based, similarly to the CSE and the patient problems utilized for PBL. Traditional examinations have perpetuated the notion that there is always a "right answer" and that making good grades on exams is sufficient for effective professional practice. It is a tremendous leap to assume that because someone knows the required information, they will perform well in professional practice. Written examinations should be based on real clinical problems, and should require students to analyze data, make recommendations, and arrive at decisions.

If written exams are used (computer- or text-based), we highly recommend scheduling test review sessions. Students should have the opportunity to argue why they chose an answer other than the one on the answer key if branching logic questions are not used! The test review should be handled like any other group discussion, with opportunities for students to direct their learning and openly discuss their points of view. When students provide a reasonable rationale for their thinking, faculty members should be receptive to accepting alternative responses. The test review can be a critical part of a successful PBL experience, allowing faculty unique opportunities to role model active listening as well as the skills and traits of a critical thinker.

Peer Evaluations

Peer evaluation is an important aspect of PBL and should be incorporated into the course, lab, or clinical grade. Peers should have the opportunity to evaluate their classmates' presentation of learning issues, incorporation of resources, preparedness for group discussion, and participation in group discussion. Peer evaluation should address both the quantity and quality of each group member's participation. Forms can be utilized to obtain peer scores and comments, which should be incorporated into student evaluations for grading purposes. Table 1-2 provides an example of a peer assessment grading form.

CRITICAL CONTENT

PEER EVALUATION

Peers should have the opportunity to evaluate their classmates' presentation of learning issues, incorporation of resources, preparedness for group discussion, and the quantity and quality of group participation.

Facilitator's Evaluation of Students

The facilitator evaluations should provide feedback on the learner's questioning skills, communication skills, learning issues, peer teaching and presentations, and critical thinking skills. The facilitator should provide this feedback at the end of each session to each student in the group. The facilitator should also offer comments regarding their role as facilitator, and seek student feedback. The facilitator should role model how to give constructive feedback, focusing on performance and behavior, not individual personalities.

If a student's performance is weak, faculty tutors should meet individually with the student to provide feedback and additional opportunities to develop the required skills. In addition, students should receive a written evaluation from their facilitator for each patient problem (case). Table 1-3 provides an example of how faculty members can provide written feedback to students during PBL courses and how it affects their grades.

Evaluation of Student Learning and Performance

A variety of different weightings and requirements should be incorporated to affect students' grades for PBL courses and curricula. One factor affecting the grade should be peer and facilitator evaluations of the learner's participation and performance in the group learning process. Other techniques for assessment of student learning can include oral and written examinations, course assignments and projects, research papers related to the problems or clinical case(s) studied, development of concept maps, clinical simulations (computerized or written as text), and numerous other ratings of group and individual participation.

For example, an introduction to PBL course might require that students perform an EBM review on a topic related to their first learning issue. Students can be graded on their search strategies and the success of their searches. Students can submit their searches by email to faculty directly

TABLE 1-2   PBL PEER EVALUATION FORM

Name of Person Evaluated:		Case Name or Number:		
Your Name:		Facilitator:		
Date:				
① POOR ② BELOW AVERAGE ③ AVERAGE ④ GOOD ⑤ EXCELLENT				
LEARNING ISSUES & RESOURCES				
Described learning issues clearly and concisely.	①	②	③	④ ⑤
Evaluated resource(s) used to research learning issues.	①	②	③	④ ⑤
Applied the information from the learning issues to the cases.	①	②	③	④ ⑤
Demonstrated adequate preparation and understanding of each learning issue.	①	②	③	④ ⑤
PEER TEACHING				
Reported information clearly and concisely.	①	②	③	④ ⑤
Used learning aid(s) to clarify the issues.	①	②	③	④ ⑤
Encouraged participation of all group members by inviting comments and responding to questions.	①	②	③	④ ⑤
GROUP PARTICIPATION AND LEVEL OF PREPARATION				
Carried a fair share of the workload.	①	②	③	④ ⑤
Came prepared to group sessions and participated with questions and answers.	①	②	③	④ ⑤
Behaved in a manner that communicated respect for all group members.	①	②	③	④ ⑤
Reconsidered decisions and suggestions based on feedback.	①	②	③	④ ⑤
COMMENTS:				

SOURCE: Department of Respiratory Therapy, Medical College of Georgia, Augusta, Georgia.

from the library or their home computers. Faculty members can assess the effectiveness of the search by reviewing the search strategies as well as the search results. Faculty can also require that hard copies of searches be printed and turned in, if that is their preference.

In subsequent PBL courses, students could be required to not only research learning issues using EBM, but to develop a critical review manuscript on a topic related to the patient problems (cases). Other projects could include participation as asthma educators in a local asthma camp or other opportu-

TABLE 1-3   FACILITATOR'S ASSESSMENT OF LEARNER'S PBL

The following items use a scale based on the student's demonstration of the appropriate PBL behaviors described below. For example, the first item evaluates the student's performance overall in presentation.

Student Name: _____   **Facilitator's Name:** _____

Date: _____

1. Poor—(Not Prepared)
2. Fair—(Minimum Effort)
3. Good—(Adequate Participation)
4. Very Good—(Exceeds Average Abilities)
5. Excellent—(Outstanding Participation and Skills)

	Not Observed	
A. Questioning Skills		
1. Formulates relevant questions.	___ 1.	① ② ③ ④ ⑤
2. Questions in a clear and consistent manner.	___ 2.	① ② ③ ④ ⑤
3. Asks questions to inform decision and actions.	___ 3.	① ② ③ ④ ⑤
4. Relies on numerous resources, not the facilitator.	___ 4.	① ② ③ ④ ⑤

Comments: _____
_____
_____
_____

B. Communication Skills		
5. Demonstrates effective listening.	___ 5.	① ② ③ ④ ⑤
6. Follows-up, expands, clarifies.	___ 6.	① ② ③ ④ ⑤
7. Yields the floor to another person.	___ 7.	① ② ③ ④ ⑤
8. Welcomes comments from others.	___ 8.	① ② ③ ④ ⑤
9. Reconsiders data, facts, opinions.	___ 9.	① ② ③ ④ ⑤
10. Asks and answers questions.	___10.	① ② ③ ④ ⑤
11. Directs feedback on the issue, not the person.	___11.	① ② ③ ④ ⑤

Comments: _____
_____
_____
_____

C. Learning Issues		
12. Describes learning issues clearly.	___12.	① ② ③ ④ ⑤
13. Evaluates and cites resource(s) used to research the learning issues.	___13.	① ② ③ ④ ⑤
14. Integrates/synthesizes the information reported in learning issues.	___14.	① ② ③ ④ ⑤
15. Applies the information from the learning issues to the cases.	___15.	① ② ③ ④ ⑤

Comments: _____
_____
_____
_____

Continued

TABLE 1-3 **Continued**

D. Peer Teaching and Presentation	Not Observed	
16. Reports information clearly.	___ 16.	① ② ③ ④ ⑤
17. Uses teaching tools to clarify main ideas.	___ 17.	① ② ③ ④ ⑤
18. Uses specific examples and resources.	___ 18.	① ② ③ ④ ⑤
19. Uses correct pronunciation and spelling.	___ 19.	① ② ③ ④ ⑤

Comments: _____

_____

_____

_____

E. Critical Thinking Skills for Respiratory Care Practice		
20. Differentiates facts from opinions.	___ 20.	① ② ③ ④ ⑤
21. Prioritizes information gathering, decision making, and actions.	___ 21.	① ② ③ ④ ⑤
22. Anticipates problems and solutions.	___ 22.	① ② ③ ④ ⑤
23. Makes appropriate decisions.	___ 23.	① ② ③ ④ ⑤
24. Uses data to support reasoning.	___ 24.	① ② ③ ④ ⑤
25. Uses reasoning to support clinical decisions and recommendations.	___ 25.	① ② ③ ④ ⑤
26. Integrates numerous perspectives.	___ 26.	① ② ③ ④ ⑤
27. Reflects on decisions and actions.	___ 27.	① ② ③ ④ ⑤

Comments: _____

_____

_____

_____

SOURCE: Department of Respiratory Therapy, Medical College of Georgia, Augusta, Georgia.

nities to engage in rural health care, community-based care, or home health care. The possibilities for implementation and evaluation of PBL are limitless, and are based on the health care resources and needs within the community and the creativity of the faculty and students.

Discussion questions relevant to the cases are particularly useful to assess the students' grasp of the content, as well as their problem-solving abilities. An overall letter or numeric grade or pass/fail grade, depending on the needs and priorities of the program of study, can determine ratings on specific assignments. Course grades can be handled in a similar fashion. Table 1-4 provides one example of a set of grading criteria using a variety of assessment tools that could be used for a PBL course. Table 1-5 provides details of how a research paper might be graded as part of a PBL course.

Assessment of the PBL Process

In addition to evaluation of student performance and learning during PBL, it is equally important to evaluate the PBL process using numerous strategies. Using the "two-minute paper" technique is particularly useful during initial implementation of PBL. Table 1-6 provides an example. This technique requires students to take 2 minutes at the end of each PBL session to briefly identify what they liked the most and what they liked the least about

TABLE 1-4   POSSIBLE GRADING FOR A PBL COURSE

The PBL courses will utilize a variety of evaluation methods to assess student learning and the PBL process. Several forms will be used to continuously assess the PBL process, the course, and student participation. The evaluation methods will be used to evaluate the course and to determine student grades. Each evaluation will count as a certain percentage of the course grade as shown below. These evaluation methods will be used:

1) Attendance and Participation (20%)

a) Daily Participation

PBL learning is based on student interaction, self-directed learning, and peer teaching. Therefore, attendance and participation are **mandatory**. You cannot participate in a discussion if you are not present! The facilitator will document your attendance and participation during each group session. If you have an excused absence for illness or personal emergency, the facilitator will not deduct from your grade provided you submit all required materials. You should call the department and either speak to the facilitator or leave a message if you are unable to attend a scheduled session. If you are absent from a class for **any** reason, you will be required to submit a typed handout covering any learning issue you were expected to teach during the session you missed. You are also required to write a paper on the learning issues discussed on that day. Unexcused absences will result in a **5% reduction** in your overall course grade.

b) The Two-Minute Paper

Each week, students will provide written feedback about the PBL sessions using the form for the two-minute paper. Students should complete the form and turn them in to the facilitator at the end of each session (one form per session). There will be a **5% reduction** in the course grade for each two-minute paper not submitted.

2) PBL Skills Evaluations (10%)

The facilitator of each group for each patient problem (case) will provide an evaluation of your PBL skills using the *Facilitator's Assessment of Learner's PBL Skills* form. The evaluation will assess your:

- Questioning skills
- Communication skills
- Learning issues
- Peer teaching and presentation
- Critical thinking skills

Students must receive a satisfactory evaluation (average of 3) to pass the course.

3) Peer Evaluations (10%)

PBL learning and clinical practice require teamwork and peer evaluations. Each student is required to evaluate the performance of each person in the group. At the end of each case, students will use the PBL *Peer Evaluation Form* to assess:

- Presentation of learning issues and resources
- Peer teaching
- Group participation and level of preparation

The overall average of the peer evaluations will determine this grade.

Continued

TABLE 1-4   Continued

4) Examinations (40%)

a) Multiple Choice Examination (Clinical Simulation Format)

A written examination will be given at the end of each session consisting of one clinical simulation per case covered during the session. For example, if the PBL course session included asthma, drug overdose, and neuromuscular diseases, there would be three cases on the exam.

b) Essay Examination

There will be one essay question on each examination. Students will be given a list of the possible essay questions to be on the test. The examination will include one of the questions from the list.

The departmental grading scale will be used to assign examination grades. The scheduled exam dates and times are noted with the significant course dates posted in the PBL handbook.

5) Evidence-Based Medicine (EBM) Research (20%)

Each student will be required to submit an EBM review based on their library search of one learning issue from one patient problem (case). The EBM search will be graded based on criteria presented in the class pertaining to that problem (case).

6) Anonymous Course Evaluations

Each student is required to submit an anonymous evaluation at the end of each case session using the form provided. One student per group will collect the forms on the last day of each case session. The forms will be turned in to the secretary by a student member of each group.

SOURCE: Department of Respiratory Therapy, Medical College of Georgia, Augusta, Georgia.

the way PBL was implemented during the session. Faculty can review this information on a regular basis to identify problem areas and make rapid and frequent adjustments as needed. Problems with faculty facilitation can be identified early to promote needed changes and enhance the faculty's awareness of their roles as facilitators. Faculty can also use student feedback to privately counsel students who may be consistently identified as nonparticipatory, unprepared, or weak overall. Faculty can also use this type of feedback as a mechanism to promote honest dialogue among peers. Teamwork requires everyone to pull his or her weight and to do a good job. Peers need experience to learn how to constructively approach peers whose performance is detrimental to the work of the group. Acquisition of these types of skills will evolve gradually, with learners having a tremendous advantage in knowing how to work with others in a group.

Student Evaluation of Faculty Facilitators

Students should have the opportunity to anonymously evaluate the PBL facilitator. The role of the teacher in PBL is to facilitate, mentor, and tutor. Students can evaluate the facilitator's effectiveness in a variety of ways, with a focus on four major areas: content, PBL process, questioning skills, and group skills. *Content:* To what extent does the facilitator probe the student's understanding of the material? *PBL Process:* Does the facilitator help students identify their learning issues and improve

TABLE 1-5 EXAMPLE FOR EVALUATION OF A STUDENT PAPER FOR A PBL COURSE

I. *Requirements for Paper:*

In this course, the student will:

Prepare an outline of the topic by the assigned date. During the first week topics must be approved by the course director and chosen from a list of available topics.

Use the standard medical databases such as: The Cochrane Library Databases, MEDLINE (Index Medicus), and Cumulative Index to Nursing and Allied Health Literature (CINAHL) for a definitive literature survey on the topic.

Use an EBM strategy to locate and retrieve medical information and submit a record of your searching strategy.

Become familiar with the use of a medical library, obtain assistance from the research librarians, and attend orientation sessions conducted by the library staff.

Observe library rules and policies.

Submit a list of references and resources including Internet sites used for your literature research.

Prepare a typewritten, double-spaced research paper about 8 to 12 pages in length.

Prepare the paper according to the format specified by the journal *Respiratory Care* (see the model manuscript and the manuscript preparation guidelines).

II. *Office Hours:*

Please observe your advisor's office hours for discussion of the research paper. Make appointments with your advisor in advance, during scheduled office hours, to review your progress and discuss any problems with your paper. Students and advisors should meet on a regular basis throughout the semester.

III. *Due Dates for Research Materials and Paper:*

NOTE: All assignments must be typewritten and double-spaced using *Respiratory Care* guidelines for preparation of manuscripts.

Date	Material Due
January 12	Topic due
February 2	Outline and list of reference materials
February 23	Rough draft
March 16	Second draft
April 6	Final paper due

IV. *Grading:*

Please turn in **all** assignments to your faculty mentor by the assigned due date. Every attempt will be made to return assignments with comments within 1 week. Please meet regularly with your faculty mentor to monitor your progress, complete assignments, and make necessary revisions. Grades for the papers will be assigned by your faculty mentor, and will be determined as follows:

Total points for paper: 200

The paper will be graded on the basis of*:

1. Content and logical discussion of the topic
2. Searching strategies and use of the best available evidence
3. Using proper format and *Respiratory Care* guidelines

Continued

TABLE 1-5   Continued

4. Neatness
5. Grammatical correctness
6. Proper use of supporting tables and graphs
7. Conclusions stated in the paper supported by data and literature cited

*Points penalized for late assignments (outline, references, rough draft): 2% deduction for each day late.
 Points penalized for late paper: 2% deduction for each day late.

Note: Please carefully follow *Respiratory Care* guidelines for typing the manuscript, preparing charts or tables, and citing references.

GRADE FORM FOR EVALUATION OF THE RESEARCH PAPER

STUDENT _____   **TOPIC**_____

	(Circle One)	
Draft in on time?	yes	no
Tables and graphs appropriate?	yes	no
Length appropriate? Number pages_____?	yes	no
Cover page included?	yes	no
Table of contents included?	yes	no
Summary included?	yes	no
Conclusion included?	yes	no
References included?	yes	no
Best evidence used?	yes	no
Grammatical errors?	yes	no
Sentence structure problems?	yes	no
Format problems?	yes	no
Continuity of thought problems?	yes	no
Followed *Respiratory Care* guidelines?	yes	no

Comments: _____

_____

_____

_____

Advisor_____   Date _____   Counseling   yes   no
_____First draft   _____Second draft   _____Final

SOURCE: Department of Respiratory Therapy, Medical College of Georgia, Augusta, Georgia.

their thinking abilities? *Questioning Skills:* Are the questions clear and geared to the learner's level of ability? *Group Process Skills:* Does the facilitator help resolve conflict within the group? Group interaction and discussion are vital to the success of the PBL approach. Therefore, facilitator and peer evaluations of performance of everyone in the group is essential and highly recommended.

TABLE 1-6   TWO-MINUTE PAPER FOR EVALUATING PBL IMPLEMENTATION

Name: _____	**Date:** _____
Problem: _____	**Facilitator:** _____

What did you like most about this PBL session?

_____

_____

_____

_____

What did you like least about this PBL session?

_____

_____

_____

_____

What suggestions do you have to improve the PBL Process?

_____

_____

_____

_____

How much time are you spending outside of class:

with the group _____   individually _____

PBL AND EVIDENCE-BASED MEDICINE (EBM)

Incorporating EBM with PBL

We advocate the incorporation of an evidence-based approach to respiratory care practice, and believe PBL courses and curricula are ideal for this integration. Figure 1-1 illustrates examples of pathways of research-based practice for health professionals, including respiratory therapists.[11] The explosion of medical information and its increased accessibility has assisted the development of EBM. Today, EBM and evidence-based health care (EBH) are utilized to express what we know about health care based on scientific evidence and outcomes data to assist in making informed clinical decisions. EBM is the judicious identification, evaluation, and application of the most relevant information to make medical decisions.[12] EBH is a comprehensive approach to systematically document achievable health care outcomes across the disciplines to inform clinical decision making.[11–13] These descriptions of EBM and EBH refer to a number of components.

First, we frame a medical or health care problem to identify the specific information needed. When the information is identified, we must retrieve

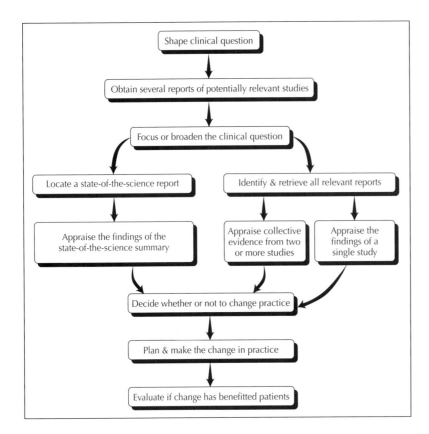

FIGURE 1-1 Possible pathways for research-based practice for health professionals. (SOURCE: From Brown.[11])

it and then evaluate it to assess its quality and validity. If we determine that the evidence is valid, then we must know how to apply it in practice.[12,15]

The research in EBM is the methodical collection of data from studies that meet strict quality criteria. All or portions of these studies can then be merged, distilled, and interpreted (metaanalysis). The "discoveries" in EBM are reviews and practice guidelines developed from this conservative evaluation of the effect and effectiveness of health care. EBM research requires adherence to specific criteria, including thorough analysis of rigorous scientific data to support approaches to health care. EBM systematically and rigorously evaluates outcomes research using methods to increase the generalizability of findings.

We advocate the use of EBM to research learning issues, using the best available data to inform knowledge, decisions, and actions in health care.

EBM approaches should be the basis for problem solving and decision making in respiratory care practice, using the best available evidence. Consequently, respiratory therapy students and their faculties must understand the types of evidence and how to use search strategies to locate and use the best available research to make informed clinical decisions. It is beyond the scope of this chapter and textbook to present research methodologies and research designs. We highly recommend incorporation of such courses into the respiratory care curricula early, in coordination with the PBL curricula.

Since PBL focuses on student problem solving, it is an ideal opportunity to incorporate evidence-based approaches to respiratory care. In addition, critical thinking skills and traits develop further whenever we closely examine and reflect on the basis for our thoughts, beliefs, and actions. Therefore, students should receive instruction on how to locate and use various forms of evidence when researching learning issues and completing PBL coursework. Furthermore, an understanding of the basics of research is essential to becoming informed consumers of medical information, including the research of EBM. Figure 1-2 illustrates the relationships between critical thinking, PBL, and EBM.

Types of Evidence

Understanding types of evidence involves knowing what constitutes evidence, methods for grading levels of evidence, and the various forms of evidence. In addition, students and faculty should evaluate the quality of evidence in the sources that they utilize, including EBM reviews, clinical practice guidelines, and clinical outcomes. An evidence-based approach to practice can gradually develop as students and faculty incorporate EBM into their research of the PBL patient problems presented in this textbook.

What Is Evidence? We all use and interpret a wide variety of resources to inform our decisions in clinical practice. The evidence we use can range from that derived from our own experience, to a colleague's opinion, to a journal article we read that gave data from a randomized controlled trial. Figure 1-3 shows a continuum of the sources of evidence.[14] There are also numerous sources of clinical knowledge beyond research, including experience, reasoning, authority, quality data, and our patient's account. Most of us draw from the evidence we believe we acquired in our formal education. We often consider things we learned as evidence without consideration of the source and validity or quality of the information. We utilize a diverse and rich reser-

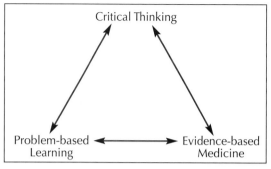

FIGURE 1-2 Supporting relationships of critical thinking, PBL, and EBM.

voir of evidence to guide our thoughts and behaviors in our clinical practice and for our own personal health care. It is critically important that each of us become educated and discerning consumers of the evidence we use to support our decisions.

You should be able to discern good evidence from bad evidence. You must know how to make judgments about the strengths and weaknesses of the evidence to critically use and appraise it, without taking what you observe, hear, or read with absolute trust. Both PBL and EBM promote reflective skepticism, which is most important in the development of critical thinking skills and traits.

EBM and evidence-based practice provide a consistent framework for evaluation of current health care and methods to improve effectiveness, without ignoring the needs of individual patients. These two contrasting needs automatically generate tension, because EBM seeks to generalize and patient health care seeks to individualize. It is not surprising that EBM has its critics. However, both

Quantitative					Qualitative
Randomized controlled trials	Nonrandomized trials	Cohort studies	Surveys	Descriptive studies	Opinion based on experience

FIGURE 1-3 Continuum of the sources of evidence.

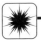

CRITICAL CONTENT

SOURCES OF CLINICAL KNOWLEDGE

- Research
- Experience
- Reasoning
- Authority
- Quality data
- Patient's account

critics and supporters of EBM would probably agree that better evidence is needed to facilitate improved health care decisions for individuals. While there has always been a need for EBM, public health agencies, health maintenance organizations, and cost-conscious hospitals have accelerated the need for and development of EBM.

Respiratory care students and their faculty should utilize EBH as one means to articulate the logic behind certain clinical practices and to evaluate CPGs, critical pathways, and respiratory care protocols. Respiratory therapists should understand and utilize EBM in their practice to expand their effectiveness in health care, providing additional opportunities for decision making and problem solving within their health care organizations. However, it is important to remember that EBM is not cookbook medicine nor is it limited to cost-cutting health care strategies.

Levels of Evidence.   Respiratory therapists and all health care providers should understand and apply a hierarchy to the levels of evidence when evaluating research regarding an intervention or therapy. EBM categorizes the research evidence into three levels, based on the design of the study. Level 1 evidence comes from a multi-site, randomized clinical trial or several single-site, randomized controlled trials. Level 2 evidence comes from a variety of quasi-experimental studies. Level 3 evidence includes correlational or descriptive studies.

Examining the levels of evidence does not provide indications of the quality of a study or the

overall strength of a body of evidence. However, examining the levels of evidence is a useful means to address the effectiveness of a study design in establishing cause and effect. The Cochrane Library and other EBM databases provide guidance for respiratory therapists and other health professionals to evaluate the levels of evidence and its quality. Respiratory therapists can be valuable consultants and members of their organizations, using EBM when developing, implementing, and evaluating CPGs, respiratory care protocols, critical pathways, and health care for individual patients.

CRITICAL CONTENT

LEVELS OF EVIDENCE

- Level 1: Evidence from a multi-site randomized, controlled study or several single-site controlled trials
- Level 2: Evidence from a variety of quasi-experimental studies
- Level 3: Includes evidence from correlational or descriptive studies

Remember: Examining the levels of evidence does not provide indication of the quality of a study or the overall strength of a body of evidence.

Forms of Evidence.   Numerous forms of evidence can inform clinical decision making. In fact, the growth of EBM has heightened the awareness of the many complexities of using research data to inform the health care of individuals. All research is susceptible to variation and not all research is equal. There are many varied examples in the literature of what constitutes evidence. The gold standard has been and continues to be the randomized controlled clinical trial. The hierarchy for characterizing evidence places the greatest emphasis on the scientific method of inquiry. However, not all of these methods are appropriate for all situations. In fact, it is often impossible to collect evidence using a randomized controlled trial. Furthermore, it is the nature of the research question that determines the most appropriate methodology.

The various forms of evidence relate to the variety of research methods and research designs. Table 1-7 provides basic descriptions of different types of research studies. Different forms of evidence derive from randomized controlled trials, case-controlled studies, cohort studies, systematic reviews, surveys, qualitative studies, and professional consensus. For example, the National Asthma Education Program (NAEP) guidelines and the clinical practice guidelines for respiratory care derive from professional consensus. If you critically review the references cited within these documents, you will understand that additional evidence from randomized trials is needed to further support recommendations and current standards of practice. EBM researchers use the three levels of evidence to conduct metaanalyses of quantitative studies. However, other forms of evidence that inform clinical decision making can be evaluated by assessment of the strength of the evidence, as shown in Table 1-8.[15,16]

TABLE 1-7　RESEARCH DESIGNS

Research design	A plan for systematically collecting and utilizing data so that a hypothesis can be properly tested or so that desired information can be accurately and efficiently obtained
Clinical trials	Pre-planned studies of the safety, efficacy, or optimum dosage schedule (if appropriate) of one or more diagnostic, therapeutic, or prophylactic drugs, devices, or techniques, selected according to predetermined criteria of eligibility and observed for predefined evidence of favorable and unfavorable effects.
Randomized controlled trials	Clinical trials that involve at least one test treatment and one control treatment with concurrent enrollment and follow-up of the test- and control-treated groups, and in which the treatments to be administered are selected by a random process, such as the use of a random-numbers table.
Metaanalysis	A quantitative method of combining the results of independent studies (usually drawn from the published literature) and synthesizing summaries and conclusions that may be used to evaluate therapeutic effectiveness, plan new studies, etc, with application chiefly in the areas of research and medicine.
Cohort studies	Studies in which subsets of a defined population are identified. These groups may or may not be exposed to factors hypothesized to influence the probability of the occurrence of a particular disease or other outcome. Cohorts are defined populations that, as a whole, are followed in an attempt to determine distinguishing subgroup characteristics.
Case-control studies	Studies that begin with the identification of a group with a disease of interest and a control (comparison, referent) group without the disease. The relationship of an attribute to the disease is examined by comparing diseased and nondiseased persons with regard to the frequency or levels of the attribute in each group.

TABLE 1-8   STRENGTHS OF EVIDENCE

TYPE	STRENGTH OF EVIDENCE
I	Strong evidence from at least one systematic review of multiple randomized controlled trials
II	Strong evidence from at least one well-designed randomized controlled trial (often multicenter) with an appropriate sample size
III	Evidence from well-designed trials without randomization, including cohort, case-control, longitudinal, and single-group pre- and postresearch designs
IV	Evidence from well-designed non-experimental studies from more than one center
V	Opinions of respected authorities based on qualitative studies, clinical evidence, descriptive studies, case reports, and reports of expert committees

SOURCE: From Muir Gray.[15]

CRITICAL CONTENT

SOURCES OF EVIDENCE

- Systematic reviews
- Randomized controlled trials (RCT)
- Case-controlled studies
- Cohort studies
- Surveys
- Decision analysis
- Qualitative studies
- Professional consensus

Students, faculty, researchers, and health care professionals must understand the various forms of evidence and how to incorporate a variety of evidence into practice. An introductory or foundational course in research methods is helpful. However, PBL provides an ideal opportunity for students to actively apply research method content with respiratory care content while solving various clinical problems. When students discuss their learning issues, it is critically important that their sources are cited and evaluated. Faculty facilitators should guide students to seek the best available evidence on the various learning issues. In addition, the PBL groups should evaluate the evidence based on its quality, thoroughness, and application to practice.

Accessing Medical Information

Accessing and using information are key components of both PBL and EBM. No one can self-direct his or her learning if they do not know how to retrieve evidence and other medical information. It is important to the success of PBL that students and faculty receive instruction on the use of the various databases available, as well as efficient searching strategies. Librarians have become a critical resource in both PBL and EBM, as well as the overall practice of health care.[17–20] We recommend that programs, faculties, and students take advantage of group and individual learning sessions provided by libraries within your university, college, hospital, and community. In addition, the self-directed learner of today must know how to use the Internet to effectively and efficiently access information. The Internet has made international resources available at home without the need to go to a library. However, do not overlook the valuable resource of librarians to help you access, locate, and use medical evidence. Library staff can provide valuable instruction and guidance, often providing specific instruction to meet learners' needs. Therefore, librarians should be actively involved in an educational program, including advisory committees and PBL steering committees. You are encouraged to view the library staff as part of your teaching faculty, who can answer questions, mentor, give advice, and role model.

Databases. There are numerous resources to use in the search for sources of evidence. It is beyond the scope of this chapter to describe the numerous searching strategies to locate, use, and evaluate medical information. One of the primary purposes of PBL is to provide students many opportunities to develop these skills while solving patient problems as they work through the various cases. This section provides an overview of some of the most common databases used for locating and retrieving medical information. Resources available to search for evidence to inform clinical decisions include The Cochrane Library, MEDLINE, EMBASE, and subject specialist databases such as HealthSTAR.

The Cochrane Library. The Cochrane collaboration is an international research initiative established to produce, maintain, and disseminate reviews of evidence. The Cochrane Library was launched in 1995 to provide evidence needed for health care decision making. The need for the Cochrane collaboration was identified because[15,21]:

- No decision maker can stay abreast of all the scientific literature.
- Textbooks quickly become out of date, especially with regard to treatment recommendations.
- Editorials and reviews often do not specify the searching strategies utilized.
- MEDLINE and EMBASE cover only about half of the world's journals.
- An expert searcher can only find about half of the randomized trials in MEDLINE.
- Even when trials can be located, they may be of low quality due to inadequate power or biases toward reporting positive results.
- Even high quality, systematic reviews can quickly become outdated.

The Cochrane Library currently maintains four databases, including controlled trials, review methodologies, systematic reviews of the effects of care, and critical assessments of effectiveness.[11,17] The Cochrane Library regularly updates its databases to facilitate the timely use of evidence in medical practice. A bimonthly publication, *Evidence-Based Medicine*, reports on recent reviews and commentaries from EBM. During PBL, students should identify and use the databases within the Cochrane Library to research learning issues. If these sources do not adequately address the learning issue then other databases should be used.

MEDLINE. MEDLINE is the National Library of Medicine's online bibliographic database for Index Medicus, which covers many disciplines including the international biomedical literature. MEDLINE also includes the allied health disciplines, the humanities, the biological and physical sciences, and information science as these relate to medicine and health care. Information in MEDLINE is indexed from approximately 4000 journals worldwide, from the US and about 70 other countries. The index includes over 11 million publications released since the mid-1960s, primarily in English. To be included in Index Medicus, a journal first must publish good science, and second its subject matter must fill a void in indexed medical science. Listing in Index Medicus/MEDLINE acknowledges a journal's legitimacy in the mainstream literature of science and medicine.

In 2000, the journal *Respiratory Care* was accepted into Index Medicus, which was an important event in the history of both the journal and the respiratory care profession. Previously, *Respiratory Care* was indexed only in the Cumulative Index for Nursing and Allied Health Literature (CINAHL). In the past, if researchers, educators, clinicians, and students did not specifically search CINAHL, they were not likely to locate manuscripts published by *Respiratory Care*. Being included in Index Medicus is a statement about the science, quality, and uniqueness of the information published. In the past, key articles often did not cite related studies published in *Respiratory Care*, largely because the authors were unaware of them. Researchers can now more readily find the studies and papers included in *Respiratory Care*, opening the journal's content to a wider audience. With exposure of the journal's contents to more readers and researchers, greater awareness of the science and clinical issues of the profession will be available, and this can further advance the art and science of respiratory care. MEDLINE can be accessed through library services or via the Internet. You can access the journal *Respiratory Care* on the Internet at www.rcjournal.com.

EMBASE.   The Elsevier Science bibliographic database covers biomedical literature from over 100 countries, with particular emphasis on drugs and toxicology. EMBASE is the shortened form of the Excerpta Medical Database, with a strong coverage of European material. EMBASE indexes approximately 3500 journals from 1974 to the present.

HealthSTAR.   HealthSTAR is a database jointly supported by the National Library of Medicine and the American Hospital Association. HealthSTAR contains citations from the published literature on health services, technology, administration, and research. HealthSTAR focuses on clinical and non-clinical aspects of health care, including topics such as administration and planning of health care facilities; health services research, health economics, finance, administration, and law; evaluation of patient outcomes and effectiveness of procedures, programs, processes, products, and services; health insurance, health policy, quality assurance, licensure, and accreditation, and other related topics.

The database contains citations and abstracts of journal articles, technical reports, monographs, abstracts from professional meetings, papers, book chapters, government documents, and newspaper articles. HealthSTAR is updated monthly and has citations from 1975 to the present.

There are numerous other databases and Internet sources for locating medical information. This section briefly described the most common databases used for locating and retrieving the best evidence and medical information for problem solving and decision making.

KEY POINTS

- PBL is a teaching-learning strategy that focuses on active learning in small groups to promote knowledge, cognitive abilities, critical thinking, and professional skills.

- PBL enables students to direct their own learning by using a variety of resources to manage and solve hypothetical work-related problems that are similar to the problems that they will encounter in the real world of professional practice.

- With PBL, the role of faculty shifts from that of lecturer to one of coach, facilitator, mentor, and tutor, because the focus is on student learning, not teaching.

- PBL allows students to have some influence over the direction, speed, and depth of their instruction.

- Most importantly, PBL focuses on the development of cognitive strategies and professional skills, including teamwork, communication, and clinical decision making.

- PBL works best when faculty members shift from their roles as teachers and become mentors, and when students shift from being passive learners and become active learners.

- PBL courses and curricula are ideal for the integration of evidence-based approaches into practice.

- Students and faculty should receive instruction on how to locate and use various forms and levels of evidence when researching learning issues and completing PBL coursework.

- An understanding of the basics of research, including the research of EBM and the goals of PBL, is essential to becoming informed consumers of medical information.

- PBL curricula promote a deeper understanding of how to efficiently retrieve, assess, and use medical information in today's complex health care industry.

- Understanding types of evidence involves knowing what constitutes evidence, methods for grading levels of evidence, and the various forms of evidence.

- Students and faculty should evaluate the quality of evidence in the sources that they utilize, including EBM reviews, clinical practice guidelines, and clinical outcomes.

- An evidence-based approach to practice can gradually develop as students and faculty incorporate EBM into their research of the PBL patient problems presented in this textbook.

REFERENCES

1. Barrows HS. *How to Design a Problem-Based Curriculum for the Preclinical Years.* New York: Springer Verlag; 1985.

2. Bruhn JG. Problem-based learning: An approach toward reforming allied health education. *J Allied Health.* 1992;21:161–173.

3. Mishoe SC, Martin S. Critical thinking in the laboratory. *The Learning Laboratorian Series.* 1994;6: 1–63.

4. Mishoe SC, MacIntyre NR. Expanding professional roles for respiratory care practitioners. *Respir Care.* 1997;42:71–91.

5. Op't Holt TB. A first year experience with problem-based learning in a baccalaureate cardiorespiratory program. *Respir Care Educ Annu.* 2000; 9:47–58.

6. Silver S. A multidisciplinary allied health faculty team: formation and first year production of problem-based learning in gerontology/geriatrics. *J Allied Health.* 1998;27:83–88.

7. Kaufman RR, Portney LG, Jette DU. Clinical performance of physical therapy students in traditional and problem-based curricula. *J Phys Ther Educ.* 1997;11:26–31.

8. Mishoe SC. Critical thinking, educational preparation and development of respiratory care practitioners. *Distinguished Pap Monogr.* 1993; 1:29–43.

9. Brookfield SD. *Developing Critical Thinkers.* San Francisco: Jossey-Bass; 1987.

10. Barrows HS. *What Your Tutor May Never Tell You: A Guide for Medical Students in Problem-based Learning.* Springfield, Ill: Southern Illinois University School of Medicine; 1997.

11. Brown SJ. *Knowledge for Health Care Practice. A Guide to Using Research Evidence.* Philadelphia: Saunders; 1999.

12. Friedland DJ. *Evidence-Based Medicine. A Framework for Clinical Practice.* Stamford, Conn: Appleton & Lange; 1998.

13. Sackett DL, Richardson WS, Rosenberg W, et al. *Evidence-Based Medicine: How to Practice and Teach EBM.* 2nd ed. Edinburgh: Churchill Livingstone; 2000.

14. Hamer S. *Achieving Evidence-Based Practice.* Edinburgh: Bailliere Tindall; 1999.

15. Muir Gray JA. *Evidence-Based Healthcare: How to Make Health Policy and Management Decisions.* New York: Churchill Livingstone; 1997.

16. McKibbon A. *Evidence-Based Principles and Practice.* Hamilton, Ontario: B.C. Decker; 1999.

17. Eldredge JD, Teal JB, Ducharme JC, et al. The roles of library liaisons in problem-based learning (PBL) medical school curriculum: A case study from the University of New Mexico. *Health Libr Rev.* 1998; 15:185–194.

18. Minchow RL. Changes in information seeking patterns of medical students: second-year students' perceptions of information management instruction as a component of a problem-based learning curriculum. *Med Ref Serv Q.* 1996;15;15–40.

19. Earl MF. Library instruction in the medical school curriculum: A survey of medical college libraries. *Bull Med Libr Assoc.* 1996;84:191–195.

20. Schilling K, Ginn DS, Mickelson P, et al. Integration of information-seeking skills and activities into problem-based curricula. *Bull Med Libr Assoc.* 1995;83:176–183.

21. Jones A. Second international Cochrane Colloquium—official annual meeting of the Cochrane Collaboration: A conference report. *Respir Care.* 1995;40:171–174.

2

CRITICAL THINKING IN RESPIRATORY CARE

Shelley C. Mishoe

With regard to excellence, it is not enough to know,
but we must try to have and use it.

ARISTOTLE
(384–322 B.C.)

LEARNING OBJECTIVES

1. Develop a personal definition of critical thinking.
2. Describe logic and how logic relates to critical thinking.
3. Describe problem solving and how problem solving relates to critical thinking.
4. Describe reflection and how reflection relates to critical thinking.
5. List, define, and give examples of the essential skills for critical thinking in respiratory care practice.
6. Describe characteristics for critical thinkers.
7. Use the THINKER approach to develop critical-thinking skills and traits.
8. Describe organizational variables that affect critical thinking in respiratory care practice.
9. Develop an awareness of the skills and traits of a critical thinker through completion of the chapter exercises.
10. Complete the exercises in other chapters to further develop critical-thinking skills and traits.

KEY WORDS

Critical Thinking
Declarative Knowledge
Dialectical Thinking
Effective Thinking
Evidence-Based
    Health Care
Logic

Logical Reasoning
Problem Solving
Reflection
Reflective Skepticism
Reflective Thinking
Reflexive Thinking
THINKER Approach

WHAT IS CRITICAL THINKING?

Critical thinking merges principles of logical reasoning, problem solving, judgment, decision making, reflection, and lifelong learning. The term **critical thinking** has become widely used and misused. There are many interpretations of critical thinking, each based on different personal agendas, purposes, beliefs, and perspectives.

To arrive at a workable definition of critical thinking, the respiratory therapist should examine the opinions of experts. Experts variously define critical thinking as "cognitive problem solving," "logical reasoning," and "rational thought," among other descriptions. Complex thinking involves various intellectual activities encompassing both creative and critical aspects. The creative aspect of thinking allows ideas and alternatives to be born, whereas the critical aspect enables the testing and evaluation of these ideas and alternatives. From this viewpoint, critical thinking involves knowing how to synthesize, evaluate, analyze, and apply.

One should not put too much emphasis on any particular definition because each definition of critical thinking has its limitations. Some definitions describe critical thinking as decision making with a major focus on intellectual activity. Other definitions relate more closely to clinical practice by acknowledging the various skills, traits, and behaviors needed for critical thinking in addition to intellect. Most recently, some investigators have coined *effective thinking* as the most suitable term to encompass the broad range of relationships among thinking skills, the dispositions to think, and discipline content.[1]

Table 2-1 shows some common definitions of critical thinking.[1–9] Examination of these definitions reveals the differences in the interpretation and relative importance of logical reasoning, problem solving, and reflection. Creativity is also important to the process of critical thinking. At the end of this chapter, you should derive your own personal definition of critical thinking, unique to your clinical setting and applicable to the many situations that arise in your respiratory care practice (Fig. 2-1).[8] The fol-

lowing sections describe critical thinking as the intellectual, social, and emotive processes of logical reasoning, problem solving, and reflection.

CRITICAL CONTENT

CRITICAL THINKING IN PRACTICE

Critical thinking merges the principles of logical reasoning, problem solving, judgment, decision making, reflection, and lifelong learning. There are many unique definitions of critical thinking, a complex topic with various meanings. Respiratory therapists should determine their own interpretation of critical thinking to enhance clinical effectiveness.

Logical Reasoning

In Western culture, critical thinking has been closely identified with the discipline of logic. Aristotle's logic and its principles were elements of education in the early history of America's colleges and universities. **Logic** covers a range of thought processes that are primarily focused on the question of rational justification and explanation. **Justification** includes

---

TABLE 2-1   COMMON DEFINITIONS OF CRITICAL THINKING

DEFINITION	REFERENCE
Political awareness and personal development	Brookfield, 1987[2]
Cognitive problem solving	Dressel & Mayhew, 1954[3]
"Effective thinking" to encompass a broad perspective of the relationships among thinking skills, the dispositions to think and discipline content	Eljamal et al. 1998[1]
Thinking in order to believe or act	Ennis, 1962[4]
Logical reasoning	Hallet, 1984[5]
Rational and purposeful attempt to use thought to move toward a future goal	Halpern, 1989[6]
Discipline-specific knowledge, skills and attitudes to solve real problems	McPeck, 1990[7]
Logical reasoning, problem solving and reflection[8]	Mishoe, 1995[8]
An understanding of and an ability to formulate, analyze, and assess the elements of thought	Paul, 1993[9]

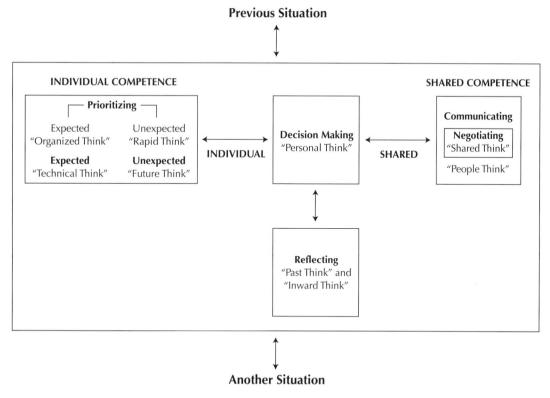

FIGURE 2-1 Critical thinking skills for effective respiratory care practice.

a set of reasons that support a conclusion. **Deduction** is reasoning in which a conclusion is supposed to follow from examination of the reasons. **Induction** is reasoning that is judged to be the best explanation that is plausible and consistent with the facts. Inductive reasoning includes **generalization**, which is the proposition that a number of things have some elements in common.

Logical reasoning is a component of critical thinking with emphasis on the cognitive aspects of thought. Because human behavior is guided by thought rather than instinct, all human thought and behavior is based on logic to some extent. In our daily activities we use logical reasoning to sort out what is relevant from what is not, what we know or do not know, what supports or goes against a belief, and what we should or should not assume.

Although logic is involved in all human thinking, the logic we use is often implicit, unexpressed, or contradictory. Most adults have not been challenged to examine and monitor their thinking in order to justify it with the standards of reason and logic. Too often we claim to offer logical reasons to justify our thoughts or actions in respiratory care practice as well as in our everyday lives. But we are usually not taught to examine our assumptions, concepts, issues, data, theories, claims, consequences, beliefs, and biases. Therefore, we operate in our comfort zones of acceptable beliefs and behavior that often have little to do with logical reasoning.[10] The realization that we often act without careful consideration of the implications and consequences of our actions can be the first step in our journey to becoming critical thinkers. This recognition often occurs during periods of reflective thinking (described later). Each of us should be challenged to examine the logic behind our thoughts and actions, an activity that will improve our critical thinking.

CRITICAL CONTENT

LOGICAL REASONING

- **Logic** covers a range of thought processes that are primarily focused on the question of rational justification and explanation.
- **Justification** includes a set of reasons to support a conclusion.
- **Deduction** is reasoning in which the conclusion is supposed to follow from the reasons.
- **Induction** is reasoning that is judged to be the best explanation that is plausible and consistent with the facts.
- **Generalization** is a proposition that a number of things have something in common.

Courses in logic aim at teaching the basics of logical operations, including inferential reasoning, categorical propositions, and syllogisms. A **proposition** is a set of words that expresses a complete thought. A **fact** is a proposition that is true. For example, it is a fact that the heart is an organ in the body that pumps blood. An **assumption** is generally thought of as a proposition of doubtful truthfulness, because it is inadequately supported by facts that establish the conclusion. For example, we assume that a vegetarian diet is good for one's health, however a diet high in fat from dairy products can actually raise blood cholesterol and increase the risk of heart attack.

Inferential reasoning involves the ability to make inferences. An **inference** is assuming that one proposition is given and guessing that another proposition follows. When you make an inference, you are drawing a conclusion based on reasons. For example, "I see a person in a lab coat placing a stethoscope on a patient's chest. Therefore, that person is a health care professional listening to heart and breath sounds." Later in this textbook, you will be given many opportunities to make inferences and clinical decisions using information from clinical cases and problems.

A logical thinker is able to use reasoning to examine the relationship between propositions in order to derive an interpretation of the truth or justification for any belief or set of beliefs. Inferential reasoning is used daily as we derive explanations and justifications, but we are not necessarily logical or critical in our examinations. Logic involves the disciplined use of rational reasoning in order to examine evidence that supports, implies, contradicts, relates, suggests, and demonstrates. Concepts, questions, language, and disciplines all have logic.

Every discipline, including respiratory care, has logic or a system of principles, concepts, assumptions, and questions that frame the discipline, activity, or practice. Although students study disciplines, most are ignorant of the logic that underlies their discipline. Students must know the logic of respiratory care in order to: 1) grasp the discipline of respiratory care as a whole, 2) think independently within the discipline of respiratory care, 3) compare and contrast respiratory care with other disciplines, and 4) apply respiratory care outside of classroom assignments. Students who fail to grasp their

CRITICAL CONTENT

INFERENTIAL REASONING

- **Inferential reasoning** involves the ability to make inferences using facts.
- An **inference** is taking one proposition as given and guessing that another proposition follows. When you make an inference, you are drawing a conclusion on the basis of reasons.
- A **proposition** is a set of words that expresses a complete thought.
- A **fact** is a proposition that is true. For example, it is a fact that the heart is an organ in the body that pumps blood.
- An **assumption** is generally thought of as a proposition that is doubtful because it is not completely supported by evidence so that the conclusion can be established.

discipline are later unable to realize their full potential as professionals.[11] Respiratory care curricula should encourage students to develop their logical reasoning skills and also understand the logic of the respiratory care discipline.

Today, evidence-based healthcare (EBH) [also called evidence-based medicine (EBM)] is one means to express what we know about health care based on scientific evidence. The explosion of medical information and its increased availability has fostered the growth of EBM, which has specific criteria including rigorous analysis of scientific data to support approaches to health care. EBM is the "conscientious, explicit and judicious use of current best evidence in making decisions about the care of individual patients."[12] You could say that EBH is a comprehensive approach to articulate the logic that underlies health care across the disciplines, and respiratory care students and their faculty should utilize EBH as one means to articulate the logic behind their clinical practices. Figure 2-2 illustrates the major components of evidence-based healthcare.[12–14]

The research done in EBM is the methodical collection of studies that meet strict quality criteria. These studies (or parts of them) are then merged, distilled, and interpreted (metaanalysis). The "discoveries" in EBM are reviews and practice guidelines developed from this conservative evaluation of the effect and effectiveness of care. The Cochrane Library is a database of controlled trials, systematic reviews of the effects of care, and critical assessments of effectiveness.[13,14] A bimonthly publication, *Evidence-Based Medicine*, reports on recent reviews and commentaries from researchers in the field. While there has always been a need for EBM, public health agencies, health maintenance organizations, and cost-conscious hospitals have increased the need for and development of EBM.

Clinical practice guidelines (CPGs), critical pathways, and patient care protocols and algorithms are useful tools that elaborate and articulate the "logic" of respiratory care. Students and faculty should examine the logic of respiratory care in their classroom, laboratory, and clinical experiences. This means we should ask: "How do we know what we know? What is it based upon? What evidence supports this practice in clinical care? Why do we practice respiratory care this way? Is there a better way? Who determined the conventional way of doing a certain respiratory care procedure or practice?" You and your faculty can come up with many more questions and examples as you reflect on the logic of respiratory care. Please review Chapter 6 for examples of how to use CPGs, protocols, and pathways to illustrate the logic of the practice of respiratory care. The following exercises are designed to help you further understand the logic of the respiratory care discipline and to enhance your logical reasoning skills.

Critical Thinking Exercise 1

EXERCISES

a. Describe inference, proposition, deduction, induction, and logical reasoning and their relationship to each other and to critical thinking.

b. Describe how logic relates to critical thinking and to respiratory care practice.

c. Describe the number and types of clinical practice guidelines (CPGs) in respiratory care and how they can be used to explain the logic of our discipline.

d. Refer to the cited references used for a specific clinical practice guideline and explain what evidence is provided to support or contradict each recommendation of the guideline.

e. Describe the propositions that were used (both stated and unstated) in the development of a clinical practice guideline.

Problem Solving

Problem solving, like logical reasoning, is perceived as cognitive, mechanical, and rational. From this perspective, critical thinking involves knowing how to think, apply, analyze, synthesize, and evaluate. Problem solving includes cognitive, affective, and psychomotor behaviors. Cognitive behaviors used during problem solving include intellectual activities such as analyzing, synthesizing, and evaluating. Affective behaviors are related to value systems, including attitudes, dispositions, and experi-

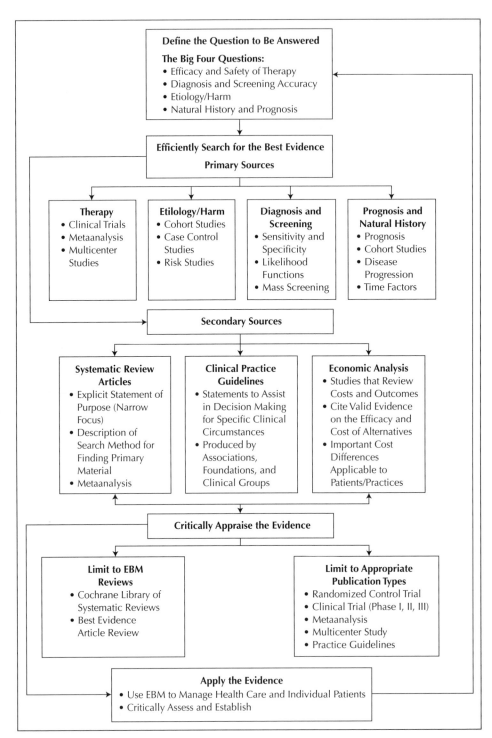

FIGURE 2-2   Major components of evidence-based medicine (EBM).

Group Critical Thinking Exercise 1

LOGIC EXERCISES

a. Use a CPG, pathway, protocol, or EBM review to explain what we know and do not know about one particular therapy or aspect of respiratory care, then explain how this information influences or reflects the logic of respiratory care.

b. Develop a clinical practice guideline, clinical algorithm, or critical pathway for respiratory care and state your evidence, assumptions, biases, concepts, issues, data, definitions, theories, and implications.

c. Develop a concept map to illustrate the logic of one aspect of respiratory care such as arterial blood gas interpretation, delivery of aerosol pharmacology, or use of oxygen devices.

ences. Psychomotor behaviors include physiologic responding and reacting during problem solving, and are interrelated with your thoughts (cognitive) and feelings (affective).

Any first-year respiratory therapy student can attest to the physiologic reactions felt while problem solving in clinic. Who has not had the sweaty palms, racing heart, and rapid breathing experienced when solving clinical problems, especially early on in one's training? Your faculty and seasoned practitioners can attest to similar physiologic reactions when their opinions and actions are questioned. A major difference is that an experienced clinician who is a role model for critical thinking will not react defensively or antagonistically to criticism or requests for further explanation. This does not mean that people like confrontation. However, a true critical thinker is open to other ideas, questions, concerns, and opinions.

What are the processes involved in problem solving? Gagne[15] identified three kinds of human processes that contribute to problem solving: intellectual skills, verbal knowledge, and cognitive strategies. He defined **intellectual activities** as capabilities stored in long-term memory that allow us to carry out procedures using symbols. Specific and general verbal knowledge of the world encompasses **declarative knowledge**, which is expressed

in verbal and written language. For example, declarative knowledge is evident when a respiratory therapy student can state the pin index safety system (PISS) for cylinders.

Declarative knowledge is an important first step, but knowing the PISS is not the same as knowing how to use cylinders and oxygen appliances. Furthermore, declarative knowledge is not sufficient when the respiratory therapist must determine whether a patient is responding to a particular oxygen delivery system. Cognitive strategies must be developed for appropriate patient assessment and delivery of respiratory care services.

CRITICAL CONTENT

Three kinds of human processes that contribute to problem solving are:

• **Intellectual skills:** capabilities stored in long-term memory that allow us to carry out procedures using symbols

• **Verbal knowledge:** declarative knowledge that is exhibited in statements using language

• **Cognitive strategies:** the abilities a person has to control his or her own learning or thinking processes in a particular situation

Gagne described **cognitive strategies** as the ability to control one's own learning or thinking processes in a particular situation.[15] Traditional education has focused on students' abilities to demonstrate their declarative knowledge without adequate attention to the development of cognitive strategies. It is important for respiratory therapy students to have opportunities to develop their intellectual skills and cognitive strategies, in addition to their declarative knowledge and psychomotor skills. For example, declarative knowledge might include the students' abilities to describe the Henderson-Hasselbach equation. Cognitive strategies would include the students' ability to utilize the Henderson-Hasselbach equation in a clinical situation when there is doubt as to the accuracy of a patient's arterial blood gas reading. Students with the most fully developed cognitive strategies are able to draw from their previous knowledge without prompting from the instructor in the application of respiratory care to patients.

CRITICAL CONTENT

MAJOR LIMITATION OF TRADITIONAL EDUCATION

Traditional education has focused on students' abilities to demonstrate their declarative knowledge without adequate attention to the development of cognitive strategies.

Problem-solving courses attempt to teach the basics of logical operation, using a problem-solving process. Problem-solving courses generally encompass the following activities as part of the **problem-solving process:** 1) recognize and define the problem; 2) select pertinent information for problem solution; 3) recognize stated and unstated assumptions; 4) formulate or select relevant or promising hypotheses; and 5) draw valid conclusions and judge validity of inferences and goals.[3]

Respiratory therapy students and practitioners must be accomplished problem solvers. Respiratory care programs and continuing education should be designed to enhance practitioners' abilities to use the problem-solving process. Problem solving is essential for respiratory therapists who are competent and valuable members of the health care team. Chapter 3 presents a discussion of how to develop problem-solving skills related to clinical decision making in respiratory care practice. The chapter also describes how to integrate various critical thinking strategies into your approach to problem solving. Please refer to Chapter 3 for further details, examples, questions, and exercises to assist in developing the problem solving and decision making skills needed in respiratory care practice.

"Problem solving" is so important for effective clinical decision making that it is often used interchangeably with "critical thinking." The authors of

CRITICAL CONTENT

The problem solving process:
- Recognize and define the problem;
- Select pertinent information for problem solution;
- Recognize stated and unstated assumptions;
- Formulate or select relevant or promising hypotheses; and
- Draw valid conclusions and judge validity of inferences and goals.

this book have a broader concept of critical thinking as it relates to clinical practice. This textbook emphasizes the importance of problem solving while also focusing on the attitudinal and practical aspects of critical thinking. The critical-thinking process encompasses logical reasoning or deductive processes, as well as creative or inductive processes.[16] Also, for thinking to be critical it is necessary that ideas, beliefs, and actions be validated through discourse with others. Merely analyzing the validity of arguments is not equivalent to critical thinking; the learner must also consider evidence found in the outside world.

Linking critical thinking with problem solving assumes that critical thinking always begins with a problem and results in a solution. However, a central element of critical thinking is the ability to raise critical questions and critique solutions, without necessarily posing alternatives. In addition, a critical thinker appreciates that there is rarely a single solution to a clinical problem. One trait of a critical thinker, the ability to appreciate multiple perspectives, frequently results in recognition that a clinical "problem" may not have a "solution," but perhaps multiple potential solutions, each with its own advantages and disadvantages. Often the best a critical thinker can do when faced with a clinical problem is point out the multiple potential solutions, and raise more questions to try and refine the list of potential solutions into a smaller number of choices. This strategy is an example of reflective skepticism, a hallmark of a critical thinker. This will be discussed in greater detail later in this chapter.

Although critical thinking is most commonly associated with tragedies or trauma called negative triggers, there are many instances when joyful, pleasing, or fulfilling experiences serve as positive triggers to critical thinking. For example, it is not uncommon for an experience such as winning an award or some other honor to trigger reinterpretation of our past actions or ideas from a new point of view. There is also an aesthetic element of critical thinking that allows the pure pleasure of playing around with ideas,[17] and playing with these ideas can stimulate your imagination. We wrote this textbook with the intention of exciting the imaginations of respiratory therapy students and their teachers so they can look at learning, teaching, and providing care in new ways. If this textbook helps respiratory therapy students take more responsibility for their careers and learning, while enjoying the learning process as true professionals should, the authors will have achieved their fundamental goals.

In summary, problem solving plays an important part in the process of critical thinking, but critical thinking is not solely problem solving. Formulating possible solutions to problems and then testing various solutions are major components of critical thinking. However, critical thinking is not only intellectual activity that involves logical reasoning and problem solving. Another major component of critical thinking is reflection, which involves emotive, behavioral, and practical aspects. This textbook gives equal attention to the practical, everyday aspects of critical thinking in our daily work and our lives.

Reflection

In addition to the problem-solving and logical aspects, critical thinking involves a reflective dimension. Reflection involves the practical aspects of critical thinking in our professional work. These practical aspects of critical thinking include communicative, experiential, and social elements. John Dewey defined **reflective thinking** as a form of thought that involves: "1) a state of doubt, hesitation, perplexity, mental difficulty, in which think-

ing originates, and 2) an act of searching, hunting, inquiring, to find material that will resolve the doubt, settle and dispose of the perplexity."[18]

The ability to maintain reflective skepticism is one of the hallmarks of critical thinking. **Reflective skepticism** allows a person to refrain from making a decision until all the evidence has been fully considered. Reflective skepticism encourages the realization that there are numerous points of reference and ways of thinking. Consequently, there can be many solutions to a problem, including multiple strategies for clinical decision making. People can step outside of their own frame of reference only by learning to think within the frame of reference of others.

It is inevitable that alternative ways of thinking will conflict with each other. **Dialectical thinking** is one aspect of critical thinking that allows you to appreciate alternative arguments or solutions to a problem. Individuals must learn how to engage in dialectical thinking in order to see both the strengths and weaknesses in opposing modes of thought. This means you can see the merits and limitations of two contrasting alternatives, an important skill for clinical practice. Frequently you will be faced with choices that require you to weigh the alternatives before making a clinical decision. Dialectical thinking will help you fairly evaluate your alternatives before making a decision, without resorting to personal bias or the other pitfalls of decision making.

Reflective thinking describes all of the intellectual and affective abilities used to explore experiences in order to lead to new understanding and deeper appreciation. **Reflexive thinking** is based on linkages in learning and is more automatic or presumed. Both types of thinking are important to clinical practice in respiratory care. For example, reflexive thinking is important to react quickly and effectively during emergency situations. Reflexive thinking is also important to our ability to prioritize. However, each of us must also reflect periodically on our automatic and habitual ways of thinking and acting in order to build our critical thinking skills.

A primary reason for facilitating critical thinking is to enhance learners' abilities to be critically reflective. Through critical reflectivity, we can

CRITICAL CONTENT

REFLECTIVE COMPONENT OF CRITICAL THINKING

- **Reflective skepticism** allows a person to refrain from decision making until all the evidence is fully considered.
- **Dialectical thinking** is one aspect of critical thinking that allows an individual to appreciate alternative arguments or solutions to a problem.
- **Reflective thinking** describes all of the intellectual and affective activities in which individuals engage to explore their experiences, leading to new insights and awareness.
- **Reflexive thinking** is based on linkages in learning and is more automatic or taken for granted.

---

become aware that our own perspectives can blind us, and therefore we can never really interpret our experiences without some degree of bias.[19] Therefore our greatest assurance of objectivity comes from exposing ideas to reflective and rational discourse. Exposing ideas to reflective and rational discourse not only requires critical thinking, but it also enhances critical thinking. Critical discourse is essential to bring together the internal and external worlds of the learner.

The reflective dimension acknowledges that being a critical thinker involves more than just intellectual exercises. Critical thinking involves more than scrutinizing arguments for assertions that are unsupported by empirical evidence. Thinking critically involves recognizing underlying assumptions that affect our beliefs and actions. It means we try to evaluate the accuracy and rationality of the justifications that we have for our beliefs and behaviors. Critical thinking in the broadest sense means that we are open to new ideas, experiences, and possibilities because we are eager to engage in the world to our fullest capacity.

Critical thinking involves calling into question the assumptions underlying our familiar and habit-

ual ways of thinking and acting. It also means that we are then ready to change our behavior on the basis of the results of our critical questioning. A critical thinker is also able to see things from someone else's perspective because he or she is aware of the diversity of values, behaviors, and social structures in the world. Critical thinking involving reflection can result in changes in assumptions made about oneself and others.

There are also the emotive aspects of critical thinking, which encompass feelings, responses, intuition, and sensations. Emotions such as depression, love, shock, elation, fear, hatred, and frustration are associated with the cognitive components of thought throughout the reflective process. Structures of thought are highly personal and emotional because they involve cherished values and beliefs, not just matters of dispassionate cognition. Critical thinking evokes powerful emotions because we are often asking painful questions about our entrenched values and behaviors. The process of critical thinking is often anxiety-producing, causing us to experience resentment, confusion, and fear, as well as joy, relief, and exhilaration. Critical thinking can enrich personal relationships, give greater meaning to our work, and result in more literate adults.[2]

In summary, the reflective dimension of critical thinking acknowledges the communicative, practical, and experiential aspects of critical thinking that guide belief and action within a social context. Reflection allows you to examine your assumptions and beliefs, which leads to new ways of thinking and acting. In short, reflective critical thinkers are not merely intellectuals solving problems, but are complex, highly developed professionals who can embrace multiple perspectives, pluralism, cultural diversity, uncertainties, change, and growth in the context of their professions and everyday lives. Critical thinking is analogous to going through life shifting gears versus driving on cruise control! Too many people go through their lives on cruise control, never calling into question what they think or feel and how both influence the way they work and live. Consequently, most of their thoughts and actions are done out of habit, and there are many missed opportunities for experiencing life and learning to the fullest.

CRITICAL CONTENT

BENEFITS OF REFLECTION

Reflection allows you to examine your assumptions and beliefs, which leads to new ways of thinking and acting. Reflective critical thinkers are not merely intellectuals solving problems, but are complex, highly developed professionals who can embrace multiple perspectives, pluralism, cultural diversity, uncertainties, change, and growth in the context of their professions and everyday lives.

Reflection Questions

1. Explain how reflection relates to your ability to develop critical thinking skills and traits.
2. Explain why critical thinking in the real world requires reflection.
3. To develop simple awareness, describe your knowledge about one aspect of respiratory care and explain how you determined you "know" this!
4. Describe how reflection can be used to help you understand your biases.
5. Describe ways you can uncover and understand your biases about particular aspects of respiratory care.

Group Critical Thinking Exercise 2

REFLECTION EXERCISES

a. Give an example of when you are going through your educational program on "cruise control" rather than challenging yourself to grow and learn.

b. Describe to your class what you intend to do in your respiratory care practice to avoid getting into a monotonous rut and why this is important to avoid.

c. Describe how feedback from your teacher or another student caused you to reflect on your respiratory care abilities. Why was this important to your learning?

d. Give an example of a clinical experience that caused you to reflect, and describe how this experience facilitated your learning and critical thinking.

SKILLS FOR CRITICAL THINKING IN RESPIRATORY CARE PRACTICE

Respiratory therapists often hear from their managers, supervisors, and even peers that they must become "critical thinkers" or that they routinely practice "critical thinking." Respiratory therapists may read journal articles that highlight the significance of critical thinking skills and may wonder about the job-related and personal significance of critical thinking.[20] Licensing and accrediting agencies stress the importance of critical thinking in respiratory care. For all medical professionals, processing information and making decisions are at the core of clinical practice. To be an effective practitioner and a vital, functioning member of today's health care team, respiratory therapists need more than just a strong knowledge base. Because of the dynamic and expanding nature of medical knowledge, the average medical professional cannot hope to survive and advance in the workplace by relying upon information gained in a formal educational setting. Mastering the thinking and reasoning skills necessary for processing both old and new knowledge is the most important task for today's respiratory therapist.

Research about critical thinking in health care comes primarily from the medicine and nursing professions. One study of critical thinking in respiratory care describes the actual critical thinking skills that are important to respiratory care practice as shown in Table 2-2.[8] Table 2-3 lists many of the situations in respiratory care practice that require critical thinking.[8] The following section describes the critical thinking skills that are essential in respiratory care practice. These skills include prioritizing, anticipating, troubleshooting, communicating, negotiating, decision making, and reflecting.[8,20–22] Figure 2-1 shows the interrelationship among these skills for critical thinking in practice. This chapter does not include exercises to develop these skills, which is a major focus of this textbook. Instead, the authors chose to focus on development of these skills in the context of solving clinical problems, a characteristic feature of problem-based learning (PBL). Learners have many opportunities to acquire and

TABLE 2-2 ESSENTIAL CRITICAL THINKING SKILLS FOR EFFECTIVE RESPIRATORY CARE PRACTICE

PRIORITIZING: "Rapid think" and "Organized think"
  The expected
  The unexpected
ANTICIPATING: "Future think"
  Problems
  Solutions
TROUBLESHOOTING: "Technical think"
  Technology
  Systems
COMMUNICATING: "People think"
  Practitioner-specific
  Situation-specific
NEGOTIATING: "Shared think"
  Responsibilities
  Medical orders for patient care
DECISION MAKING: "Personal think"
  Individual
  Joint
  Consultative
REFLECTING: "Inward think" and "Past think"
  The patients
  The decisions
  The profession

SOURCE: Reprinted from Mishoe.[8]

further develop these skills when working on the specific patient problems presented in this textbook.

Prioritizing

Prioritizing is the ability to arrange work according to the importance of the task. Prioritizing may be defined as "rapid think," and it is a critical thinking skill fundamental to respiratory care practice, needed to organize work according to importance, and to respond rapidly to emergencies and problems. Prioritizing requires respiratory therapists to not only make decisions or judgments, but also to act quickly in emergencies, a skill respiratory therapists describe as being quick on your feet or responsive.

Prioritizing the expected work is "organized think," while prioritizing the unexpected problems and emergencies is "rapid think." Prioritizing the expected work generally involves the logical reasoning dimension of critical thinking. The problem-solving dimension of critical thinking is involved when practitioners prioritize handling of unexpected emergencies and problems. Prioritizing is most important in settings in which respiratory therapists have significant responsibility for airway and ventilator management.

Respiratory therapists must be able to organize a plan and then make rapid adjustments according to the changing demands of the situation in order to function safely and effectively. This means that therapists have to be both organized and flexible so they can respond to patient care needs and situations relative to their importance or urgency. Therapists cannot respond with the same speed and urgency to every situation and be safe and effective clinicians. They must continuously assess their patients and clinical situations in order to determine when and where to concentrate their time and effort. The therapist's ability to prioritize impacts how he or she handles emergencies, and this affects their ultimate effectiveness in patient care.

Respiratory therapists are often faced with conflicting demands and emergencies, requiring them to act quickly in making the proper judgment. There are many instances when patients, nurses, other respiratory therapists, and physicians will simultaneously call on the therapist, and he or she must adequately cope with these demands. The therapist has to determine in an instant which aspect of a situation requires immediate attention.

In a typical clinical situation respiratory therapists perform many routine tasks, but they must also respond in emergencies. In both types of situations, after an initial judgment has been made about a patient's treatment, adjustments in task order must be made as conditions change. Because patients' conditions may change often during the course of the day, the therapist must constantly reprioritize as the day unfolds. Patient lives may depend on the ability of the respiratory therapist to properly prioritize work. Assessing and maintaining the airway is the foremost priority in acute respiratory care practice.

In a busy intensive care unit, for example, a respiratory therapist may be performing routine suc-

TABLE 2-3 OBSERVED SITUATIONS THAT REQUIRE CRITICAL THINKING IN RESPIRATORY CARE PRACTICE

Technology

Equipment malfunction	Alarms activated
Shortages of equipment	Recommend technology or therapy
Selecting and gathering equipment and supplies	Modifying equipment for novel care
Equipment not easily located	Equipment not set-up or available when needed in an emergency
Evaluating, using, and troubleshooting new technology	

Patients

Rare diseases	Unexpected response to respiratory care
Emergencies:	Problems with patient management:
Cardiac arrest	Patient fighting the ventilator
Respiratory failure	Patient not adequately oxygenated and/or ventilated
Inadvertent extubation	Multiple patient problems or situations demanding the therapist's time simultaneously
Emergency intubation	
Patient transports and admissions	
Novel approaches to respiratory care	
Neonatal delivery and transports	Responding to patient questions and reactions
Patient assessment	Mistakes or problems with patient care
Coaching, reassuring, and instructing patients	Modification in respiratory care

Other Clinicians

Questions from nurses, physicians, clinicians	Unclear or inappropriate medical order
Medical order does not coincide with patient care or with proposed care plan	Another clinician's behavior threatens the patient
Making suggestions and recommendations	Multiple persons talking to or asking for the respiratory therapist at the same time
Conflicting requests/demands from other clinicians	Asking questions
	Share in decision making with other clinicians

SOURCE: Reprinted from Mishoe.[8]

tioning on a patient receiving mechanical ventilation. At the same time, a patient in a nearby bed may suddenly go into cardiac arrest. The respiratory therapist must quickly and safely stop the suctioning procedure and resume mechanical ventilation on this patient before attending to cardiopulmonary resuscitation for the other patient. More than 1 hour may be required to complete the resuscitation. While attending the resuscitation, the respiratory therapist's beeper may show a message that an emergency intubation is needed for a patient with bleeding in the mouth and upper airway. A few minutes later, the radiology department may call to say that another patient's ventilation-perfusion scan is complete and he can be transported back to the ICU. During this time, multiple trauma patients from a car accident may arrive in the emergency department (ED). The respiratory therapist must quickly prioritize responsibilities and tasks so that all these patients receive optimal care. The therapist must also communicate quickly and effectively with others, including nurses, physicians, and other respiratory therapists, to obtain necessary assistance and to make others aware of any delays or reassignments in patient care.

CRITICAL CONTENT

PRIORITIZING

Prioritizing the expected work is "organized think," while prioritizing the unexpected problems or an emergency is "rapid think." Respiratory therapists must be able to organize a plan and then make rapid adjustments according to the unexpected demands of the situation in order to function safely and effectively. This means that therapists have to be both organized and flexible so they can respond to patient care needs and situations relative to their importance or urgency.

Anticipating

Anticipating involves the ability to think ahead and envision possible problems. Not only do respiratory therapists need to prioritize their work, they also need to exercise foresight in an effort to stay a step ahead and prevent potential problems. Anticipating is "future think," and it is an important element in resolving situations and evaluating patient care on a continuous basis. Anticipating differs from prioritizing, because when anticipating, the emphasis is to either avoid a problem entirely, or if that is not possible, to be prepared to quickly and decisively act.

The ability to anticipate is necessary whenever respiratory therapists make modifications in a patient's respiratory care, such as extubation, intubation, or ventilator changes; after making such changes, the therapist should be able to anticipate the patient's response. This foresight helps the therapist to evaluate the efficacy of the intervention. By mentally comparing the patient's response to the expected response, the therapist is able to prevent problems from occurring, rather than merely responding to problems after they occur. The primary aspects of anticipating are making recommendations for respiratory care and evaluating the outcomes to improve patient care.

Anticipating enables the therapist to "see the big picture," and the skills of anticipating and pri-

oritizing are interrelated. The ability to anticipate influences the therapist's ability to prioritize and vice versa. Therapists are better able to prioritize and respond appropriately to urgent or routine aspects of their work when they are also able to anticipate the results of their actions. On the other hand, the ability to prioritize allows therapists to use their time more effectively. Respiratory therapists can thus have greater opportunity to avoid problems through anticipation.

Anticipating problems and their solutions requires respiratory therapists to continuously and holistically assess their patients, a skill often described as being able to sense impending doom, pick up on subtle changes, and predict what will happen. Anticipating is useful when respiratory therapists make modifications in patient care or in respiratory care; when they are expecting a new patient or facing a new situation; when they plan ahead for equipment needs and actions they will take; when they prepare topics that they need to discuss with physicians; and when they notice subtle a change in their patient's condition that might indicate a problem. Anticipating in respiratory care practice involves a therapist's ability to continuously and holistically assess the patient, the data, the technology, and the situation, in order to either prevent problems or at least find solutions early when problems do develop. The skill of anticipating requires global or gestalt thinking in order to get a grasp of the whole situation and effectively come up with plans and solutions that prevent problems from occurring in respiratory care practice.

CRITICAL CONTENT

ANTICIPATING

Anticipating involves the ability to think ahead and foresee possible problems. Anticipating is "future think." This activity relates to a continuous and total approach to resolving a situation and includes the ability to "see the big picture."

Troubleshooting

Respiratory care is a highly technical profession, so it is not surprising to find that critical thinking in clinical practice involves troubleshooting. Troubleshooting is "technical think" and refers to the ability to locate and correct technical problems. Respiratory therapists should be able to introduce new equipment and methodology, modify and adapt new technology for particular needs and situations, and identify and correct equipment malfunctions or breakdowns in the process of delivering respiratory care. When there are shortages of equipment, malfunctioning equipment, or if equipment cannot be located quickly, these situations can rapidly become real emergencies. Troubleshooting includes all the technical aspects of respiratory care that require critical thinking.

CRITICAL CONTENT

TROUBLESHOOTING

Troubleshooting is "technical think" and refers to the ability to locate and correct technical problems. Respiratory therapists should be able to introduce new equipment and methodology, modify and adapt new technology for particular needs and situations, and identify and correct equipment malfunctions or breakdowns in the process of delivering respiratory care.

Troubleshooting equipment involves the ability to locate, process, and correct technical problems. Logical thinking and problem solving are integral components of troubleshooting. Resources respiratory therapists may find helpful include manufacturers' manuals, on-line technical assistance, and other respiratory therapists who are more familiar with the equipment. Troubleshooting may range from simple problems (Is the machine turned on?) to more complex problems (Why does an error message continue to appear after proper corrective steps have been taken?). Nurses and physicians may not understand that a laboratory result like an arterial blood gas measurement has been delayed due to a machine error. Respiratory therapists are expected to properly maintain and use their equipment for therapeutic and diagnostic procedures. Proper maintenance and quality controls (another aspect of anticipating) will help to avoid equipment malfunctions. Nurses and physicians rely on the respiratory therapist's technical expertise and expect him or her to respond knowledgeably to alarms or problems involving mechanical ventilators, pulse oximeters, capnographs, transcutaneous oxygen monitors, and other respiratory care devices.

Not only is the therapist responsible to respond immediately to technical problems, he or she needs to have a calm, systematic approach in assessing, identifying, and correcting the malfunction. No matter what the technical problem, a basic principle is to always assess the patient as well as the equipment. For example, it is easy to get absorbed when attending to all the alarms and controls on a ventilator when called to the bedside, but your first action should be to check the patient, and make sure that someone manually ventilates the patient while you systematically troubleshoot the mechanical ventilator.

Communicating

Critical thinking in practice requires the respiratory therapist to gather and disseminate information through verbal and nonverbal communication with nurses, physicians, patients and their families, other respiratory therapists, and other clinicians. Communicating is the ability to exchange information with others; communicating is "people think." Gathering appropriate and sufficient information to analyze, evaluate, and make judgments in clinical practice depends on effective communication. Effective communication is also dependent on having good working relationships with other members of the health care team. Therefore it is not surprising that critical thinking in actual clinical practice not only requires effective communications skills, but it is also influenced by personality traits.

Communicating in respiratory care practice is practitioner-specific and situation-specific. There is a tremendous amount of skill involved in knowing what to say, how to say it, and when to say it, based on the specifics of each situation. Each respiratory therapist communicates in a way that is comfortable for him or her and is appropriate for both their personality and the situation. It is not surprising that being able to communicate clearly, concisely, and convincingly is considered by many to be the single most important skill in professional practice.

CRITICAL CONTENT

COMMUNICATING

Communicating is "people think." Gathering appropriate and sufficient information to analyze, evaluate, and make judgments in clinical practice depends on effective communication. Effective communication is also fostered by good working relationships with others.

Communication style, duration, and frequency varies greatly depending on the key players involved, including the therapists, the patients and their families, the nurses, the physicians, other clinicians, and other respiratory therapists. In practice, information gathering is not merely selecting items from a list of possibilities as it is presented on a clinical simulation examination. Critical thinking in clinical practice is very much dependent upon communications with others as a primary means of exchanging the information that is needed for moment-to-moment patient care. Respiratory therapists need to be able to share information with other members of the health care team easily and efficiently.

If respiratory therapists cannot precisely communicate clinical parameters and their meaning to physicians and nurses, effective patient care may be limited or even jeopardized. Respiratory therapists may obtain anomalous or conflicting patient data such as unusual lab results and need to speak with a physician or nurse to ascertain the patient's clinical condition or diagnosis. If a respiratory therapist cannot communicate competently, then he or she will be unable to think critically in their clinical practice. The goal in communicating is obtaining

more information as well as sharing information. If an insufficient amount of information is exchanged, the respiratory therapist may be unable to interpret, analyze, and evaluate the patient's condition. A respiratory therapist may be able to critically analyze data or troubleshoot technical problems, but if the individual cannot communicate effectively, he or she cannot perform critical thinking in the real world.

Communicating effectively with patients is also essential to critical thinking in respiratory care practice. Respiratory therapists communicate with patients in order to obtain information, make assessments, explain, coach, or reassure. Offering reassurance is often the major purpose for communicating with patients in the ICU. Since many critically ill patients are intubated and cannot speak, communications with these patients is necessarily nonverbal. Respiratory therapists usually become adept at reading lips, facial expressions, and body gestures. Very often, the therapist will ask a patient direct questions that can easily be answered by a nod or shaking the head from side to side. Novice therapists need to learn how to ask simple yes or no questions in order to get appropriate responses from their patients.

It is common to see a respiratory therapist holding a patient's hand or patting the patient's arm or shoulder to offer reassurance when using nonverbal communication. In coronary care units, recovery units, and surgical ICUs, respiratory therapists often ask patients to squeeze their hand in order to assess the patient's level of awareness and ability to cooperate. Respiratory therapists use this information to assist them in making decisions about extubation, ventilator management, oxygen therapy, and other aspects of respiratory care.

To summarize, not only is communicating an essential skill for critical thinking in practice, but critical thinking is also essential for effective communication. Communicating is essential to obtain information required for critical thinking and critical thinking is essential in determining how to best communicate with others, including patients. Critical thinking in clinical practice requires therapists to gather and share the information needed for proper patient care through verbal and nonverbal communications with nurses, physicians, patients, families, and other clinicians. Critical thinking in clinical practice is not possible unless therapists can communicate effectively during clinical situations and exchange critical information at the bedside. Effective communication skills include the awareness of subtleties such as tone of voice, body language, and personality attributes of other health care workers and patients, all of which are important when using critical thinking in clinical practice.

Negotiating

Critical thinking in practice also requires the respiratory therapist to be able to negotiate patient-care medical orders and responsibilities. Negotiating is carrying on discussion in an attempt to influence others. Respiratory therapists negotiate with others when they do not have sole authority in determining patient care; negotiating is "shared think." Although negotiating requires communicating skills, not all communicating is negotiating. Negotiating differs from communicating because its intent is to impart information and ask questions in an effort to influence the decisions and actions of others.

Performance on a clinical simulation examination requires the respiratory therapist to make the right clinical decision after assessing the necessary data. However, in actual clinical practice, the respiratory therapist must negotiate to obtain the power he or she needs to do what they believe is best for the patient. Negotiating is exchanging information through discussion in a way as that will enhance overall patient care by influencing respiratory care.

Respiratory therapists may feel at times that they have little control over patient care, but as responsible health care providers and critical thinkers, they may be able to negotiate the medical order to provide the best possible health care for the patient. For example, respiratory therapists often interact with physicians to discuss changes in mechanical ventilation or to make recommendations regarding the appropriateness of respiratory care therapies.

To negotiate effectively, respiratory therapists need good communication skills and the ability to make suggestions and clearly explain them. Successful negotiators often phrase their suggestions

as questions, or make indirect implications and inferences about possible alternative actions. Effective listening is important to any communication, but it is essential for negotiations.

If the respiratory therapist is unable to negotiate, there will be limited access to that therapist's expertise. In order to negotiate effectively, respiratory therapists need effective communication skills and the ability to make rapid judgments. They must also be able to explain how they came to their conclusions. The ability to effectively communicate enhances the therapist's opportunities to negotiate patient care decisions, which are ultimately controlled by the physician via the medical order. It is only through negotiations that respiratory therapists can expand their opportunities for improving patient care based on their unique expertise.

CRITICAL CONTENT

NEGOTIATING

Negotiating is "shared think." Although negotiating requires communicating skills, all communicating is not negotiating. Negotiating differs from communicating in that the intent is to impart information and ask questions in an effort to influence the decisions and actions of others.

In summary, negotiating patient care responsibilities and orders for medical care is essential for critical thinking in clinical practice in order to achieve the best decisions and outcomes of patient care. One study found that the criteria for negotiating in respiratory care practice include: the seriousness of the patient's problem; whether it is a cardiopulmonary problem; the need for assistance or backup; the extent to which a particular solution is evident; the need to clarify medical orders or obtain assistance; the particular physician or physician service; and the therapist's feelings at the time and his or her confidence in their ability to influence medical orders or patient care decisions.[8,22] Chapter 4 provides further criteria for the skills of communicating and negotiating as well as additional questions and exercises.

Decision Making

Every aspect of respiratory therapy practice is impacted by the decisions we make individually in each of our situations and collectively within our profession. Respiratory therapists must be able to make smart clinical decisions if they are to deliver safe and effective patient care. Therefore, decision making is fundamental to critical thinking in respiratory care practice. Decision making is the ability to reach a judgment or conclusion or to decide on a course of action. Decision making is "personal think."

Respiratory therapists make clinical decisions on their own, by conferring with nurses and physicians at the bedside, and by consulting with other clinicians. Therapists and nurses continuously ask one another questions, exchange information, and share in the responsibility for decision making about patient care. Respiratory therapists often have the opportunity to participate in making clinical judgments and decisions. Respiratory therapists are certainly able to make decisions about their own work flow by exercising three of the above described aspects of critical thinking: prioritizing, anticipating, and troubleshooting.

When a unique problem is encountered, respiratory therapists can pursue consultation beyond bedside interactions and seek additional opinions

CRITICAL CONTENT

DECISION MAKING

Decision making is "personal think." Decision making is the ability to reach a judgment or conclusion; to decide on a course of action. Respiratory therapists must be able to make good clinical decisions if they are to deliver safe and effective patient care. Therefore, decision making is fundamental to critical thinking in respiratory care practice.

from other respiratory therapists, supervisors, the medical director, physicians, and even with clinicians at other hospitals and institutions. Respiratory therapists can also search the literature and use the Internet to inform their decisions.

Nurses and physicians also consult with respiratory therapists and other clinicians to share patient care decisions. Respiratory therapists share decision making with nurses and physicians regarding patient care overall, including various aspects of respiratory care. Respiratory therapists share decision making during rounds with physicians, during emergencies, when handling novel cases, and when physicians, nurses, and other therapists seek their opinions and guidance. Respiratory therapists are often the best informed about the various indications, contraindications, hazards, and limitations of various diagnostic and life-support technologies.

Others rely on the respiratory therapist's decision-making abilities in choosing among the numerous strategies and technologies for providing quality respiratory care services.[8,22] They may also seek feedback or advice regarding their experience, unique problems, and new strategies. Respiratory therapists are able to derive greater satisfaction and a sense of accomplishment from their work when sharing decision-making responsibilities for patient care.[8,20–22]

Reflecting

Reflecting is the ability to "think about thinking" in order to explore one's own assumptions, opinions, biases, and decisions. Reflecting may be considered introspective or "inward think." If the reflecting is retrospective in nature, then reflecting becomes "past think." Respiratory therapists may reflect on their work, their patients, their decisions, and their profession. Reflection helps respiratory therapists to learn from previous mistakes and problems; to handle the pain of errors in judgment; and to gain satisfaction from their work and contribution to health care and their profession.[8,21,22]

Reflection changes as respiratory therapists grow in their careers and assume different roles and responsibilities. Generally speaking, as respiratory

CRITICAL CONTENT

REFLECTING

Reflecting is the ability to "think about thinking" in order to explore one's own assumptions, opinions, biases, and decisions. Reflecting may also be considered introspective or "inward think." If the reflecting is retrospective in nature, then reflecting becomes "past think." Respiratory therapists may reflect on their work, their patients, their decisions, and their profession.

therapists become more experienced and make fewer errors, they begin to reflect more on the wider context of their profession and health care in general.[8] One of the most profound outcomes of reflection is that practitioners realize the multiple perspectives of circumstances, the gray areas of decision making, and the many levels of interpretation. Put more simply, we become aware that there is usually more than one correct interpretation of reality. Therefore, reflection is important to help respiratory therapists develop the disposition of a critical thinker, which is important for the implementation of critical thinking in actual practice.

Each respiratory therapist must acquire and develop the essential skills described in this part to be able to use critical thinking in respiratory care practice. Please refer to Part II of this textbook where there are several questions, exercises, and sample problems to help you develop these critical thinking abilities. You should refer to the present chapter to assist you in the completion of the Critical Thinking exercises.

CHARACTERISTICS OF CRITICAL THINKERS

Critical thinkers show distinct characteristics. No matter which definition of critical thinking is used, certain common attributes emerge that help to distinguish the critical from the uncritical thinker. The critical thinker has perfected the ability to adeptly

TABLE 2-4 ATTRIBUTES OF A CRITICAL THINKER

The critical thinker has an understanding of and an ability to formulate, analyze, and assess the following elements:
1. The problem or question at issue;
2. The purpose or goal of thinking;
3. The frame of reference or point of view involved;
4. Assumptions made;
5. Central concepts and ideas involved;
6. Principles or theories used;
7. Evidence, data, or reasons advanced;
8. Interpretations or claims made;
9. Inferences, reasoning, and lines of formulated thought;
10. Implications and consequences involved.

SOURCE: Reprinted from Paul.[23]

use the elements of thought shown in Table 2-4.[23] The uncritical thinker, on the other hand, is usually perceived as vague, shallow, illogical, unreflective, inconsistent, or inaccurate.[2,9]

General Traits of Critical Thinkers

Critical thinkers also show common affective qualities or traits. The critical thinker usually has these characteristics: inquisitiveness; a concern about being well-informed; alertness to opportunities to use critical thinking; trust in the process of reasoning inquiry; self-confidence in their own ability to reason; open-mindedness; flexibility; is tolerant of the opinions of others; fair-mindedness; honesty; is prudent and suspends judgment until all the facts are in; and is willing to reconsider his or her position.[8,24]

No matter what the profession, an extensive list of characteristics seems to indicate that there are differing degrees of critical thinking, and that most adults appear to possess some of the attributes, qualities, and abilities of critical thinkers. Table 2-5 shows the characteristics of critical thinkers in contrast to those of uncritical thinkers. It is important that respiratory therapy students and practitioners

TABLE 2-5   CHARACTERISTICS OF CRITICAL VERSUS UNCRITICAL THINKERS

CRITICAL THINKERS	UNCRITICAL THINKERS
Clear	Confused
Precise	Unrefined
Specific	Vague
Analytical	Shallow
Logical	Illogical
Reflective	Unreflective
Thorough	Superficial
Consistent	Inconsistent
Accurate	Inaccurate
Valid	Invalid

be given many diverse learning experiences to help them develop critical thinking skills.

Critical Thinking Traits of Respiratory Therapists

A study of respiratory therapists in the health professions revealed the following common traits related to critical thinking: 1) willingness to reconsider; 2) appreciation of multiple perspectives; 3) willingness to challenge someone else regardless of the power structure; 4) understanding of how other therapists' behavior impacts them and their profession; 5) responsibility for their own learning and understanding; and 6) openness to continuing change in their personal and professional lives.[6,25] Consequently, words that describe the traits of respiratory therapists who are critical thinkers include: open-minded, sensitive, engaging, responsible, accountable, passionate, outspoken, dedicated, caring, disciplined, and fair. These characteristics greatly impact the respiratory therapist's ability to use critical thinking in clinical practice. These personal traits of therapists enable them to keep a fresh perspective and look for new ways to improve their work performance. Therefore, critical thinking can be evident even during routine aspects of our work.

Respiratory therapists' capacity to reconsider and to appreciate multiple perspectives contribute to their ability to communicate and negotiate more effectively. Both the willingness to reconsider and the appreciation of multiple perspectives are critical thinking traits that influence every aspect of the therapist's practice. When respiratory therapists (or anyone else, for that matter) can listen to others' opinions and reconsider their own position, it helps them avoid mistakes, allows them to give better patient care, and they often learn something in the process.

Clinicians who are open to multiple perspectives are generally more eager to learn from others and prefer using collaborative approaches to solving problems in their practice. Most professionals who are critical thinkers come to realize just how little they, or anyone else, really know. Over time, respiratory therapists learn from experiences in which patient outcomes were improved when an approach was taken that was different from their recommendation. Consequently, a respiratory therapist's ability to appreciate multiple perspectives develops with increased experience and contributes to even greater openness. Therefore, critical thinkers appreciate multiple perspectives and use them to provide better patient care and to improve their practice. Also, it appears that the ability to appreciate the patients' perspectives motivates clinicians to use critical thinking to find ways to improve patient care. The attitudes and traits of respiratory therapists affects their ability to keep a fresh perspective. Therapists should continuously look for ways to improve their work performance and patient care.

Respiratory therapists who are willing to reconsider and can appreciate multiple perspectives can be more willing to challenge others. The willingness to challenge others is particularly evident when therapists use the skills of communicating and negotiating, which are essential to critical thinking in practice. Respiratory therapists are able to maintain reflective skepticism, and therefore they realize that there is no single right answer to many of the problems in professional practice. Consequently they are more likely to confront and challenge others in an attempt to participate in patient care decisions via negotiations and recommendations. The flip side of the coin is that respiratory therapists with this broad perspective will also be more willing to apologize for their mistakes. Again, the ability to see multiple perspectives enables you to see when your decisions or behaviors are less than perfect.

The willingness to make patient care recommendations is related to the ability to appreciate the patients' perspectives.[8] For example, it appears that because therapists are able to put themselves in their patients' shoes and can appreciate their patients' perspectives, they are more willing to go to bat for their patients. There are many situations in respiratory care practice when respiratory therapists must question others and make recommendations regarding patient care. For example, respiratory therapists who are critical thinkers will negotiate with physicians in order to delay extubation of patients who they believe are too unstable.[8,25] Respiratory therapists' critical thinking skills and traits help determine when, how, and why they make patient care recommendations and try to negotiate the medical order.

Another common critical thinking trait among respiratory therapists' is their understanding that the actions of other therapists impact them and their profession. Consequently, this trait affects the communicative aspect of critical thinking in their practice. More-experienced respiratory therapists must mentor less-experienced therapists and technicians because any practitioner's mistake hurts the patient, the department, and the entire profession. Students in respiratory care are encouraged to seek positive role models and to have a sounding board when suboptimal behaviors are evident in clinical practice.

Respiratory therapists who are critical thinkers are able to see the broader perspectives of the department, the organization, and the profession. Consequently, respiratory therapists should look out for other respiratory therapists, in order to mentor them or to apply peer pressure when necessary. Thus, there is a relationship between the traits of the therapists and their tendency to use the skills of communicating and negotiating in order to mentor and/or apply peer pressure. Respiratory therapists should be able to demonstrate and give examples when they challenge other therapists to do a better job for their patients and their profession. Respiratory therapists should apply peer pressure to persuade other therapists and clinicians to perform at a high level of quality in clinical practice.

Continuing to learn is another critical thinking trait. Respiratory therapy students and clinicians must assume responsibility for their own learning and growth. Even respiratory therapists with 10, 15, or 20 years of experience must continue to grow and learn. The technology and innovative approaches to patient care change rapidly. In general, respiratory therapists who are critical thinkers are eager and enthusiastic about their work and their patients.

There are educational opportunities from learning on the job, through in-service programs, and at professional meetings. Respiratory therapists should seek answers in resources like books and journals or on the Internet if they have questions or want more specific information. Much of our continuous learning occurs on the job by asking questions and interacting with others. In respiratory therapists, motivation and responsibility for their continued learning contributes to further development of related critical thinking skills. Furthermore, respiratory therapists can be more effective when communicating and negotiating in their practice because they can give specific reasons or build stronger arguments as a result of their continued learning.

Openness to continuing change in our personal and professional lives is also related to our critical thinking abilities. The ability to initiate and embrace change is a characteristic trait of expert respiratory therapists, which influences critical thinking in their practice.[8,25] Not only are these therapists more open to change, they are also most likely to initiate change. Respiratory therapists who are critical thinkers will look for ways to implement change to improve patient care. They will also continuously evaluate and improve the way respiratory care is practiced at their institutions. The most developed critical thinker will also try to influence other respiratory therapists to welcome or accept change, which can solve problems and lead to improvements in their practice. It appears that the therapists' realization that they can initiate change evolves over a period of time and is related to experience, confidence, and commitment. The motivation for initiating change comes from the therapists' sense of responsibility to be their best, and they are equally motivated to do the best work they can.

CRITICAL CONTENT

CRITICAL THINKING TRAITS THAT ARE IMPORTANT TO RESPIRATORY CARE PRACTICE

- Willingness to reconsider
- Appreciation of multiple perspectives
- Willingness to challenge someone else regardless of the power structure
- Understanding of how behavior of other respiratory therapists impacts them and their profession
- Taking responsibility for their own learning and understanding
- Openness to continuing change

The affective dimensions of thought significantly influence critical thinking in clinical practice and everyday life. The following section provides a novel strategy to facilitate critical thinking using the THINKER approach. Part II of this textbook includes numerous questions and exercises for respiratory therapists to help in developing critical thinking skills and traits using the THINKER approach.

SEVEN BASIC COMPONENTS IN THE PROCESS OF CRITICAL THINKING: THE THINKER APPROACH

The process of critical thinking is complex, involving many large and small steps. The critical thinker has the ability to formulate, analyze, and assess several elements using the thought processes shown in Table 2-4. This chapter introduces the THINKER acronym to help learners at every level to improve their critical thinking. The acronym **THINKER** is used in this textbook to help students remember the important components in the process of critical thinking. The THINKER process for critical thinking involves: **T**ime-out, **H**esitation, **I**nference, **N**o-

tions, **K**nowledge, **E**xpression, and **R**eflection. You are challenged to learn these important steps and then to use the acronym THINKER to critically evaluate your own thinking in your professional work as respiratory therapists and in your everyday life.

Time-Out

The first thing to do when dealing with any situation is to take time-out to ascertain the main problem, issue, point, or question. You can waste a lot of time and misdirect your energies if you don't focus on the real problem, issue, or question. You should ask yourself questions such as "What is this all about?" "What is really going on here?" "What is important here?" "What matters the most in this situation?" "What am I trying to accomplish (or prove)?" "What does the other person(s) hope to accomplish or gain here?" You should take a time-out and ask yourself these and similar questions whenever you approach a situation using critical thinking. Take time-out to focus on the real matter at hand to enhance your skills as a critical thinker.

In high-stress situations, a realistic time-out may only be a few seconds to collect your thoughts and frame the problem. Whenever possible, take sufficient time to think about what you are thinking! In today's fast-paced world, we have accelerated the rates at which we respond, reply, react, and resolve. In my opinion, we must remember the importance of a pause or time-out to assess our position and consider our next move. Furthermore, a time-out will increase your awareness of how you communicate and respond to problems. This will help you enhance and reinforce your use of reflective thinking, rather than reflexive thinking.

CRITICAL CONTENT

TIME-OUT

In high-stress situations, a realistic time-out may only be a few seconds to collect your thoughts and frame the problem. Whenever possible, take sufficient time to think about what you are thinking!

Hesitation

Once you take time-out to focus your thoughts and related emotions, you should hesitate. You should hesitate before making any hasty conclusions and maintain reflective skepticism. This means you should call into question your reasons for thinking what you think. When you are formulating your argument you should formulate your own reasons. When making a decision, you should search for reasons to support as well as contradict your initial inferences and premises. This means you can identify your reasons and the reasons of others when focused on a particular problem, issue, question, or point before coming to a conclusion. Hesitation does not mean you are slow and inefficient; it means you realize the impact of your actions and behaviors on a particular situation, and allows you to move forward with confidence.

CRITICAL CONTENT

HESITATE

You should hesitate before making any hasty conclusions and maintain reflective skepticism.

Inference

Inference refers to the process of going from a valid (true) reason to a conclusion. Once you have taken time-out to focus on the real issues and then identified the reasons, you must then evaluate those reasons. When you hesitate, you are determining the reasons and ascertaining whether they are true. When you go on to make inferences, it means that you have accepted the reasons as true and now are determining if the reasons are adequate to reach the conclusion. You need to ask yourself "Since my reasons are true, is it logical or reasonable to now reach the conclusion that I have come to?" For example, if A and B are true, does this mean that it is reasonable to conclude (or infer) that C is also a true? Inferences are made after examining evidence to support reasons.

CRITICAL CONTENT

INFER

An inference should be made only when you have valid reasons to support a conclusion.

Notions

Notions are any form of beliefs, opinions, views, plans or intentions. We generally form notions after making inferences. Our notions are usually based on a particular situation, context, or circumstance. The context includes the people and environment that influence what the thinker is doing or judging.

CRITICAL CONTENT

NOTIONS

Notions are any form of beliefs, opinions, views, plans, or intentions. We generally form notions after making inferences.

Each context has certain implicit (unstated) and explicit (stated) rules that influence the thinking process. The people we interact with in a certain situation have their own beliefs, experience, knowledge, emotions, predispositions (including prejudices and biases), interests, and purposes. The environment includes the physical and social variables such as government, religion, social norms, families, and institutions, to name a few.

It is useful to think of our beliefs, opinions, views, and intentions as notions because it emphasizes the vagueness of our mental imagery. This allows us the freedom to maintain multiple perspectives and to question what we think.

Knowledge

Knowledge is achieved after we carefully examine our notions. Knowledge can be described as the state of knowing or understanding. Knowledge includes learning and enlightenment, both for individuals and for all of humanity. In the broadest sense, knowledge is the body of facts and principles accumulated by a civilization over time. Sharing our notions and determining the factual basis for what we think individually and collectively is how we acquire knowledge.

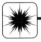

CRITICAL CONTENT

KNOWLEDGE

Knowledge is the body of facts and principles accumulated within a society over time. We acquire knowledge by individually and collectively examining the factual basis for what we think.

Expression

Critical thinking involves clearly expressing what you know. Validation of knowledge requires expression and critical discourse with others. Critical discourse involves evaluation of our arguments and the arguments of others, which requires clear expression. Expression of our ideas, thoughts, and beliefs is necessary because it is through interaction with others that a body of knowledge is obtained. Critical discourse forms the basis of our knowledge, therefore it is important to be precise when you write

CRITICAL CONTENT

EXPRESSION

Validation of knowledge requires expression and critical discourse with others. Critical discourse involves evaluation of our arguments and the arguments of others, which requires clear expression. Expression of our ideas, thoughts, and beliefs is necessary because it is through interaction with others that a body of knowledge is obtained.

and speak. This means that you must clearly and plainly say what you mean. You must also be able to persuade others to clearly express themselves to you so you can know what they are really saying.

Communication and negotiations are important components of critical thinking in our everyday lives. Chapter 4 presents a discussion of how to develop the communication and negotiation skills needed for effective respiratory care practice. The chapter also describes how to integrate the process of critical thinking to improve your thinking, communication, and negotiation skills. Chapter 4 also presents further details, examples, questions, and exercises to assist the learner with further development of communication and negotiation skills. We suggest you practice these skills to improve your effectiveness in respiratory care practice.

Reflection

The concept of reflection is described earlier in this chapter. You are encouraged to read the section on reflection and to think again about how it relates to your critical thinking skills and traits. Reflection is one of the most important of the abilities of a critical thinker, and you should make a conscious effort to make yourself more reflective. It is fortunate that the acronym THINKER ends with the letter R! Reflection should be the end point of your thinking process, and the beginning of the critical thinking process.

CRITICAL CONTENT

REFLECTION

Reflection should be the end point of your thinking process and the beginning of the critical thinking process.

As you become more critically reflective, you will be better able to take time-out (the beginning of the THINKER process) and to improve every aspect of your critical thinking. Critical thinking is a continuing growth process related to our thoughts, experiences, behaviors, attitudes, and environment. The THINKER process can aid students and faculty in developing awareness, commitment, and abilities to become more effective thinkers and professionals.

CRITICAL CONTENT

THE THINKER APPROACH

- **Time-out:** The first thing to do when dealing with any situation is to take time-out to ascertain the main problem, issue, point, or question.
- **Hesitation:** Once you take time-out to focus your thoughts and related emotions, you should hesitate before reaching any hasty conclusions and maintain reflective skepticism.
- **Inference:** Once you have taken time-out to focus on the real issues and then identified the reasons, you must then evaluate those reasons. Inference refers to the process of going from a valid (true) reason to reaching a conclusion.
- **Notions:** We generally form notions after making inferences. Our notions are any form of beliefs, opinions, views, plans, or intentions, usually based on a particular situation, context, or circumstance.
- **Knowledge:** Knowing is achieved after we carefully examine our notions. Knowledge can be described as the state of knowing or understanding.
- **Expression:** Critical thinking involves clearly expressing what you know. Validation of knowledge requires expression and critical discourse with others.
- **Reflection:** Reflection should be the end point of your thinking process, and the beginning of the critical thinking process.

In summary, students are encouraged to adopt the THINKER strategy to assist them in understanding and gaining critical thinking skills and traits. The THINKER process for critical thinking provides a practical method to gain awareness and expertise, while it provides students and faculty with a simple tool for focusing on desirable behaviors to enhance critical thinking.

Critical Thinking Exercise 2

USING THE THINKER APPROACH

a. You are asked to recommend home oxygen therapy for a patient with chronic obstructive pulmonary disease (COPD) who has carbon dioxide retention and severe hypoxemia. Formulate a recommendation using an example of each of the seven processes of the THINKER approach to decide what you will recommend.

b. You are using a weaning protocol to manage mechanical ventilation for a patient with Guillain-Barré syndrome. Describe how the THINKER approach can assist you with your assessment of your patient.

c. Use the THINKER approach when working through other chapter exercises throughout this textbook and in your clinical practice. Include examples of when and how the THINKER approach helped you develop the skills and attitudes of a critical thinker.

ORGANIZATIONAL VARIABLES AFFECTING CRITICAL THINKING

Organizational factors also impact critical thinking in actual practice. Although a description of essential skills and traits for critical thinking can explain how it is used in clinical practice, the explanation is incomplete. To adequately describe critical thinking as it is implemented in professional practice, it is equally important to discuss the contextual variables. Where the practitioner works affects the degree to which critical thinking is encouraged, expected, or even tolerated. Organizational variables affect when, how, and why critical thinking is evident in respiratory care practice. Figure 2-3 shows the interrelationship among the skills, traits, and organizational variables

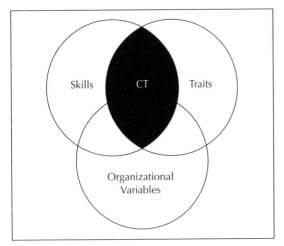

FIGURE 2-3 Interrelationship among the skills, traits and organizational variables for critical thinking in practice.

for critical thinking in clinical practice. Critical thinking in practice depends on the therapists' skills and traits as well as organizational variables. The potential for critical thinking in practice is greatest in organizations that encourage critical thinking among its professionals possessing the necessary skills and traits. Figure 2-4 shows that critical thinking is not evident in practice if organizational vari-

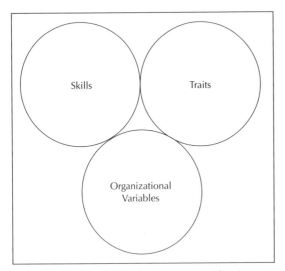

FIGURE 2-4 Critical thinking is not evident in practice if organizational variables are lacking and professionals do not possess the necessary skills and traits.

ables are lacking and professionals do not possess critical thinking skills and traits.

Numerous organizational factors affect critical thinking in respiratory care practice, such as: involvement and level of support from the medical director; departmental administration and climate of the respiratory care department; the scope of the practice, duties, and responsibilities of therapists; and role delineations between entry level respiratory therapists (CRTs) and advanced level respiratory therapists (RRTs). The following sections describe how each of these organizational variables affects critical thinking in respiratory care practice.

Role of the Medical Director

The role of the medical director in respiratory care departments either facilitates or inhibits critical thinking by respiratory therapists. A supportive medical director can facilitate critical thinking in respiratory care practice, whereas an unsupportive medical director can stifle it.[8,25] It appears that the medical director's support or lack of support influences respiratory therapists' communications and negotiations with physicians. The type and frequency of recommendations made to physicians varies in correlation with the level of support given by the medical director. Respiratory therapists are most likely to use critical thinking and make recommendations regarding patient care at institutions where there is strong involvement and support from the medical director and other physicians.[25,26]

Contextual variables within the organizations where we work influence critical thinking in actual practice. A description of the skills and traits essential for critical thinking in respiratory therapists can define the use of critical thinking in clinical practice. Nonetheless, it appears that the setting where the respiratory therapist works is another factor that can either facilitate or inhibit critical thinking in respiratory care practice.

Respiratory therapists appear more relaxed and at ease when making recommendations for patient care at hospitals where there is frequent, supportive involvement from the medical director.[8] Respiratory therapists can compare and contrast their roles in patient care and how they change under different medical directors. When the medical director is involved and supportive, respiratory therapists play a bigger role in patient care decisions. Consequently, respiratory therapists have greater opportunities to use critical thinking in their practice.

When the medical director is involved and supportive, respiratory therapists will demonstrate greater confidence when they make recommendations. The therapists are also more likely to challenge physicians and stand behind their positions.[8,25] Knowing that the medical director encourages therapists to express their opinions, thoughts, and suggestions can only serve to encourage critical thinking in clinical practice.

Many medical directors are not only supportive of the respiratory therapists at their institution, they and other physicians are also supportive of the respiratory care profession in general. Position statements and letters of support from physician organizations such as the American College of Chest Physicians (ACCP), the American Society of Anesthesiologists (ASA), and the California Thoracic Society (CTS) state the important role respiratory therapists play in health care.[26–30] In addition, the ACCP has issued a position statement supporting the use of respiratory care protocols.[26] Support from national professional associations and physicians at the local level and in our workplaces can facilitate critical thinking in respiratory care practice. Several medical directors and many physicians are involved in state and national professional associations for respiratory care, including the National Association for Medical Direction of Respiratory Care (NAMDRC). Recently, NAMDRC issued a statement of support, stating that respiratory care practitioners are the nonphysician caregivers best qualified to render respiratory services.[26] Many physicians have also supported state licensure of respiratory therapists and were instrumental in promoting approval of their state licensure bills by the legislature.

It is difficult to sort out how much of communications and negotiations are a matter of personal characteristics versus organizational factors. Although it is difficult to separate how much critical thinking is determined by dispositions versus orga-

nizational factors, the findings from one study clearly indicate that a supportive medical director can facilitate critical thinking in clinical practice.[8] It appears that when there is little support from the medical director, respiratory therapists will make recommendations less often, unless they are more assertive or the situation is clearly life threatening. It was apparent that the therapists working in settings where there was strong support from the medical directors were more outspoken and involved in patient care decisions,[8,25] therefore there are greater opportunities for critical thinking in their practice. Increased opportunities to participate in decision making can lead to the development of therapists' critical thinking skills and traits. Chapter 6 provides a detailed discussion on the important role of medical director and physician support for development of clinical protocols.

Climate of the Respiratory Care Department

Departmental administration and the climate of the respiratory care department also affect critical thinking in respiratory care practice. Respiratory therapists are aware of the level of support and expectations from department administrators. Respiratory therapists' willingness to take risks or initiate change is related to the climate of the respiratory care department. The climate or culture of a respiratory care department can be categorized as follows: progressive and innovative (ahead of the times), current and satisfactory (up to date), and status quo (behind the times).

A status quo department is one in which there are standardized ways that therapists interact with physicians and the medical director is generally uninvolved and unsupportive.

The majority of departments can be described as current and up to date. In these departments, therapists have access to the latest technology and are instrumental in introducing the newest approaches to respiratory care. Respiratory therapists are more likely think critically, make recommendations, and initiate change when department administration provides opportunities for therapists to learn and grow.

Some respiratory care departments can be described as progressive. At these institutions, there are formal and informal opportunities for the staff to participate in the administration of the department.[8,25,26] Collaboration between department management and the staff is evident and everyone is open to trying out new ideas and strategies for improving patient care, the department, and the profession. In progressive settings, it is evident that critical thinking is encouraged. Respiratory therapists are more likely to think critically to initiate change if they can see that their recommendations for innovative solutions to problems may be implemented.

Strong departmental leadership is needed to establish standards of practice that facilitate rather than inhibit critical thinking. A single therapist is not solely responsible for how physicians interact with respiratory therapists throughout the entire organization. The department's climate partly determines the expectations placed on therapists, such as how they interact with physicians and how much their opinions are valued, that ultimately impact critical thinking in practice.

The hospitals with the most progressive respiratory care departments tend to be the same settings in which support from the medical director and hospital administration is the strongest.[8,25] The most progressive departments also have a history of strong support from the medical director, department management, and hospital administration. It is difficult to determine the exact interrelationship of these organizational factors. Are the department directors more effective because of supportive relationships with hospital administration and the medical director? Or is the organizational support present in the first place because the department directors are effective?

The most progressive departments have had well-established respiratory care departments in place for 10 to 20 years. Further study is needed to attempt to answer the questions posed above; however, critical thinking is enhanced in respiratory care practice when the climate of the department is progressive and there is leadership from the department administrators, physicians, and medical directors.

Scope of Practice

Opportunities for critical thinking in respiratory care practice are determined in part by the respiratory therapist's scope of practice at each institution. Every institution is different regarding the exact duties and responsibilities of respiratory care practitioners. Scope of practice determines which patient care duties and responsibilities are handled solely by respiratory care practitioners, and which are shared with nursing staff or handled by other health care professionals, including physicians. The opportunities to perform certain duties and responsibilities either facilitate or inhibit critical thinking in respiratory care practice. Chapter 5 offers numerous examples of an expanded scope of practice in respiratory care practice, including the role of physician extender.

Performing technical duties in and of itself does not necessarily facilitate critical thinking in respiratory care practice. For example, if respiratory therapists are expected to draw arterial blood samples, but there is little opportunity to discuss results with physicians, then the skill itself does not promote critical thinking. Once a manual or psychomotor skill is mastered, the activity itself does not necessarily promote critical thinking. However, if respiratory therapists are able to perform certain tasks, and as a result they have increased opportunities to participate in decision making, then critical thinking is enhanced.

In most departments there are opportunities for respiratory therapists to make patient care decisions within certain limitations. At some institutions, there are patient care protocols for therapies such as oxygen, aerosol, humidity, incentive spirometry, and chest physical therapy with percussion. Protocols specify guidelines the therapists can follow to make changes in patient care without consulting with the physician. In some institutions, protocols per se are not used, but there are guidelines, parameters, policies, and procedures that are used by therapists to make decisions. The opportunity for respiratory therapists to manage respiratory care within specified guidelines requires them to develop strong patient assessment skills to coincide with their expanded scope of practice. Please refer to Chapter 6 for a complete discussion of this topic.

It is becoming common for respiratory therapists to shoulder major responsibilities for airway and ventilator management. Critical thinking is facilitated in practice when respiratory therapists have greater responsibility for airway and ventilator management. At the institutions with the most progressive departments, respiratory therapists are able to intubate, ventilate, wean, and extubate patients at their discretion. Ventilator flow sheets should be modified to allow more detailed assessment by respiratory therapists, who can then assume a greater role in patient management. Organizational factors including improvements in the control and dissemination of information (such as ventilator flow sheets) can increase the therapist's scope of practice, which can facilitate critical thinking in practice.

Respiratory therapists should continue to develop and modify protocols to increase their role in patient assessment and decision making. Therapists should also seek out opportunities to increase their interactions with physicians and their participation as part of the health care team. All of these factors can facilitate critical thinking in respiratory care practice.

The scope of practice for respiratory therapists at various hospitals either inhibits or facilitates critical thinking in respiratory care practice. Technical or psychomotor skills, in and of themselves, do not facilitate opportunities for critical thinking. However, opportunities for critical thinking can be enhanced through improved technology and the use of protocols. Furthermore, the role of respiratory care departments and respiratory therapists in obtaining and disseminating clinical information facilitates critical thinking in respiratory care practice.

Role Delineations between Entry Level and Advanced Practice

Critical thinking in respiratory care practice is also affected by whether or not the role delineations between therapists credentialed for advanced (Registered Respiratory Therapists; RRTs) or entry level

practice (Certified Respiratory Therapists; CRTs) are implemented. At hospitals where there are specific role delineations between advanced and entry level therapists, advanced therapists have greater opportunities for critical thinking in their work.[8,25] When there is little distinction between the duties of RRTs and CRTs, the level of practice is limited, more along the lines of entry level practice. Although not studied, it is speculated that CRTs probably have greater opportunities for critical thinking in these settings where roles of RRTs are limited.

When there are clear and distinct roles for RRTs and CRTs, all therapists seem to enjoy "blanket credibility." Blanket credibility refers to the established performance and scope of practice of a particular group of health care professionals. When blanket credibility is not evident, each individual therapist must prove him- or herself and establish individual credibility. At some hospitals individual credibility determines how assignments are made. It is also well established what each individual therapist can or cannot not do. The Committee for Accreditation of Respiratory Care (CoARC) is the organization that administers accreditation of educational programs in respiratory care. Previously, the Joint Review Committee for Respiratory Care Accreditation (JRCRTE) was the organization that administered accreditation of educational programs in respiratory care. JRCRTE had different criteria and mechanisms for accreditation of respiratory therapy programs and respiratory therapy technician programs. Furthermore, the National Board for Respiratory Care (NBRC) had separate role delineations and credentialing systems for RRTs and certified respiratory therapy technicians (CRTTs). However, in respiratory care practice, the differences between therapists and technicians and their separate role delineations were not necessarily implemented.

One study found that almost half of the sample worked at hospitals where there was little distinction in practice between RRTs and CRTTs (now renamed CRTs).[8] It was not unusual to find technicians working in critical care performing the same duties as the respiratory therapists. This was especially true at hospitals that had status quo departments. There were no differences in pay or responsibilities between RRTs and CRTTs at many hospitals. In other hospitals, although there were differences in pay between RRTs and CRTTs, technicians often performed work similar to that of therapists. In these settings, no distinctions were made between technicians and therapists, and the technicians were also called therapists. This scenario has limited opportunities for critical thinking in respiratory care practice since most professions are judged by their "least common denominator."[31] In many health care settings, physicians have little knowledge of the differences in accreditation, education, training, and credentials between entry level and advanced practice.

The same hospitals with role delineations tend to have strong support from administration, the medical director, and physicians.[8] Therefore, it is difficult to separate which organizational factor has the greatest influence. Are there greater differences between the roles of therapists and technicians when there is strong support from the medical director? Or is strong support from the medical director and other physicians greater when there are role delineations between therapists and technicians?

In 1998, the NBRC implemented new credentialing examinations based on task analysis and eliminated the technician category. The NBRC now recognizes two levels of respiratory therapists: the entry level examination credentials Certified Respiratory Therapists (CRTs) and the advanced level examination credentials Registered Respiratory Therapists (RRTs). By January 1, 2001, all new students entering programs will have to graduate with a minimum of an associate's degree. This essentially will eliminate the technician level in respiratory therapy. These changes acknowledge the need for more extensive education, to cover the additional content, expanded role, and greater expectations placed on today's respiratory care professionals. Although the technician certification has been discontinued, the respiratory care profession can further promote critical thinking by not blending the roles of CRTs and RRTs, so that advanced practice can flourish, promoting the growth of the profession.

Respiratory therapists have the greatest opportunities for critical thinking in practice when there is a supportive medical director, strong departmental leadership, a liberal scope of practice, and role delineations between RRTs and CRTs. The essential skills, personal traits, and organizational factors illustrate the multidimensional nature of critical thinking in actual clinical practice.

KEY POINTS

- This chapter describes critical thinking and problem solving, giving a basic introduction to the concepts of thinking, logic, problem solving, reflection, and lifelong learning.

- The chapter elaborates on the essential skills and traits needed for critical thinking in respiratory care practice.

- The essential skills for critical thinking in respiratory care practice include prioritizing, anticipating, troubleshooting, communicating, negotiating, decision making, and reflecting.

- The traits of respiratory therapy critical thinkers include: 1) willingness to reconsider; 2) appreciation of multiple perspectives; 3) willingness to challenge someone else regardless of the power structure; 4) understanding of how other therapists' behavior impacts them and their profession; 5) responsibility for their own learning and understanding; and 6) openness to continuing change in their personal and professional lives.

- This chapter describes and advocates the THINKER approach for helping students and respiratory therapists remember the important components in the process of critical thinking.

- In addition, the chapter discusses the organizational or contextual factors that influence critical thinking in respiratory care, which include involvement and level of support from the medical director; departmental administration and the climate of the respiratory care department; scope of practice, duties, and responsibilities; and role delineations between entry level and advanced respiratory therapists.

- Respiratory therapy students and their faculties can enhance their critical thinking abilities and dispositions by carefully reading the chapter and completing questions and exercises in this chapter and throughout the textbook.

- Critical thinking is a complex construct to understand, and even more difficult to implement in the delivery of respiratory care.

- Students, faculty, and indeed all respiratory therapists must continuously strive to improve their professional abilities to be effective health care professionals throughout their careers.

REFERENCES

1. Eljamal MB, Sharp S, Stark JS, Arnold GL, Lowther MA. Listening for disciplinary differences in faculty goals for effective thinking. *J Gen Education.* 1998;47:117–148.

2. Brookfield SD. *Developing Critical Thinkers.* San Francisco: Jossey-Bass; 1987.

3. Dressel P, Mayhew LB. General education: Explorations in evaluation. Final report of the Cooperative Study of Evaluation in General Education. Washington, DC: American Council on Education; 1954.

4. Ennis R. A concept of critical thinking. *Harvard Educational Rev.* 1962;32:81–111.

5. Hallet GL. *Logic for the Labyrinth: A Guide to Critical Thinking.* Washington, DC: University Press of America; 1984.

6. Halpern DF. *Thought and Knowledge: An Introduction to Critical Thinking.* 2nd ed. Hillside, NJ: Erlbaum; 1989.

7. McPeck JE. *Teaching Critical Thinking: Dialogue and Didactic.* New York: Routledge; 1990.

8. Mishoe SC. Critical Thinking in Respiratory Care Practice. *Dissertation Abstr Int.* 1995;55:3066A (University Microfilms No. 9507227).

9. Paul RW. *Critical Thinking: What Every Person Needs to Survive in a Rapidly Changing World.* Rohnert Park, Calif: Center for Critical Thinking and Moral Critique; 1993.

10. Janoff-Bulman R. *Shattered Assumptions: Toward a Psychology of Trauma.* New York: Free Press; 1992.

11. Resnick LB. Learning in school and out. *Educational Researcher.* 1987;16:13–20.

12. Sackett DL, Rosenberg WMC, Gray MJA, et al. Evidence-based medicine: What it is and what it isn't. *Br Med J.* 1996;312:71–72.

13. McKibbon A, Eady A, Marks S. *PDQ Evidence-Based Principles and Practice.* Hamilton, Ontario, Canada: B.C. Decker; 1999.

14. Jones A. Second international Cochrane Colloquium—official annual meeting of the Cochrane Collaboration: A conference report. *Resp Care.* 1995; 40:171–174.

15. Gagne R. Learnable aspects of problem solving. *Educational Psychol.* 1980;15:84–92.

16. Garrison DR. Critical thinking and adult education: A conceptual model for developing critical thinking in adult learners. *Int J Lifelong Education.* 1991; 10:287–303.

17. Meyers C. *Teaching Students to Think Critically: A Guide for Faculty in All Disciplines.* San Francisco: Jossey-Bass; 1986:5.

18. Dewey J. *How We Think: A Restatement of the Relation of Reflective Thinking to the Educative Process.* Boston: D. C. Heath; 1933.

19. Mezirow J. A critical theory of adult learning and education. *Adult Education.* 1981;32:3–27.

20. Mishoe SC, Martin S. Critical thinking in the laboratory. *Learning Laboratorian Series* 1994;6:1–63.

21. Mishoe SC, Courtenay B. Critical thinking in respiratory care practice. Proceedings of the 35th Annual Adult Education Research Conference. Knoxville: University of Tennessee; 1994:276–281.

22. Mishoe SC. Critical thinking in respiratory care practice. *Respir Care.* 1996;41:958 (abstract).

23. Paul RW. A proposal for the national assessment of higher-order thinking at the community college, college and university levels. ERIC Document Reproduction Service No. ED 340 762, 1991.

24. Facione PA. Critical thinking: A statement of expert consensus for purposes of educational assessment and instruction. ERIC Document Reproduction Service No. ED 315 423, 1990.

25. Mishoe SC. The effects of institutional context on critical thinking in the workplace. Proceedings of the 36th Annual Adult Education Research Conference. Edmonton, Alberta: University of Alberta; 1995:221–228.

26. Mishoe SC, MacIntyre NR. Expanding professional roles for respiratory care practitioners. *Respir Care.* 1997;42:71–91.

27. American College of Chest Physicians, accessed December 15, 2000 http://www.aarc.org/advocacy/resources/physician_letters/accp_letter.gif

28. American Society of Anesthesiologists, accessed December 15, 2000 http://www.aarc.org/advocacy/resources/physician_letters/asa_letter.jpg

29. ACCP Supports Respiratory Care Protocols, accessed December 15, 2000 http://www.aarc.org/advocacy/resources/physician_letters/protocols_accp.html

30. California Thoracic Society, accessed December 15, 2000 http://www.aarc.org/advocacy/resources/physician_letters/cts_paper.html

31. Kacmarek RM. Respiratory care practitioner: Carpe diem! Program Committee Lecture. *Resp Care.* 1992; 37:264–269.

3

CLINICAL
PROBLEM SOLVING

Melvin A. Welch, Jr.

*There is no reward for the fastest guess
in clinical problem solving.*

MEL WELCH
2000

LEARNING OBJECTIVES

1. Give a working definition of clinical problem solving.
2. Identify steps of a systematic approach to problem solving in respiratory care.
3. Explain how problem-solving and decision making relate to critical thinking in respiratory care practice.
4. Identify and explain how problem-solving skills relate to advanced practice credentialing in respiratory care.
5. Identify the relationship between problem solving and decision making.
6. Describe what is known about base knowledge and clinical experience and their impact on the ability to problem solve.
7. Describe the role of using an evidence-based approach to solving clinical problems in respiratory care practice.
8. Identify common barriers to respiratory therapists acquiring clinical problem solving skills and methods to overcome these barriers.
9. Describe the characteristics of the novice problem solver.
10. Cite a variety of examples in which problem solving is applied in clinical respiratory care practice.
11. Identify the characteristics of the problem-solving respiratory therapist.

KEY WORDS

Adherence
Ambiguity
Cognitive Strategy
Cues
Hypothesis

Novice
Precipitously
Problem Solving
Spectrum
Synergistic

INTRODUCTION

This chapter presents ideas about how to develop problem solving skills related to clinical decision making in respiratory care practice. This task, once accomplished, will go a long way toward facilitating your development as a respiratory care professional. Although the information contained in this chapter would probably be useful to almost anyone involved in practicing respiratory care, we have written it with the new graduate or novice respiratory therapist in mind. For this reason we will not focus much attention on the very complex issues related to how "experts" solve problems.

We begin this journey with a brief working definition of what we mean by *problem solving,* and then proceed to a discussion of its relationship to decision making and critical thinking. Next follows an overview of the relationship of problem solving to advanced practice credentialing, and shall end with a brief discussion of the common approaches to problem solving.

Clinical Problem Solving Defined

In order to better learn to become a problem solver, it seems appropriate to first answer the question: What is clinical problem solving? Problem solving can be defined in many different ways. Although there are many other definitions of problem solving, from a respiratory care practice standpoint problem solving could be defined as: *the recognition that a problem exists, followed by a systematic process during which a solution, or often solution(s), to the problem are then determined, implemented, and evaluated.* When we insert the word "clinical" in front of problem solving, we are simply defining the context in which the process will be applied (ie, the problem to be solved pertains to the clinical care of a patient).

At first this definition may appear simple and straightforward. On the other hand, it may not initially make sense to you. Through the use of examples and discussion in this chapter, the chosen definition should become clear to you. As it turns out, there is nothing that simple and straightforward about developing the skills to carry out this task. Even what would seem to be the simple act of recognizing and defining what problems are to be solved does not come easily. As a result, the identification of the problem to be solved is actually the first stage of the problem solving process.

The next logical question may be: What is the nature of, or what types of problems are we talking about recognizing? In a traditional medical setting the *problem* is often equated with the *medical diagnosis.* This is certainly one type of problem, but it is not the *only* type, and it is not the primary type of problem we must solve as respiratory therapists. A *problem* for our purposes is any situation that presents itself that requires decision(s) to be made in order for care to proceed in a manner that ultimately leads to an improved outcome for our patient. This is a very broad use of the word, but one that does suit our purpose of trying to assist you in developing your clinical skills to aid in making decisions, as problematic situations present themselves to be solved.

Sometimes the problem is very straightforward (eg, a leak in a ventilator circuit causing loss of volume, or a hypoxemia that requires initiation or adjustment of some form of therapy). Sometimes, however, the problem is much more subtle, as in the following example.

As a new graduate respiratory therapist you will be constantly facing situations that involve making decisions. Some of these situations (problems) will be relatively minor and will appear to be easily resolved. In fact, you probably do not even recognize that you are problem solving when you first head to the clinical area after obtaining the shift report from the outgoing respiratory therapists.

Your first clinical problem as you begin your shift typically involves deciding how you will proceed in the delivery of respiratory care to the patients assigned to you. You will probably think "First I will go check on my two patients who are receiving mechanical ventilation in the ICU, then I will proceed to the less critically ill patients." This seems like a pretty simple and routine decision to make. But wait, upon **reflection** you recall that during the shift report you were told that Ms. Smith in room 546 has been very short of breath and wheezing most of the night. In fact, she has called for her treatment earlier than scheduled a couple of times during the night. Although Ms. Smith is not due for her next bronchodilator treatment for another hour, perhaps should you stop by and take a quick look at her before heading off to the ICU?

A few questions quickly run through your head. Should you have asked for a bit more detail about her response to the most recent treatment? Just how bad is her asthma, you wonder. Has Ms. Smith been intubated previously for her asthma? Was she appearing worse as the night progressed, or was she starting to improve? Oh well, mechanical ventilation patients *always* have priority over non-ICU patients, don't they? At least that is what you recall one of your clinical instructors once told you. Have you figured out yet that this was a *generalization,* and that of course there will be exceptions? Do you recognize that applying the critical thinking skill of *prioritizing* is, in fact, a form of problem solving? Maybe if you had gathered a bit more data during the shift report, you would be more comfortable making the decision you have to make right now. As you gain experience you will refine and develop these skills to assist you as you try your best to provide quality respiratory care.

The above scenario is commonplace and it called for critical thinking before you even saw your first patient of the day! As a respiratory therapist you will have numerous opportunities on a daily basis to make decisions that affect the care your patients receive. Becoming aware of the process you are using to arrive at your decisions is likely to result in better quality decision making. Perhaps you can also become a better problem solver and ultimately make decisions that lead to better outcomes. In fact, as a *professional* you are committed to make decisions based on what the latest research shows (ie, having a research-based practice) whenever there is outcomes research to help support your decisions.[1] This is known as using evidence-based medicine (EBM), and it is the way a therapist "makes an effort to integrate research findings into clinical thinking and decision making while recognizing that effective health care practice is more than the mere application of scientific knowledge."[2] Using an EBM approach will be particularly important whenever you are faced with recommending some form of diagnostic or therapeutic procedure to either assist you in further defining the problem, or to treat the problem you have identified. This will be discussed further, later in this chapter.

Problem Solving, Critical Thinking, and Decision Making

Just what is the relationship between problem solving, critical thinking, and decision making? First, it is important to recognize that there are many points in the problem solving process at which decisions have to be made. For example, you have to decide if a piece of data is relevant, what additional data to collect, and if the data you have are valid and reliable, among other things. These are all decisions that, though important, could be referred to as "mini-decisions." These decisions are all important small steps made while following the problem solving process. However, when most people think of "decision making," they are more likely thinking of the more obvious, major decisions, such as "What are you going to do to solve the problem with the patient's worsening condition?"

I propose that making these major decisions also occurs at a specific point along the problem solving process. One of the steps in our proposed strategy for problem solving is formulation of solution(s) to the problem. However, before you can proceed to the next step in the problem solving process, you must make a particularly important decision. Ultimately, you must select one of the proposed solutions you have identified and give it a try. This is the decision that most people would think you are referring to when you discuss problem solving and decision making, making the major decision about treatment. It is at this stage of the problem solving process that you make, and then implement, this decision.

How does critical thinking fit into this problem-solving process that we are introducing? Critical thinking is what should be practiced during each step in the problem-solving process. All of the traits and characteristics of the critical thinker, as well as the affective and cognitive strategies that promote critical thinking, must be applied during each step of the problem-solving process. To assist you in this task, the THINKER strategy described in Chapter 2 can be implemented during various steps in the problem-solving process to remind you to utilize critical thinking processes as you work through the steps to solve the problem.

Relationship of Problem Solving to Advanced Practice Credentialing

The attainment of the Advanced Practice credential offered by the National Board for Respiratory Care (NBRC), the Registered Respiratory Therapist (RRT) credential, has always been one of the goals for the career-minded graduate therapist. The second part of the examination process for this credential, the clinical simulation examination (CSE), requires the therapist to overtly make two fundamental types of decisions. You are asked to decide what information is relevant to a particular situation, referred to as *information gathering,* and then, based on your assessment of the relevance of that information, you must decide what action would be most appropriate at that point in time, for instance, selecting options in the section entitled "Decision Making."

You may not realize it at the time you are doing it, but you are in fact following the basic stages of a medical problem-solving process as you work through the CSE. These two phases, the sections on information gathering and decision making, are basically identical to the two major phases of decision making that characterize medical problem solving, according to Connelly and Johnson.[2] These researchers described medical problem solving as being characterized by "designation of the correct diagnosis and selection of a therapy that positively affects the patient's problem."

What the NBRC CSE does not always explicitly have you do is pause to present your assessment of the meaning of the data you have selected. You are *not* specifically asked to identify the diagnosis or problem, you are simply asked to select a course of action to remedy the problem as you understand it, based on your interpretation or assessment of the data you have selected. This lack of formally identifying the problem should not be viewed as a fault or weakness of the exam, merely recognized as a test design practicality. The fundamental assumption made by the exam designers is this: if you were able to select most of the relevant information and not much irrelevant or unnecessary data (ie, made good small decisions) and you

made a reasonable decision of what to do next (ie, made a good major decision), then you must have made a reasonable assessment for problem identification. After all, you picked an acceptable solution! Thus, it is presumed that you have properly identified the problem(s).

You may have noticed by now that I have avoided saying you picked the right or correct solution. This is a critical point in understanding the nature of medical decision making. The NBRC "experts" understand that there is often more than one reasonable solution to a medical decision. This is why there are varying degrees of acceptable responses to many of their decision making sections. There is no one correct pathway of decision making through the simulated problems, just as there is not one acceptable pathway of care for our patients in real life; thus the NBRC exam system simulates the complexity of reality.

The skills needed to successfully make these CSE decisions rely a great deal on the application of critical thinking, and both very much depend on your problem solving abilities. Focusing on, and ultimately defining, the problem by examination of relevant data, followed by picking an acceptable action to take in the decision making section are basic components of what I have proposed to be our working definition of problem solving.

Common Approaches to Problem Solving

When it comes to solving problems in everyday life, there are a limited number of strategies. Some of the most commonly used problem-solving strategies are trial and error, intuition, experimentation, and some form of the scientific method.[3] Trial and error and experimentation are not practical approaches for the novice problem solver and hence will not be discussed further here.

Interestingly, intuition, although not widely accepted or advocated as a preferred method of solving problems, does seem to play a role in describing how some experts arrive at their solutions. Intuitive reasoning has been researched in the nursing profession with some indications that intuitive processes may be combined with other information processing methods to assist in solving problems.[4] The focus of this chapter, however, is on the development of problem solving skills in the novice respiratory therapist, therefore the role of intuition is beyond the scope of this chapter.

The scientific method, or more accurately a quasi-scientific method, has most often been advocated as an organized process that can be followed to solve problems. Novices who are unfamiliar with the content and the context should utilize the scientific method and EBM approaches to solve problems while gaining experience and expertise. The scientific method follows a step-by-step process that ultimately leads to a proposed hypothesis or solution(s) to the problem presented. Many proposed models for following a systematic problem solving process in medicine appear to be variations of a process most often called the *hypothetico-deductive model* (HDM), which was described by Elstein and colleagues in 1978.[5] This process involves initial hypothesis generation followed by data gathering to modify, refine, reject, and/or replace the hypothesis. This process proceeds until the problem solver is satisfied that the problem has accurately been identified and an acceptable solution has been found. This strategy is the foundation for the proposed model that follows.

A PROBLEM-SOLVING STRATEGY FOR RESPIRATORY THERAPISTS

Although no single model or reasoning strategy has been demonstrated to be superior to others, there is evidence that using some form of systematic approach offers advantages over not following a systematic process.[6] What this means to the therapist seeking to develop these skills is that you should approach problem solving by having a basic strategy or process that you intend to follow as you work through problems. You can think of this as having a "cognitive strategy" for how to deal with problem solving, as described in Chapter 2. The following is proposed as a reasonable process to follow when problem solving in respiratory care:

1. Initial problem recognition
2. Problem definition and analysis
3. Formulation of solution(s)
4. Implementation
5. Evaluation

Problem solving runs the gamut from the simple to the very complex. As a consequence of this, the model strategy suggested above must allow for considerable variability in how thoroughly each step is followed. For a simple problem, the first three steps may be quite short, and the last couple of steps may be so short as to be barely recognizable as discrete steps at all. On the other hand, a clinical problem that involves the need to develop a respiratory care plan with therapeutic interventions will require more thorough coverage of each step of the problem-solving process.

Problem-Solving Step 1: Initial Problem Recognition

The first stage of problem solving is to review the initial data. For example, the initial data when approaching a patient-assessment type of problem can consist of data such as current complaints, physical examination data, patient background factors, and other historical data. These bits of data are often referred to as *cues*. Cues are stimuli that can trigger the problem-solving process. The more obvious cues are often referred to as signs (objective data) and symptoms (subjective data from patient). From these initial presenting signs and symptoms must come an initial recognition that there is, in fact, a problem that exists.

At this initial stage it may not be clear precisely what is wrong, but the key point is that the problem solver recognizes something is amiss. It may be an abnormal physical examination or lab finding, or perhaps noticing a trend of increasing pressure on a mechanical ventilator over the course of the previous shift. At this stage a problem is recognized, but just what the specifics are or their significance is not clear. The next step in the problem-solving process will refine and eventually define the problem in more specific terms. It is at this next step that the problem solver will **infer** meaning to the initial data.

Problem-Solving Step 2: Problem Definition and Analysis

The data that are already present should be verified for accuracy if possible. Sometimes this involves a re-measurement, or personally gathering the data again instead of relying on someone else's report or recording of data. For example, a nurse reports to you that patient Mr. Jones' SpO_2 is 85%, or a student assigned to work with you reports that Mr. Smith has "no breath sounds on the right." In situations like these your first reaction should be to quickly verify the data before taking other actions. These are not situations in which you are not trusting the data from your colleague; however, it is critical that the data be verified whenever possible before decisions are made based on them.

The next step is interpretation of the data. Their most likely meaning must be established. Part of this process is to make a judgment about the significance and relevance of the data. It is at this point that **inferences** are made about the meaning or importance of specific cues or pieces of data. The critically thinking problem solver is going to be cautious at this stage of the problem-solving process. This is a very critical stage of the process, because it is tempting to accept the most obvious possible meaning of data that comes to mind, and to not maintain the reflective skepticism that is so important to being a critical thinker. Remember, the critical thinker always utilizes cognitive strategies such as suspending judgment, refining generalizations, and avoiding oversimplifications. Remember the "H" in the THINKER approach to critical thinking: *hesitate*—do not jump to conclusions derived from your initial impressions!

The critical point here is that making **inferences** about the meaning of data must be done with caution and with as much background information as possible. To give you an opportunity to further develop this concept, see Critical Thinking Exercise #1: Inferring Meaning to Data. The clinician may also infer relationships among some cues and

Critical Thinking Exercise 1

MAKING "INFERENCES" FROM INITIAL DATA

Let's take the two examples just identified in the text. Recall that the initial data reported are: Mr. Jones' SpO_2 is 85% and Mr. Smith "has no breath sounds on the right." Given these initial data, each student should do the following:

a. Identify what your first action would be once this information was reported to you.

b. Identify what you would infer that the data most likely mean.

After each student has completed this exercise individually, the entire class (or if feasible, in groups of 6 to 8 students) should discuss what each student came up with for the answers to this exercise. The discussion should be held in an environment that encourages diverse interpretations and is nonjudgmental. The instructor should serve as a facilitator to keep the discussion going, but should ensure that the students do most of the talking!

cluster them together (see Critical Thinking Exercise #2: Clustering Data).

Based on your preliminary interpretation of the data, (*inferring* meaning and relevance, and formation of data clusters), one or more hypotheses (proposed explanations) are formulated. These hypotheses should be consistent with your interpretation of the initial data and must explain the abnormality noted.

These hypotheses serve an essential function. They form the context within which further data gathering takes place. After hypothesizing, the problem solver applies the critical thinking skill of **anticipating**. With each hypothesis you would have certain findings that would be *anticipated* (predicted to be present), and other findings that would not be expected (or should be absent) (see Critical Thinking Exercise #3: Anticipating Findings).

Collection of additional data now proceeds with the intent of testing the proposed hypothesis or hypotheses. The additional data are gathered to determine if a patient's findings are consistent with

Critical Thinking Exercise 2

CLUSTERING DATA

The act of clustering data is one in which you take different pieces of data that you think are all pointing to, or are consistent with, the same interpretation. These pieces of data, when taken individually and not in context of the clustered group, may not be a very strong basis on which to infer a specific interpretation. However, *when considered as a group*, with all of them consistent with the proposed inference, they take on synergistic strength, and enhance the likelihood of the inference ultimately proving to be a valid or correct one.

Practice clustering data: Patient Mr. Williams:

You are given the following data: Mr. Williams, a 58-year-old male, is admitted to the emergency department (ED). The patient reports being very short of breath for the past 2 days, increasingly so over the past 12 hours. He is observed to speak in very short phrases and reports coughing up large quantities of yellow/green sputum. Initial data are as indicated below:

On room air: f 30/min, temp. 38.3° C, pulse 118, BP 144/88, SpO$_2$ 84%.

On nasal cannula at 3 L/min: f 24/min, temp. 38.2° C, pulse 100, BP 136/84, SpO$_2$ 88%.

a. What would be the most likely hypothesis for Mr. Williams' diagnosis?

b. Which data do you feel can be clustered to lead to this diagnostic inference (explain your answer)?

c. How would you evaluate this patient's response to oxygen, using clustered data?

The above CT exercises could be assigned to be completed individually, or by small groups working together. After time has been permitted to perform the exercise, (as either an out-of-class assignment or as an in-class exercise) the faculty member should facilitate a discussion by the entire class of the responses that were developed.

the proposed explanation (hypothesis). The additional data that are gathered are compared to those that would be anticipated to see how well the hypothesis fits the data in the specific situation.

From this process, the hypothesis is accepted as the proper explanation, modified, or perhaps even replaced completely by a new hypothesis that is more consistent with the interpretation of the current data. This process can potentially go through a number of cycles of hypothesis modification and data collection until the problem solver is satisfied that the problem(s) have been accurately identified.

Critical Thinking Exercise 3

ANTICIPATING CLINICAL FINDINGS BASED ON THE HYPOTHESIS

Once initial data have been verified and initial meaning assigned (**inferences** have been made about the meaning and relevance of the data), one or more hypotheses are usually formulated. The next step is to decide what new or additional data would be useful to obtain and review to assist in accepting, modifying, or rejecting the proposed explanations for what is going on.

Exercise:

Assume you have looked over some initial data in a couple of different situations and have come up with the following hypotheses to explain what you think the initial data indicate:

Hypothesis situation #1: There is a leak around this patient's artificial airway cuff.

Hypothesis situation #2: This patient (on a mechanical ventilator) has developed a tension pneumothorax on his right side.

For each of these hypotheses, perform the following exercise:

a. Identify at least 4 clinical findings that you would anticipate to find that would be consistent with the hypothesis. (These findings, if found, would support the hypothesis as a correct explanation.)

b. Identify at least 3 findings that would be inconsistent with the hypothesis. (These findings would *not* support the hypothesis.)

Your instructor may assign additional hypotheses for you to use when performing this exercise. After completion of this exercise (either individually or in small groups) the class should have a facilitated discussion of the students' responses.

Problem-Solving Step 3: Formulation of Solution(s)

Once the problem has clearly been identified, a plan to solve the problem can be proposed. The nature of the solution will necessarily depend considerably on the type of problem identified. Knowledge of what solution should be proposed for each problem comes from a variety of sources, including textbook and classroom learning as well as practical experience, to name the most common traditional sources. Health care practices are changing, however, and so too must respiratory care practice. Decisions or recommendations made by respiratory therapists should no longer just be based on what seems reasonable to the therapist, or what is usually done.

In respiratory care, as in most medical sciences, there has been a growing recognition that many decisions should not be based on personal preferences, past experience, or anecdotal information, but rather on research findings whenever possible. Certainly all the major decisions, such as choosing a therapeutic plan, but also some of the mini-decisions, such as deciding whether an expensive or invasive diagnostic procedure is really needed, call for an EBM approach. In clinical problem solving, the EBM approach is most likely to impact decisions that deal with recommending diagnostic or therapeutic procedures when developing a care plan. An evidence-based approach should be the therapist's first choice when selecting the most appropriate solution to a problem.

In an effort to assist therapists in their goal to practice evidence-based care, professional organizations like the American Association for Respiratory Care (AARC) have developed and published clinical practice guidelines (CPGs).[7] These research-based practice guidelines were developed by a diverse group of individuals, using all literature available at the time of publication, and were widely circulated to provide maximum opportunity for other practitioners' input. Basing clinical decisions on CPGs whenever possible is highly recommended. In addition to CPGs, other tools have been developed to assist the clinician in decision making. As discussed in Chapter 2, critical pathways, patient care protocols, and algorithms are also useful tools that can assist in decision making. Examples of protocols are also available in Chapter 7.

To develop your decision-making skills at this stage of the problem-solving process, be sure to recall some of the critical material from Chapter 2. Remember to practice **reflective skepticism** and **dialectical thinking**. Recall that reflective skepticism allows a person to refrain from decision making until all the evidence has been fully considered. Reflective skepticism encourages the realization that there are numerous points of reference and ways of thinking. Consequently, there can be many solutions to a problem. In addition, dialectical thinking allows you to appreciate alternative arguments or solutions to a problem. Dialectical thinking will help you fairly evaluate your alternatives before making a decision, without resorting to personal bias or other pitfalls of decision making. In the end, after weighing the alternative solutions, you may even decide to propose multiple solution(s) to a colleague or the physician if you are providing recommendations. Having a list of proposed solutions discussed and debated within a group (if practical) before deciding on the final solution is often a good idea in decision making.

Although EBM should be practiced whenever possible, not all clinical problems encountered are going to have research-based evidence available to assist in the decision-making process. Simple problems may be resolved with straightforward and simple solutions. For example, a leak from a hole in the ventilator circuit may simply call for the ventilator tubing to be replaced. Unfortunately, many of the problems that arise are not so straightforward in their resolution. If the leak turns out to be from around the artificial airway cuff, the solution may appear simple, but is it really that straightforward? (See Critical Thinking Exercise 4: Is the Obvious Solution Always the Right Solution?)

Problem-Solving Step 4: Implementation

Implementation is a critical step in the problem-solving process. The effectiveness of implementation of a solution will vary widely with the skills

Critical Thinking Exercise 4

IS THE OBVIOUS SOLUTION ALWAYS THE RIGHT SOLUTION?

Sometimes, after a problem has been identified with reasonable certainty, there is a tendency to quickly adopt the usual or expected solution, often without a second thought. Remember to practice **reflective skepticism** and **dialectical thinking** whenever possible. This is consistent with the cognitive strategy of suspending judgment as long as is practical before making an important decision.

Exercise:

Place yourself in the clinical situation in which you have concluded that there is clearly an air leak around your patient's artificial airway. This is evident from a variety of data, that once clustered, make a pretty solid conclusion that air is indeed getting by the cuff.

a. Identify the usual "fix" (solution) for this problem.

This should be rapidly done by the entire group or class. Afterwards, poll the students and record what solution the majority of the class determined to be the usual, quick fix. Now, as a group, debate, discuss, and answer the following:

b. Have the group identify at least 3 "special circumstance" situations where the usual solution would not be the most desirable solution.

c. For each special circumstance situation, what would the most desirable solution be?

and knowledge of the person doing the implementing. The skills required can be from any of the three learning domains: psychomotor skills, knowledge, or interpersonal skills (communication effectiveness, empathy, etc). This needs to be kept in mind as one evaluates the effectiveness of the implemented solution. If the solution appears to fail, was it because the solution did not fit the problem, or was the shortcoming in the implementation of the solution? This will be carefully analyzed in the next step of the problem-solving process.

Implementation of a solution can be extremely simple, or it can be very complicated, depending on the nature of the problem(s) and the solution(s). If the problem was simple and the solution simple,

then the implementation will in all likelihood be simple. For example: (a) problem: leak from a hole in a ventilator circuit; (b) solution: replace defective tubing; (c) implementation: the simple task of replacing the defective tubing is performed.

When the problem(s) are more complicated, the solution(s) become more complicated, and thus the implementation will often become more complex. For example, in the situation in which the problem calls for implementation of a therapeutic procedure as a solution, we are really using our problem-solving process as a respiratory care planning process. If formulating a care plan in response to the problem, it is important to first use an EBM approach to select a solution that has a scientific basis (if the research literature has addressed the topic), and secondly to identify specific therapeutic objectives, to aid in evaluation of effectiveness of the chosen therapy. If the therapeutic objectives are stated in terms of expected outcomes, the therapist will be able to determine more clearly the degree to which the objectives have or have not been achieved (and if the problem has or has not been solved). See Chapter 7, Table 7-12 for excellent examples of outcomes measures that are appropriate for various therapeutic interventions that may be recommended in a care plan.

Problem-Solving Step 5: Evaluation

The final step of problem solving is evaluation. As with the other steps in our problem-solving model, the complexity of the evaluation will depend on the nature of the problem. Some problems may be simple enough that the evaluation process will consist of simply gathering new data and examining them to see if the problem still exists. Let's first look at our previous example of a leak in a ventilator circuit (problem), in which we implemented the solution of changing the ventilator circuit tubing (solution). When we gather new data, and see that the measured exhaled tidal volume is now back to matching the ventilator setting, our assessment is that the problem has been solved, thus, end of evaluation!

On the other hand, if our identified problem(s) had called for development of a respiratory care plan and implementation of therapeutic procedures, the evaluation phase would be considerably more involved. Vitale and Nugent[8] have described the evaluation process for an implemented care plan as having four steps:

Step 1: Evaluation begins with a reassessment that involves collecting new information. Once the care plan is implemented, the patient is reassessed, new clusters of data are identified, and the significance of these new data is determined. These activities allow you to accurately identify the patient's responses to the care provided.

Step 2: Now you must compare the patient's actual response(s) to the expected outcomes. (It should be apparent why it is essential to have identified the expected outcomes!) Consider this dilemma: If you cannot identify the expected response(s) of a patient to bronchodilator therapy during an asthma attack, how will you know if the patient did or did not respond appropriately? (See Critical Thinking Exercise 5: Identifying Expected Outcomes to a Therapeutic Intervention.)

Step 3: Analyze factors that affected the actual outcomes for the purpose of drawing conclusions about the success or failure of specific interventions. Was the intervention ineffective because it was not properly or consistently administered? Was the implemented solution the correct one for this patient? Are there variations in the solution that you considered, but did not try yet? Did you accurately identify the problem? Was the outcome measurable?

This step of evaluation requires going back to the beginning of the problem-solving process to attempt to determine why the plan did not work. This **reflection** on the problem-solving process that was used may help identify areas in which alternate interpretations could be made that could provide new insight into the problem or its possible solution(s). It may well be that an alternate solution should now be tried. Rarely is there only one approach to treating a problem.

Step 4: Modify the plan of care that you implemented, based on your analysis performed during Step 3. If the failure was in the quality or consistency of the implementation, this would need to be addressed with the personnel involved. If the analysis provided new insights into alternate

solution(s), the plan of care should be modified accordingly.

The extent of the evaluation needs to be appropriate for the complexity of the problem and the implemented solution(s). Simple problems and solutions may be rapidly evaluated, whereas complicated clinical problems may require evaluation over a prolonged period of time, using multiple measures of data to determine success or failure of the problem-solving process.

Critical Thinking Exercise 5

IDENTIFYING EXPECTED OUTCOMES TO A THERAPEUTIC INTERVENTION

Providing bronchodilator therapy is one of the more common respiratory care procedures performed. In order to evaluate if an implemented plan of bronchodilators was effective, a therapist has to evaluate the patient's response to therapy and compare it to the expected response.

a. Use an EBM approach to identify as many potential positive responses as possible to bronchodilator use.

b. Identify the potential negative responses (side effects).

Present your responses to a group or the whole class for feedback and discussion. Faculty will function as a facilitator for the discussion. After the class discussion, answer the following two questions:

c. What are some of the difficulties with identification of the anticipated response?

d. How does your answer to this exercise relate to the ongoing controversy over bronchodilator use?

THE ROLE OF KNOWLEDGE BASE AND CLINICAL EXPERIENCE IN PROBLEM SOLVING

There is no question that knowledge base and clinical experience are important variables that can affect one's problem-solving ability. It has been proposed that physicians learn largely by gaining insights from clinical experience.[9] In addition, problem-solving skills are largely attributed to clinical experience that helps to develop pattern recognition processes in experts.[10] Although these are interesting theories about how experts solve problems, the focus of this chapter is to lay the groundwork to allow the novice to strengthen problem-solving skills. There has been very little research into how the novice (student) gains from early clinical experiences. The following is an interesting proposition for your consideration.

There appears to be some substance to the perception that there are different qualities of experience. Some students and therapists appear to gain much from their clinical experiences, while others do not appear to gain the same amount of insight or knowledge. This is probably a function of the degree to which the person internalizes their experience by organizing or storing what they have learned in a manner that allows them to recall it when they face a similar situation in the future. It is one thing to simply perform a task; it is quite another to be mentally active during the process. To be "mentally active" is to reflect on what you are doing while you are doing it.

Much of what you learn from a clinical experience when you are a student comes from bedside instruction by other therapists. During clinical instruction, you are shown and told what steps to follow to perform a procedure, but how often are you asked why you are doing it, or what alternatives exist to a given procedure? Are you ever asked why a procedure is not done another way or what complications to watch for while you are doing it? If you ask yourself these questions while performing procedures, you will have an enriched clinical experience, and will more likely be able to transfer what you are learning to new or similar situations. This is the essence of being mentally active as you learn to perform your duties as a respiratory therapist.

When it comes to problem solving, there appears to be a significant benefit from **reflecting** on how problems are solved in the actual clinical setting. How often have you stopped, while still at the bedside, and actually reconstructed the process by which you or a colleague just solved a problem? If you want to be a problem solver, this may be the single most important thing you can do to develop this skill. Learn from your experiences by reflecting on what has happened, thus internalizing the knowledge in such a manner that you can recall it when confronted with a similar situation.

Knowledge base is yet another variable that plays a role in problem-solving ability. A number of researchers have proposed knowledge-driven problem-solving models that are based on the assumption that students typically try to understand new information based on their existing knowledge. There is no disputing that knowledge base is important, but it appears to be an oversimplification to conclude that mere content knowledge leads to problem-solving ability.

Research reveals that successful problem solvers must possess comprehensive knowledge, but what is even more important is the way in which they organize their knowledge.[11] The manner in which the knowledge is structured or organized in one's mind is apparently quite critical. An expert problem solver is thought to have their knowledge structured in such a way that it can easily be retrieved from memory and applied to the case at hand.[12] Still other researchers have emphasized that an expert's diagnostic superiority should be attributed to the organization of their knowledge rather than to variables associated with the problem-solving process.[13] It is clear that both clinical experience and knowledge base, or more precisely knowledge organization, are important components of an expert problem solver.

What is not so clear is how a novice therapist learns to organize their knowledge such that it can be more easily accessed when needed. Some believe that this is one of the potential benefits of the PBL process. It is thought by some PBL advocates that learning information in the context of a clinical problem may lead to an improved ability to recall that information when it is needed in the future. Although this seems logical, it remains to be proven if this is indeed true.

BARRIERS TO ATTAINMENT OF PROBLEM-SOLVING SKILLS

To become an expert problem solver, you must overcome the many barriers to problem solving.

One of the most important steps you must take as a respiratory therapist is to become a more critical thinker; hence a better problem solver is more **reflective** in their thinking. The THINKER approach presented in Chapter 2 can improve your reflective abilities and contribute to development of critical thinking traits, which should improve your ability to solve problems in practice. It is our hope that using the THINKER strategy may help overcome some of the barriers to problem solving by giving you a process to follow that will help you avoid the common mistakes made by the novice.

To stop and actually "think about your thinking" is not that easy to do, but the benefits can be enormous. This point is brought up now, just as we begin a discussion of behaviors and characteristics of the novice problem-solving therapist, for good reason. As each characteristic or behavior is discussed, ask yourself: Do I ever do that? Does that describe me? This retroactive form of reflection may begin to raise your awareness of traits that interfere with or prevent critical thinking, thus inhibiting your problem-solving ability.

Now comes the hard part! In addition to reflecting back on your past behaviors, you need to develop the ability to stop in *real time*, and **reflect** on the thinking process you are following *as you confront decisions* you must make. With very little analysis, you will often find that you are actually about to make a decision based on an absent or inadequate critical thinking process.

Emotional Barriers

It has been said that fear and anxiety are the greatest emotional barriers to problem solving.[14] As students, which of you hasn't asked yourself: What if I make a mistake? A student's anxiety is understandable. Provision of health care is obviously very important and nobody wants to make mistakes when a patient's health could be affected. Although the concern is real and appropriate, the environment created by instructors or even colleagues in practice can have a significant impact on the level of anxiety created by a particular situation. A calm, reassuring environment is desirable and should be the goal of anyone who is helping a novice to develop the skills and traits needed for critical thinking in respiratory care practice.

Characteristics of the Novice Problem Solver

The novice problem solver is frequently (although not always) someone new to their profession. Therefore, the novice starts off at a disadvantage attributable to a much smaller base of content-specific knowledge, as well as considerably less clinical experience. The importance of these issues has already been discussed. Although these reasons could be considered convenient excuses for all their difficulties with problem-solving behavior, it is probably only a partial explanation at best.

I propose that the novice respiratory therapist has difficulty with problem solving not only due to their lack of knowledge base and experience, but also due to two other factors. First, many novices do not appear to follow a systematic strategy to solve problems. Second, as they work their way through the problem-solving process, they often display a number of behaviors or characteristics, that act as barriers to successful resolution of the problem. It is our hope that by learning a strategy to follow, and by recognizing barriers that inhibit problem solving, the novice can avoid these mistakes and will strengthen their problem-solving skills.

Now as we examine each step of the problem-solving process, we will identify behaviors often seen in novices that are thought to inhibit critical thinking, and thus function as barriers to their ability to solve problems. As we review each step look for any characteristics that might describe your behavior! To become a more effective problem solver you must **reflect** on your own typical behaviors and compare them to the examples below. Recognition of ways in which you are inhibiting your own critical thinking will assist you in improving your problem-solving skills.

Novice Characteristics at the Problem Recognition Stage.   The obvious novice mistake here is inability to recognize that something is amiss. A novice will often just not recognize a problem when it confronts them! Obviously, recognizing that data are *abnormal* starts with knowledge of what is *normal*. At first this seems like an extremely straightforward assessment, but as you will see, it is not that simple! Making a comparison of actual data from a given situation to textbook normal data is not so easy.

First, we must acknowledge that in human physiology the definition of "normal" often varies according to a number of factors, including such variables as age and/or gender. All therapists learn that the normal respiratory rate for a newborn is different than that for a child or an adult, and of course even this "normal" number is given as a range of values. How would you answer this simple question: What is a normal blood pressure? Is age a factor? How about gender? Of course, to most correctly respond to the question you would have to factor in both age and gender, and even then you really should identify a range of values due to human variability. By now I hope you are willing to accept the premise that even identifying what is normal is not without some challenge.

Let's suppose you gave this answer: Normal BP is 120/80 mm Hg for a 70-kg adult male. Patient Mr. Smith is a 70-kg adult male and his BP is 130/86. Is it *abnormal*? Now we get into interpretation of this question: Is the difference between this patient's actual value and what I know to be normal significant enough to be considered *abnormal?* We may reach back and try to remember, now what was the *range* of normal? Even if we judged it in this case to be "slightly abnormal" (what ever that means), is it abnormal enough to be relevant to our assessment of this situation? What a mess! Trying to make this distinction has confused students (and some faculty members) for years.

The truth of the matter is that this type of assessment is done by all clinicians, on multiple pieces of data, all the time! What I should say is that people will **infer** meaning to this data when they look at it (ie, interpret it as "slightly abnormal" or "normal"). The difficulty here is that even experts would have difficulty without knowing the full context of the situation just exactly what to **infer.** Without actually being there and having a complete picture of the patient's situation, it is difficult to

know exactly how to interpret this deviation from normal. Until the patient's BP reading reached some specific number we learned as the lower value for hypertension, we may just **infer** that it is, in fact, normal. In fact, it is most likely the BP of 130/86 mm Hg would have to be judged as normal if this piece of data was assessed out of context, with only textbook normal values for comparison. It does not deviate significantly enough from textbook *normal* to warrant a label of hypertension.

Now comes the real complexity to this situation. What if we knew Mr. Smith's history? What if it was well established that *his* usual BP was 110/68 mm Hg? It had been this value for years. Now what do we think of his current BP of 130/86? In the context of this additional information, we may very well infer a different meaning to the same piece of data.

What adds complexity to inferring meaning to data is that often the problem solver should be looking at data more to assess if it is *atypical* for the particular situation, not just if it is *abnormal* or not. This adds a whole new layer of complexity to the situation. The concept of looking for the *atypical* more than for the *abnormal* is for some a difficult concept to grasp. *Typical* is what you would expect given the circumstances the patient is in. *Atypical* is when you find something is not what you expected given the circumstances. If the circumstances are ones of a healthy, disease-free, resting person, then *typical* probably means *normal*. Let's examine another couple of examples to help to clarify this point.

In a situation in which you can establish what is typical for a given patient regarding physical examination findings, lab tests, and so on, this is very useful. A patient's data should not just be compared to *normal* values, but should be compared to what would be expected for this patient given the circumstances they are under at the time (ie, what is typical for that patient). We often refer to this as establishing the patient's **baseline** for that particular parameter. With this in mind, let's examine two potential situations in which respiratory therapists may find themselves.

The first is when you may have some personal background information on what is typical for a given patient. In the example above of Mr. Smith, if you have an actual history of what the patient's blood pressure has been, you have a frame of reference (baseline) with which to compare the current data. If you had known his BP was well established as stable at 110/68 mm Hg, you most likely would have **inferred** the BP of 130/86 as atypical. If it is atypical it is a potential problem!

In the second situation, in which you have no personal background (baseline) information, you will have to rely on what you understand to be typical. This means relying on what you have learned through textbook and classroom instruction, or through clinical experience. You would have some expectation as to what would be typical for this type of patient, keeping in mind whatever circumstances the patient is currently in. Inferring meaning to data without personal background information will be more difficult for the novice.

The novice will be unable to use the subtle cues that an expert can use to help interpret the meaning of data. For example, let's say our patient had been Ms. Smith, a woman who appears to be about 20 years of age, who presents with no visible signs of distress. The novice would probably compare the BP of 130/86 to the most likely normal numbers they remember (120/80), and may very well **infer** that the BP is "normal." An expert would more likely consider age, gender, and clinical situation (no apparent distress) as "clustered cues" that would cause him or her to not **anticipate** that the BP would be as high as 130/86. This BP value does not fit well with the situation taken as a whole. It is more likely that the expert would **infer** a different meaning (ie, hypertension) to the same data.

So what does all this mean? It clearly means that base knowledge and clinical experience will influence how data are interpreted, that is, what **inferences** will be made about the data. As a result, the novice may not even recognize a problem when confronted with it! It also means that the novice needs to **reflect** on how they assign meaning to data in order to learn how to apply critical thinking skills like **anticipating** to their clinical situations. This would likely result in improved ability to recognize a problem when it is encountered.

What then should a novice do if he or she detects something they think might be *atypical* for a given clinical situation? The answer is simple: Do what any good critical thinker would do and ask someone! A carefully considered and well-stated question is often appreciated by co-workers and often leads to a great learning experience. You don't have to be sure that something is a problem or is atypical to simply make a statement like "I see Ms. Smith appears to be using her accessory muscles of ventilation; is that unusual in this situation?" (See Critical Thinking Exercise 6: Problem Recognition: What's "Normal" Anyway?)

Critical Thinking Exercise 6

PROBLEM RECOGNITION: WHAT'S "NORMAL" ANYWAY?

Knowing what to expect in a given situation is critical if one is to recognize when the data are *not* what you would expect! At first, it would seem simple to know what to expect in a given situation; the novice would say: "Things should be just whatever I memorized as 'normal,' shouldn't they?"

The following CT exercise can be assigned to be completed individually, or by small groups working together. After the exercise has been performed (either as an out-of-class assignment or as an in-class exercise), the faculty member should facilitate a discussion by the entire class of the responses that were developed.

Exercise 6.1: Patient Thompson's $PaCO_2$ has just come back 40 mm Hg! Dr. Carr is very upset! Given only this small amount of information, please answer the following two questions:

a. Describe at least 2 situations in which Dr. Carr is upset because the $PaCO_2$ is too low.

b. Describe at least 2 situations in which Dr. Carr is upset because the $PaCO_2$ is too high.

Exercise 6.2: You administer an aerosol bronchodilator to a patient and notice wheezing after the therapy that wasn't present before you started the treatment.

a. Is this a problem?

b. What would your next, most immediate action be?

Novice Characteristics at the Problem Definition and Analysis Stage.   There are a number of

potential characteristics displayed by the novice problem solver that appear during this step in the problem-solving process. Refer to Table 3-1 for a list of some of these non-problem-solving behaviors. When examining them as a group, there are obvious overlaps with a constant theme. The non-problem solver is displaying a lack of tolerance for ambiguity. According to Taylor, "Ambiguity-intolerant individuals experience psychological stress or threat when confronted with ambiguous situations. They tend to come to premature closure, thus reaching conclusions that often are based on inadequate stimulus sampling."[15]

Students and novice therapists often display behaviors in which they appear to treat clinical situations like they are dealing with flash card problems. The novice needs to know that it is often desirable to ask a number of probing questions and perhaps to gather additional data before providing a proposed answer. There is no reward for the fastest guess in clinical problem solving!

It would appear that much of this behavior is learned by students who perceive (sometimes quite correctly) that their instructors want them to just regurgitate the textbook answer. This perception that they should respond with *the* answer in a flash card reflexive manner leads to students becoming very uncomfortable with ambiguity. It is incumbent upon educators in particular, but really all clinicians, to combat the tendency to oversimplify situations and to resort to generalizations as a quick response to ambiguous clinical situations.

An additional explanation is given by Henry[14] for some of the difficulty the novice displays when performing an analysis of a problem. There are so many flowcharts, algorithms, and protocols already available and used in clinical practice that the novice is not forced to experience the process of deciding which data are needed in a given situation. Novice clinicians may be good at gathering data, but they have not learned which data are needed for what purpose. If asked why a specific piece of data is gathered in a protocol, they will often not be able to cite the rationale. Being able to cite the reasons for an action is one of the cognitive strategies displayed by a critical thinker. As

TABLE 3-1 CHARACTERISTICS OF THE NON-PROBLEM SOLVER DURING THE PROBLEM DEFINITION AND ANALYSIS STAGE OF PROBLEM SOLVING

- Does not recognize the scope of the problem (can't see the whole picture)
- Often focuses on one thing at a time, and bases the hypothesis on a single cue
- Often skips the step of gathering more data and jumps to a conclusion, generating a hypothesis early and sometimes ignoring cues that are not consistent
- Jumps right into solution development before problem is clearly defined

Critical Thinking Exercise 7

USING THE THINKER APPROACH TO OVERCOME BARRIERS TO PROBLEM SOLVING

The following exercise can be assigned individually, or for small groups to work through. After completion of the exercise, it is recommended that a facilitated discussion be held with the entire class to review the results of performing this exercise.

Exercise:

You enter a patient's room to give Mr. Karl his "aerosol treatment." You notice his neighbor, a new admit in the next bed, looks like he may be in trouble. The patient is sitting in a chair and appears to be sleeping (you have no background on this patient). His fingertips are blue, he is using accessory muscles to breathe, and you hear a slight audible wheeze from across the room. What would be your first, immediate action?

a. First, perform the exercise based on your normal, honest reaction: What would be your first, immediate action?

b. Now use the THINKER approach to work your way step by step through this clinical situation. Is there any difference in how you approach this situation? Was your action the same? What part of the THINKER approach, if any, did you find helped you think your way through this situation?

recommended at the beginning of this section, **reflecting** on what steps are done and the reasons for each action will go a long way toward developing your critical thinking and thus your problem-solving skills. (See Critical Thinking Exercise 7: Using the THINKER Approach to Overcome Barriers to Problem Solving.)

Novice Characteristics at the Formulation of Solution(s) Stage.

Much of what was said for the problem definition and analysis step also applies here. The novice goes for the quick answer and often proposes standard textbook solutions. These are fine, if they fit the particulars of the individual and the diagnostic data. The problem is that often the solution is one designed to fit all problems of the kind. Although there are limited choices for therapeutic solutions to problems that call for a care plan, there is room for some individualization of therapy. Review the array of available treatments in Chapter 7 in Table 7-11.

The second major concern is the novice's fixation on selection of the single appropriate solution. As one gains experience and develops problem-solving skills it becomes evident that in medical practice there is rarely only one approach to solving a problem. Not every clinical situation is a multiple choice problem with a single best response. A good problem solver will often come up with a number of proposed solutions and then narrow these down to the one to be implemented. When practical, the proposed solutions should be presented to other colleagues in order to allow for the collective wisdom of the group to be brought to bear in making the final selection. (This is consistent with the THINKER approach, in which the **"E"** is for **express your opinions** in discourse with others.) The alternatives should be kept in mind pending the results of the evaluation phase of problem solving.

Novice Characteristics at the Implementation Stage.

Implementing a solution is often not a problem area; if the novice has the technical skills, he or she can usually perform a task. The weakness of the non-problem solver will show if the solution requires some modification as it is being implemented. For example, assume the problem is a patient's $PaCO_2$ is unacceptably high, and the solution agreed upon is to increase the tidal volume on the patient's mechanical ventilator. This seems straightforward enough. However, when the novice increases the tidal volume, the peak inspiratory pressure increases precipitously. The novice may have expected the pressure to rise, so it does not occur to him or her that the rise in pressure was greater than anticipated, and indicates a severe decrease in compliance. The lung is being overdistended and the tidal volume increase turns out to be an unacceptable solution. The solution needs to be changed or at least modified. The problem is that the novice will often not have the skills to correctly interpret the outcome, and thus is unaware of the need to suggest modification of the solution.

Novice Characteristics at the Evaluation Stage.

Evaluation of an implemented solution to a problem requires a clear idea of the expected outcome(s) of the intervention. Often the novice does not possess the skill to adequately interpret the results of the solution. The non-problem solver is unable to relate the actual outcome with the desired one. For example, oxygen therapy may be applied to a patient, resulting in what is perceived as only a minimal gain in the patient's SpO_2. The novice may interpret this as a failure to attain the desired goal. Upon closer inspection it is noted that the patient's pulse dropped 15 beats/min, and the respiratory rate is now only 20/min compared to 28 before oxygen therapy was begun. It is also noted that the SpO_2 actually did increase from 88% to 91%. Apparently the novice is unaware of the multiple goals of oxygen therapy (to decrease myocardial and ventilatory work in addition to treating hypoxemia), as well as the significance of the shape of the oxyhemoglobin dissociation curve (a 3% increase in SpO_2 represents a more substantial improvement in PaO_2 than the novice apparently recognizes). When all of the above factors are put together, many clinicians would assess that a reasonable response to therapy has occurred.

The non-problem-solving novice is going to have a difficult time evaluating responses to solution implementation in the complicated medical world. At first glance the difficulty in evaluation in the example above may seem to be primarily attributable simply to a lack of knowledge base. Although there is no denying that this may be part of the problem, it is an oversimplification to come to this conclusion. The non-problem solver is a non-critical thinker, and thus looks for a simple, quick answer. Usually no single cue is enough for the novice to make an informed decision.[16] To recognize that the totality of the data, once all the cues are clustered together, points to a different conclusion than that reached by focusing on only a single piece of data requires a critical thinking approach to data analysis! Just as it often takes clustering of data to assist in definition of the problem, this same type of skill is required when analyzing the response to implementation of a solution.

Evaluation often requires one to go through the entire problem-solving process from the beginning. Review the four-step process for evaluation recommended earlier in the chapter. Although not identical, this four-step evaluation process is very similar to our model strategy for problem solving. All of the shortcomings of novices will become evident again as they attempt to proceed through the evaluation process. All the skills required to work through a problem are re-challenged as you attempt to evaluate how effective your solution was at resolving the problem. The end of the problem-solving process is truly just the beginning of the next cycle of problem solving!

THE SPECTRUM OF PROBLEM SOLVING IN RESPIRATORY CARE

The range of problems encountered by respiratory therapists in their clinical work is very broad. In order to appreciate some of the types of clinical problems therapists will be expected to solve, you should review Table 2-3, "Observed Situations That Require Critical Thinking in Respiratory Care Practice." This table not only identifies three categories of situations in which critical thinking may be required, it provides a convenient way of thinking about the various situations in which clinical problem solving may be encountered.

Using these three categories, we will now identify examples in which problem solving can occur in clinical practice and in addition, we will underscore the importance of using other critical thinking skills to accomplish implementation of your proposed solution(s).

Technology

Locating and correcting technical problems has long been a skill expected of the respiratory therapist. This skill, commonly referred to as **troubleshooting,** is actually a perfect example of clinical problem solving. The key factor that puts it under the subcategory of troubleshooting is that technology (equipment) is involved. All of the steps recommended in our problem solving strategy can be followed; to first recognize, then define the problem, propose solution(s), implement a fix, and then evaluate if the solution has solved the problem.

What will really challenge your critical thinking skills will be to determine if the problem that is occurring is actually a technology-based one, or if it is based on clinical deterioration of the patient. This can best be illustrated by an example. The "high pressure" alarm on your ventilator begins to sound. The patient appears anxious and is struggling to breathe. As you approach solving this clinical problem you will have to rule out equipment malfunction (ventilator or airway) as well as patient deterioration (eg, acute pulmonary edema, pneumothorax). Who ever said problem solving was going to be easy?

Patients

Many, perhaps even most, of the clinical problems therapists encounter begin here. Assessing if the intubation tube is correctly placed, evaluating the cause of an unexpected response to a procedure, determining why the patient does not seem to be understanding the instructions you are giving—these are all examples of where problem solving may be required. Of course assessing a patient to determine their respiratory care needs and developing an evidence-based respiratory care plan is one of the more common situations that call for application of your problem-solving skills.

As identified earlier, the skill of **prioritizing** is considered to be a major critical-thinking skill, yet it can also be viewed as a form of problem solving. You are presented with the data on all your patients, including their physician orders, diagnoses, latest clinical findings, the last time they received care, and their next scheduled time for receiving care. This typically occurs during a shift report in which the person who has provided care passes on this key information. You also need good **communication** skills to obtain all the necessary information to help you prioritize your work for the day. As you can see, everyday practice demands a mixture of problem solving with many other critical-thinking skills!

Other Clinicians

Frequently, after you have done your initial prioritization, you may find the need to reprioritize. This often occurs when you have several other health care practitioners all asking for your assistance with a patient, and of course they all need it NOW! Your **communication** and **negotiation** skills are going to be put to the test as you interact with the many other health care practitioners in your clinical practice. Communicating with, and sometimes negotiating with, other health practitioners is extremely common in clinical practice.

Problems with patient management could have been listed in the previous section, but because they so often lead to interaction with others, most often nurses and physicians, it has been listed here, under our discussion of interaction with other clinicians. After you have applied the problem-solving strategy to a clinical patient management problem like those listed in Table 2-3, ("patient fighting the ventilator" or "patient not adequately oxygenated or ventilated"), you will now have developed one or more solutions that you want to present to the patient's physician. You will be most effective in **communicating** and **negotiating** your recommendation(s) if you have done a good job of **anticipating** the physician's likely concerns, and have incorporated them into your solution formulation.

Your efforts to problem-solve a patient management situation will not be effective if you are unable to utilize your other critical thinking skills to ensure that your solution(s) are implemented. Problem solving indeed covers a broad spectrum of the therapists' interactions and clinical activities, and involves many of the other elements of critical thinking that have been identified and discussed in the first few chapters of this book.

CHARACTERISTICS OF THE EFFECTIVE PROBLEM-SOLVING THERAPIST

It is clear from reading the previous sections that the effective problem-solving therapist is one who has developed more than just their problem-solving skills. In fact, it is impossible to develop your problem-solving skills without possessing many of the characteristics of a critical thinker that are described earlier in this book. Each step of the model problem-solving strategy requires application of many different critical-thinking skills, as well as demonstration of critical-thinking traits, and utilization of many of the affective and cognitive strategies that promote critical thinking. These skills, traits, and strategies that are most prominent in problem solving are identified in Tables 3-2 and 3-3. Although clinical

TABLE 3-2   CRITICAL-THINKING SKILLS AND TRAITS THAT ARE PROMINENT IN EFFECTIVE PROBLEM SOLVERS

SKILLS	TRAITS
• Prioritizing	• Willingness to reconsider
• Anticipating	
• Troubleshooting	• Appreciation of multiple perspectives
• Communicating	
• Negotiating	• Broad perspective of health care
• Reflecting	
• Decision making	• Lifelong learner
	• Adaptable

TABLE 3-3 AFFECTIVE AND COGNITIVE STRATEGIES THAT PROMOTE CRITICAL THINKING AND ARE PROMINENT IN EFFECTIVE PROBLEM SOLVERS

- Refining generalizations and avoiding oversimplifications
- Comparing analogous situations
- Evaluating credibility of sources of information
- Generating solutions
- Comparing and contrasting ideals with actual practice
- Noting similarities and differences
- Examining or evaluating assumptions
- Distinguishing relevant from irrelevant facts
- Making plausible inferences, predictions, and interpretations
- Recognizing contradictions
- Exploring consequences and implications
- Giving reasons and evaluating evidence and alleged facts
- Suspending judgment

problem solving may be thought of as a separate, discrete skill, it is quite evident that it overlaps with, and relies upon, the use of many other critical-thinking skills. Effective critical thinkers are good problem solvers, and effective problem solvers are adept at it because they are good critical thinkers!

KEY POINTS

- Problem solving can be defined as *the recognition that a problem exists, followed by a systematic process during which a solution, or often solution(s), to the problem are then determined, implemented and evaluated.*

- Decision making occurs at a number of levels throughout the problem-solving process, but the major decision is usually selection of a solution for implementation.

- All of the traits and characteristics of the critical thinker, as well as the cognitive strategies that promote critical thinking, must be applied during each step of the problem-solving process.

- The NBRC advanced practitioner examination simulates the complexity of clinical reality and tests important aspects of your problem-solving skills.

- A model problem-solving strategy in respiratory care contains the following steps: Initial problem recognition, problem definition and analysis, formulation of solution(s), implementation, and evaluation.

- The key point in the initial stage of problem solving is when the problem solver recognizes something is amiss.

- A novice often does not know what to anticipate in a given situation, hence he or she may have difficulty recognizing a problem when it arises.

- An evidence-based approach should be the respiratory therapist's first choice when selecting the most appropriate solution to a problem.

- The final step of the problem-solving model calls for evaluation.

- Simple problems and solutions may rapidly be evaluated, whereas complicated clinical problems may require evaluation over a prolonged period of time, using multiple measures of data to determine success or failure of the problem-solving process.

- The THINKER strategy may help overcome some of the barriers to problem solving by giving you a process to follow that will help you avoid common mistakes made by novices.

- Fear and anxiety are the greatest emotional barriers to problem solving.

- The non-problem solver displays a lack of tolerance for ambiguity, and thus often fails to suspend judgment, a key critical-thinking strategy.

- Rarely is there just a single solution to a clinical problem.

- Effective critical thinkers are good problem solvers, and effective problem solvers are adept at it because they are good critical thinkers!

REFERENCES

1. Brown SJ. *Knowledge for Health Care Practice, A Guide to Using Research Evidence.* Philadelphia: WB Saunders; 1999.

2. Connelly DP, Johnson PE. The medical problem solving process. *Hum Pathol.* 1980;11:412–419.

3. Taylor C. Problem solving in clinical nursing practice. *J Adv Nurs.* 1997;26:329–336.

4. Radwin LE. Research on diagnostic reasoning in nursing. *Nurs Diagn.* 1990;1:70–77.

5. Elstein AS, Shulman LS, Sprafka SA. *Medical Problem Solving: An Analysis of Clinical Reasoning.* Cambridge, Mass: Harvard University Press; 1978.

6. Neame RL, et al. Problem solving in undergraduate medical students. *Med Decision Making.* 1985;5: 311–324.

7. American Association for Respiratory Care Clinical Practice Guidelines. http://www.rcjournal.com/online_resources/cpgs/cpg_index.html. Date of access 2/11/01.

8. Vitale BA, Nugent PM. *Test Success: Test-Taking Techniques for the Healthcare Student.* Philadelphia: F.A. Davis Company; 1996.

9. Slotnick HB. How doctors learn: The role of clinical problems across the medical school-to-practice continuum. *Acad Med.* 1996;71:28–34.

10. Norman GR. Problem-solving skills, solving problems, and problem-based learning. *Med Educ.* 1988; 22:279–286.

11. Mandin H, Jones A, et al. Helping students learn to think like experts when solving clinical problems. *Acad Med.* 1997;72:173–179.

12. Chowlowski KM, Chan LK. Knowledge-driven problem-solving models in nursing education. *J Nurs Educ.* 1995;34:148–154.

13. Custers EJFM, Boshuizen HPA, Schmidt HG. The influence of medical expertise, case typicality, and illness script component on case processing and disease probability estimates. *Mem Cogn.* 1996;24: 384–399.

14. Henry JN. Identifying problems in clinical problem solving. *Phys Ther.* 1983;63:526–529.

15. Taylor PA. Strategies for enhancing student learning by managing ambiguities in clinical settings. *Nurs Educator.* 2000;25:173–174.

16. Taylor C. Clinical problem-solving in nursing: Insights from the literature. *J Adv Nurs.* 2000;31: 842–849.

4

COMMUNICATION AND NEGOTIATION

Shelley C. Mishoe

*The most important thing in communication
is to hear what isn't being said.*
PETER F. DRUCKER

LEARNING OBJECTIVES

1. Identify and explain the basic concepts of effective communication, including common expressions, levels of communication, principles, and assumptions.
2. Explain the factors that affect communication, including environmental, emotional and sensory, verbal expressions, nonverbal cues, interpersonal, physical appearance, and status.
3. Identify barriers to communication and ways to overcome these barriers.
4. Explain the ways people communicate and the importance of conveying believability for effective communication and negotiation.
5. Identify common miscommunication problems and ways to avoid them.

6. Identify and explain how the skills of the sender and the receiver affect communication and negotiation.
7. Describe and illustrate effective questioning strategies and techniques.
8. Elaborate on the effective use of questioning strategies and techniques in the practice of respiratory care.
9. Explain how communication and negotiation relate to critical thinking in respiratory care practice.
10. Describe the characteristics and qualities of collaborative relationships in health care.

KEY WORDS

Active Listening	Collaborative	Effective	Leading
Adherence	Compound	Communication	Questions
Affective	Questions	Empathy	Negotiation
Assertive	Confidentiality	Encoding	Nonverbal
Aggressive	Confrontation	Facilitation	Communication
Closed-Ended	Decoding	Feedback	Open-Ended
Questions	Defensive	Jargon	Questions
Cognitive	Dialogue	Kinesics	Personal Space

CHAPTER DESCRIPTION

One of the major advantages of PBL is the opportunity it provides for the development of effective communication skills and traits. A basic premise of this textbook is that effective respiratory therapists are effective communicators! The purpose of this chapter is to emphasize the importance of effective communication and negotiation in respiratory care practice, and to provide exercises to develop these skills. Health care is highly interactive, requiring frequent and sometimes serious communication among patients, their families, health care professionals, and support personnel. Therefore, to be an effective respiratory therapist it is essential to have the interpersonal skills and traits needed to communicate and negotiate with others.

Communication has been identified as a skill standard for all health professionals and an essential component of any respiratory care curriculum.[1,2] Unfortunately, professional preparation and continuing education programs in respiratory therapy may not adequately facilitate this important professional skill. Often we merely pay lip service (pun intended) to the importance of communication. When educational programs include communication in their curricula, the focus may be on theory or information, without providing actual experiences with feedback and evaluation. Consequently, respiratory therapists may not be able to apply the concepts of effective communications in their clinical practice. This chapter and many chapters throughout the textbook include specific exercises to facilitate acquisition of effective communication skills. Facilitation of effective communication is an integral part of the overall PBL process.

INTRODUCTION

Effective communication is one of life's most crucial skills. If communication is not effective, the result can be serious errors, misfortune, misunderstanding, disagreement, and conflict. Ineffective communication in the workplace also contributes to misuse of time and other resources, which can be costly. Communication is a complex and dynamic process that is at the heart of all human interactions. It has universal application and has been identified as one of the most daunting challenges confronting any human encounter. The importance of effective communication cannot be overstated. The critical nature of health care and the frequent need for urgency in so many cases makes it more vulnerable to the devastating consequences and repercussions of poor communication. In spite of the inherent difficulties, it is possible to learn how to communicate in confident, caring, and competent ways, all of which will make you a much more effective health care provider.

The evolving role of today's respiratory therapist requires a greater degree of understanding and appreciation for meaningful communication. In addition, respiratory therapists must be able to negotiate. Respiratory therapists have become more than technical clinicians and diagnosticians. They are technical experts, patient assessors, decision makers, consultants, case managers, and patient educators. All of the traditional and emerging roles in respiratory care, as well as the changes in how people work, require respiratory therapists to be proficient in the finer points of effective communication. In addition, the need for and importance of negotiation has never been greater in the health care industry, partly due to the increased workloads, accountability, and emphasis on improved resource allocation.

The key to meaningful patient education is effective communication. It is clear that satisfaction, compliance, and clinical outcomes depend on how health care professionals interact with patients. The basic purposes for communication in health care are to establish rapport with the patient and family, to obtain or provide information, to give instructions, and to persuade patients to change their behaviors.[3] Many factors, such as attitudes, values, and cultural backgrounds, influence opinions and determine thoughts, and can affect communication. Feelings of fear, anxiety, or pain can hinder effective learning. In addition, the timing and the environment in which the interaction takes place can affect communication.

We live in a time when access to information and communication has never been greater or faster, including the use of cellular phones, email, voice mail, pagers, scanners, computers, and the

Internet. Consequently, it is more important than ever before that health care professionals are effective communicators who can use a variety of mediums in various settings.

Respiratory therapists, both novice and expert, must enhance and strengthen their interpersonal communications with other respiratory therapists, physicians, nurses, allied health professionals, patients, family members, and the community. Of particular importance are communications related to health care assessment, disease management, patient education, and multidisciplinary collaboration.

HOW COMMUNICATION AND NEGOTIATION RELATE TO CRITICAL THINKING IN RESPIRATORY CARE PRACTICE

The reflective dimension of critical thinking acknowledges the communicative aspect of critical thinking that guides beliefs, decisions, and actions within a social context. Critical thinking in practice is very much dependent on communications with others as a primary means for giving and receiving information needed for patient care. Although cognitive skills are important, information gathering in practice is not merely selecting data from a list of possibilities as presented on a clinical simulation examination. Respiratory therapists must be able to communicate effectively in order to gather the appropriate information to interpret, analyze, evaluate, infer, judge, or explain. If a respiratory therapist cannot communicate effectively, he or she will be unable to think critically during a given situation in clinical practice. In other words, although a respiratory therapist can have well-developed cognitive skills to critically analyze data, critical thinking in practice is not likely to be effective unless the person is able to access and share information with others. Effective communications are dependent on good working relationships with others. Therefore, it is not surprising that critical thinking in actual practice not only involves the skill of communicating, but also is affected by personal traits.

Communicating in respiratory care practice is practitioner-specific and situation-specific. Communication style, duration, and frequency vary greatly depending on the key players involved, including the therapists, patients, nurses, physicians, and other respiratory therapists. The major ways that respiratory therapists communicate with these key players can be described as "reassuring the patients," "respecting the nurses," "knowing the doctors," and "mentoring new clinicians."[4–6]

Critical thinking in practice also requires respiratory therapists to be able to negotiate patient care medical orders and responsibilities. Negotiating is initiating discussion in an attempt to influence others. Respiratory therapists negotiate when they do not have sole power or authority to do what they think is best for the patient, the department, their institution, and their profession. There is an intimate relationship between the skills of communicating and negotiating. Although negotiating requires communicating skills, all communicating is not negotiating.

Negotiating differs from communicating because the intent is to impart information and ask questions in an effort to influence others' decisions and actions. Practitioners negotiate when they do not have sole power or authority to do what they believe is best in a specific situation in their practice. It is rare in health care, or life, that a single individual has sole authority for decision making. Therefore, every health care professional should realize how collaborative teamwork requires negotiation.[7]

Health care professionals and respiratory therapists should not think of negotiations as confrontations, because this implies a negative intent with poor outcome. In the same vein, the terms argumentative reasoning, argument, and critical thinking should be perceived in a positive light. *Argumentative reasoning* requires logic and skilled reasoning used to draw a conclusion or choose a solution to a problem. People approach problems and situations from many perspectives, therefore differences of opinion are likely to occur. The skilled negotiator understands the value of multiple perspectives and the need to keep personal biases in check, while relying only on the evidence. It is through shared dialogue and effective communications that the best solutions to problems, including those in patient care, can be realized.

Cognitive performance on a clinical simulation examination requires the respiratory therapist to make the right clinical decision after assessing appropriate data. However, in actual practice the respiratory therapist must negotiate power through the medical order to obtain the opportunity to do what they believe is right or best for the patient under specific circumstances. Negotiating patient care responsibilities and medical orders is essential for critical thinking in clinical practice in order to collectively solve problems. If respiratory therapists are unable to negotiate, then there is limited access to the therapists' professional expertise and cognitive critical thinking skills.[4-6] Respiratory therapists must be skilled negotiators in order to participate in decision making and influence patient care medical orders regarding the management of respiratory care. If the respiratory therapist is unable to negotiate, there will be limited access to that therapist's expertise.

In order to negotiate effectively, respiratory therapists need adequate communication skills and the ability to make judgments. They must also be able to explain how they came to their conclusions. The ability to effectively communicate enhances the therapist's opportunities to negotiate legitimate power for patient care decisions, which are ultimately controlled by the medical order. It is through negotiations that respiratory therapists can expand their opportunities for improving patient care based on their unique expertise. Ultimately, these types of experiences will facilitate the growth and development of the critical thinking skills and traits (described in Chapter 2) essential for effective practice.

BASIC CONCEPTS

Communication is such a complex human behavior that it is difficult to explore thoroughly in a single chapter. However, there are basic concepts, assumptions, and strategies that can provide a solid foundation on which to build your skills.

Basic Goals of Communication

Communication has been defined as the sending and receiving of a message.[8] It has also been defined in terms of encoding and decoding, where information in the form of words, symbols, actions, pictures, numbers, and gestures are transformed into ideas and feelings.[9] Communication is obviously an interactive process that uses a set of common rules.[10] It is continuous, dynamic and transactional,[10] and can be written, verbal, or nonverbal as well as therapeutic. Human psychology and psychiatry utilize the therapeutic aspects of communication. This is also true for much of the communication that occurs in respiratory therapy and other health professions. In its therapeutic context, communication will entail an exchange that culminates in helping someone to overcome stress, anxiety, fear, or other emotional experiences. It can also express support, provide information and feedback, correct distortions, and give hope.[10]

The purpose of communication is to transmit a message from one person to another that is mutually understood. The sender (the person conveying a message) attempts to persuade the receiver (the person receiving the message) to respond to the sender's request. The basic goals of communication are for the sender to request: (1) understanding, (2) action, (3) information, and/or (4) comfort from the intended receiver.[7] Requests can be either direct or indirect.

Basic Goal of Negotiation

For purposes of this chapter and textbook, the term *communication* refers to the exchange of mutually comprehensible messages for the purposes of sharing understanding, information, or comfort. When the purpose of communication is to influence another person toward a specific action, using the term *negotiation* makes the distinction. In reality, we are always trying to influence others when we communicate, whether it is to share information, comfort, or understanding. However, when our specific goal is to attempt to influence another's actions, we refer to this type of communication as negotiation. By using the term *negotiation*, respiratory therapists can increase their awareness level about the intent of their communication (to influence someone else), which may facilitate effective communication and negotiation. As you become a skilled communicator, your ability to negotiate and contribute more to patient care will improve.

CRITICAL CONTENT

COMMUNICATION AND NEGOTIATION

Communication: the exchange of mutual messages for the purposes of:

• Understanding
• Information
• Comfort

Negotiation: communication with the specific intent to influence another's action, beliefs, or attitudes

The Communication Process

Communication is best described as a process involving separate and distinct components that are essential for the communication to be successful. The process of communication can be expressed this way: "The *sender* transmits the *message*, which is *encoded* and sent through the *channel* for *decoding* by the *receiver* who then sends *feedback*."[8] It is through feedback that the sender of a message determines if the receiver grasped the intended message. Without feedback, it is not possible to have effective communication because there will be no information to verify that the communication served its intended purpose. Feedback is essential to effective communication, serving as a bridge between the sender and the receiver. Skilled communicators not only know how to send good messages, they are competent at soliciting honest feedback to evaluate the effectiveness of any communication process.

The sender, or the source, is the person or group initiating the interaction. The sender can be a single individual such as a department chairperson who is attempting to supervise his or her department. The sender can be a patient educator attempting to communicate instructions to the patient or family prior to discharge. The sender can be a clinician or diagnostician attempting to collaborate with a physician, nurse, or fellow health care practitioner. It can also be an institution or organization attempting to communicate its mission or philosophy.

Encoding is the transformation of ideas and perceptions into symbols that can be transmitted to the other person(s) in a communication encounter. The message consists of the conveyed information, facts, data, ideas, thoughts, feelings, or attitudes. It is the content to be communicated. The message is encoded in the form of words, symbols, actions, pictures, numbers, or gestures. The message is transmitted through a channel or medium that can be verbal, nonverbal, or a combination of both. Messages can be transmitted through sound (speaking and listening), sight (seeing), touch (feeling), smell, and taste. Decoding is similar to encoding and entails transforming the words, symbols, actions, pictures, numbers, or gestures back into the thought, feeling, or attitude that makes up the message.

The receiver is the recipient of the sender's message or the person or group for which the communication was intended. The receiver could be a respiratory therapy student attempting to learn an important concept such as acid-base balance and its application to arterial blood gas analysis. It could be a respiratory therapist attempting to receive directions from the day shift lead therapist regarding his or her workload. It could even be a patient or family member attempting to receive information, education, or training regarding treatment. Feedback is the final component in the process, and it occurs when the receiver and sender verify each other's perception of the message. It entails the receiver encoding a return message, either verbally in the form of words or nonverbally through body language. A breakdown in the communication process can occur at a number of points along the communication process. There are many characteristics that are essential in nurturing effective communication. Table 4-1 describes some competencies for effective communication.

In most interactions, persons are both the receivers and senders of messages, both verbal and nonverbal. The effective communicator is able to simultaneously fulfill the roles of both sender and receiver. While sending a message, an effective communicator will respond to verbal and nonverbal messages to adapt the messages he or she is sending

TABLE 4-1   EFFECTIVE COMMUNICATION COMPETENCIES

Accountability	Ask and expect others to be responsible for their behavior
Assertiveness	Respect your own interests and the interests of others
Believability	Achieve congruent verbal and nonverbal communications
Caring	Consider the needs of others and facilitate their goals
Confrontation	Ask others to examine how their behavior affects others
Collaboration	Work with others to solve problems and achieve goals
Confidence	Feel free to express yourself—say "No" when necessary
Confidentiality	Let the person know you will respect their confidence
Expression	Know when and how to express your opinions
Empathy	Interact with others in a way that they know you understand
Genuineness	Say what you think and feel
Honesty	Say what you mean and mean what you say
Humor	Use comical or amusing interactions to build relationships
Respect	Show others they are worthwhile and important
Self-disclosure	Know when and how to relate your thoughts and feelings
Supportiveness	Seek support you need from others, especially colleagues
Specificity	Be clear so others can understand your meaning
Trust	Show others they can believe in your integrity and honesty

to achieve their intended purpose(s). In addition, they will ask questions and solicit feedback to determine if there is a mutual understanding.

EFFECTIVE COMMUNICATION

Effective communication is more than posting a message or sending an email. Effective communication implies a shared meaning between the sender and the receiver.[7] When you post a memo on the department bulletin board or send an email message to everyone on the institution's mailing list, you have no way of knowing if the person received the intended message. There is no feedback and therefore no assurance that the intended receiver actually read the memo or received the email. The classroom and the patient education setting are other situations in which communication problems can occur. Teachers will often employ written examinations and clinical competency assessments as means to assure this shared meaning.

Patient education usually incorporates questioning techniques and patient demonstration to assure understanding and to verify the effectiveness of the educational strategies or materials. In short, communication will not be effective unless and until both the sender *and the receiver* share the same meaning. Table 4-2 provides characteristics of effective patient educators who are skilled communicators.[11]

The Components of Communication

Over three decades ago, Dr. Mehrabian wrote landmark articles on communication, and was one of the first to describe the importance of body language.[12,13] However, even during ancient times there was acknowledgement of the importance of nonverbal communication, which is reflected in several quotations. For example, Herodotus said, "We are less convinced by what we hear than by what we see." The verbal component or the actual spoken words comprises only 7% of the communication process. Appearance and body language, the visual component, account for 55% of the way in which a person interprets a message. Tone of voice, the vocal component, accounts for 38% of the message, as shown in Fig. 4-1.[13]

In other words, nonverbal communication, including body language and tone of voice, determines 93% of our communication! The implication

TABLE 4-2 CHARACTERISTICS OF EXCELLENT PATIENT EDUCATORS

Confidence
Prepares and selects the necessary teaching content/materials
Provides an appropriate learning environment
Prepares an appropriate teaching-learning plan

Competence
Decides what is important to teach
Provides individualized patient instructions
Ensures the patient's safety
Determines the patient's understanding

Communication
Establishes rapport
Alleviates patient anxiety
Gives clear directions
Uses simple pictures, models, or demonstrations
Speaks the patient's language
Uses verbal communications that are consistent with nonverbal cues

Caring
Has empathy and is responsive to the patient's communications
Recognizes patient's concerns
Provides encouragement and coaching
Allows sufficient time

SOURCE: Adapted from Rankin et al.[11]

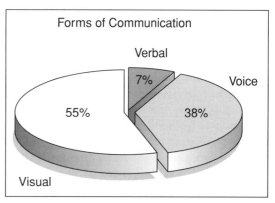

FIGURE 4-1 Dr. Mehrabian was the first to describe the importance of nonverbal communications, showing that only 7% of communication is determined by the verbal component, the actual words we use. About 55% of communication depends on the visual component, the body language; and 38% is affected by the tone of voice, the vocal component. Consequently, 93% of our communication is nonverbal, with the smallest portion, only 7%, determined by the verbal component. (*Source: Mehrabian.*[12,13])

is that the great majority of how the communication is interpreted is determined by the nonverbal, or the way the message is delivered, while only 7% is determined by the actual content. Furthermore, research indicates that when there is inconsistency in the message, the receiver is more inclined to believe the visual and vocal rather than the verbal.[11] Any communicator will achieve believability and sincerity when the nonverbal communication is consistent with the spoken words, the verbal component.

Nonverbal Communication

Nonverbal communication includes the use of body language as well as tone of voice, accounting for a large percentage of our communications. In

fact, if there is a discrepancy between the non-verbal and the verbal communications, another person will more likely believe your nonverbal message than the verbal one. There are gender and cultural differences in the use of verbal and non-verbal communications. However, it is possible to generally discuss some commonalities of nonverbal communications.

What you are speaks so loudly that
I cannot hear what you say.
RALPH WALDO EMERSON

Nonverbal cues are defined as a form of communication without words, and include messages created through body motion (*kinesics*), the use and interpretation of space (*proxemics*), the use of sounds (*paralinguistics*), and touch.[8] Nonverbal communication is powerful and it is learned. We develop the ability to understand nonverbal cues through modeling or imitating the actions or gestures of our parents and peers. Nonverbal communication is considered an extremely reliable index of the real meaning of what is being said or communicated.[8,13] A person is generally unable to exert as much conscious control over the nonverbal content of their communication.

Respiratory therapists should be encouraged to examine their communication style, including the nonverbal and verbal aspects, and obtain feedback from peers, faculty, and other health care professionals, including their medical director. The critical thinking exercises in this chapter and throughout the textbook can facilitate respiratory therapists' skills to become effective communicators.

Body Language. Body language includes gestures, posture, facial expressions, and positioning. The study of body language, or *kinesics*, involves nonverbal movements such as shifts of posture and muscle tone, and gestures of the hand and eye as well as other facial expressions. The least controversial aspect of body language is the use of facial expressions, which is the most easily observable. Charles Darwin in his classic book *The Expression of Emotion in Man and Animals* asked his colleagues around the world to observe human beings to help him determine if the expressions and gestures are consistent in all the races of humankind.[14] Darwin found that their responses showed a great deal of similarity worldwide in communication of humans through facial expressions.

The study of gestures can be very difficult when they are separated from their context. However, a complex and complete message can be inferred when gestures are fitted together. A single expression or gesture can be misinterpreted, because a static gesture may be contradicted by a previous or subsequent gesture or expression. To accurately perceive nonverbal communication, it is necessary to understand the congruence of a cluster of gestures and expressions.

Table 4-3 provides examples of the implied meaning of various facial expressions, body positions, hand gestures, and head gestures. Respiratory therapists should study these cues to increase their awareness of how they affect human communication. This list is far from comprehensive, and entire courses and peer-reviewed journals such as the *Journal of Nonverbal Communication*, are devoted to this important aspect of communication. Although this list provides some information on the use of nonverbal cues, it is a cluster of gestures,

expressions, and positioning that determines nonverbal communications.

Touching is another means of nonverbal communication. In medicine, touching can be used to communicate caring, comforting, closeness, empathy, and trust. Lightly touching the shoulder of a patient is an extremely effective and powerful form of nonverbal communication. This simple gesture can communicate that "I'm here to help you" or "I understand." Nonverbal communication is usually an important determinant in winning others' cooperation, understanding, and acceptance. Being genuine and using nonverbal communications appropriately will enhance the effectiveness of the respiratory therapist.

The use of space, called *proxemics*, varies with the type of interaction and whether it is public, social, personal, or intimate. During public events and lectures, interactions generally occur at great distances. The typical work setting interaction is at a minimum distance of 4 feet. When interacting in the work setting, it is important that you do not become too personal by invading an individual's personal space. The perception of one's personal space varies in different cultures.[15] In the US, most people feel like their personal space is invaded if others stand closer than an arm's length (about 3 feet). Personal conversations or friendly work interactions occur within a person's personal space, but at a greater distance than intimate interactions.

CRITICAL CONTENT

TYPICAL DISTANCES FOR HUMAN INTERACTIONS

Public	12 to 25 ft	Lectures or presentations
Social	4 to 12 ft	Business and work settings
Personal	1½ to 4 ft	Personal conversation with a friend
Intimate	Within 1½ ft	Limited to more intimate relationships; patient care, and comforting patients

TABLE 4-3   NONVERBAL COMMUNICATIONS

Facial Expressions

Acknowledgment	Upper smile showing top teeth only to say "How do you do?," a slight tip of the head with or without an upper smile
Analysis (deep)	Wrinkle of the skin below the lower eyes, frown, muscles below the eyes are relaxed so that the mouth is open, tongue may protrude
Anger or antagonism	Eyebrows close together, eyes drawn downward in a frown, wrinkled forehead, lips turned downward and tightly closed, jaws clenched, teeth not showing, maybe flaring nostrils or grinding teeth, fixed eye contact (stare), pupils dilated
Astonishment/shock	Eyes and mouth opened wide, eyebrows raised
Contentment	A simple smile with corners of the mouth turned up, without showing teeth
Coyness	Upper smile with the lower lip curled in and possibly down
Deceit	Eyes blink, look up and away, pupils dilated
Defiance	Similar to anger, but the head and jaw are often thrust forward, direct eye contact without blinking or looking away
Embarrassment	Slight flush to the facial skin and possibly moving down to the neck and chest
Defensiveness	Pursing of lips (tight-lipped)
Disbelief or envy	Raised eyebrow
Discomfort or guilt	Avoid eye contact (gaze aversion)
Frustration	Roll eyes upward as if to say "Please stop!"
Happiness	A broad smile showing upper and lower incisors with depth, without eye contact
Interest	"Giving someone the eye," eye contact more than 60% of the time
Listening	More eye contact than when talking, looking between 30% and 60% of the time, various gestures of consideration or evaluation
Pretentiousness	Oblong smile, with the lips drawn back from upper and lower teeth without depth, like a polite grimace or a smirk
Shyness	Gaze aversion, often looking down and back up, possibly with an embarrassment flush

Walking Gestures

Arrogance	Strutting walk, deliberately self-conscious, chin raised, exaggerated swing of arms, legs somewhat stiff
Critical and secretive	Walk with hands in pockets, even in warm weather
Dejected or sad	Walk with head down, stooped shoulders, and dragging feet
Goal-oriented adult	Brisk walk with arms swinging freely and comfortably
Hands on hips	"Burst of energy" depicts a sprinter versus steady goal-oriented person
Happy child	Quick walking, light on feet, maybe even skipping
Problem solving	Move slowly with a meditative pose, looking down slightly, hands clasped behind the back
Setting the pace	In every organization, the leader sets the walking pace with subordinates keeping in step behind

Continued

TABLE 4-3 Continued

Hand and Head Gestures	
Affection	Use of various touching gestures and leaning in towards a person
Anger	Angry facial expressions possibly with clenched fists, pointing the index finger at the person, or the vulgar "giving the finger" or other obscene gestures
Agreement	Nodding head up and down, with or without a smile
Approval/congratulations	Pat on the back or shoulder
Attraction	Various preening gestures, such as combing hands through the hair, adjusting a tie or scarf, moistening the lips, glancing at a self-reflection as if "to check things out"
Boredom	The blank stare, or droopy eyes and head-in-the-hand gesture, maybe drumming fingers
Confidentiality	A quick wink as if to say "this is between you and me."
Closure/termination	Person may stand up to indicate the meeting is ended, or a person may point their feet or body towards the door or exit while remaining seated
Confidence	Direct eye contact, straight posture, square shoulders, but relaxed
Consideration	Chin-stroking evaluation or fingers on forehead or chin (as depicted by Auguste Rodin's sculpture "The Thinker")
Critical	Hands blocking parts of the face or hands crossed, leaning away
Deceit	Rubbing end of nose or hands hidden (something to hide), eyes blink and look away
Decision making	When seated, males may tug at their pants and fidget in their chair, males and females will adopt various consideration and evaluation postures before making a decision
Defensiveness	Hand to the back of the neck (defensive beating gesture) or fingers under the collar of a shirt (hot under the collar), or arms crossed tightly across the chest (this can mean the person feels the temperature is cold and is trying to warm him- or herself)
Delaying	Gestures involving eyeglasses, pipes, and other objects, in which the person engages with the object for pause or procrastination; may indicate more time is needed for consideration, evaluation
Dislike	Turning up one's nose or the oblong smile
Dominance/ownership	Putting feet up on things such as a desk, leaning on things such as your car or your desk
Doubt	Touching eyes, as if to say "I don't see it"
Disagreement	Raising eyebrows, shaking head from side to side
Disapproval or loss	Thumbs-down sign
Encouragement or win	Thumbs-up sign
Evaluation (positive)	Index finger on chin or forehead, leaning forward, putting hands over eyes and even closing eyes as if deep in thought (similar to consideration)
Evaluation (negative)	Peering upward or over the top of eyeglasses, raising eyebrows
Expectation	Rubbing the palms together
Hiding something	Speaking from the side of the mouth (like convicts or gangsters) or speaking through hands covering the mouth

TABLE 4-3   Continued

Honesty	Open, upward palms, hands above the table or hand to the chest, with eye contact
Hurried	Avoidance of eye contact with brisk walking if possible, pointing away from the person toward the exit as if to make a getaway
Interest	Head cocked to one side, impression of listening intently
Listening	Maintaining eye contact, showing concentration and aspects of consideration and evaluation
Making a point	Possibly pointing the index finger, but not at another person, or counting off fingers with each point the person emphasizes
Reassurance	Use of various touching gestures
Self-assured	Steepling (joining the tips of fingers together like a church steeple) while speaking or listening; subtle steepling indicates confidence
Stress	Fidget in the chair, inability to sit or stand still, possibly drumming the fingers
Superiority	Both hands clasped behind head and leaning back in the chair, or standing over anyone to indicate you want them subordinate
Support	A-okay sign
Tense	Hands tightly clenched or wringing hands together
Wanting to interrupt	Tugging on your ear or touching on the forearm or elbow of the person speaking
Wanting to speak	Raised hand
Wishing	Crossed fingers (index finger with middle finger)

Tone of Voice. The tone of voice is another form of nonverbal communication because it communicates to another individual more than the actual content of the words. To some degree, the tone of our voice is genetically determined based on the anatomy and physiology of the larynx. However, persons consciously and unconsciously change their tone of voice when communicating with others as an important component of the communication process. Respiratory therapists should examine their vocal tone and take the time to work on improving it if it is inhibiting or limiting effective communications. For example, a person with a high-pitched or squeaky tone of voice (think of Mickey Mouse) can improve their vocal tone through awareness, practice, and experience, to change the rate, volume, and pitch of their voice.

The rate and volume of the words spoken is a powerful component of communications. A depressed patient will generally speak slowly, at a low pitch, and tolerate longer periods of silence than one who is not depressed. Aggressive persons will generally speak loudly and rapidly, enunciating their words precisely. Aggressive persons also will often interrupt another speaker, or they may ridicule, tease, joke, and even insult others.[2] You should be careful to avoid aggressive or inappropriate communications by examining your words and tone of voice, in addition to your body language. Many consider a deep-pitched, slow, breathy, enunciated voice to be sensual (such as the way Marilyn Monroe sang "Happy Birthday" to President John F. Kennedy). A gruff, stern, low-pitched, rapid voice can indicate impatience or disapproval. A high-pitched, shaky, breathless voice can show insecurity or fear. A quiet, raspy voice can mean shyness. A robust, loud, light, and cheerful voice can indicate friendliness or happiness. A flat, monotonous, low voice can indicate depression or a person's unwillingness to engage with another. Using a smooth, mellow tone of voice in a medium pitch and volume can convey confidence.

CRITICAL CONTENT

NONVERBAL COMMUNICATION

- Facial expressions
- Hand and head gestures
- Walking gestures
- Tone of voice
- Rate and volume of the spoken word
- Space/distancing
- Touching

Verbal Communication

Verbal communication involves the language, choice of words, questions, jargon, and feedback. Language is the basis of communication and words are the tools or symbols for the exchange. Words are symbols used to convey thoughts and are open to interpretation. As previously described in the patient education chapter, highly technical medical jargon is rarely appropriate for patient/therapist interaction. Using jargon increases the chance that your patient, student, co-worker, or anyone you communicate with will not grasp the information or the intent. In addition, if you use jargon, acronyms, or highly technical language, you will have missed an opportunity to build rapport.[15] As a general rule, use the simplest, most common words that can adequately convey your thoughts so the receiver will comprehend your message. For communications to be most effective, the words should coincide with the vocal tone and body language. Your credibility and believability are decreased if your body language or the tone of voice is inconsistent with your message.

CRITICAL CONTENT

VERBAL COMMUNICATION

- Choice of words
- Rate and volume of the spoken word
- Jargon
- Language
- Questions
- Feedback
- Use of silence

Critical Thinking Exercise 1

COMMUNICATION STYLES AND THEIR EFFECTIVENESS

Consider the two examples below detailing differences in communication styles and describe how each respiratory therapist will most likely affect their patient's respiratory care. Please note that in the following scenarios each patient is ready to wean based on evidence-based criteria for weaning from mechanical ventilation.

Nathan, a respiratory therapist who is a new graduate, approaches the attending physician during patient rounds to report a patient's weaning criteria and discuss alternatives. His nonverbal communication reflects uncertainty because he has a slumped posture, he holds his hands stiffly at his sides without using gestures, and he speaks in a low voice with an audible quiver and hesitation, and an abundance of qualifiers such as "aah" and "mmm." While Nathan is speaking, he looks at the data in front of him, without making eye contact with the physician. Nathan says in a low voice, "I guess this patient is ready to wean; the data look good."

a. What does the nonverbal communication say and how do you think the physician will respond to the information?

At the same time, in another intensive care unit, Jesse, another new graduate from the same program, is also interacting with a physician during patient rounds to discuss weaning criteria and possible alternatives. Jesse approaches the physician with an air of confidence, but without arrogance or self-importance. After giving a friendly smile with eye contact, Jesse tells the physician, "I have the weaning criteria for Ms. Smith—I think she's ready; she looks good!" His voice is clear, calm, and deliberate without any fillers like "you know," "um," or "uh." When he states that the patient is ready he gives a thumbs-up gesture, a smile, and brief eye contact, indicating his confidence in his interpretation of the data and his patient assessment skills.

b. Describe the differences in verbal and nonverbal communication between Nathan and Jesse.

c. What do the nonverbal communications of each respiratory therapist convey?

d. How do you think the physician will respond to each respiratory therapist?

e. Reflect on these examples and decide which example best describes your communications with physicians.

 Group Critical Thinking Exercise 1

ASSESSING COMMUNICATION STYLE

Each student in the class should independently prepare an oral response to this question: How can respiratory therapists contribute to improvements in patient care and health care delivery? The group should convene and each student will have 5 minutes to present their response. If possible, the faculty or support personnel should videotape each person during his or her presentation, and give the video to the student so they can perform a self-evaluation of both their verbal and nonverbal communications. The class will provide feedback regarding each student's verbal and nonverbal communication style and its effectiveness or limitations after each oral response.

Feedback

An important component of communication is feedback. In addition, feedback is essential to critical thinking because our thinking is only critical when we examine it through discourse with others! Feedback is an important tool in assuring understanding and in building rapport. It helps us see our behavior from another person's perspective, and

 Group Critical Thinking Exercise 2

VERBAL AND NONVERBAL COMMUNICATIONS

a. *Verbal Skills*: Divide the class into teams of 2. For a minimum of 1 week each pair should sit down once a day and practice active listening skills. Each person should speak for 10 minutes and then listen for 10 minutes. Use body language to show you are listening intently and reflect back to the person what you think they are saying and feeling.

b. *Nonverbal Skills*: Once a day for the next 30 days, each student should observe the nonverbal behavior of those around them. Do not judge or form conclusions; simply observe. After 1 week, pick a specific person to observe. How does he or she walk? What about facial expressions and other gestures the person uses? What do the nonverbal cues tell you? If possible, share these observations with the person or with the entire class, to build self-awareness and observational skills that are essential for effective communication.

---

this information tells us how someone else is reacting to our communication. During any interaction, each person utilizes the skills of the sender and the skills of a receiver. By gauging the feedback we receive, we modify the messages we send to enhance our communication effectiveness. For example, vague responses or squinting eyes may be the kind of feedback that indicates uncertainty.

An effective communicator is able to request and to accept feedback. When requesting feedback, be sure you are ready to receive it, be specific in your request, show appreciation, and think about the feedback you receive.[8] Whenever respiratory therapists detect uncertainty in a patient, a student, or a co-worker, they should seek feedback so they can clarify the communication. Table 4-4 shows common interviewing mistakes to avoid when conducting a patient interview.

There is a difference between giving feedback and giving advice. Giving feedback is merely a reflection of how another person's behavior is affecting us, without any pressure to change the person's behavior. Feedback should be given in the

TABLE 4-4   COMMON ERRORS WHEN CONDUCTING AN INTERVIEW

- Overdirecting the interview
- Asking leading questions and/or compound questions
- Speaking too much, without allowing sufficient time for a response
- Giving little or no effort to active listening
- Leading the person's responses either verbally or nonverbally
- Using medical jargon and/or acronyms
- Making judgmental statements
- Giving insufficient time or effort to allow a response
- Paying little attention to any barriers to communication

form of perceptions, to increase the likelihood that the other person will be receptive to the information. When giving feedback, consider: 1) your reasons for wanting to give feedback, 2) whether the person wants your feedback, and 3) if the place and time are appropriate. Keep in mind these considerations: it is important to be specific, convey your perspective, speak genuinely, and determine how the feedback is received by inviting comments.

CRITICAL CONTENT

Requesting Feedback	Giving Feedback
Be sure your are ready	Gain permission to give feedback
Be specific in your request	Be specific in your perception
Be sincere and open	Be sincere and open
Understand the person's perspective	Convey your perspective
Show appreciation for the feedback	Show appreciation for the listening
Think about the feedback	Think about the person's reaction to the feedback

Questioning Techniques

Asking appropriate questions at opportune times is fundamental to effective communications in respiratory care practice. Effective questioning is especially critical in the patient interview, a cornerstone of patient assessment. When respiratory therapists become skilled in asking questions, they can obtain more useful information, saving time, money, and other resources.

Why Is the Information Needed? Questions asked usually focus on the why, who, what, how, when, and where. Before making any inquiries, consider why you need the information. It is a useful strategy to let someone know why you are asking the questions because they are more likely to give you the information you are seeking. For example, in your follow-up examination of a child with asthma, you may want to learn about the caregiver's understanding of the signs and symptoms of asthma, as well as the treatments. Before asking specific questions, you may want to explain your motives: "I would like to ask you some questions about your understanding of asthma and its management. Your responses will help me to determine your needs and ways to help you cope with your child's asthma. Is that okay with you?"

Who Can Provide the Information? Who you will ask is another important consideration. Sometimes asking questions will lead you to other individuals who can provide the information you seek. In some cases, you must ask questions to even determine who is the best person to question. On many occasions patients cannot answer some of the questions, and it may be important to ask family members. For example, a person may not be aware of their snoring and cessation of breathing during the night, and it is appropriate to question other family members to help determine the need for a sleep study. Whenever a health care professional confers with family members, it is respectful to inform the patient and to question the family in the patient's presence. Many of the patients seen by respiratory therapists are intubated and cannot speak because of the artificial airway. In these cases, it is important to find other means to communicate with the patient and to ask family members questions as well.

Types of Questions. Next, you should determine what to ask, to ensure your intentions are clear, and how to ask it, to invite an open response. There are several types of questions, including closed-ended, open-ended, clarifying, compound, and leading questions. It is usually best to ask open-ended questions, such as, "Tell me how you take your medications" or "What can I do to help?" However, closed-ended questions are best when specific information is needed, such as, "Did you go to the doctor's office today?" or "Did you send the arterial blood gas sample to the lab?"

Closed-ended questions yield a limited array of possible answers, and will generally be answered with a simple "yes" or "no." These types of questions have value in some cases; however, they have limited value during the initial patient interview or assessment. Open-ended questions are considered the most valuable form of questioning during the initial patient interview. They yield the broadest amount of information and allow more freedom of response. Open-ended questions generally involve short probes followed by periods of silence in which the interviewee is permitted more in-depth and personal responses. They almost always begin with "what," "why," or "how." Examples are "What brings you to the hospital?" or "Tell me about your SOB."

A clarifying question attempts to correct ambiguity and to clear up the meaning of confusing responses. Patients or other interviewees are asked to elaborate on the issue that is ambiguous or uncertain. Examples are "What do you mean by the statement: 'I have a cold'?" or "What exactly do you mean by SOB?"

Leading questions are questions phrased in such a way that a predetermined or expected response is inevitable. Such questions reflect the bias of the interviewer and should be avoided because they can produce useless, unreliable, or inaccurate responses. Examples are "You've never smoked, have you?" or "You're feeling better today, aren't you?" This type of question may lead a patient to give you the response he or she thinks you want to hear rather than what they are really feeling or thinking.

Compound questions entail asking more than one question at a time and not allowing adequate time for each reply. These questions are usually confusing and do not yield clear results. When asked a compound question, a person generally responds to the last part of the question. An example of a compound question to a colleague: "Did Dr. Jones make rounds and did he recommend the weaning protocol for Ms. X, Mr. Y, and Ms. Z? And what about Dr. Smith?" An example of a compound question to a patient: "Have you ever had, TB, HIV, asthma, used drugs, smoked cigarettes, or had breathing problems?"

Silence. When you ask someone a question, it is critical that you allow a long enough silent period for the person to formulate and offer a response. A common communication mistake is to ask questions, but never really wait and listen to the responses. The THINKER strategy presented in Chapter 2 is useful to help you improve your communication effectiveness, especially in the area of waiting and carefully formulating your response. The THINKER strategy can be equally useful to help you develop appropriate silent time when eliciting responses from others!

When and Where Should You Ask Questions?
Finally, the when and the where of questioning are also important. You can have the best reason, attitude, and questions, but if the place or time or both are inappropriate, you are not likely to receive the information you seek through questioning. For example, it is best to question a colleague about a problem in a private place at a predetermined time when both of you agree to discuss the matter. If you spring unexpected questions on a patient, colleague, or even a friend, you will likely meet with silence or resistance in answering. Effective communications require sufficient time. Unfortunately, in today's climate of managed care, time is frequently in short supply, making it even more critical for respiratory therapists to develop and improve effective communication skills.

CRITICAL CONTENT

THE VALUE OF SILENCE

A common communication mistake is to ask questions, but never really wait to listen to the response. The THINKER strategy can be useful to help you improve your communication effectiveness by allowing the respondent sufficient silent time for them to formulate a response to your question. The THINKER strategy can be useful to promote the skill of active listening.

Confrontation and Assertiveness. Confrontation is a tricky aspect of questioning because it requires the right timing, tone, and nonverbal and verbal communications. Otherwise, confronting shuts down communication rather than providing the information you seek. Confrontation does not have to be problematic if communications are assertive and responsible, not passive or aggressive. *Assertiveness* is the ability to confidently and comfortably express thoughts and feelings while respecting the legitimate rights of others.[8] Assertion is not continual confrontation; it is a conscious choice of knowing the who, what, where, how, and when of effective communications, and dealing with positive and negative circumstances.

Confrontation is sometimes necessary when you want to bring a patient's behavior or emotional state to their conscious awareness. Responsible and assertive confrontation is necessary when dealing with unacceptable behavior from another person, such as a peer, patient, or student. For example, you may ask a colleague, "Did you tell me that you replaced the supplies on the crash cart? I could not find an 8 endotracheal tube when I needed one on my shift last night." Here is an example of how you might confront a patient with your questioning: "You said your breathing was fine, yet I noticed your rate was quite high and your breathing is labored" or "You said you are not angry, yet I observed you raising your voice and clenching your fists."

CRITICAL CONTENT

COMMUNICATING ASSERTIVELY REQUIRES SPECIFIC SKILLS AND SELF-CONFIDENCE

• Skill in a variety of communication strategies is useful to express thoughts and feelings.
• Keep a positive attitude about communicating honestly and fairly.
• Skill at keeping a balance between your rights and the rights of others fosters effective communication.
• Feeling comfortable with your level of self-control over negative feelings such as fear, shyness, anger, guilt, and doubt will improve your communications.
• Feel confident and behave with respect for yourself and others.

Facilitation. Facilitation is a technique whereby words, postures, or actions encourage respondents to give more detail. The nonverbal aspects of communication are essential to facilitating with sincerity and genuineness. Facilitation can be as subtle as encouragement by saying "Please go on," or it

CRITICAL CONTENT

USEFUL QUESTIONING TYPES AND TECHNIQUES

• Closed-ended questions
• Open-ended questions
• Clarifying questions
• Facilitation
• Silence
• Support and reassurance

POOR QUESTIONING TECHNIQUES

• Confrontation
• Leading questions
• Compound questions

could be expressed as an "uh huh," or an encouraging nod of the head. Nonverbal actions that display sincerity, genuine interest, and attentiveness include sitting forward and looking at the patient with interest (remember how the head cocks when a person is intently listening). A facilitating communicator knows how to build and maintain rapport through careful monitoring of their skills as both sender and receiver. Table 4-4 shows common errors made when conducting an interview.

SKILLS FOR SENDING AND RECEIVING COMMUNICATIONS

During any interaction a person is both a sender and receiver of information. Communication is a highly complex and interactive process, one that requires numerous speaking, listening, and other affective abilities. The next two sections will elaborate on the skills of the sender and the receiver. Effective communications require a person to be able to send and receive verbal and nonverbal messages, ask and answer questions, elicit feedback, and evaluate the interaction on a continual basis.

Skills of the Sender

The sender should ask him- or herself what they want to accomplish prior to sending a message to someone else. This is followed by choice of a time and an appropriate setting for the interaction. For example, the goals of a patient education session are to assess learning needs, provide instruction, and evaluate understanding and performance. The choice of time and setting should minimize interruptions and distractions in an area that is quiet, comfortable, and furnished with appropriate resources (eg, blackboard, audio-visual aids, written materials). Such an environment may be found in the patient's room or a designated conference area. The same would hold true for a staff performance appraisal, a student clinical competency assessment, or an employee interview.

The second measure is to speak clearly, slowly, and deliberately. Managed care has seriously restricted the time that health professionals spend with patients. Often, the respiratory therapist is in a hurry and may have a tendency to speak too quickly, or to miss important cues as the receiver, focusing on the sending. This is especially problematic when communicating with the elderly, who may need the added time to absorb and process what is being said. It is equally important not to speak too softly, abruptly, or impatiently.

A third measure would be to notify the receiver of the importance of the communication. For example, prior to a patient education session, it is wise to tell the patient that they will be discharged in a few days and will be responsible for self-administration of their metered dose inhaler. This information provides motivation for them to learn the procedure, and you are more likely to gain their attention and cooperation. Additionally, it is good practice to indicate the time required for the exchange, and keep them informed about it as you proceed through the teaching process. Finally, it is best to conclude with a summary of the key points, highlighting the most important considerations.

A fourth measure is to solicit feedback. Again using the patient education session as our example, it is prudent to open the dialogue with a general statement, inviting them to stop you at any point should they have a question or concern. Periodically, it might be wise to stop and ask, "Do you understand what I am saying?" Requiring the patient to demonstrate the method or technique is an extremely effective way to assure the patient has mastered it and solicit feedback.

The fifth measure is to eliminate the unnecessary. Most people use 30% more words than necessary.[16] Attempt to be as clear and concise as possible. When in doubt, say it and wait for feedback.

The sixth measure is to concentrate on the reception. Your focus as the sender should not be on yourself, but rather on the interaction between you and the other person. This will instill an attitude of collaboration, rather than one of superiority and authority. Whenever possible, share information rather than lecturing. Finally, providing simple written or visual instructions can be useful, as are follow-up telephone interviews.

CRITICAL CONTENT

SKILLS OF THE SENDER

- Decide what you want to accomplish and the questions you will ask.
- Choose an appropriate person, time, and place.
- Speak clearly, slowly, and deliberately, utilizing the skills listed in Table 4-1.
- Assess the receiver's nonverbal and verbal communications.
- Monitor your own nonverbal communication and emotions.
- Listen effectively and without making hasty judgments.
- Determine why, when, and how to become the receiver.
- Request feedback.

Skills of the Receiver

Hearing is a physical act in which sound is detected, while listening is an intellectual and emotional act that includes understanding and requires active involvement. These are the skills of the active listener: (1) listen to the content, (2) listen to the intent, (3) assess the sender's nonverbal communication, (4) monitor your nonverbal communication and your emotional filters, and (5) listen with empathy, without making judgments.[17]

CRITICAL CONTENT

ACTIVE LISTENING

- Listen to the content.
- Listen to the intent.
- Assess the sender's nonverbal communication.
- Monitor your nonverbal communication and your emotional filters.
- Listen with empathy, without making judgments.

Listening to the content means giving your full attention to the speaker. Eliminate internal and external distractions, and if necessary be prepared to take notes and to physically move closer to the sender. Do not prepare your responses while the sender is communicating. Stop talking and listen to the verbal and nonverbal messages!

Listening to the intent is a challenging skill. It means attempting to hear the whole message, not just what is implied. The intent will include the content and the nonverbal cues, as well as the sender's background, biases, and any other factors that have bearing on the issue at hand. When you listen to the intent, you are listening to *why* he or she says something, rather than just the *what*. You may need to paraphrase or seek clarification of the sender's intention. You should not use your emotions to interpret the intent. For example, one of your staff respiratory therapists may call to say, "I cannot come in today because my child is sick." A busy and harried supervisor may only hear the first part of the communication and prematurely pass judgment that the respiratory therapist is trying to get out of work. However, with effective listening, the supervisor may hear that the child and the family are in the emergency room because they suspect meningitis and the child will be undergoing a spinal tap.

The third skill is the ability to assess the sender's nonverbal communication. Nonverbal cues are expressed through body language as well as tone of voice, and represent over 90% of the message. They also represent the "how" rather than the "what" of the message. The nonverbal cues are considered a true reflection of the sender's innermost thoughts. When there is incongruity between what is seen and what is heard, the nonverbal cues usually indicate the correct interpretation. Astute respiratory therapists will notice the inconsistency in the communication and will ask appropriate questions, seeking clarification and understanding. The RT may also perceive and respond to the nonverbal messages. For example, a respiratory therapist was asked by a colleague: "What do you think of the recommendations I made during the staff meeting this morning?" Before giving honest feedback, the astute therapist may pick up on the defensive posturing and unwillingness to listen on the part of the sender (see Table 4-3). If the colleague immediately started heading for the door after asking the question, without making eye contact, thereby sending a defensive message, it may be wise to withhold feedback for the moment.

Skillful listeners monitor their own nonverbal cues and control their emotional filters. This simply means that just as the sender is sending nonverbal messages, so is the receiver. The receiver's messages could be supportive and encouraging, such as, "Yes, I'm with you, go on," or they could be saying, "Oh please continue (*sarcasm*), don't let me interrupt!" The receiver should try to not discourage communication with nonverbal cues of disapproval or rejection. The receiver should also maintain neutrality and listen to the whole message.

Both sender and receiver have a particular mindset which has been developed over years. This mindset consists of the personal biases, experiences, and expectations held by each of us. Everyone has these deep-seated feelings and beliefs, and it is best to use self-control when receiving. A mindset might be expressed like this: "Critical thinkers are open-minded and flexible. Joe was not open-minded or flexible when I suggested we change the staffing schedule during the holidays. Therefore, Joe is not a critical thinker." While this is obviously a ridiculous conclusion, it shows how our biases, opinions, and conclusions affect each other, often interfering with good communications. Listeners should control their emotional filters and not allow them to interfere with receiving the entire message.

Listening empathetically involves a commitment to immerse yourself in another person's perspective in order to understand the situation from their point of view, and then communicating that you understand. Empathetic listening means you are able to provide feedback that reflects that you care about the other person and that what they have to say is important. Empathetic listening is essential to patient care and patient education. Furthermore, the ability to understand something from another person's point of view is a major component of critical thinking in the workplace.

Being nonjudgmental means being open-minded and not entering a situation with preconceived thoughts, opinions, or decisions. In essence, you

CRITICAL CONTENT

SKILLS OF THE RECEIVER

- Listen empathetically to the content and the intent.
- Assess the sender's nonverbal and verbal communication.
- Monitor your own nonverbal communication and emotions.
- Listen effectively and without making hasty judgments.
- Determine why, when, and how to become the sender.

Group Critical Thinking Exercise 3

Each student should be given 15 to 30 minutes to make a presentation on one of the following to the entire class, along with the faculty, medical director, and other physicians. Each presentation should be videotaped. Following the oral presentation, each student should be given the opportunity to review the videotape with the class and receive feedback regarding their verbal and nonverbal communications.

a. Using a clinical practice guideline, clinical algorithm, or critical pathway for respiratory care that you developed for Chapter 2, state your evidence, assumptions, biases, concepts, issues, data, definitions, theories, and implications.

b. Describe a concept map you developed for Chapter 2 to illustrate the logic of one aspect of respiratory care, such as arterial blood gas interpretation, delivery of aerosol pharmacology, or use of oxygen devices.

c. Make recommendations for respiratory care when given a case scenario and clinical data, choosing any example from Part II of this textbook.

are reflecting on the whole message and allowing the person to communicate what they think and feel. Table 4-4 shows common mistakes made during an interview, and these should be kept in mind when conducting patient interviews.

Levels of Communication

There are also different levels of communication that every sender and receiver should perceive.[15,17] The five levels of communication range from Level 1 communication, the most intimate, to Level 5, the lowest form of communication.

Level 5 communications are the lowest level of human interaction and are characterized by meaningless statements and clichés. There is no genuine sharing because Level 5 comments are intended to be superficial. This type of communication is more of an acknowledgment, such as, "Hello, how are you?" Most people expect to hear, "I'm fine," nothing more and nothing less. If the person does not respond at all, we may wonder if they are okay or if they were deliberately ignoring us, which communicates something else. If the person responds with a lengthy account of what they did over the weekend, we may become impatient, because we intended a simple acknowledgment. Usually we expect to hear a Level 5 response when we offer a cliché or simple acknowledgement.

Level 4 communications are also relatively shallow forms of interaction, in which neutral topics are discussed. Level 4 interactions are characterized by small talk. This includes talking about the news, the weather, or sports scores. Neither party shares anything personal and the interaction remains impersonal, safe, and noncontroversial. An example of Level 4 communications could be a situation in which you are waiting for the elevator and you see your medical director and say, "Hi! How are you?" He responds with a Level 5 comment, "Fine, thanks." There is silence for a minute as you both continue to wait for the elevator. Should either choose to enter into a Level 4 communication, one might say, "It is nice to see the sun again after all the rain we had last week." While still shallow and without risk, it is more engaging and entails a higher level of communication. If you offer this type of Level 4 comment, the medical director has the option of engaging you in Level 4 or providing a short response, which essentially says that he wishes to stay at a Level 5. Now you will need to make the decision whether to ask another question, hoping to engage him, or to accept his initial indication of not entering into a deeper conversation.

If a person enters into Level 3 interactions, he or she will begin to share some personal ideas, opinions, or judgments. The information is usually guarded and monitored very closely. In fact, if the listener indicates disapproval, boredom, or confusion, the sender may become hesitant to continue sharing. In Level 3, more risk is taken because there is self-disclosure and an attempt to begin to build a relationship. It will also require some degree of trust and time to develop the relationship. In order for Level 3 communications to take place, both parties must participate in the exchange. Should you find yourself expressing your views and the other person is either silent or evading the issue, it may be that you are in a Level 3 interaction and the other person is still at a Level 4. At this point you may want to end the conversation or move back up to Level 4. For example, Level 3 communications can occur between you and a fellow therapist when you are both willing to share personal views on controversial health-related issues or work-related problems.

If the relationship continues, you can enter into Level 2 communications, in which there is more self-disclosure. During Level 2 interactions each person begins to share the more personal and emotional aspects of their lives. Individuals who have spent a considerable amount of time together exhibit Level 2 communication. At this level individuals share their deeper thoughts, fears, joys, and emotions, and have developed a solid foundation of trust. Level 2 communications are shared between persons who enjoy a true friendship.

The highest level of communication is Level 1. This level of communication is limited to a select few and restricted to married partners, family members, and intimate friends. Significant sharing, empathy, and mastery of a deep relationship characterize this level of communication.

While the five levels of communication do not have universal application to all health care encounters, they have been addressed in the literature and have value in therapeutic relationships.[5] In any therapeutic relationship, it is important that the respiratory therapist go beyond Level 4 and 5 in order to establish a rapport, and get the patient to open up and gain trust and cooperation. This can be especially tricky during the interview and physical assessment process because the therapist must maintain a professional demeanor and yet not be too distant or impersonal and impede the flow of valuable health-related information. Equally important is the need to avoid displaying any inappropriate emotion. During patient education and interaction, it is usually not appropriate to move to Level 2 communications.

When faced with a hostile or emotionally charged encounter, it is more productive to stick to the facts and not succumb to useless name-calling or other forms of conflict. Finally, developing and maintaining a good rapport between other members of the health care team can be invaluable in creating a congenial, productive, and satisfying work climate. The important point is to develop and maintain a relationship built on honesty, trust, and respect.

Communication can move to higher levels when persons have good questioning techniques, effective listening skills, and the characteristics outlined in Table 4-1. An assertive and responsible communication style is the most desirable, allowing you and others to move to the highest and most effective levels of communication.

CRITICAL CONTENT

LEVELS OF COMMUNICATION

Level 5	Cliché conversations
Level 4	Reporting facts
Level 3	Personal ideas and judgments
Level 2	Feelings and emotions
Level 1	Most intimate communication

AGE-SPECIFIC ASPECTS OF COMMUNICATION

The Elderly

Aging affects the various aspects of communication, with those on the healthy end of the continuum having markedly less deterioration than those at the opposite more extreme deterioration. The majority of interaction skills acquired over the years remains intact in the healthy older person.[18] However, aging does affect vision, hearing, voice, kinesics, and cognition, presenting specific communication limitations and needs. Diseases compound the limitations of aging, presenting additional communication needs as well as problems. For instance, normal voice production can be compromised through a variety of pulmonary, cardiac, and neurological diseases. Patients with COPD can become short of breath, resulting in disruption of airflow, reduced intensity and duration of phonation, and alterations of voice frequency.

Communication may be the single most important skill to maintain or improve in the elderly to help adaptation to the aging process as much as possible.[19] Hearing impairments rank second after arthritis as the impairment that most limits functioning in the elderly.[18] A hearing impairment can become a hearing handicap if it deteriorates sufficiently that it affects a person's ability to perform the activities of daily living. Even slight high-frequency hearing loss can affect perception of words. Speaking slower, louder, and using gestures can improve your communication with elderly people with hearing loss.

Visual changes can also affect the elderly. Whenever possible, use health-related materials printed in larger type. When giving demonstrations, make an effort to be sure that the patient can see and hear the demonstration. Asking questions and requesting feedback, the hallmark of effective communicating, are absolutely essential when working with elderly patients.

Some elderly people may have changes in communication practices in these four areas: maintaining the focus of the conversation, conveying semantic meaning via language, reminiscing, and self-disclosing. When two people speak, they convey shared meaning by attempting to stay on the same topic as they talk. Healthy elders are able to maintain focus on the topic of conversation. However, changes in cognition with diseases such as Alzheimer's cause breakdowns in communication under these four conversational circumstances: 1) at points of real or apparent topic change, 2) when there are competing conversational foci, 3) during attempts to track the focus of a lengthy discussion and, 4) when returning to the main topic.[20] Specific strategies to use when interacting with patients with Alzheimer's include restating the topic of conversation, using props, avoiding pronouns, and sticking to one topic. Health professionals should make it clear when the focus shifts to another topic, and use these strategies.

Several strategies can be used to facilitate improved communication to overcome hearing loss, poor eyesight, and other changes associated with normal aging or diseases of the elderly, as shown in Table 4-5.[19,20] In addition, creating an external environment conducive to sending and receiving messages is essential.

Children

The communication needs of children focus on their developmental stage, ability to understand, and their ability to use language.[11] There is wide variation in children's abilities to communicate, and this is affected by their intellectual skills and developmental level. Children are generally strong auditory communicators who respond more favorably to less formal, more casual interactions. However, some children may be visual learners who often may have auditory perceptual disability. Consequently, a variety of strategies must be utilized to meet the needs of children, with or without disabilities. Children are generally more comfortable with technological equipment and enjoy communications that incorporate pictures, games, and simulations.

TABLE 4-5   WAYS TO IMPROVE COMMUNICATION WITH ELDERLY PERSONS

- Analyze possible motivations for any changes (fiscal, physical, social, emotional, and so forth) in interaction patterns.
- Keep the topic of conversation clear. If the person makes irrelevant comments, clarify the topic.
- Arrange the furniture, environment, and circumstances to promote interaction.
- Listen actively. If miscommunication occurs, repeat ideas using different words, phrases, or examples.
- Accommodate the hearing- or visually-impaired individual with a quiet, well-lit, slow-paced, relaxed environment.
- Allow the person to reminisce and self-disclose positive and negative life events to promote rapport, trust, understanding, and insight.
- Determine if the person is experiencing emotional isolation and offer assistance.
- Motivate elderly persons to communicate by asking them to problem solve or make meaningful contributions to the discussion.
- When dealing with an elderly person in an emergency, offer to contact next of kin for family support.
- Involve the family and caregivers in the communication and patient education processes to facilitate the person's care and quality of life.
- Determine if the primary caregiver (usually the spouse or a daughter) of the frail elderly person needs assistance to deal with tasks and the stress of caring for the elderly patient.
- Ask the person to repeat the health care instructions and to demonstrate proper performance of activities of daily living, including meeting health care needs.

There is a pressing need for new methods to adequately assess health-related quality of life in children.[21] Children who have chronic diseases such as asthma can have a different perception of their own quality of life than their parents.[22] The same can be said of the child with chronic disease and the caregiver. Consequently it is important to communicate as much as possible directly with the pediatric patient to build their knowledge of their disease, improve their self-esteem and self-management abilities, and foster adherence to care plans. Use of pictures, symbols, colors, reward systems, reassurance, and games can build rapport and understanding in children. Sick children are especially in need of caring, effective communications. Respiratory therapists have an important role in helping children with chronic cardiopulmonary disease to build their self-management skills through effective communications and education.

Adolescents

The adolescent presents unique communication challenges because he or she is neither a child nor an adult. Physical and emotional maturation combined with intellectual ability will greatly determine the adolescent's ability to communicate with peers, teachers, parents, and health care personnel.[23] When providing instructions or other forms of patient education to the adolescent it is generally advisable to include the primary caregiver. However, the effective communicator will gauge the level and direction of the instruction to meet the patient's needs, relying heavily on nonverbal cues from the adolescent. It is important to respect the adolescent's need for individual recognition, as well as their dependence on a parent or caregiver. The respiratory therapist should form a partnership with the adolescent and the parent(s) to build trust, rapport, understanding, and foremost, patient adherence.

The peer group particularly influences adolescents and most feel awkwardness about their changing body, emotions, and thoughts. Consequently, it is important to provide opportunities for adolescents to interact with peers who face similar acute or chronic illness. Peer support, inter-

action, and identification with others facing similar circumstances can improve the health care and quality of life for all patients. In addition, adolescents need mechanisms to cope with their illness in a way that can help them fit in with peers who do not have similar circumstances. Patient adherence in the adolescent age group is more challenging than with other age groups. Effective communication and patient education address the needs and concerns of adolescents, particularly their need for peer acceptance and approval.

 Critical Thinking Exercise 2

a. Develop 3 sets of patient education materials on the use of asthma medications and tailor each to the pediatric, the adolescent, and the geriatric patient.

b. Modify question 2a to develop 3 sets of patient education materials on a topic of your choice, tailoring each to the pediatric, the adolescent, and the geriatric patient.

 Group Critical Thinking Exercise 4

Utilize the materials developed for the previous exercise (#2) to actually provide patient education to a child, teenager, or geriatric patient. This exercise can utilize real patients, standardized patients, or role playing. The faculty should divide the class into manageable groups, depending on the time allocation and numbers of students and patients.

WHAT IS THE PATIENT'S ABILITY TO COMMUNICATE?

In addition to age-specific aspects of communications, patients may have limitations such as the inability to read or an endotracheal tube that prevents speaking. In health care, communication challenges are unique, diverse, and critically important. Table 4-6 shows the most common communication

T A B L E 4 - 6   FREQUENCY OF COMMUNICATION PROBLEMS REPORTED BY PATIENTS

DESCRIPTION OF PROBLEM	PATIENTS REPORTING THE PROBLEM (%)
Not told about daily routine	44.9
Not told who to ask for help if needed	31.8
No doctor or the doctor in charge not available to answer questions	22.6
Doctor or nurse did not explain how much pain to expect before a test	21.1
Not told things they should have been told before admission	10.3
Did not get understandable answers from nurses in response to important questions	7.2
Did not get understandable answers from doctors in response to important questions	6.4
Not given enough privacy while receiving important information about condition	4.5
Information about condition given in a way that upset patient	3.9

SOURCE: From Cleary et al.[24]

problems reported by patients.[24] Limitations of speech, hearing, and sight can compound these problems and also present unique challenges. The following sections briefly describe ways to overcome patient fears by improving health care communications and therapeutic communication.

Speech, Hearing, and Vision Limitations or Impairments

Many patients in critical care have limitations such as impairment of verbal functioning. Impairment of speech or language may result from altered physical condition (such as removal of the larynx), medications (such as paralyzing agents or narcotics), or the use of technology (such as intubation and mechanical ventilation). It is established that intubated patients experience negative emotions when they are unable to speak. Research has shown that both men and women report moderately intense feelings of anger and fear about being unable to speak.[25] These emotional responses appear to be closely related to a patient's inability to speak. Interventions are needed to decrease patient distress and facilitate communication.

Careful assessment of patient communication abilities and attempts to match them to one or more communication methods are important. It is equally important to allow sufficient time so that

patients can express their physical and emotional needs.[26] Ideally, alternate communication methods should be discussed and selected prior to surgery that might affect hearing, speech, vision, or any other component of communication. Alternative methods of communication can include lip reading, use of picture boards, paper and pencil or magic slates, eye blinks, hand squeezes, note cards, American Sign Language, and computer-aided communication. To choose the communication system, it is necessary to assess the patient's level of consciousness, language, fine motor skills, gross motor skills, and any paralysis. It is best to talk with a patient when providing care, whether they appear alert, disoriented, or even comatose.

The astute health care professional will utilize a variety of communication strategies and carefully assess nonverbal cues when communicating with any person. Sensory communication issues, whether in the patient care area or the classroom, can be overcome by having the sender employ multiple senses in the sending of the message. Multiple sense learning may entail showing pictures (visual) as well as explaining something with words (auditory).

Interpersonal Factors

Intrapersonal factors are elements within the individual that affect communication, such as world-view, developmental stage, language mastery, reading comprehension, attitudes, values, cultural heritage, religious beliefs, convictions, preoccupations, experiences, feelings, interests, and relative perception of illness or wellness. These intrapersonal factors influence medical choices and decisions. Interpersonal factors involve how two or more people interact and communicate.

The developmental stage includes cognitive abilities as well as psychosocial development. Specific aspects of developmental stages include thinking ability, comprehension, attention span, maturity, and independence. The developmental stage of the very young will require that they receive assistance from family members and/or other caregivers. The elderly may also need assistance, as their mental acuity will diminish over time.

Illiteracy and Reading Comprehension. Illiteracy is an important element affecting communications, especially in health care. Approximately 20% of American adults are illiterate and another 34% are functionally illiterate.[26] Furthermore, the average reading level of the adult population in the United States is at the eighth grade level.[27] With the complexities and technicalities of health care, it is questionable whether or not patients understand what is being communicated when such limitations exist. Illiteracy and low reading comprehension can seriously undermine effective communication under any circumstances. Keep in mind that the patient may not wish to admit to having difficulty reading, which compounds the problem. Complex medical language and the intimidating health care environment further compound the problem, posing significantly greater challenges to communication, education, and follow-up care.

Cultural Considerations. Mastery of the language is another concern, especially since many patients do not use English as their primary language. This cultural diversity issue is becoming quite significant. The 1990 census data indicated that over 21% of the US population is made up of minorities, and the number continues to rise. The belief systems of various racial and ethnic groups can be considerably different. Western cultures are largely biomedical in their health care beliefs, while Eastern cultures may believe in religion, mysticism, or natural healing.[27] Many cultures such as Native American, Hispanic, and Chinese utilize home remedies and complementary health care practices. These cultural beliefs greatly affect communication.

Eastern and Hispanic cultures are generally male dominated in terms of hierarchy, have a strong family structure, and demonstrate considerable respect for their elderly. These cultural beliefs heavily influence communication between respiratory therapists, the patients, and their families. For example, a recommendation to place an elderly, ailing parent in a nursing home may seem like a reasonable suggestion, but it can create anxiety and even resistance in certain cultural groups. Interacting with patients from different cultures can be challenging because eye contact, the use of words like "no" and "yes," and touch can all have different meanings than we are used to. Health care providers must relate to the patient's culture so these patients do not feel intimidated or frightened when they seek medical care. Understanding various cultures can enhance communication, satisfaction, and ultimately the health care of diverse groups of patients.

ADDITIONAL FACTORS AFFECTING COMMUNICATION

Physical Appearance and Status

Physical appearance is a major component of the first impression made by anyone. Elements of physical appearance and status include age, gender, race, body size, shape, body movements, posture, dress, hair, jewelry, adornments, body smell, role, position, organizational status, influence, and professionalism. With regard to body size and shape, there is a perception that large physical size will generally convey dominance, power, authority, and control. It is well known that tall, attractive people are generally perceived as more intelligent and have a natural advantage in receiving promotions. It is also well known that morbidly overweight people are judged by others to be lazy or slow, which often makes them victims of job discrimination and social ridicule. Posture and body movement also factor into communication because acting stern, distant, and holding the body rigid can send a message of being unapproachable. Posture and body movement can also convey openness and receptivity, such as is exhibited when one freely walks around the room with arms extended, or sits back in one's chair with hands behind the head.

Dress is an especially important point because people are generally making judgments about others based on their attire. Proper professional dress is a critical component of professional behavior. You only have a few moments to make a favorable first impression. Proper attire can make or break you in a professional job interview or patient interview. This aspect of professional communication is so important that entire books are dedicated to the topic. If a respiratory therapist enters a patient's room wearing soiled scrubs and shoes and having a 2- or 3-day growth of beard, this does not make a positive impression. On the other hand, if a respiratory therapist enters a patient's room wearing clean clothing and a pressed, white lab jacket and name badge, they often receive immediate attention and credibility. Whether you accept it or not, patients and other health care professionals respond more favorably to a positive professional appearance. Therefore, respiratory therapists have to dress and act professionally to be recognized and treated as professionals.

It is advisable to maintain a well-groomed appearance with minimal body adornments. Long nails, heavy cologne, and ornate jewelry do not communicate professionalism. Heavy cologne or perfume can, in fact, elicit adverse respiratory responses in sensitive individuals. Respiratory therapists have to be sensitive to this and refrain from any behavior that may cause actual harm or discomfort to their patients.

A person's role relates to their position and organizational status, which is often communicated by professional attire. Patients and subordinates may be intimidated by individuals having higher status and may curtail or refrain from any purposeful communication with them. Therefore, dressing for patient care differs from dressing for a professional interview because the purpose and goals differ. In patient care, physical appearance and dress should communicate professionalism, without unnecessary formality, which can distance some patients. Tables 4-7A and 4-7B give an overview of proper attire for a job interview and for patient care settings.

There is also the white lab jacket phenomenon.[23] This tenet says that wearing a white lab jacket will generally create an aura of instant credibility, acceptance, recognition, and stature. The white jacket is associated with health care, which affords the wearer the opportunity to ask intimate questions and perform physical assessments. Patients will answer questions and instantly trust the health professional in a white jacket. The aura of the white jacket or white coat denotes power and responsibility. The initial trust fostered by the white lab jacket can open the door to a trusting patient-therapist relationship. Respiratory therapists must recognize and respect the credibility society gives health care personnel, symbolized by the white jacket phenomenon.

Physical appearance and status have a significant bearing on communication. Therefore, respiratory therapists should do as much as possible to maintain a positive appearance and professional status within their organization and the community.

CRITICAL CONTENT

PHYSICAL APPEARANCE AND STATUS
- Age/gender/race
- Body size and shape
- Body movements and posture
- Dress, hair, and body adornments
- Body smell
- Role/position/titles
- Organizational status and influence

TABLE 4-7A   DRESSING PROFESSIONALLY FOR JOB INTERVIEWS

	EVERYONE	MEN	WOMEN
General appearance	Pay attention to first impressions, details, and neatness, and project a professional image. Wear neutral colors such as gray, navy, tan, and white.	Nothing trendy in clothing, hairstyle, or shoes. Clean, manicured hands with trim nails.	Nothing trendy in clothing, hairstyle, make-up, shoes, or jewelry. Neat nails with light polish or no polish.
Clothing	Research the company's culture and dress code, choose traditional styles.	Clean and pressed suit, dress shirt and tie or sport coat, slacks, and tie.	Clean and pressed suit with skirt or dress, slack suits okay in some instances.
Shoes	Polished dress shoes; no athletic, casual shoes or sandals.	Dark colored dress shoes and socks.	Dress shoes with a modest heel and stockings.
Hair	Combed hair with a professional, traditional cut and style.	Short hair preferred, long hair neatly tied back.	Neat, simple hairstyle. Long hair pulled back from the face.
Accessories	Avoid cologne; wear minimal jewelry; no visible tattoos or body piercing.	A ring and watch is sufficient, no earrings.	A ring, watch, and pair of earrings is sufficient.

TABLE 4-7B   PROFESSIONAL DRESSING FOR PATIENT CARE

General appearance	Neat, clean, professional, conservative
Clothing	Required dress code may include scrubs with a lab coat, casual business dress with a lab coat, or other specified uniform with ID
Jewelry, cologne	Wear none except a watch if needed
Accessories	No visible tattoos, body piercing
Hair	Clean, neat, and either short or tied back
Shoes	Polished, comfortable walking shoes

Environmental Factors

Communication does not occur in a vacuum and environmental conditions affect it. Environmental factors influence the degree and manner in which a person chooses to communicate. It also sends many nonverbal cues that people interpret. These interpretations affect a person's behavior either consciously or unconsciously. For example, the degree of formality and sensed pace will affect how people communicate. A formal, highly structured atmosphere will tend to alienate persons who are unfamiliar with the setting. If accompanied by nonverbal cues that further limit interaction, people will withdraw and communication will be limited. A casual, more relaxed atmosphere, combined with friendly nonverbal gestures such as a smile, will put others at ease, promoting interaction.

The pace of the environment also affects the way and amount people communicate. If there are many people scurrying about involved in different tasks, it will discourage communication. Consequently, a busy, formal setting is not suited for effective communications such as patient interviews. First impressions are tremendous facilitators or inhibitors of communication. Therefore, it is important that the physical appearance and the environment make a good first impression that welcomes interaction, comfort, trust, and openness.

CRITICAL CONTENT

ENVIRONMENTAL FACTORS AFFECTING COMMUNICATION

- Lighting
- Formality
- Physical space
- Architecture
- Furniture
- Familiarity
- Noise
- Temperature
- Privacy
- Pace

Sensory and Emotional Factors

Emotional or sensory factors have a major impact on communications. Emotional or sensory factors can consist of fear, stress, anxiety, pain, and limited or compromised mental acuity, sight, hearing, or speech. The health care environment is a place where considerable stress and anxiety exist. Patients, students, practitioners, and other heath care providers can exhibit negative emotions because of feelings of loss of control, frustration, low self-esteem, and inadequacy. Patients will often exhibit fear for their own well being as well as that of their family. For example, a patient suspecting he has a terminal illness may be so distraught that his ability to communicate can be significantly impaired.

The stress and burden of patient care needs can significantly affect respiratory therapists' and other health care providers' interactions with the patient. Students today also experience considerable pressure to achieve program requirements and demonstrate clinical competency in our high-stress health care environment. Pain can also serve as a source of distraction to communication, and is common in our patients. Significant physical pain, as well as the numbing effect of pain medication, creates numerous communication problems and challenges.

ADDITIONAL FACTORS AFFECTING NEGOTIATION

Power

The ability to influence another's behavior to attain a desired result is the basis of any negotiation. Examples of negotiations done by respiratory therapists include: 1) getting a patient to comply with a treatment plan, 2) having a physician consider your recommendation, 3) developing and implementing a respiratory care protocol, 4) obtaining a schedule change to meet your personal or professional needs, and 5) introducing a state law for regulation, credentialing, and/or reimbursement for respiratory care. Generally, one uses power bases with effective communications to successfully negotiate.

Take a moment to consider and evaluate your influence skills. Think of a time when you wanted to influence a person with decision-making authority in your life. How did you influence this person? What did you do or say? How did you feel? Were you successful (ie, did you get what you needed)? Pay attention to your answers. Ideally, you did your homework (research) and developed strategies ahead of time (ie, you anticipated the encounter and considered how to be most effective). To become skilled at negotiating, you must think about the needs of the persons you interact with and then choose a strategy that you believe will be most successful.

There are many ways to approach influencing skills. One useful approach is to understand and utilize your power bases. These are the types of power bases that people share.[7,28]

1. *Coercive power* is based on the ability to punish. If you can create fear in another, you have coercive power.

2. *Connectional power* is based on your connections with other people in the organization, community, and broader audiences. If people respond to you because they perceive you have influence on other prominent influential people, you are using connectional power.
3. *Expert power* comes from knowing how to get things done because of your expertise.
4. *Informational power* comes from having the inside track to the most current information, causing others to rely on you.
5. *Legitimate power* comes from your position within an organization, such as a position of authority as manager, administrator, or supervisor.
6. *Referent power* is the power that comes from personality, having a dynamic, charismatic personality that inspires people.
7. *Reward power* comes from the ability to reward others and is often related to one's legitimate power within an organization.

It is the other person's perception of your power that causes others to respond to you during any negotiation. In other words, the power bases you have and use determine your influence strategies and success at negotiating. Power sharing is essential to the whole process of collaboration. It is the other person who lets us influence him or her. You can improve your ability to negotiate various aspects of respiratory care by understanding and expanding your power bases.

Collaboration

Society is demanding new approaches to coordinating health care, requiring reevaluation of the independent and interdependent roles of the health professions. Consequently, collaboration has become a major need and focus. *Team* and *teamwork* are other common terms for *collaborators* and *collaboration*. It is through collaboration that disparate individuals or organizations are able to act in ways they could not on their own to solve problems they cannot solve on their own.[28]

The interdependence and effective functioning of any team requires shared power or shared authority. In health care, collaboration involves a negotiating process that builds on the contributions of various health professionals to form a new conceptualization of a problem.[28] Negotiation requires effective communication in order to develop and nurture a true collaboration. Furthermore, the style of communication must be one of openness, trust, and mutual respect between two or more persons who are valued for their expertise and competence. Thus, respiratory therapists must be effective communicators and negotiators who understand their interdependence. Respiratory therapists must know how to use power bases to achieve positive outcomes for their patients, their profession, and their organizations. Respiratory therapists function as true collaborators when they understand and acquire the needed skills and attitudes.

 Critical Thinking Exercise 3

a. Think about how you use your power bases to influence people around you.
b. Which power base is your strongest? Which is your second strongest?
c. Which power bases do you normally not use? Which are the ones you avoid? How does this limit you?
d. What power base(s) did you use the last time you influenced a decision maker?
e. Ask others how they perceive you and why or when they have allowed you to influence them. Try to obtain feedback from others you trust to help you learn what is it you did (or did not do) that allowed them to respond to you.

WRITTEN COMMUNICATION

It is beyond the scope of this chapter to present detailed information about written or electronic forms of communication. Each medium for commu-

T A B L E 4 - 8   AN EXAMPLE OF A RÉSUMÉ FOR GRADUATING RESPIRATORY THERAPISTS

Any Graduate
100 Professional Place
City, ST 12345
(123) 456-7890
agraduate@internetprovider.net

PROFESSIONAL AND CLINICAL SKILLS:

Neonatal/pediatric care	Chest x-ray assessment	Classroom and lab teaching
Oxygen therapy	Arterial puncture	Medical records
Chest physiotherapy	Patient assessment	Telemedicine training
Patient education	Traditional therapies	Netscape Communicator
Ventilator management	Medication administration	MS Word 7.0
Waveform analysis	Intubatient airway management	WordPerfect 6.0
Cardiopulmonary rehabilitation	Infection control	MS Internet Explorer
ABG and electrolyte analyses	Hemodynamic monitoring	PowerPoint 2000
Pulmonary rehabilitation	Pulmonary function testing	Word Excel and Access

WORK HISTORY:

Respiratory Therapy Student, Clinical Experience: 1000 hours, January 2000–May 2001.
Certified Respiratory Therapist, ABC Clinics, January–May 2001.
Emergency Room Transporter, September 1998–February 2000.
Volunteer Asthma Educator, Champ Camp by Georgia Lung Association, July 1999.
Customer Service/Technical Support Representative, Medical Systems, January 1996–June 1998.
Purchasing Assistant, Medical University, Any State, September 1994–January 1996.

EDUCATION:
Medical College of ABC, City, State
 June 1998–May 2000, B.S. Respiratory Therapy, GPA 3.8
State University of XYZ, City, State
 September 1995–August 1997, Biology Major, GPA 3.5
University of ABC, City, State
 August 1993–May 1995, Biology Major, GPA 3.2

CREDENTIALS:
Certified Respiratory Therapist as of January 2001
Registry-Eligible Respiratory Therapist as of May 5, 2001
Advanced Cardiac Life Support (ACLS) Provider, 2000
Neonatal Resuscitation Program (NRP), 2000

ACHIEVEMENTS:
Honor graduate of the Medical College of ABC respiratory therapy program, May 2001
Dean's List numerous semesters, June 1995–May 2001
Secretary of respiratory therapy class, June–August 2000
Recipient of Lambda Beta Scholarship, 2000
Member of the American Association for Respiratory Care, 1998–present
Recipient of National Volunteer Award from American Lung Association for Asthma Education, 2000
Invited and attended roundtable leadership meeting for student government, 2000
State championship for Future Business Leaders of America, 1995

nication has its unique challenges, requirements, limitations, advantages, and disadvantages. Respiratory therapists must be skilled at reading and writing medical records, including physician orders, care plans, discharge summaries, treatments, and assessment. Specific exercises to build written skills are interwoven throughout this textbook.

In addition, respiratory therapists must be skilled at writing professional letters, résumés, and reports. There are numerous resources on the Internet and in traditional textbooks to guide professionals to make a positive first impression in the written component of any job search. Table 4-8 provides an example of a résumé for a graduating respiratory therapist. Table 4-9 provides an example of a cover letter for the résumé for a job application. It is equally important to make a good impression in writing, paying attention to details and using traditional styles. The résumé and cover letter should be printed by a laser printer on light colored, high-quality bond paper. All documents should be thoroughly examined to check for neatness, spelling, correct grammar, and typographical errors.

Electronic Forms of Communication

With regard to the channel or medium used for communication, respiratory therapists must be aware of the extensive and increasing use of electronic media. Meetings and phone discussions are increasingly limited, having been replaced by electronic forms of interaction. In addition, memos, letters, directives, and other more formal written formats are being replaced by voice mail, e-mail, and electronic forums such as chat rooms and bulletin boards. Electronic forms of communication offer the advantages of high speed and low cost. However, it is important to choose the communication medium that is most appropriate for the circumstances and situation at hand.

Electronic forms of communication have facilitated the speedy access to numerous types of patient data, allowing for greater use of telemedicine and long-distance learning. Physicians, nurses, respiratory therapists, and others can access various types of patient data for clinical decision making and con-

sultation. However, electronic communication does not always allow for the type of interaction required. For example, it has been shown that telephone interviews can be an effective means to follow-up with patient education needs and provide comfort or reassurance. But keep in mind that although it is often not practical in today's world, in some cases there is no substitute for face-to-face communication, in which verbal and nonverbal communication can clarify meaning as well as nurture a relationship.

CRITICAL CONTENT

INTRAPERSONAL FACTORS AFFECTING COMMUNICATION

- Developmental stage
- Literacy/illiteracy
- Reading comprehension
- Language mastery
- Experiences
- Attitudes/values
- Cultural considerations
- Religious beliefs/convictions
- Motivations/feelings/interest
- Level and perception of illness or wellness
- Independence/dependence

BARRIERS TO COMMUNICATION AND NEGOTIATION

Numerous factors must be addressed to achieve effective communication and negotiation, including awareness of barriers. Table 4-10 highlights some of the most common barriers to effective communication and negotiation. The choice of words should always be carefully considered in any communication. Use of language that consists of abstract words, slang, and medical jargon can result in confusion and misunderstanding. It is equally important to separate your own emotional feelings from the message. Anger, anxiety, stress, strange-

TABLE 4-9   AN EXAMPLE OF A COVER LETTER FOR JOB A APPLICATION

Any Graduate
100 Professional Place
City, ST 12345
(123) 456-7890
anygraduate@internetprovider.net

June 24, 2001

Dr. Respiratory Manager
XYZ Hospital and Clinics
Department of Respiratory Therapy
City, ST 12345

Dear Dr. Manager,

I am seeking a full-time position as a registered therapist with the XYZ Hospital and Clinics. I will graduate from the Medical College of ABC on May 5, 2001. Upon graduation, I will have a Bachelor of Science Degree in Respiratory Therapy and will be RRT-eligible. I will be available for immediate employment upon graduation. The position you advertise in the respiratory therapy journal (specify name of journal, typed in *italics*) fits well with my education, experience and interests.

Your position requires someone who can rotate into various critical care units, including adults and pediatrics. I have critical care experience working with adults and children using the latest technologies to provide and monitor respiratory care. I have Advanced Cardiac Life Support (ACLS) Provider, Certified Respiratory Therapist (CRT), and Neonatal Resuscitation Provider (NRP) credentials. I have extensive exposure using clinical practice guidelines and protocol-based care during my clinical rotations and work as a certified respiratory therapist. I am competent and comfortable working with adult and pediatric patients in a variety of settings, including intensive care units and asthma camps for children. My enclosed résumé provides more details on my qualifications.

I believe I will be a genuine asset to your team of respiratory therapists because I am capable of competently handling a full workload. I have a sound understanding and clinical experience with most aspects of respiratory care. I consider myself a responsible team member who possesses a strong work ethic. I am finishing my clinical externship at this time. I am available during the day for a job interview to further discuss my qualifications and to learn more about this opportunity.

I am thoroughly impressed with the respiratory therapy program at the XYZ Hospital and Clinics. The responsibilities of the respiratory care staff and the wide application of protocol-based care in your facility make it a unique environment. Please contact me by phone or email to arrange a suitable time to discuss this position. I look forward to hearing from you. Thank you for your consideration.

Sincerely,

Any Graduate

Enclosure

ness, denial, fear, isolation, lack of control, boredom, or other negative emotions will be apparent in your nonverbal communication and will obstruct meaningful interaction. Glib statements such as, "Everything will be fine, you'll see," may be untrue, and therefore such statements are usually annoying rather than comforting.

Lack of sensitivity or awareness contributes to other communication barriers. For example, using the wrong timing is a common mistake when communicating. If you say something important when the person is upset or ill, he or she will be unable to actively listen. Being too opinionated by giving advice and expressing unnecessary disapproval or criticism will inevitability result in miscommunica-

tion or poor communication. Inappropriate confrontation or belittling a person's feelings can bring dialogue to an abrupt halt. Other destructive tendencies include acting defensively, interrupting the person, or correcting someone in front of others. A common barrier to communication occurs when people try to infer meaning by interpreting behaviors, rather than obtaining feedback through effective questioning. Respiratory therapists should consciously direct their efforts toward enhancing relationships and fulfilling the purposes of their communication as much as possible.

TABLE 4-10   BARRIERS TO COMMUNICATION

- Interrupting or abruptly changing the subject
- Conveying negative feelings
- Misusing facts or data
- Introducing unrelated information
- Offering premature explanation or counseling
- Using improper timing such as saying something important when the person is upset
- Making glib statements offering false hope, or insincere reassurance
- Using clichés, jargon, technical terms, trite expressions, and/or empty verbalisms
- Expressing insincere approval or undue disapproval
- Using forceful mannerisms to express strong opinions
- Giving advice, stating personal experiences, opinions, or value judgments
- Giving pep talks, telling another person what to do or that you know how they feel
- Probing with persistent "yes" or "no" questions
- Challenging or asking in a confrontational way; demanding explanations or proof
- Belittling the person's feelings or thoughts
- Defending or protecting someone or something

KEY POINTS

- Effective communication is essential for professional respiratory care practice.

- Communication can be written, verbal, or nonverbal, and it can be therapeutic.

- Every health care professional should understand that collaborative teamwork requires effective communication and negotiation; therefore, these skills must be acquired.

- Respiratory therapists can continually add to their learning and expertise to communicate effectively in a variety of situations.

- Nonverbal communications include the use of body language as well as the tone of voice, and these make up the largest percentage of our communications.

- If there is a discrepancy between the nonverbal and the verbal communications, another person will more likely believe what you say nonverbally.

- Asking appropriate questions at opportune times is fundamental to effective communications and respiratory care practice.

- Effective questioning is especially critical in the patient interview, a cornerstone of patient assessment.

- An effective communicator is able to request and accept feedback.

- Physical appearance and status have a significant bearing on communication. Therefore, respiratory therapists should do as much as possible to maintain a positive appearance and professional status within their organizations and the community.

- First impressions count! Therefore, learn to put your best foot forward in professional practice, including job interviews and collaborative and patient interaction situations.

- Respiratory therapists must actively and deliberately work to evaluate and improve their active listening, interviewing, communication, and negotiation skills through practice and feedback.

REFERENCES

1. Cullen DL, Sullivan JM, Bartel RE, et al. Delineating the educational direction for the future respiratory care practitioner. Proceedings of a National Consensus Conference on Respiratory Care Education. Dallas: American Association for Respiratory Care; 1992.

2. National Health Care Skill Standards Project. Quality and excellence: national health care skill standards. San Francisco: Far West Laboratory for Educational Research and Development; 1995.

3. Arnold E, Boggs K. *Interpersonal Relationships: Professional Communication Skills for Nurses.* 2nd ed. Philadelphia: Saunders; 1995.

4. Mishoe SC. Critical thinking in respiratory care practice. *Dissertation Abstr Intl.* 1995;55:3066A (University Microfilms No. 9507227).

5. Mishoe SC, Courtenay B. Critical thinking in respiratory care practice. Proceedings of the 35th Annual Adult Education Research Conference. Knoxville: University of Tennessee; 1994:276–281.

6. Mishoe SC. Critical thinking in respiratory care practice. *Respir Care.* 1996;41:958 (abstract).

7. Ulschak FL, SnowAntle SM. *Consultation Skills for Health Care Professionals. How to Be an Effective Consultant within Your Organization.* San Francisco: Jossey-Bass; 1990.

8. Balzer-Riley JW. *Communication in Nursing.* 4th ed. St. Louis: Mosby; 2000.

9. Northouse LL, Northouse PG. *Health Communication: Strategies for Health Professionals.* 3rd ed. Stamford, Conn: Appleton & Lange; 1998.

10. Schuster PM. *Communication: The Key to the Therapeutic Relationship.* Philadelphia: F.A. Davis Company; 2000.

11. Rankin SH, Stallings KD. *Patient Education: Issues, Principles, Practices.* 3rd ed. New York: Lippincott; 1996.

12. Mehrabian A, Williams M. Nonverbal communication of perceived and intended persuasiveness. *J Personality Soc Psych.* 1969;13:37.

13. Mehrabian A. *Silent Messages.*, Belmont, Calif: Wadsworth; 1971.

14. Darwin, C. *The Expression of Emotion in Man and Animals.* Chicago: University of Chicago Press; 1965.

15. Purtilo R. *Health Professional and Patient Interaction.* 4th ed. Philadelphia: Saunders; 1990.

16. Dellinger S, Deane B. *Communicating Effectively: A Complete Guide for Better Managing.* Radnor, Pa: Chilton Book Company; 1980.

17. Dugger J. Listen Up: Hear What's Really Being Said. West Des Moines, Iowa: American Media Publishing; 1995.

18. Huntley RA, Helfer KS. *Communication in Later Life.* Boston: Butterworth-Heinemann; 1995.

19. Lubinski R, Higginbotham DJ. *Communication Technologies for the Elderly: Vision, Hearing and Speech.* San Diego: Singular Publishing; 1997.

20. Webb LM, Schreiner JM, Asmuth MV. Maintaining effective interaction skills. In: Huntley RA, Helfer KS, (eds). *Communication in Later Life.* Boston: Butterworth-Heinemann; 1995.

21. Christie M, French D. *Assessment of Quality of Life in Childhood Asthma.* Chur, Switzerland: Harwood Academic Publishers; 1994.

22. Baker RR, Mishoe SC, Harrell LM, et al. Assessment of caregiver's knowledge of asthma and quality of life. *Am J Respir Dis Crit Care Med.* 1996;153:A754.

23. Neitch SM, Mufson MA. *Becoming a Clinician: A Primer for Students.* New York: McGraw-Hill; 1998.

24. Ryan ME, Collins FJ, Dowd JB, Pierce PD. Measuring patient satisfaction: A case study... data collection instrument entitled the Picker-

Commonwealth Survey on Patient-Centered Care. *J Nurs Care Quality.* 1995;9(2):44–53.

25. Menzel LK. A comparison of patients' communication-related responses during intubation and after extubation. *Heart Lung.* 1997;26:363–371.

26. Williams M. An algorithm for selecting a communication technique with intubated patients. *Dimensions of Critical Care Nursing*—1992; 11:222–229.

27. Boyd M, Graham B, Gleit C, et al. Health Teaching in Nursing Practice: A Professional Model. 3rd ed. Stamford, Conn: Appleton & Lange; 1998.

28. Sullivan TJ. Collaboration: A Health Care Imperative. New York: McGraw-Hill; 1998.

5

HEALTH CARE DELIVERY SYSTEMS AND RESPIRATORY THERAPISTS ACROSS THE CONTINUUM OF CARE

Kathleen M. Hernlen

The unexamined life is not worth living.
SOCRATES
(470–399 BC)

LEARNING OBJECTIVES

1. Define the continuum of care and factors that have changed the continuum of care in recent years.
2. Compare the traditional and nontraditional roles of respiratory therapists.
3. Discuss the role of the respiratory therapist in each area of the continuum of care, including skills, rewards, and areas of concern.
4. Discuss why the respiratory therapist is qualified for nontraditional roles.
5. Discuss the history of home health and how federal legislation has affected the role of the respiratory therapist.
6. Describe the role of case manager and the criteria for certification.
7. Define the types of subacute care.
8. Discuss the cost effectiveness of respiratory therapists in subacute care.
9. Discuss the role of pulmonary rehabilitation, disease prevention, and wellness programs in relation to managed care.
10. Discuss the various roles of respiratory therapists in industry.
11. Describe the role of respiratory therapists in diagnostics.
12. Define "physician extender" and discuss why the respiratory therapist is qualified for this role.

KEY WORDS

Managed Care	Pulmonary Rehabilitation
Subacute Care	Industry Consultant
Home Health	Polysomnography
Medicare Program	Physician Extender
Case Manager	Myocardial Infarction
Wellness Programs	Coronary Artery Bypass Graft

TRADITIONAL AND NONTRADITIONAL ROLES FOR RESPIRATORY THERAPISTS

History of Traditional Respiratory Therapist Roles

Respiratory therapists can trace their roots to 1798 in Bristol, England. Thomas Beddoes established the Pneumatic Institute, where he applied oxygen to patients to treat heart diseases, asthma, and opium poisoning. The modern use of oxygen began in earnest at the turn of the 20th Century. During the first 2 decades of the century, oxygen devices such as nasal catheters, oxygen tents, and oxygen masks were developed and used in clinical settings. This created a need for knowledgeable people who could administer oxygen; thus the field of respiratory therapy was born.

In the 1940s a group of physicians and "oxygen technicians" in Chicago began meeting to discuss oxygen therapy. These discussions lead to the creation of the Inhalational Therapy Association in 1946.[1] Over the next few years the membership grew, and in 1954 the group was renamed the American Association of Inhalation Therapists (AAIT). For a complete list of common abbreviations used in this chapter, see Table 5-1.

The 1960s saw much advancement in technology, including the development by Leland Clark and John Severenghaus of electrodes that allowed for clinical blood gas analysis. The Bird Mark 7 and the Bennett PR-1 pressure-limited ventilators were also used clinically. This lead to the need for better-trained, knowledgeable specialists. In 1968 the first certification board was established and the first certification examinations for inhalation therapy were given in 1969.[1]

The 1970s saw even more advancements in the field of respiratory therapy as air/oxygen blenders, pulse oximetry, oxygen concentrators, portable liquid oxygen systems, and intermittent mechanical ventilation (IMV) were developed and incorporated into clinical practice. In 1978 the National Board for Respiratory Therapy developed entry-level criteria that set the standards for entry into the field.[1] In 1979 the first clinical simulation examination for advanced practitioners was administered, replacing the previously used oral examination.[1]

As technology continued to improve in the 1980s and 1990s, advancements in the profession included the development and use of pressure control ventilation, continuous flow ventilation, extracorporeal membrane oxygenation (ECMO), and home care ventilators. Respiratory therapy was recognized as a profession by the government according to the guidelines laid out under the Public Health Service Act, Title VII, Section 701.[2] The respiratory care profession saw tremendous growth, especially among specialty fields. The certified pulmonary function examination was first administered in 1984. This was followed in 1987 by the advanced pulmonary function examination. In 1991, the first perinatal pediatric examination was given.[1]

The development of the respiratory care profession emphasized the importance of providing respiratory care by highly trained persons in the hospital setting. As new trends in health care emerged, respiratory therapists quickly responded in order to best meet patient needs and establish the new profession. This adaptability has been an asset in recent years as health care technology continues to develop at a rapid rate. The respiratory care profession now required personnel who had advanced technical training and experience in clinical decision making and critical thinking. Departments capitalized on the therapist's skills in clinical decision making by implementing protocol based care.[3]

CRITICAL CONTENT

HISTORY OF RESPIRATORY THERAPY

- In 1798 oxygen was first used in the clinical setting.
- The first certification examination was given for inhalation therapy in 1969.
- The National Board for Respiratory Therapy developed entry-level standards for the profession in 1978.
- Respiratory therapy was recognized as a profession by the government in the 1990s.

Traditional Services Provided by Respiratory Therapists. Since its birth, the primary or traditional setting for the delivery of respiratory therapy has been in the hospital. Typically, a centralized respiratory therapy department provided a variety of respiratory services. Services provided were usually divided into two major areas: general patient care and critical care. The services provided by respiratory therapists were categorized as 1) oxygen therapy, such as routine oxygen administration, transport, and hyperbaric oxygen administration; 2) therapies, including jet nebulizers, metered dose inhalers (MDIs), intermittent positive-pressure breathing (IPPB), and chest physiotherapy (CPT);

TABLE 5-1 ABBREVIATIONS

American Association for Respiratory Care (AARC)
Professional society for respiratory therapists committed to enhancing the profession of respiratory care

Balanced Budget Act of 1997 (BBA)
Law enacted in 1997 that made significant changes to the Medicare system

Durable medical equipment (DME)
Health care equipment for home care patients

Food and Drug Administration (FDA)
An agency of the US government under the Department of Health and Human Services responsible for assuring the safety of food and drugs

Health Care Financing Administration (HCFA)
A division of the US Department of Health and Human Services that is responsible for overseeing the Medicare program

Health maintenance organization (HMO)
An example of a managed care organization. A group practice health care program providing comprehensive prepaid medical care

Joint Commission on the Accreditation of Healthcare Organizations (JCAHO)
An organization that evaluates and accredits hospitals, health care networks, managed care organizations, and health care organizations providing home care, long-term care, behavioral health care, and ambulatory services

Long-term acute care hospitals (LTAC)
Licensed hospitals that are exempt from the Medicare prospective payment system as long as they keep their average patient length of stay greater than 25 days

Occupational Safety and Health Administration (OSHA)
A branch of the US Department of Labor whose mission is to save lives, prevent injuries, and protect the health of America's workers

Prospective payment system (PPS)
A method of payment for services provided to Medicare patients

Preferred provider organization (PPO)
An example of a managed care organization. An agreement in which arrangements are negotiated between a third-party payer, usually a self-insured company, and a group of health care providers, usually physicians and hospitals, who furnish services at lower-than-usual fees in return for prompt payment and an increased volume of patients

Skilled nursing facility (SNF)
Identified beds certified by the Health Care Financing Administration (HCFA) to participate in the Medicare program for servicing its long-term care benefit recipients

3) physiologic monitoring such as arterial blood gas sampling and interpretation, pulmonary function testing, pulse oximetry, and capnography; 4) ventilator management, including adult, pediatric, infant, and noninvasive ventilation; and 5) specialized skills such as transports, cardiopulmonary resuscitation (CPR), and airway care.[4] While many of these services were delivered in both general care and critical care, others such as ventilator management were seen only in critical care.

CRITICAL CONTENT

TRADITIONAL RESPIRATORY THERAPY SERVICES

- Hospitals developed centralized respiratory therapy departments.
- The departments offered services in general care and critical care units.
- Services provided by respiratory therapy departments included oxygen therapy, medication delivery and airway clearance, physiological monitoring, ventilator management, and specialized skills.

Why Nontraditional Roles Are Emerging For Respiratory Therapists

The past few years have seen many changes in the delivery of health care. The traditional delivery system, with the acute care hospital providing the majority of health care, has been replaced with a system that has broadened the continuum of care. This system, while still in the process of defining itself, has already seen the emergence and increased significance of subacute care facilities, home health agencies, and prevention/wellness programs. In the future, patients may spend more time in these nontraditional care settings. Private and public sector factors are precipitating these changes.

Private Sector. The change in emphasis from hospitals to other health care settings has been brought about by several factors in both the private and public sectors. Private sector forces such as managed care and the emergence of health care as a

major social issue, along with public sector policy and regulatory changes to the Medicaid and Medicare systems, have had tremendous impact on the delivery of health care. Changes to the health care system are occurring rapidly and require all health care professions to adapt and be flexible in order to keep up.

The health care system has come under criticism from both the public and private sectors who are no longer willing to financially support a system that continues to have such high rates of inflation. This has fueled the managed care industry and instigated a vigorous debate about national health care reform. Because of the increased costs of health care, employers have cut the amount of money they are willing to spend for employee health benefits. Consequently, insurers are seeking ways to offer the same services at lower costs. Managed care can be defined as "structures and interventions to control the price, volume, delivery site, and intensity of health services provided, the goal of which is to maximize the value of health benefits and the coordination of health care management for the covered population."[3]

Managed care companies such as health maintenance organizations (HMOs) and preferred provider organizations (PPOs) provide enrollees with medical and hospital care in exchange for an agreed-upon fee. The goal is to assure that the patient will receive adequate care in the appropriate health care setting. Requirements for continuation of stay for each setting are set and reviewed by utilization reviews. When a patient no longer meets the acuity level required, the patient is transferred to a less costly setting. With managed care, the hospital receives a set fee per diagnosis on each patient covered. If health care providers can provide care for less than this set fee, they pocket the difference. This type of reimbursement is called **prospective payment**.

Prospective payment systems (PPS) have become increasingly popular as a replacement for the more traditional **fee-for-service**. Fee-for-service was the system in which each item or service provided had a set price that was charged each time the item was used or the service provided. This old system was felt by many to encourage overutilization of resources. There was no incentive (at least not a financial one) to limit utilization or health care costs, because under fee-for-service, the more services provided, the higher the charges to the patient's insurance company, and the more profit for the health care provider. Under this system, health care costs and utilization of services continually escalated. Hence the prospective payment system was born. With PPS, health care professionals provide whatever care they feel is appropriate, and they make a profit if the care provided costs less than the set fee. The fee with PPS is often based on the diagnosis (e.g., the federal government's Medicare system's diagnosis related groups [DRGs]) or a fee per day the patient is hospitalized. Payment can, however, be based on a fixed amount of reimbursement per person per year, in a given geographic area. Fixed payment is referred to as "capitated" payment. Under any of these systems the health care provider has an incentive to carefully scrutinize the delivery of services and minimize inappropriate or excessive utilization.

CRITICAL CONTENT

MANAGED CARE

- The private and public sectors have helped create a larger continuum of health care.
- The goals of managed care are to control the cost of health care and at the same time provide adequate care.
- Examples of managed care include physician provider organizations (PPOs) and health maintenance organizations (HMOs).
- Prospective payment systems have replaced the traditional fee-for-service system.

Public Sector. With the inception of Medicare and Medicaid in the 1960s, health care flourished. Medicare is now the nation's largest payer for health services, covering a total of approximately 37 million beneficiaries.[5] The reimbursement policies allowed consumers to choose their own providers in a fee-for-service agreement. Under

fee-for-service agreements, an individual or an insurance carrier made payment at the time services were rendered. Consequently the utilization and costs of health care skyrocketed in the United States. There were few limitations or constraints under the fee-for-service system, which was based on retrospective payment (i.e., the payment occurring after the service is provided). This system greatly increased inflation, with health care costs consuming ever larger amounts of the gross domestic product.

In an effort to bring the health care system under control and streamline costs, Congress passed various pieces of legislation in an attempt to address the runaway increases in health care costs. The first of these was the creation of professional standards review organizations (PSROs) in 1972, that set up peer review groups in which physicians reviewed the length of stay (LOS) and level of care (LOC) of patients in acute care hospitals. The intent was to reduce the length of hospital stays and to transfer patients to lower-cost settings as soon as medically reasonable. In response to the loss of revenue resulting from shorter stays, the costs of other nonregulated services started increasing. Health care providers simply increased the cost of the other services they provided to make up for the lost revenue. This so called "cost shifting" is blamed by many for the unrealistic charges for many items in the hospital environment (including respiratory care services).

The next congressional action to control costs was the Tax Equity and Fiscal Responsibility Act of 1982 (TEFRA), that mandated the development of a PPS for Medicare and led to the development of the DRG system that so profoundly affected hospital reimbursement. Most recently, Congress passed the Balanced Budget Act (BBA) of 1997 to address continuing health care cost concerns. The BBA reduced the amount of money for services provided for respiratory services in the home health and subacute care arenas. The Balanced Budget Act included provisions for a five-year plan to decrease Medicare expenditures by $115 billion.[6] Home health expenditures were decreased by $16.2 billion, with significant cuts to home medical equipment and oxygen.[6] Other health care professions experienced similarly drastic reductions in reimbursement for their services. Reductions in health care reimbursement were much greater than intended. Consequently, numerous reforms to the BBA of 1997 have been proposed and some have been implemented as of the time this chapter was written.

Managed care is becoming increasingly popular among Medicare and Medicaid beneficiaries. Recent data from the Health Care Financing Administration (HCFA) indicated that almost 4 million Medicare beneficiaries and more than 11 million Medicaid recipients participate in managed care programs.[7] This increasing use of managed care among Medicare and Medicaid patients, along with the reductions in payments for respiratory services in the home health and subacute care arenas, has contributed to the changes currently being seen in the health care delivery system.

CRITICAL CONTENT

US GOVERNMENT HEALTH CARE POLICY CHANGES

- Medicare is the nation's largest payer for health care services.
- A growing number of Medicare beneficiaries are enrolled in managed care plans.
- PSROs were created in 1972 to reduce LOS and LOC of hospitalized Medicare patients.
- Congress passed TEFRA in 1982 to implement PPS (DRGs), which reduced payment to acute care hospitals.
- Congress passed the BBA in 1997, which directs the HCFA to reduce the amount of money provided for respiratory therapy services in home health and subacute care.

Population. While public and private sector changes have been responsible for many of the changes in the health care delivery system, perhaps the factor that will have the biggest impact on the future of the delivery of health care is the changing demographic makeup of the US. The population is

aging and living longer than ever before. By 2010 the estimated average life expectancy will be 77.9 years.[8] The total US population of persons over 65 is expected to be 69 million by 2050.[9] The number of people needing respiratory care is expected to increase with this increase in the aging population.

Another reason for the development and expansion of outpatient and subacute care is the number and types of patients, especially those with chronic problems. According to the Centers for Disease Control, chronic obstructive pulmonary disease (COPD) is the fourth leading cause of death, killing over 100,000 people annually, and pneumonia is the sixth leading cause of death, killing 80,000 people annually.[10] The number of Americans with asthma exceeded 14.8 million in 1995.[11] The prevalence of diseases such as asthma, chronic bronchitis, pneumonia, and congestive heart failure, especially among the elderly, will continue to present a challenge for respiratory care practitioners in the 21st Century. According to the National Heart, Lung and Blood Institute, in 1998 the annual cost to the nation for COPD was $26 billion, including $13.6 billion in direct health care costs.[12]

CRITICAL CONTENT

POPULATION CHANGES INCREASING THE NEED FOR RESPIRATORY THERAPY

- An aging American population
- Increased life expectancy
- Increased incidence of chronic pulmonary diseases, such as bronchitis, emphysema, and asthma
- Technological advances
- Increased focus on health promotion, wellness
- Better-informed public with greater access to medical information

Hospital Changes. The increased use of managed care, changes in reimbursement strategies, and the aging population have challenged acute care hospitals to develop means to decrease their costs. Hospitals have undergone restructuring and reorganization in the past decade. A recent survey of the American Association of Respiratory Care (AARC) found that 67% of its members worked in organizations that had restructured in the past 5 years.[3] Recent changes include decreasing the levels of management, labor substitution, decentralization of respiratory care departments, patient-focused care, and use of alternative or contract employees.[3]

Many respiratory care departments in the US have undergone some form of decentralization. With total decentralization, respiratory care practitioners are no longer assigned to a respiratory department, but instead are assigned to a nursing unit and report directly to nursing supervisors.[3,13] Other hospitals have adopted a partially decentralized structure in which some of the respiratory duties or personnel have become decentralized, while other duties, usually the more technically advanced, are provided by a core respiratory department.

Labor substitution has proven to be a double-edged sword for respiratory care practitioners in the traditional setting. With the use of protocols, respiratory therapists have been able to expand their skills by providing assessments and choosing treatment plans for patients. On the other hand, nurses or other health care personnel have assumed selected respiratory therapist duties in some settings. There has been considerable concern about the competency of these alternative personnel. Studies have shown that respiratory therapists demonstrate better technique in the delivery of respiratory procedures than other personnel.[3,14,15] Hospitals utilizing respiratory therapists under respiratory therapy–directed treatment protocols have significantly less overutilization of respiratory therapy treatments.[16] Many hospitals have hired contract or alternative employees through agencies, instead of hiring them directly, as a means of cost control.

In theory, patient-focused care involves restructuring staff and services to better meet the needs of the patient. Services and resources are brought to the patient's bedside whenever possible,

in contrast to the old method of transporting patients and their families to the services. Advocates of this model of health care delivery feel that this creates a more "patient friendly" atmosphere and decreases the number of staff members that interact with the patient. Labor substitution is often implemented in this model of health care delivery. Employees are cross-trained in a variety of tasks in order to be able to provide the needed services at the patient's bedside.

The cost of caring for patients is greater in the acute care setting, due to the number of fixed costs such as staff and equipment. Therefore, cost containment concerns have lead to the development of postacute care delivery sources such as home health, subacute care, and outpatient programs, where the cost of caring for patients is lower. The estimated cost of caring for a patient in a hospital (nonintensive care) ranges from $300 to $800/day with the cost of intensive care ranging from $800 to $2000/day. The cost of subacute care ranges from $600 to $700/day.[17]

According to the American Healthcare Association, during the 1990s the number of subacute care beds increased dramatically. At the end of the decade there were between 35,000 and 45,000 subacute care beds in the US.[18] The National Subacute Care Association predicts that within 5 years, subacute care will account for 40% of all Medicare expenditures.[19]

CRITICAL CONTENT

HOW HOSPITALS HAVE CHANGED IN THE US

- Restructured many respiratory therapy departments
- Greater emphasis on cost containment
- Expanded continuum of care
- Decreased number of acute care hospital beds
- Increased number of subacute beds
- Greater use of patient-focused care, labor substitution, contract, per diem, and part-time employees

Roles Emerging in Nontraditional Respiratory Therapy

In order to adapt to the changes in the health care system, respiratory therapists have had to change as well. The development of nontraditional arenas for care has offered new, challenging opportunities. Respiratory therapists have taken advantage of this enlarged continuum of care to create new niches for themselves. This includes new roles in areas such as postacute care (including subacute and long-term facilities), home health, case management, industry, rehabilitation programs, and physician offices.

Respiratory therapists have put their educational skills to work in rehabilitation, wellness, and disease prevention programs. Their clinical skills have been expanded into areas such as cardiopulmonary diagnostic testing and polysomnography. Respiratory therapists, who have benefited from strong relationships with physicians, have created new roles by becoming physician extenders. Areas such as research, medical writing, and industry now employ respiratory therapists. The doors of opportunity in respiratory therapy are wide open.

CRITICAL CONTENT

EMERGING ROLES FOR RESPIRATORY THERAPISTS: NEW OPPORTUNITIES

- Home health
- Subacute care
- Cardiopulmonary rehabilitation
- Disease prevention
- Wellness/education programs
- Medical writing
- Research
- Industry
- Sales
- Physician extenders

Why Respiratory Therapists Are Qualified for Nontraditional Roles

Respiratory therapists have been able to capitalize on this new way of thinking, because they have the skills needed to thrive under managed care.

Respiratory therapists have strong, specialized backgrounds in the diagnosis, treatment, and prevention of cardiopulmonary diseases. Treatment of cardiopulmonary diseases constitutes a large portion of the high health costs for chronic diseases that create challenges for managed care companies. Respiratory therapists have strong assessment skills and the ability to create treatment plans that can lower the cost of caring for chronic pulmonary patients. Please refer to Chapter 6 for a complete discussion of care plans/protocols and Chapter 7 for a detailed study of patient assessment. These are critical components of respiratory care, especially in nontraditional roles. Respiratory therapists are the experts on respiratory equipment, products, and medications. Because of their knowledge of cardiopulmonary diseases, respiratory therapists make excellent patient educators, and they have been able to utilize these skills in prevention and wellness programs such as pulmonary rehabilitation.

Respiratory therapists have capitalized on their strong clinical backgrounds and assessment skills to create new careers in nontraditional settings. While 80% of all respiratory therapists are employed in hospitals, recent studies conclude that many of the job opportunities for respiratory therapists in the next few years will be in nontraditional settings.[3] In order to make this transition more complete, respiratory therapists must add to their existing skills. They must prove their cost effectiveness, adapt to new practice settings, and focus on dealing with the chronic aspects of disease management and not just the acute phase. They must be willing to take on new responsibilities and be open to taking risks.[3] Respiratory therapists will need to expand their skills in communication and patient education, and increase their knowledge of managed care and reimbursement.

Respiratory therapists have always been valued for their clinical expertise, knowledge, and management of respiratory diseases; however, working in nontraditional roles requires development of a new set of skills. What was important in an acute care setting may not be as important to a respiratory therapist working in a subacute care or home health setting. The professional and personal skills needed change from environment to environment.

CRITICAL CONTENT

WHY RESPIRATORY THERAPISTS ARE QUALIFIED FOR NEW ROLES

- Strong clinical backgrounds in the diagnosis, treatment, and prevention of cardiopulmonary disease
- Patient assessment skills and the ability to create effective treatment plans
- Excellent patient educators, and teaching self-care is increasingly important in today's health care environment
- Excellent candidates for training as new practices emerge due to their backgrounds and adaptability
- Technology specialists with computer skills

RESPIRATORY THERAPISTS IN HOME HEALTH CARE

Definition and History of Home Health Care

At the turn of the 20th Century, the majority of health care was provided in the home. Due to the advancement of medical knowledge and technology, this soon became impossible and hospitals became the best sites for providing health care. During the past century, most patients have recovered from illnesses in acute care hospitals. They did not return to their homes until they were able to care for themselves. There has been a recent change in this thinking. The financial incentives realized by managed care companies, coupled with the desire of more patients to recover in their homes, has resulted in the increasing use of home health care. Home health care has been defined as "the provision of services and equipment to the patient in the home for the purpose of restoring and maintaining his or her maximal level of comfort, function and health."[20]

Home health care traces its roots as far back as 1893 when 2 nurses in New York, Lillian Wald and Mary Brewster, created the Henry Street Settle-

ment.[21] They provided health and social services to the poor in the home. This eventually led to the creation of the Visiting Nurses Association (VNA). The VNA primarily provided care to the poor and was funded through both public and philanthropic contributors. In 1947 the nation's first hospital-based home health care department was established at Montefiero Hospital in New York City.[21]

Home health benefited from the creation of the Medicare program in the 1960s. Medicare part A, which provides hospital benefits, contained a mechanism to reimburse for intermittent skilled visits provided to homebound patients. At that time, respiratory therapy, as a profession, was in its infancy and was not included in the reimbursable services in part A of Medicare. Medicare part B partially reimbursed for items of medically necessary equipment and supplies provided for use in the home. Because of this legislation, from 1966 through the 1990s the number of home health care agencies grew rapidly.

CRITICAL CONTENT

HISTORY OF HOME HEALTH CARE

- Home health care began in New York in 1893.
- Medicare part A reimburses for intermittent skilled visits.
- Medicare part B partially reimburses for items of medical necessity, such as equipment and supplies.
- Respiratory therapy is not included in the reimbursement for skilled visits.
- Recognition for the value of respiratory therapists in home health care, including reimbursement for services, is needed.
- Home health care costs are generally less than acute care costs.

Types of Home Health Care Services

Today, home health care services can be provided to patients with acute illnesses, exacerbations of chronic illnesses, or those with long-term disabilities who do not require hospitalization. Home health care services fall into 5 different categories: home health agencies, hospice, home medical equipment, home infusion therapy, and homemaker services/private duty nursing.

Home health agencies provide visits by skilled health care professionals on an intermittent basis. These providers must be licensed by the state and certified under Medicare Conditions of Participation if Medicare reimbursement is sought. When Medicare was developed, respiratory therapy was in its infancy, and it was not recognized as one of these services. The American Association for Respiratory Care (AARC), along with other health care professionals and consumer advocates, are working to ensure adequate medical services for Medicare beneficiaries. The AARC is working with others to convince Congress of the need to reverse the health care cuts that resulted from the Balanced Budget Act of 1997. The AARC is also working with HCFA to include respiratory therapy services as reimbursable professional services. While respiratory therapists were not recognized as a covered service under Medicare regulations, that did not mean they have not been involved in home health care.

Home "durable medical equipment" has been the main means of providing respiratory services to the home patient. Companies arrange for the selection, delivery, setup, use, and ongoing maintenance of medically necessary equipment in the home. Durable medical equipment (DME) companies are reimbursed for the sale and rental of equipment. In most cases 80% of the cost is covered and 20% is the patient's responsibility.

With the development of sophisticated medical equipment that could be used in the home, respiratory therapists were initially recognized primarily as equipment experts. Respiratory therapists soon emerged as important members of the home health care team because of their expertise in patient assessment, disease management, and intervention. Home health care companies have seen the benefit of having respiratory therapists on staff, because patients who receive comprehensive ongoing education and services provided by respiratory thera-

pists are less likely to be readmitted to the hospital. The DME companies have been able to hire and pay for a respiratory therapist out of the money generated by medical sales and rentals. While recent cuts under the BBA have reduced the reimbursement structure for DME equipment rental and sales, managed care companies have recognized and established the importance of respiratory therapists in this arena by seeking home health companies who provide respiratory expertise.

The opportunities for the growth of respiratory therapy in home health care are great. The JCAHO has been accrediting home health programs since 1988.[22] In 1995, over 4600 had received their accreditation status.[22] By 1996 there were an estimated 5000 to 10,000 respiratory care practitioners working in a home health care setting.[22]

CRITICAL CONTENT

HOME HEALTH SERVICES AND RESPIRATORY THERAPY

- Types of home health care services include home health agencies, hospice, home medical equipment, home infusion therapy, and homemaker/private duty nursing.
- Respiratory therapists in home health care primarily work for DME companies.
- The Balanced Budget Act of 1997 significantly reduced the reimbursement for DME sales and rentals.
- Medicare does not include respiratory therapy as a directly reimbursable skilled service.

Respiratory Therapy Home Health Care Services

Respiratory therapists in the home setting deliver services to diverse patient populations with varying ages and disease processes. Patients range from premature infants requiring supplemental oxygen and monitoring, to elderly patients on mechanical ventilation. Oxygen therapy may be provided to patients with chronic hypoxemia or COPD. Patients with reversible airway disease, such as asthma, may receive education on self-care for such things as trigger avoidance and bronchodilator administration. Airway clearance techniques may be taught to children with cystic fibrosis, or patients with tracheostomies. Noninvasive positive pressure ventilation (NPPV) may be provided for patients with obstructed sleep apnea or COPD. Patients who cannot be weaned from ventilators may live at home, receiving care provided by home health respiratory therapists. In addition to these therapies, diagnostic tools and monitoring equipment such as pulse oximeters and apnea monitors may be used in the diagnosis, treatment, and prevention of diseases such as obstructive sleep apnea (OSA) and sudden infant death syndrome (SIDS).

The duties of a home health respiratory therapist include initial and ongoing assessments, patient and caregiver education and training, follow-up home visits, as well as liaison activities between the patient and physician. The initial assessment of a home health patient often begins before the patient returns home. Unlike hospitals, which have strict safety codes for medical equipment, individual homes must be inspected by the respiratory therapist to ensure the physical environment of the home meets safety standards. This involves making sure the house has working smoke detectors, the electrical outlets are grounded, and there are enough exits in case of fire. The respiratory therapist must coordinate the type of equipment needed and the delivery and setup of the equipment.

When the patient arrives home, an actual physical assessment of the patient must be performed. A respiratory therapist must have strong clinical assessment skills in order to do this. Unlike working in a hospital, a home health respiratory therapist is expected to make assessments using only a stethoscope, a blood pressure cuff, and a pulse oximeter. The therapist may then make recommendations to the physician concerning the treatment and equipment needed by the patient.

The therapist must also determine if the patient or their family is capable of providing the care needed by the patient. Even though prior instruction often occurs, the reality of the responsibilities of caring for someone does not become clear to potential caregivers until they are in the home setting. If the caregiver is incapable of providing adequate care, the therapist must work with the family, physician, and case manager to develop a plan of care that meets the needs of the patient.

Education of the patient and the caregiver(s) is one of the most important responsibilities of the home health therapist. They must be trained on the safe and proper use, storage, cleaning, infection control techniques, and maintenance of all equipment. They must also be trained in what to do when the equipment fails or malfunctions. Backup plans for such an event must be established beforehand and completely understood by the patient and caregivers. Education about disease management, medications, and signs and symptoms of disease must be covered. The patient, family, and respiratory therapist create a treatment plan working together.

Often, patients may not have had time to fully come to terms with their disease while in the hospital, or may not have had the opportunity to ask questions about their disease or medications. The hospital setting may act as a deterrent to asking such questions, because many people often find it to be a foreign and intimidating environment. Being in their own homes makes patients more comfortable, and this often leads them to ask more questions. The home health respiratory therapist becomes the educational resource for these patients. While many people have a good understanding of their disease process from information received from their physician or hospital personnel, they often still have questions for the home health respiratory therapist.

The respiratory therapist must be able to answer questions about cardiopulmonary diseases, management of these diseases, anatomy, treatments, and medications. For instance, a patient is often sent home with numerous prescriptions. The patient may have questions concerning the type of medicine: When do I take it? Why do I need it? How do I take it? How will I pay for it?

The respiratory therapist may conduct follow-up visits monitoring the progress of the patient while at home. The number of follow-up visits will depend on the severity of the patient's disease. Based on the patient's progress (or lack of progress), the therapist may make suggestions to the physician about the care of the patient. The follow-up visits may also be required to make sure the provided services and equipment are still needed. The patient may need to meet some specific qualifications for the continued use of home health care. For example, in order to qualify for HCFA Medicare part B reimbursement for oxygen, a patient must have a PaO_2 of 55 or less, or a SaO_2 of 88 or less, and a pulmonary diagnosis, or must meet other very specific criteria; see Chapter 12 for details.

CRITICAL CONTENT

SERVICES AND DUTIES OF THE HOME HEALTH RESPIRATORY THERAPIST

- Services provided by the home health respiratory therapist include oxygen therapy, bronchodilator therapy, airway clearance techniques, invasive and noninvasive positive pressure ventilation, and diagnostics.
- The duties of a home health respiratory therapist include initial and ongoing assessments, patient and caregiver education, follow-up visits, and liaison activities between patients and physicians.

Durable Medical Equipment

The equipment used by respiratory therapists in the home differs in many ways from respiratory equipment used in a hospital setting. Homes do not have piped-in oxygen; instead patients are provided with oxygen conservers, concentrators, and small cylinders. Air compressors often provide medication delivery. Home ventilators are generally smaller and less sophisticated, and offer fewer modes than hospital ventilators. They must be durable, portable, and less intimidating because nonmedical personnel will be using them. They also do not

have as many alarms as hospital ventilators. Apnea monitors often have recording equipment so the therapist can document usage and trends for their later analysis or so the physician may do so. Home health companies often have a variety of oxygen devices on hand for the patient to try, such as oxygen conserving cannulas, and various lightweight portable systems. The therapist works with the patient to find the right devices for each person. Currently, the home health industry is so strong that many companies are now developing products primarily for the home market.

CRITICAL CONTENT

HOME HEALTH EQUIPMENT

- Home health equipment is simpler and more portable than hospital equipment.
- Many manufacturers develop products and equipment strictly for use in the home

Skills Needed by the Respiratory Therapist in Home Health Care

While the home care setting is not like an acute or intensive care setting, and less time management and organizational skills may be needed, strong interpersonal skills are essential. A good home health therapist must truly love working with all types of people in many different surroundings. A typical day may take the respiratory therapist from the most expensive subdivision to government housing projects, and from the cleanest home to the most unkempt; therefore, the respiratory therapist must be adaptable and ready to work in any environment. Being able to relate to the patient in a nonjudgmental manner helps build the relationship between the patient and the therapist. Therapists must exhibit empathy and understanding, and be prepared to use negotiating and sometimes motivational skills in working with their patients.

Many people have difficulty adjusting to the permanent presence of the oxygen equipment or the need for lifelong medication usage. Although they may have often been informed of this in the hospital, the reality often does not hit them until they return home and begin day to day life. While the respiratory therapist cannot force a person to use oxygen, they can give examples of how using the oxygen will improve their quality of life and allow them to pursue activities that interest them. The therapist may offer suggestions for dealing with potential problems, such as the need to plan outings in advance to ensure the patient will have an adequate supply of oxygen. Many times patients decide not to use their oxygen or take their medications because they feel better or because they have begun to deny that they still have problems. Respiratory therapists must use their persuasive powers to educate the patient about the consequences of this choice. Having established a good relationship helps when trying to convince a patient why he or she should stick to the treatment plan.

Therapists in the home care setting also need a thorough knowledge of reimbursement policies and case management. Many times, physicians will order prescriptions or treatments for patients thinking they are using the most cost-effective means, but in reality they are costing the patient more money. For example, a metered dose inhaler may be the most cost-effective method of delivering bronchodilator therapy in the hospital, but not in the home. In some states, Medicare may not pay for the MDI, but will pay for the unit dose albuterol for nebulization. Therefore the role of the respiratory therapist is critical in reducing the cost of care for the health care provider as well as the patient.

CRITICAL CONTENT

SKILLS NEEDED BY THE HOME HEALTH RESPIRATORY THERAPIST

- Strong interpersonal skills
- A nonjudgmental attitude
- Ability to work in various environments
- Ability to educate patients and family members
- Knowledge of reimbursement policies

Rewards for the Home Health Respiratory Therapist

Despite the concerns about reimbursement, home health therapists find many aspects of their jobs rewarding. Many respiratory therapists enjoy the flexibility of being able to set their own schedule. They also report the job is less stressful than working in acute care settings and having to deal with frequent emergency situations. Home health respiratory therapists enjoy the ability to have personal interactions and build stronger relationships with patients and their families. Being able to follow a patient for a significant amount of time is another reward. The chance to teach patients about their disease, equipment, and ways of improving their quality of life is one of the most rewarding aspects of home health care.

CRITICAL CONTENT

REWARDS OF HOME RESPIRATORY THERAPY

- Flexibility to set your own schedule
- Ability to have more personal interaction
- Opportunity to build stronger relationships with patients and their families
- Teaching patients about their disease, equipment, and care
- Improving the quality of life for patients and their families

RESPIRATORY THERAPISTS AS CASE MANAGERS

Goals of Case Management

The Certification of Insurance Rehabilitation Specialist Commission (CIRSC) defines case management as "a collaborative process which assesses, plans, implements, coordinates, monitors, and evaluates the options and services to meet an individual's resources to promote quality, cost-effective outcomes."[23] The goals of case management include the following: achieving optimum patient outcome, early intervention, coordination and continuity of care, a safe transition from one facility to another, and containment of costs to conserve limited benefit dollars.[24] Accomplishing these goals is no small task and requires skills in organization, communication, and knowledge of managed care reimbursement policies. In order to meet these goals, the case manager must be flexible and able to work with other disciplines, the patient, and the patient's family.

CRITICAL CONTENT

GOALS OF CASE MANAGEMENT

- The goals of case management include the following: achieving optimum patient outcome, early intervention, coordination and continuity of care, a safe transition from one facility to another, and containment of costs.
- The case manager relies on family members and other interdisciplinary team members to help in the assessment, implementation, and evaluation of the care plan.

Each patient must be assessed to identify any risk factors that would interfere with providing care. For example, will a patient be able to independently perform all activities of daily living upon returning home? If not, who will be able to help the patient? Once the assessment of risk factors has been completed, a plan of care that is focused on the patient must be developed.[23] The case manager relies on family members and other interdisciplinary team members to help in the assessment, implementation, and evaluation of the plan of care.[23] For instance, if the patient cannot perform all activities of daily living, will a family member be able to help? If not, what facility would best suit the patient? Will this be a short-term stay or will the patient require long-term care? These are the types of questions many case managers deal with on a daily basis.

CRITICAL CONTENT

QUESTIONS FREQUENTLY ASKED OF A CASE MANAGER

- Will a patient be able to independently perform all activities of daily living upon returning home?
- If the patient cannot perform all activities of daily living, will a family member be able to help?
- What facility will be best for the patient if home care is not acceptable?
- Will this be a short-term stay or will the patient require long-term care?

Respiratory Therapist Case Managers

Case management has become an essential component of all health care professions. There are two components of case management related to respiratory care. The first is the incorporation of case management into the daily duties of the respiratory therapist. The second is the respiratory therapist acting in the capacity of case manager for patients.

Many hospitals, insurance companies, HMOs, and PPOs have utilized respiratory therapists as case managers in an effort to provide quality care and remain cost effective. Respiratory therapists are qualified to become case managers because of their experience in patient assessment, patient education, care planning, implementation, monitoring, and evaluation of the course of therapy.[25] The number of respiratory therapists functioning in the role of case manager has increased, especially those dealing with patients who have chronic pulmonary diseases. Chronic pulmonary diseases are often difficult to supervise under managed care. Respiratory therapists are experts in dealing with patients with chronic pulmonary problems because of their knowledge and management of the disease, the equipment, and treatment services needed.

A recent study by the AARC found that within the previous 5 years, 27% of the respiratory therapists questioned had added case management to their duties. Twenty-four percent of the respondents already felt case management was an ongoing or constant duty.[3] For these respondents, case management had become a routine part of the their daily activities. It is expected that these numbers will grow with the continuing emphasis on reducing costs for cardiopulmonary care. By using these new skills, respiratory therapists have created new opportunities, because many hospitals have incorporated disease management programs into services provided by respiratory therapy departments.

Another way respiratory therapists have utilized case management is in the development and implementation of protocol-based care. Hospitals have seen the benefit of using protocols in the reduction of LOS and the cost savings enjoyed when treating patients with pulmonary diseases.[3]

Hospital-based case managers have varied job duties. They must work closely with insurance companies to assure that the patient still meets requirements for acute care. They perform clinical reviews of the patient on a daily basis. They must coordinate discharge planning and function almost as social workers in working with patients and their families. They may also be involved in the prevention of disease, as one of their goals is to decrease readmissions to the hospital.

HMOs and other managed care entities have financial incentives to keep patients healthy and out of hospitals. Some have begun to realize the fiscal benefits of having respiratory therapists deal with patients who have respiratory diseases. HMOs that employ respiratory therapists as case managers tend to utilize them for education and provision of clinical services.[3]

Case managers who work for managed care companies receive referrals from physicians concerning patients who are enrolled in their plan. The case manager performs an assessment of the patient and develops, implements, and coordinates a plan of care. The patient is monitored on an ongoing basis as long as case management services are needed. Case managers also review hospital daily censuses to identify hospitalized case management patients and interface with the hospital-based case manager. Together, the two case managers work to coordinate discharge planning. The managed care case manager is responsible for confirming patient eligibility and authorizing referrals for home health care and equipment.

Physicians have also seen the additional benefits of having respiratory therapists as case managers in their offices. Primary care physicians are not reimbursed for services such as asthma education and many do not have the time to provide their patients with the extensive education they may require. Physicians who participate in managed care plans often have their patient outcomes monitored by the managed care companies. If their outcomes are not appropriate, they could be in jeopardy of losing managed care contracts. This has led some physicians to hire respiratory therapists as case managers. Physician groups have employed respiratory therapists as case managers to help them make decisions about which pulmonary tests are most beneficial for each patient. Physicians have utilized respiratory therapy case managers to help with the education of their patients on topics such as disease processes and medication delivery.[3]

In most cases, it is possible to obtain reimbursement for patient education provided by a respiratory therapist in the physician's practice because it can be billed as a level 3 visit. Unfortunately, many respiratory therapists incorrectly believe that that they must change professions and become a physician assistant (PA) if they wish to provide primary care under direction of a physician, but this is not the case. There are currently no state licensure laws that prohibit respiratory therapists from working as physician extenders. Increasingly, physician practices, outpatient clinics, HMOs, and acute care settings are employing respiratory therapists as physician extenders who are qualified to provide primary care, including patient assessment and education.[26]

CRITICAL CONTENT

RESPIRATORY THERAPY CASE MANAGEMENT

- A recent study by the AARC found that within the past 5 years, 27% of the respiratory therapists questioned had added case management to their duties.
- Many hospitals, insurance companies, HMOs, and PPOs have utilized respiratory therapists as case managers in an effort to provide quality care and remain cost effective. Managed care companies realize the fiscal benefits of having respiratory therapists deal with patients who have respiratory diseases such as asthma and COPD.

While utilizing respiratory therapists in the role of case managers is a new concept, some areas of health care delivery are more open to the idea than others. Areas of nontraditional respiratory care, which emerged and grew in part because of managed care, are more open to hiring respiratory therapists as case managers. Nursing homes and home health organizations are 4 times more likely to utilize respiratory therapists as case managers than hospitals.[3]

Certification Criteria for Case Managers

Although many entry-level case management positions do not currently require certification, case manager certification is highly recommended. Case managers may become certified by the Commission for Case Manager Certification by meeting certain requirements. "An applicant's license or certification must be based on a minimum educational requirement of a post-secondary program in a field that promotes the physical, psychological, or vocational well being of the persons being served."[27] The examination is voluntary and is administered by the Commission for Case Manager Certification. Respiratory therapists are qualified to apply for certification based on the requirements

of the commission. They must also demonstrate practical experience in case management. These 5 core components of case management must be met to be eligible to sit for the examination: coordination of services, physical and psychological factors, benefits and cost analyses, case management concepts, and community resources.

Coordination of services may be as simple as arranging for the continuance of respiratory treatments or oxygen when a patient is discharged home. Physical and psychological factors could involve procuring equipment such as wheelchairs or arranging for a house to become wheelchair compatible. Benefits and cost analysis is used in an effort to ensure the patient receives quality care at a reasonable cost. Knowledge of community resources involves knowing what services are provided in the general area in which the case manager is located; for instance, knowing what programs or services hospitals, equipment companies, and home health companies provide. The case manager must be familiar with resources provided by service and volunteer organizations in the community, such as churches and the United Way. If the community does not provide a needed service, the case manager must find a way to provide the patient with the service.

CRITICAL CONTENT

CORE COMPETENCIES NEEDED FOR CERTIFICATION AS A CASE MANAGER

- Ability to coordinate health care services
- Knowledge of patients' physical and psychological factors
- Ability to determine patient benefits and perform cost analyses
- Understanding of case management concepts
- Knowledge of community resources

Applicants must also have a minimum of 12 months of full-time experience under the supervision of a certified case manager, 24 months of full-time experience without supervision from a certified case manager, or 12 months of full-time experience as a supervisor overseeing individuals who provide direct case management services. A candidate who successfully completes the examination is credentialed as a Certified Case Manager (CCM). This certification must be renewed every 5 years.

CRITICAL CONTENT

REQUIREMENTS FOR CASE MANAGEMENT CERTIFICATION

- Applicants must have a minimum of 12 months of full-time experience under the supervision of a certified case manager; or
- 24 months of full-time experience without supervision of a certified case manager; or
- 12 months of full-time experience as a supervisor overseeing individuals who provide direct case management services.

Skills Needed by the Respiratory Therapy Case Manager

A respiratory therapist's entry into case management requires a bachelor's degree and registered respiratory therapist (RRT) credential. Respiratory therapists who want to be case managers should have strong clinical backgrounds, knowledge of the diagnosis and treatment of pulmonary diseases, and outstanding patient assessment skills. They should also have effective social, organizational, and communication skills. In addition, respiratory therapists should have a thorough knowledge of reimbursement and health plan benefits, patient care settings, support services, and current legislation. Respiratory therapist case managers must be able to work independently and prioritize.

Respiratory therapists working as case managers must be able to deal with many different health care disciplines and be flexible in their thinking. They must look at the patient as a whole person and not just as a patient with respiratory illness. Case management entails social work, dis-

charge planning, and disease management. The respiratory therapy case manager must be able to wear different hats and juggle many aspects of the job at one time.

Case managers often have to deal with sensitive issues, such as the decision to place a patient in a nursing home. Therefore, they need highly refined empathy skills and tact. In hospital settings, case managers can become intimately involved with the patient's family. The respiratory therapist functioning as a case manager must sometimes discuss uncomfortable or unpleasant issues with patients or families. In order to foster communication and understanding, he or she must be able to balance the needs of the patient and family with the needs of the managed care company. The case manager often meets with family members daily to update them on the plans for the patient, and at times he or she becomes the liaison between the family members, the physician, and the managed care company. Case managers sometimes also serve as intermediaries between the insurance company and the physician, so effective communication skills are a must.

CRITICAL CONTENT

SKILLS NEEDED BY CASE MANAGERS

- Empathy
- Tact
- Flexibility
- Strong assessment skills
- Knowledge of reimbursement practices
- Organizational skills
- The ability to work independently
- Prioritization skills
- A broad perspective of the health care field

Areas of Concern and Future Roles

Future concerns for respiratory therapists as case managers include educating managed care entities about the roles of respiratory therapists as case managers. This area of opportunity will expand by proving the cost effectiveness of respiratory therapists as case managers. In order to market themselves to HMOs, respiratory therapists should market themselves as disease specialists.[3] They should promote themselves as educators with specialized clinical knowledge.

Many managed care entities do not view respiratory therapists as cost effective.[3] Additional research must be conducted and published to help overcome this problem. A final concern is that many respiratory therapists are unaware of this career opportunity. Further study and promotion of this subspecialty of respiratory therapy must be done within the respiratory care community.

CRITICAL CONTENT

DEVELOPING THE CASE MANAGER ROLE OF RESPIRATORY THERAPISTS

• Many respiratory therapists are unaware of this career opportunity.
• Case managers face difficulties in educating managed care entities about the use of respiratory therapists as case managers.
• Respiratory therapists face difficulties in proving the cost effectiveness of respiratory therapists as case managers.

Rewards for the Respiratory Therapist as Case Manager

The ability to work with patients to help them improve their quality of life is one of the rewards reported by case managers. Patients often develop strong relationships with their case managers. This relationship often leads patients to make changes in their lives because they have someone motivating them. Another reward is coordinating the total care of the patient instead of only the cardiopulmonary component of care.[3]

CRITICAL CONTENT

REWARDS OF CASE MANAGEMENT

• Working with patients to help them improve their quality of life
• Coordinating the total care of the patient
• Focusing on health care delivery and total care
• Expanding health care knowledge and experiences

RESPIRATORY THERAPISTS IN SUBACUTE CARE

Definition of Subacute Care

As hospitals look for ways to decrease the number of patient days per stay, postacute care has become more popular. Subacute care attributes its growth to the Medicare prospective payment system. Managed care sets limits on the amount of money provided to hospitals for patient care. It also utilizes strict review criteria to make sure that patients meet the requirements for acute care.[17] Though still in the process of defining itself, subacute care has become a feasible alternative for patients who no longer require acute care. Subacute care is often an intermediary between the acute care hospital and returning the patient to the home.

There has been some confusion in the health care delivery system about what constitutes criteria for subacute care. This situation is further complicated by Medicare reimbursement policies. The American Subacute Care Association defines subacute care in this manner: "subacute patients are sufficiently stabilized to no longer require acute care services, but are too complex for treatments in a traditional nursing center. Subacute care centers and programs typically treat patients who present with rehabilitation and/or medically complex needs and require physiological monitoring."[28] All subacute care facilities require respiratory care services. The type of subacute care facility and the acuity of the patient determine the degree to which they require respiratory therapy services. The Joint Commission on Accreditation of Healthcare Organizations (JCAHO) has specifically identified respiratory care as a necessary component of accreditation for subacute care.[28]

Subacute care is experiencing rapid growth due to several factors. Managed care and Medicare reimbursement policies and our aging population are among the top reasons. In 1994, subacute care was a $1 billion industry.[28] Within 5 years it is projected that subacute services will account for 40% of Medicare expenditures, generating revenues of approximately $20 billion.[29] Subacute facilities have 20% more revenue from managed care than nursing homes and 14% more revenues from managed care than rehabilitation centers.[3]

CRITICAL CONTENT

SUBACUTE CARE

- Subacute care is often an intermediary between the acute care hospital and returning the patient to the home.
- The Joint Commission on Accreditation of Healthcare Organizations (JCAHO) has specifically identified respiratory care as a necessary component for accreditation for subacute care.
- Within 5 years it is projected that subacute services will account for 40% of Medicare expenditures, with revenues of approximately $20 billion.

Services Provided by Respiratory Therapists in Subacute Care

The type and amount of services provided by respiratory therapists will vary depending on the setting and patient acuity. In most cases, if ventilator man-

agement is offered in the subacute facility, respiratory therapists are available 24 hours a day. If ventilator management is not a component of care, respiratory therapists may be available daily. Respiratory therapists working in hospitals have become more specialized in recent years, while respiratory therapists working in subacute care have become more generalized in the services they provide. Ironically, many administrative supervisors of subacute care facilities value respiratory therapists for their respiratory specialization.

Services provided may be complex and are often similar to duties performed by therapists in hospitals. These services include assessment, treatment, care planning, diagnostics, airway management, pulse oximetry, capnography, and other traditional therapies. As respiratory therapists are seen as the experts in subacute care, they provide more of the airway care such as tracheal care and suctioning, than in traditional settings. The patients in subacute care are generally medically stable and do not require extensive diagnostic workups. For this reason, there is less emphasis on diagnostic procedures. There is less physician interaction in subacute care, so respiratory therapists rely on the use of protocols for weaning patients from oxygen or ventilator management.

Another difference between subacute care and hospital care is the increased emphasis on teamwork and collaboration. There is more interdisciplinary care in subacute care, because each practitioner uses their expertise to achieve goals set by the team for the patient. As pulmonary experts, respiratory therapists in-service the health care staff on respiratory diseases, equipment, and procedures. Respiratory therapists must coordinate their services closely with nurses, as well as occupational, physical, and speech therapists. Because of this collaborative effort, there are stronger relationships between the disciplines and a heightened awareness of the treatment plans and goals. For instance, if a respiratory therapist is in the process of weaning a patient from a ventilator, he may need to coordinate with the physical therapist to arrange the best time for physical therapy so it does not fatigue the patient and interfere with the weaning process.

Two critical members of the interdisciplinary team are the patient and the patient's family. In subacute care, they play a vitally important role in the planning and implementing of care plans. One aspect of care that is emphasized in subacute care is education. The patient and caregivers rely on the respiratory therapist for education about the disease process, its management, treatment interventions, and equipment. Working closely with other disciplines helps to ensure that patients receive the information they need to help them achieve their treatment goals.

CRITICAL CONTENT

RESPIRATORY SERVICES PROVIDED BY SUBACUTE CARE

- The type and amount of services provided by respiratory therapists will vary depending on the setting and patient acuity.
- Services include assessment, treatment, care planning, diagnostics, airway management, pulse oximetry, capnography, and other traditional therapies.
- There is more interdisciplinary care in subacute care as compared to hospital care.

Types of Subacute Care

There are different types of subacute care facilities, including long-term acute care facilities (LTAC), skilled nursing facilities (SNF), specialty hospitals, rehabilitation hospitals, and respiratory units within an acute care hospital. The types of postacute care settings are defined by these criteria: nursing hours per day, rehabilitation requirements, length of stay, and cost within a particular institution.

Long-term acute care facilities (LTAC) are licensed hospitals that are exempt from the Medicare prospective payment system as long as they keep their average patient length of stay greater than 25 days. LTAC hospitals receive payment from Medicare on a reasonable cost basis, and they usually specialize in patients who have pulmonary problems or medically complex problems. The patients no longer require extensive diagnostic work-ups, but do need additional therapy and nursing support. Nursing services are generally provided 5 to 7 hours per day. Occupational therapy, physical therapy, and respiratory therapy are offered daily. If the LTAC has ventilator patients, respiratory therapy is offered 24 hours per day. Patients usually stay an average of between 10 and 60 days. The cost averages $600 to $700 dollars per day.[17]

Skilled nursing facilities (SNF) are identified beds certified by the Health Care Financing Administration (HCFA) to participate in the Medicare program for servicing its long-term care benefits.[17] One way to differentiate skilled nursing facilities from LTACs is the number and amount of services provided. SNFs generally provide fewer services than LTACs. SNFs offer an average of 2 to 3 nursing hours per day; occupational therapy, physical therapy, and respiratory therapy are offered on an as needed basis. The length of stay for patients averages more than 60 days with an average cost of $100 to $150 per day.[17] Skilled nursing facilities may be freestanding or hospital-based. As a general rule, the cost of caring for a patient is higher in a hospital-based SNF.

Many hospitals have created their own SNFs to deal with patients who require long-term ventilation or who have medically complex problems. These units were among the first subacute care programs in the country,[3] and they have been proven to be cost effective in many cases. For instance, Shawnee Mission Medical Center implemented a SNF with respiratory therapists providing services, and found it improved health care outcomes. The LOS for pneumonia patients decreased from 8 days to 4 days, which decreased the costs of caring for pneumonia patients by 50%.[30] The American Health Care Association sponsored a study that concluded that Medicare could save at least $142 million per year if ventilator-dependent patients were treated in SNFs instead of being transferred to acute care facilities.[3]

CRITICAL CONTENT

DIFFERENTIATING SNFS AND LTACS

- Long-term acute care facilities (LTAC) are licensed hospitals that are exempt from the Medicare prospective payment system as long as they keep their average patient length of stay greater than 25 days.
- Skilled nursing facilities (SNF) are identified beds certified by the Health Care Financing Administration (HCFA) to participate in the Medicare program for servicing its long-term care benefits.

CRITICAL CONTENT

A STUDY OF MEDICARE BENEFICIARIES TREATED BY RESPIRATORY THERAPISTS IN SNFS REVEALED:

- Patients had a 3.6-day shorter length of stay
- Patients saved Medicare $97.9 million
- Mortality rate was reduced

Cost Effectiveness of Respiratory Therapists in Subacute Care

The AARC recently commissioned a study to determine the cost effectiveness of respiratory therapists providing services to patients with respiratory diagnoses in the skilled nursing facility. This study compared outcomes and costs between patients who received respiratory services from respiratory therapists and patients who received respiratory services from nonrespiratory personnel. The analysis revealed that Medicare beneficiaries treated by respiratory therapists had better outcomes and lower costs than those not treated by respiratory therapists.[31] Patients who were treated by respiratory therapists had a 3.6-day shorter length of stay with a projected annual cost savings of $97.9 million to Medicare in 1996.[31] About 31% more beneficiaries who were treated by a nonrespiratory therapist during an initial SNF visit required subsequent services in a hospital emergency room or outpatient setting. Medicare spent 23% more to treat these patients.[31] In addition, Medicare beneficiaries who were treated by respiratory therapists had a 42% lower mortality rate at their next encounter with the Medicare system compared to a similar group who received respiratory care from non-RT caregivers.

Skills Needed by Respiratory Therapists in Subacute Care

While many of the skills used in subacute care settings are the same as those used by respiratory therapists in traditional hospital settings, there are some important differences. Respiratory therapists who work in subacute settings have less physician interaction so they must be self-directed, willing and able to make decisions, and able to implement treatment plans for their patients. For example, they must possess strong critical thinking and problem solving skills. They must have strong clinical backgrounds with disease management skills. They should have experience working with protocols and care plans as these are used more in subacute care. Please refer to Chapter 6 for a complete discussion on working with protocols and their increasing role in respiratory care.

Subacute care respiratory therapists find there is more of an educational component involved in their job. Therefore, they must have excellent communication and teaching skills. Respiratory therapists need the ability to relate to people from all backgrounds, and with various literacy levels, as they will be involved in the education of the patient and caregivers concerning the pulmonary component of the patient's medical condition. As the respiratory experts, they will also be responsible for the continued training of the subacute care staff in matters regarding respiratory therapy, as well as a primary patient educator.

Subacute care places an emphasis on interdisciplinary care planning and teamwork. In addition to working independently as a respiratory therapist, the respiratory therapist in subacute care must also function as an interdisciplinary team member. A thorough knowledge of the skills and services provided by other allied health professionals is essential, as is a cooperative nature and strong communications skills. A good background in the development and implementation of care plans, outcomes assessment, and discharge planning is needed.

The availability of many tests or diagnostic procedures is often limited in subacute care. Many diagnostic tests that are available within a manner of minutes in a hospital are not readily available in subacute care. Obtaining results can take longer because services are often contracted. In order to deal with this situation, the respiratory therapist must have exceptional physical assessment skills with a good clinical background, especially in chronic cardiopulmonary diseases.

While patients in subacute care are hemodynamically more stable than patients in hospital ICUs, they may require more specialized hands-on care and attention. Patients in intensive care units are often subjected to invasive procedures, advanced monitoring, and pharmacological treatments. Patients in subacute care are subject to fewer invasive procedures and monitoring, but do require specialized services from many allied health professionals. These patients often require treatment from such disciplines as occupational therapy, physical therapy, and speech language pathology. Many patients in subacute care settings who are receiving mechanical ventilation have been on mechanical ventilators for a long period. Overcoming not only the physical factors of the disease, but also the emotional and psychological factors takes special skills. The respiratory therapist is often required to work one on one with patients in order to establish a trusting relationship. Respiratory therapists must have good people skills and be willing to become involved not only with the physical aspects of the disease, but also the emotional and psychological components of chronic diseases. Patience and the ability to empathize with patients and families helps to deal with the disease process as a whole.

CRITICAL CONTENT

SKILLS NEEDED BY THE RESPIRATORY THERAPIST IN SUBACUTE CARE

- Respiratory therapists working in subacute care need strong clinical backgrounds with good assessment skills, strong communication skills, patience, and the ability to work with teams.
- Respiratory therapists must have good people skills and be willing to become involved in the emotional and physical impact of the disease process.

Areas of Concern and Future Roles

The primary concern for respiratory therapists working in subacute care facilities is reimbursement for their services. Many skilled nursing facilities have decreased the number of respiratory therapists utilized by their facilities due to decreased reimbursement from Medicare. Many have cross-trained nursing or support personnel to provide respiratory therapy services. A recent study demonstrated the cost effectiveness of respiratory therapists in SNFs. The AARC hopes to use the results of this study to demonstrate the need for respiratory therapists in SNFs.

Managed care plans have shown a trend toward increased use of subacute care because more patients are discharged from acute care hospitals quicker than before the implementation of managed care. If the trend continues, the number of LTAC and rehabilitation hospitals needed will increase, providing more opportunities for respiratory therapists.

Rewards for the Respiratory Therapist in Subacute Care

Many patients in subacute settings are long-term or chronic patients. Respiratory therapists who work in this area find satisfaction from improving the patient's quality of life. Being able to wean a patient from mechanical ventilation who has been ventilated for weeks or months is just one of the rewards. Other respiratory therapists enjoy being able to become more involved and spend more time with their patients. They enjoy the less hurried, one-on-one contact with their patients. Many respiratory therapists who work in subacute care enjoy the opportunities they have to get to know not only the patients, but family members as well. They feel this helps them see the patient as a whole person. Other respiratory therapists enjoy the opportunity to be self-directed by the use of protocols. Respiratory therapists are able to make assessments of their patients and implement the care they feel is needed. The opportunity to work closely with other disciplines also appeals to respiratory therapists who work in subacute care.

RESPIRATORY THERAPISTS IN DISEASE PREVENTION AND WELLNESS MANAGEMENT PROGRAMS

Pulmonary Rehabilitation

With greater emphasis being placed on education and the prevention of diseases as a means of controlling costs, many hospitals have developed pulmonary rehabilitation centers and wellness programs for chronic diseases. Pulmonary rehabilitation, while not a new concept to respiratory care, has become more important in recent years. The American College of Chest Physicians Committee on Pulmonary Rehabilitation defined the pulmonary rehabilitation concept in 1974.[32] This definition of pulmonary rehabilitation specified the need for individual patient assessment and education from a multidisciplinary team that focused on the physiological and psychological problems associated with chronic lung problems. The National Institute of Health defines pulmonary rehabilitation as "a multidimensional continuum of services directed to persons with pulmonary disease and their families, usually by an interdisciplinary team

of specialists, with the goal of achieving and maintaining the individual's maximum level of independence and functioning in the community."[32]

The goals of pulmonary rehabilitation are achieved by helping patients increase their activity through exercise training and education. Pulmonary rehabilitation programs are usually divided into 3 phases. Phase one is the pretesting portion of the program, in which the candidate performs tests such as a pulmonary function test, stress test, and the 6- to 12-minute walking test. Patients are asked to complete questionnaires that assess their nutritional, psychological, and vocational needs.

The second phase of the program includes education and exercise. Educational topics include lung anatomy, breathing and pulmonary hygiene techniques, nutritional guidelines, medications and equipment, and the importance of exercise conditioning. Patients are monitored for oxygen saturation levels, breathing techniques, pulse and rhythm rates, and blood pressure while performing exercise. The exercise may be very simple such as walking or riding a stationary bike. As the patient progresses through the program, the workload is gradually increased.

The final phase of the program includes follow-up care and long-term maintenance. The patient is taught how to monitor his or her progress and encouraged to develop an individual exercise program. The need for continued lifelong exercise is stressed.

CRITICAL CONTENT

PULMONARY REHABILITATION

- Is an effective means of controlling costs for patients suffering from chronic lung disease
- Includes assessment, education, exercise training, and long-term maintenance
- Uses a multidisciplinary approach to focus on the psychosocial aspects of chronic pulmonary diseases

Wellness Programs

Managed care has placed an emphasis on providing education and programs not only for individuals who are ill, but also for individuals who are currently healthy, in order to maintain their good health. This approach is used with the expectation that it will decrease long-term health care costs, because healthy people require less health care. In order to accomplish this goal of keeping people healthy, hospitals and managed care companies have established wellness programs. Wellness programs include classes that educate consumers so they can maintain, and possibly even improve, their quality of life. They cover topics such as the benefits of diet, exercise, sleep habits, relaxation techniques, diagnostic screenings, and the psychosocial aspects of health. The emphasis is placed on preventing disease and establishing and maintaining healthy habits for life.

Building on the pulmonary rehabilitation concept, many hospitals have started other wellness programs such as cardiac rehabilitation, smoking cessation programs, and asthma education programs. Community wellness programs covering a wide variety of topics are increasingly popular among hospitals. Respiratory therapists have been able to expand their job descriptions by providing education through these programs.

Hospitals are not the only facilities offering wellness programs. Managed care companies offer wellness programs to their enrollees as a means of keeping readmissions to hospitals low. By reducing admissions to hospitals, managed care companies benefit financially, while at the same time improving the health of their clients. Many managed care companies now employ respiratory therapists as disease managers or case managers, realizing they can provide expert education to clients with asthma, COPD, and other pulmonary diseases. Instead of waiting for an acute episode, this approach addresses the chronic aspect of the disease by providing the patient with an individual treatment plan and an expert to help guide them in their care.

Disease specialists develop treatment plans for enrollees in conjunction with physicians. They monitor the enrollee's progress, either by telephone or during home visits. They evaluate the enrollee's progress and offer moral support and expert education.

Entrepreneurial respiratory therapists have seized this opportunity to either work for managed care companies, or they have started their own businesses selling educational programs to managed care companies or directly to physicians. Many physicians do not have the time or up-to-date information to provide for their patients' education. Respiratory therapists have been able to step into the niche created by this need.

CRITICAL CONTENT

WELLNESS PROGRAMS

- Managed care companies that employ respiratory therapists in wellness and disease prevention programs have been able to reap financial rewards.
- Hospitals offer additional services including disease prevention and wellness programs.

Skills Needed by Respiratory Therapists in Pulmonary Rehabilitation and Wellness Programs

Respiratory therapists who work in pulmonary rehabilitation or wellness programs require well-developed educational skills. They need to have a strong background in the pathophysiology and treatment of pulmonary diseases, as well as a good understanding of pulmonary function testing. They need strong interpersonal and communication skills and the ability to motivate people. A strong background in geriatrics is suggested, but the ability to work with individuals of all ages is needed.

Rewards for Respiratory Therapists in Rehabilitation and Wellness Programs

Respiratory therapists who work in pulmonary rehabilitation and wellness programs enjoy building positive relationships with patients and their families. They often have the opportunity to get to know them as individuals much better than the traditional therapist. In many cases they become the primary source of health education for patients and their families, so a strong bond may become established.

These therapists are able to help motivate individuals to make positive lifestyle changes to improve their health. They are also able to provide hope and encouragement to people who have seen their lives change due to chronic illnesses. Many rehabilitation therapists enjoy their job because the patients are committed to learning and want to benefit from the program. The patients are not there because of acute care needs, but because they want to learn how to manage their disease. Making a difference in the quality of life of patients rewards therapists working in these types of programs.

Areas of Concern and Future Roles

With the increased use of managed care, the future of pulmonary rehabilitation and wellness programs is bright. The increasing emphasis on disease management and prevention, along with the aging population, has created a demand for these types of programs. One of the goals of managed care is to reduce the number of readmissions to acute care facilities by patients with chronic pulmonary diseases. Many managed care companies have found that the investment of money in this area pays off by lowering costs overall, due to the decreased need for more expensive acute care. Pulmonary rehabilitation and wellness programs can help attain this goal. The number of patients suffering from pulmonary disease is increasing as the population ages. This will create a need for more programs that are able to help educate patients on how to manage their diseases.

CRITICAL CONTENT

PULMONARY REHABILITATION AND WELLNESS PROGRAMS

- Respiratory therapists working in pulmonary rehabilitation and wellness programs need strong educational skills and a background in cardiopulmonary disease management.
- Respiratory therapists working in these programs have the opportunity to get to know their patients better.
- The growing use of managed care has created a greater demand for respiratory therapists working in pulmonary rehabilitation and wellness programs.

RESPIRATORY THERAPISTS IN INDUSTRY

Respiratory therapists have been able to pursue new roles in the medical industry. In fact, many respiratory therapists have made the transition in recent years from staff therapists to therapists employed by different types of industry. Companies that once relied on respiratory therapists in minor roles are now utilizing them in jobs such as technological design, consulting, product development, marketing, and sales. As technological advances are made in respiratory therapy, companies realize that respiratory therapists should be involved in the planning, design, and marketing of the equipment they use. Respiratory therapists have also found creative outlets in expanding fields such as medical writing and research. While these fields are just beginning to realize the contributions respiratory therapists can make to their industries, they offer hope for the future growth of respiratory therapy.

Industry Consultant

Many industries, such as the pharmaceutical and biotechnical industry, hire respiratory therapists to aid in market development. These companies realize the benefits of having respiratory therapists, with their strong backgrounds in health care, anatomy, physiology, and cardiopulmonary disease management, involved in the market analysis for new or existing products.

Respiratory therapists assess the market by communicating with the physicians, researchers, and respiratory therapists in their geographic areas. They educate physicians and research scientists about the company's current products and provide updated research outcomes and studies. By interacting with the medical community, they help in determining the research necessary to market a product, and assist in the recruitment of research participants. Consultants often coordinate educational programs or present lectures at educational programs. In return, clinicians share their impressions of the products, results of clinical studies, and give their input on the need for future products.

Skills Needed by Respiratory Therapists Working as Industry Consultants.   Respiratory therapists who work as industry consultants need strong backgrounds in the basic sciences with an emphasis on anatomy and physiology. Industry consultants must know about the experts in their field in their geographic area. They must have extensive knowledge of research methodologies, the research performed on their product in the past, current research, and proposed research needs.

Respiratory therapy industry consultants enjoy autonomy in their work so they must be self-directed and motivated, and they should have strong organizational and prioritization skills. A major portion of their job involves communication so they must have well-developed interpersonal skills and be able to develop strong professional relationships. Market consultants deal with frequent changes as the market for their products changes. They should be adaptable and flexible because their territories and products can change quickly.

Technology Development

Manufacturers of respiratory therapy equipment require the clinical expertise that can be provided

CRITICAL CONTENT

INDUSTRY CONSULTANTS

- Many industries, such as the pharmaceutical and biotechnical industries, hire respiratory therapists to aid in market development.
- Respiratory therapists who work as industry consultants need a strong background in the basic sciences, with an emphasis on anatomy and physiology.
- A major portion of industry-related positions involve communication.
- Respiratory therapists working in industry must have well-developed interpersonal skills and be able to develop strong professional relationships.

by respiratory therapists. Respiratory therapists are their best resources to let manufacturers know what clinicians need in their products. Respiratory therapists employed in the technological aspect of industry help in the development and engineering of new or existing products. They often meet with focus groups of other respiratory therapists and physicians to determine the needs of the market.

Once the needs have been established, respiratory therapists work with engineers to design the product. As a team they must not only design a product that meets the user's needs, but also addresses regulatory issues and meets Food and Drug Administration (FDA) guidelines as well.

Once the product has been approved by the FDA, respiratory therapists help with the marketing of the product. They often work with marketing departments to develop marketing strategies. Respiratory therapists provide the needed clinical expertise to the sales force, many of whom may also be respiratory therapists. They can provide the technical education the sales force needs in the marketing of the product. Respiratory therapists may also be involved in contract negotiations with distributors and purchasing groups.

Skills Needed by Respiratory Therapists Working in Technology Development. Respiratory therapists working in product design and development need to be self-directed, with well developed time management skills. They must be cognizant of the different working environment that exists in industry. The hours are often long and unpredictable with traveling often required. Although there is often no patient contact, respiratory therapists working in industry need strong clinical backgrounds. They also need the ability to transfer the knowledge they have gained from their clinical backgrounds into a vision of the future. They must be visionaries who provide guidance in the development of respiratory therapy products that will help to provide quality care to patients.

Respiratory therapists in technology development need to be able to communicate well with people with no clinical background, such as purchasing agents or upper management personnel. A basic knowledge of business trends and terminology helps. The therapist must be able to think analytically in order to promote their products, contribute to product design, and interact with others in business.

CRITICAL CONTENT

RESPIRATORY THERAPISTS WORKING IN PRODUCT DESIGN AND DEVELOPMENT

- Provide expertise and assistance in the development and engineering of new or existing products
- Work with engineers to identify and design products
- Provide clinical expertise to the sales force, many of which may also be respiratory therapists
- Need to be self-directed with well-developed time management skills
- Provide no direct patient care and rarely have patient contact

Sales

Many companies employ respiratory therapists as sales or marketing representatives for their products. Because these products are sold to respiratory therapists and pulmonary physicians, it only makes sense that respiratory therapists are the best people to market these products. Respiratory therapist marketing representatives have a better understanding of the product and the environment in which it will be used, and can answer technological questions from therapists, physicians, and other clinicians. Therapists working in marketing positions involving sales are often assigned their own territories. Travel is often required with sales positions as these territories can cover several hundreds miles and several states. International travel may also be required.

Skills Needed by Respiratory Therapists in Sales. Respiratory therapists involved with sales must be excellent communicators with the ability to establish professional relationships. Strong interpersonal skills and self-motivation are two qualities of a successful salesperson. Respiratory therapists involved with sales should have knowledge of current business concepts, especially in the area of managed care and negotiated contracts. They must be able to educate all members of the medical community about their product.

Research

The idea of conducting respiratory therapy research is intimidating to many respiratory therapists. They may feel they are not qualified or do not have the background required to perform research, but this is not always the case. Many prominent respiratory therapists in the research realm are also practicing clinicians. In fact, most of the research reported today by respiratory therapists resulted from questions that these therapists encountered in their day-to-day jobs. All respiratory therapists should be interested in research because it validates and promotes the growth of the profession.

Respiratory therapists interested in conducting research should start small. They can often begin with their daily activities. What questions do they have concerning the outcomes or cost effectiveness of therapies? They should choose research in an area in which they have some clinical expertise. The opportunities for performing research are greater in colleges, universities, and large hospitals that are associated with educational institutions, but research can and has been performed at all levels of care.

Before undergoing a research project, the researcher should find a mentor. The mentor should be someone who has experience in conducting and presenting research. Research mentors should be experienced and familiar with research techniques and publication criteria.

Many seasoned researchers suggest new researchers begin with an abstract presentation, since they take less time. Abstracts may be case reports, device evaluations, or original studies. Another research technique is presentation of clinical papers, which are written for submission to peer-reviewed journals.

Most research conducted at this level does not need outside funding. If funding is needed, there are several sources available. Often industries will provide funding for projects. It is suggested that a contract be negotiated before the project starts so funding cannot be withdrawn if the industry is not pleased with the preliminary results. Other organizations such as the American Association for Respiratory Care, the American Respiratory Care Foundation, and the American Lung Association offer competitive grants and monetary awards to promote research.

Skills Needed by Respiratory Therapists in Research. Many respiratory therapists feel they need advanced degrees to enter the research field, but this is not always the case. However, a background in statistics is very useful. Research in all aspects of respiratory therapy is needed. The main requirement is a background in the area of respiratory therapy in which you seek to pursue research. Respiratory therapists interested in research must be willing to work on their own time, because research can be time consuming. Projects usually take many months to complete, given the time

needed to conduct research, collect data, analyze it, and publish the results.

Respiratory therapists interested in conducting research must be self-motivated. While there are some respiratory therapists involved in research on a full-time basis, most therapists performing research are doing so either in conjunction with their full-time jobs, or as an independent endeavor. Respiratory therapist researchers should also be able to withstand criticism and rejection. Research results undergo extensive peer review, much of it critical, before the work is published. It is not uncommon for an article to be rejected more than once or require several rewrites before it is published.

CRITICAL CONTENT

RESPIRATORY THERAPISTS IN RESEARCH

- Many prominent respiratory therapists working in the research realm are also practicing clinicians.
- Seasoned researchers suggest that novice researchers begin with an abstract presentation since abstracts require less time to complete than an entire manuscript.
- Research is time consuming, taking many months to conduct the study, collect and analyze data, and publish findings.
- Research undergoes extensive peer review and constructive criticism before it can be published. It is not uncommon for an article to be rejected more than once and require several rewrites before it is published.

Medical Writing

Another avenue open to respiratory therapists is the field of medical writing. Respiratory therapists have an extensive background in cardiopulmonary anatomy and pathophysiology, making them ideal candidates for medical writing. Medical writers may work in a variety of venues, including journal articles, research articles, and textbooks. Medical writers not only do their own writing, but also assist other authors in their writing or serve as editors. They also create and edit tables and graphs and present statistical information.

Medical writers are needed to write and edit material that is presented at professional conferences or symposiums, such as pamphlets, brochures, slides, and handouts. Medical writers also serve in the process of obtaining FDA approval of drugs. Before the FDA approves a drug, extensive documentation must be presented. Medical writers are charged with the task of completing the application, which requires extensive writing skills. Managed care has created new opportunities for medical writers to educate patients, create clinical pathways, and document research outcomes.

Skills Needed by Respiratory Therapists in Medical Writing. Respiratory therapists interested in medical writing need a strong background of English grammar and spelling, with a master's degree preferred. The writer must be able to work alone, and computer skills are a must. Anyone interested in medical writing should contact the American Medical Writers Association. This association educates people about medical writing and offers certification programs.

CRITICAL CONTENT

MEDICAL WRITING

- Medical writers may work in a variety of venues, including journals, research reports, and textbooks.
- Managed care has created new opportunities for medical writers to educate patients, create clinical pathways, and document research outcomes.
- Anyone interested in medical writing should contact the American Medical Writers Association

Rewards for the Respiratory Therapist in Industry

Respiratory therapists involved in the design and development of technology find the chance to look at patient care from a different angle rewarding. Respiratory therapists working in industry also enjoy the ability to make a difference in the lives of patients and fellow respiratory therapists. Therapists working in industry enjoy the prospect of making sure the products used provide the patient with the best quality care.

Respiratory therapists involved in research get a sense of accomplishment from performing research, and researchers enjoy the chance to support or reject research hypotheses. Respiratory therapy researchers also enjoy the rewards of helping the respiratory therapy community to grow and improve as a profession.

CRITICAL CONTENT

TECHNOLOGY REWARDS

- Respiratory therapists involved in the design and development of technology find the chance to look at patient care from a different angle rewarding.
- Respiratory therapists involved in research get a sense of accomplishment from performing research.

RESPIRATORY THERAPISTS IN DIAGNOSTICS

Polysomnography

History of Polysomnography. Sleep has always fascinated scientists, but it wasn't until the second half of the 20th Century that significant research was done on the study of sleep. In 1953, the discovery of rapid eye movements (REM) during sleep lead to further study on the subject.[33] The first sleep disorders center was established to perform objective evaluations of sleep disorders in 1971.[33] The study of sleep has yielded not only medical benefits, but social benefits as well. According to the National Highway Transportation Safety Administration, drivers falling asleep at the wheel resulted in over 200,000 crashes and 1550 deaths.[34,35] According to the National Center on Sleep Research, over 40 million Americans suffer from sleep disorders.[36]

Sleep Testing.   During the last 2 decades, the study of polysomnography has witnessed tremendous growth as medical professionals and the public have become more aware of the importance of sleep. Sleep centers that perform special testing have become more important in recent years in the diagnosis and treatment of sleep disorders. Sleep studies are indicated for patients who report excessive daytime sleepiness of unknown medical origin that does not improve with 2 weeks of increased sleep time. Sleep studies include 2 main tests: polysomnography and the multiple sleep latency test (MSLT). These tests, which may be used separately or together, incorporate activity-based monitoring of motility patterns. These tests are used to diagnose disorders such as narcolepsy, sleep apnea, and restless leg syndrome. Please see Chapter 15 for more comprehensive information on sleep disorders and respiratory problems.

The testing requires the use of various types of equipment to monitor body movement during sleep. Typical sleep studies involve placing electroencephalograph electrodes on the scalp to monitor brain activity for sleep staging, placing electrodes near the outer canthus of the eye to monitor eye movement, placing electromyograph electrodes to monitor limb movement, use of belts or strain gauges to monitor abdominal and chest wall movement, and use of nasal and/or oral air flow sensors.[37] In addition to these items, pulse oximeters and electrocardiograph electrodes are used to monitor oxygen saturation levels and cardiac rhythms.

Many hospitals have developed their own sleep laboratories. However, due to the expensive equipment needed, other hospitals have contracted

with independent sleep laboratories. The majority of sleep testing is performed in an outpatient setting, and many labs now perform sleep studies in the patient's home. In order to perform these in-home tests, the equipment is altered so that it is more portable.

CRITICAL CONTENT

TESTING FOR SLEEP DISORDERS

- The first sleep disorders center was established in 1971 to perform objective evaluations of sleep disorders.
- Sleep studies include two main tests: polysomnography and the multiple sleep latency test (MSLT).
- Testing requires the use of various equipment that is used to monitor body movements, vital signs, and other parameters.
- Many hospitals have developed their own sleep labs. However, due to the expensive equipment required, other hospitals have contracted with independent sleep laboratories.

Skills Required for Polysomnography

Many respiratory therapists have the basic background needed to begin working in sleep laboratories. They require additional training in the operation of the equipment and procedures related to sleep testing. This can be achieved in a number of ways. There are a variety of educational programs available to individuals wanting more education in polysomnography, ranging from 2-year programs to 1- to 2-week courses on sleep-related subjects.

Advancing in the field requires further education that allows one to score sleep studies. Scoring the study requires interpretation of data obtained during the testing. The scoring of polysomnography may be performed any time after the testing is completed. Many sleep labs employ polysomnographers who provide scoring services only and do not perform the tests. This allows some polysomnographers to work during the day.

The Board of Registered Polysomnographic Technologists offers an examination that is designed to assess the competence of individuals performing polysomnography. In order to apply for the examination, candidates must meet these conditions: completion of 18 months' experience in polysomnography, or completion of 12 months' experience and proof of credentialing in a health-related field. All candidates must be certified in basic cardiac life support. Upon successful completion of this exam, the credential of registered polysomnographic technologist (RPSGT) is awarded.

Respiratory therapists interested in polysomnography should be skilled in performing and evaluating diagnostic procedures, as the majority of the tests require constant monitoring. They should be able to operate a variety of different equipment, enjoy working night shifts, and prefer quiet environments. One particularly useful skill is the ability to put patients at ease. The testing procedure itself is intimidating to patients as it involves the application of many electrodes and monitors to the body. Many patients also feel ill at ease with the prospect of someone watching them sleep. The polysomnographer needs strong people skills in order to calm patients so they feel comfortable and can complete the test.

Cardiopulmonary Laboratories

Types of Testing.   One of the areas the AARC has identified as a field with the opportunity for expansion of the scope of practice for respiratory therapists is cardiopulmonary diagnostics.[38] Blood gas analysis, pulmonary function testing, and cardiac testing are already a part of the scope of care of therapists in many acute care settings. However, the growing trend is to perform these tests in outpatient settings or through independently contracted services. Many subacute facilities do not have laboratories on site, but contract with outside labs for these services. Respiratory therapists have a clinical background in cardiopulmonary diseases, which make them ideal candidates for working in cardiopulmonary diagnostic laboratories.

CRITICAL CONTENT

POLYSOMNOGRAPHY

- Many respiratory therapists have the basic backgrounds needed to begin working in sleep laboratories.
- Advancing in the field requires further education that allows one to score sleep studies.
- The Board of Registered Polysomnographic Technologists offers an examination that is designed to assess the competence of individuals performing polysomnography.
- Upon successful completion of this exam, the credential of registered polysomnographic technologist (RPSGT) is awarded.
- One particularly useful skill is the ability to put patients at ease.

Many therapists have seized upon this opportunity to establish new entrepreneurial ventures by establishing their own labs. Respiratory therapists have created companies that offer laboratory services such as pulmonary function and sleep study testing. They have contracted with managed care companies to provide services for clients enrolled in managed care programs. Other respiratory therapists have focused on providing diagnostic testing in industrial settings. Industries are required by federal law to provide safe workplaces for employees. Tests required by the Occupational Safety and Health Administration (OSHA) for industries include testing respirators for proper fit, asbestosis testing, and audiometric testing for noise levels.

Skills Needed for Cardiopulmonary Testing. Respiratory therapists working in diagnostic testing require technical abilities. They should enjoy working with and maintaining equipment, and they also need strong computer skills, especially with hardware, software, and telecommunication technology.[39] They should be familiar with the various organizations that accredit laboratories and the various government rules regulating them. Those therapists who service industries will need to be familiar with standards and testing requirements for OSHA. They may need to complete additional continuing education courses in order to meet OSHA compliance levels.

Rewards for the Respiratory Therapist in Cardiopulmonary Diagnostics

Many respiratory therapists involved in diagnostics enjoy the satisfaction of providing a needed service to patients, and also enjoy diagnosing disease. As opportunities for new ventures expand in the field, many respiratory therapists have fulfilled their dreams of owning their own businesses. Diagnostics has provided new markets for these respiratory therapists and allowed them to utilize their creative and business skills.

CRITICAL CONTENT

CARDIOPULMONARY DIAGNOSTICS

- The AARC has identified cardiopulmonary diagnostics as another opportunity for expansion of the scope of practice for respiratory therapists.
- Respiratory therapists have created companies that offer laboratory services such as pulmonary function and sleep study testing.
- Respiratory therapists working in diagnostics should be familiar with the various organizations that accredit laboratories and the various government rules regulating labs.

THE RESPIRATORY THERAPIST AS PHYSICIAN EXTENDER

Duties of the Physician Extender Outside of Acute Care Settings

Respiratory therapists have often functioned as physician extenders in acute care and traditional hospital settings. Another avenue recently opened to respiratory therapists, due in part to the growth in managed care, is the therapist as a physician extender in other settings. Managed care emphasizes treating patients before acute situations occur, and the best place to do this is the physician's office. In order to meet the goals of decreasing ER visits and hospital admissions, many physicians have employed respiratory therapists in their offices to provide the services their patients need. The respiratory therapist has the necessary clinical background and expertise needed to fill the role of physician extender.[2]

Therapists working in physician offices often perform many of the same duties they did in acute care settings, but they may also have the opportunity to expand these skills by providing services such as spirometry, pulmonary function testing, arterial blood gas punctures and analysis, assisting with bronchoscopies, and assisting physicians with other procedures. In addition to these duties, physician extenders spend a large portion of their time providing patients with education about their disease, treatment techniques, and medications. They have the time to spend with patients that the physician does not. They often follow-up with patients about their care and become an important liaison between the patient and the physician. They may also be involved with the arrangement of home care services and negotiations with HMOs and insurance companies for providing care and certification of care.

Skills Needed to be a Respiratory Therapist Physician Extender

Respiratory therapists who wish to function as physician extenders in primary care should have excellent clinical competencies with several years' experience in the acute care setting. They should possess strong educational skills and the ability to teach at all levels, because a good portion of their time will be spent educating patients and their families. While physician extenders work under the authority of a physician, they enjoy a good degree of autonomy. Respiratory therapists working as

CRITICAL CONTENT

RESPIRATORY THERAPISTS AS PHYSICIAN EXTENDERS

- Many physicians have employed respiratory therapists in their offices to provide the services their patients need.
- Physician extenders may have the opportunity to expand their skills by providing services they do not provide as traditional therapists.
- Physician extenders spend a large portion of their time providing patients with education about their disease, treatment techniques, and medications.
- Physician practices can be reimbursed for primary care and education provided by respiratory therapists during office visits.

physician extenders can assume a variety of duties and responsibilities that overlap with those of other health care professionals. A physician extender is able to assume a wide scope of practice, including medical technology, radiological services, and nursing and physician assistant responsibilities in most states because licensure laws are nonrestrictive. This means that the scope of practice for providing health care services is not restricted to any single health care profession. Appropriately-trained personnel from a number of disciplines can provide health care.

Respiratory therapists who wish to provide primary care as physician extenders should feel comfortable working alone. They will also need good organizational skills to function in a busy medical practice. Above all, they need a high level of professionalism since they are functioning as an extension of the doctor.

Rewards for the Respiratory Therapist Physician Extender

Respiratory therapists who work as physician extenders enjoy the opportunity to expand not only their

skills but their profession as well. They enjoy better relationships with staff and patients. They report the ability to make a greater or more positive impact on the lives of their patients as one of the most rewarding aspects of the job. While the work may be similar to that done in an acute care setting, one of the perks of being a physician extender is the chance to spend more time with patients. Many therapists enjoy the added autonomy the job provides.

CRITICAL CONTENT

SKILLS NEEDED BY PHYSICIAN EXTENDERS IN PRIMARY CARE/PHYSICIAN PRACTICES

- Excellent clinical competencies
- Several years' experience in the acute care setting
- A high level of professionalism
- Respiratory therapy credentials plus additional training or skills in related health care professions

INTRODUCTION TO THE CASE STUDY

Now you proceed into the most exciting part of this chapter, that of working through a case. Your instructor will assign you to work on specific critical thinking exercises, and possibly group critical thinking exercises depending on the available time, types of patients you are likely to encounter in your clinical rotations, and resources available. Please check with your instructor to verify which cases and exercises you should complete, either individually or working in groups. Your instructor may also assign you to develop the learning issues as part of your problem-based learning (PBL) process, or you may be assigned specific predetermined learning issues that have been developed for this chapter. Please check with your program faculty before proceeding with the following case.

CASE STUDY 1: MULTIPLE SETTINGS OF PATIENT CARE

BEA CONTINUED

Acute Care Hospital

Bea Continued is a 66-year-old white female with COPD and a history of smoking 1.5 packs/day since she was 16 years old. One month ago she was admitted through the ED of a hospital with an acute myocardial infarction (MI), which required coronary artery bypass grafting (CABG). Her post-operative stay was complicated by pneumonia and respiratory failure requiring mechanical ventilation. Over the past month, she had failed several attempts to wean from the ventilator. She has been transferred to a long-term acute care (LTAC) facility for further ventilator management.

Long-Term Acute Care Hospital

Jane, the respiratory therapist, is performing her initial assessment. She notices that Mrs. Continued has dark circles under her eyes, difficulty paying attention, and a sad appearance.

Later that day, the medical team, consisting of Jane, the doctor, nurse, occupational therapist, physical therapist, speech therapist, and case manager, meets with the patient's husband and daughter to develop a plan of care for Mrs. Continued. Her husband, Earl, states, "I don't understand why she needs that breathing machine. She's never been sick before. Sometimes Bea had to stop and catch her breath, but she is always on the go. She volunteers for our church and she and her friends get together and play bingo at least twice a week."

Her daughter, Ann, says, "I think she has given up. She seems to just want to lie in bed. I wish she could talk to me. I know I could help her if I just knew what she was thinking."

The next morning, while you are performing trach care you notice that the stoma is red and inflamed. Several days later Mrs. Continued's ventilator settings are SIMV 6, VT 650 cc, FIO_2 30%, PS 20. Her pulse oximetry is 94% and her PS tidal volume is 500 cc. Dr. Carter asks you to assess Mrs. Continued for weaning trials. She is later placed on a T tube at 40%. Thirty minutes after

Critical Thinking Exercise 1

COMMUNICATION

a. How can the medical team best communicate with Mrs. Continued?

b. In order to work together as a team, the medical staff must have effective communication. What can the medical team do to facilitate communication among team members and with Mrs. Continued and her family?

being placed on the T tube, Mrs. Continued becomes anxious and starts pulling at the tube. She says, "I can't breathe. Put me back on the machine." Her saturation is 95% and her spontaneous tidal volume is 450 cc. After being returned to ventilation she immediately calms down. Mr. Continued tells you, "This is what happened at the other hospital. Every time they took her off the breathing machine she'd go crazy."

Critical Thinking Exercise 2

ANTICIPATION

The weaning process may be frightening and intimidating to patients. What can be done to help Mrs. Continued when she becomes anxious during further weaning trials?

A week later, Mrs. Continued has been weaned to a 30% T collar with saturations of 92%. The speech therapist asks the respiratory therapist to help monitor the patient while she performs a modified swallow study. After receiving the results of the study, Mrs. Continued is started on a liquid diet with orders to advance to a pureed diet as tolerated.

Two days later, the respiratory therapist performs trach care on Mrs. Continued's #8 nonfenestrated trach tube and notes the stoma is pink and without inflammation. She suggests to Dr. Carter that they begin initiating the protocol for decannulating of Mrs. Continued's trach.

Critical Thinking Exercise 3

NEGOTIATING

Suppose Dr. Carter is reluctant to begin the decannulation process. What arguments can you make to support this procedure?

Three days later, Mrs. Continued's trach has been pulled and she is on a 2 L/min nasal cannula with saturation of 92%. The team feels Mrs. Continued is ready to go home and begins preparations for her discharge. She will require oxygen, metered dose inhalers, and physical therapy. The home health company requests lab work for qualification for oxygen reimbursement for Medicare. They ask the respiratory therapist to help in the coordination and delivery of the equipment. The home health respiratory therapist arranges to meet Mr. Continued at their house so she can complete an environmental safety check.

Home Health

Mrs. Continued is discharged from the hospital. The respiratory therapist soon arrives to talk with her about the oxygen concentrator and cylinders. "This stuff looks dangerous. What if something goes wrong?" asks Mr. Continued. The respiratory therapist explains about the equipment, including back-up procedures and infection control techniques. While she is undergoing an initial physical assessment, Mrs. Continued asks the RT, "How long will I have to wear oxygen?" Before leaving, the respiratory therapist promises to check back with them in a couple of days.

On her follow-up visit, the respiratory therapist smells cigarette smoke when she enters the house. Mrs. Continued is in the kitchen, but is not wearing her oxygen. Mrs. Continued tells the RT: "I feel funny wearing that in front of my friends. Besides they can't smoke when they visit me if I have it on."

Critical Thinking Exercise 4

NEGOTIATION

a. How can the respiratory therapist convince Mrs. Continued to wear her oxygen?
b. What will happen if Mrs. Continued decides not to wear her oxygen?

A few weeks later the home health respiratory therapist receives a phone call from Mrs. Continued. She says: "My doctor wants me to do something called pulmonary rehab? What is that?"

Pulmonary Rehabilitation

Mrs. Continued begins pulmonary rehabilitation at the local hospital. The RT has Mrs. Continued complete a health and lifestyle questionnaire. Several of the questions deal with smoking. Mrs. Continued admits she still smokes. "I only smoke 5 or 6 cigarettes a day. It's so hard to quit, especially when I get together with all of my friends who smoke," she says. The respiratory therapist also performs a pulmonary function test. The respiratory therapist asks Mrs. Continued what goals she hopes to accomplish with pulmonary rehabilitation. Mrs. Continued asks the respiratory therapist, "If I do this program, will I be able to get rid of the oxygen?" The respiratory therapist starts Mrs. Continued on an exercise regimen that includes walking on a treadmill and lifting small weights. Mrs. Continued is reluctant to start exercising and asks, "How is this going to help my breathing?" Mrs. Continued completes a 6-minute walk on the treadmill and walks 400 feet.

Over the next few weeks, Mrs. Continued continues to work with the RT 3 times a week in

CASE STUDY 1: MULTIPLE SETTINGS OF PATIENT CARE *(continued)*

the pulmonary rehabilitation program and joins the smoking cessation class offered by the hospital. Mr. Continued and his wife also begin to take walks around the neighborhood every other morning. At the end of the pulmonary rehabilitation program Mrs. Continued is able to walk 800 feet during her 6-minute walk on the treadmill.

Home Health

After completing the pulmonary rehabilitation course, the home health respiratory therapist visits Mrs. Continued. She is wearing her oxygen and playing bingo with two of her friends. Her saturation is 94% on 2 L/min and 85% on room air. She

Critical Thinking Exercise 5

TROUBLESHOOTING AND ANTICIPATING

a. Is it possible for Mrs. Continued to travel to her grandson's graduation on oxygen? What arrangements will need to be done in order to allow her to attend?

b. What instructions and suggestions would you give Mrs. Continued so she is prepared to troubleshoot any problems?

c. Is Mrs. Continued a candidate for LVRS?

tells the respiratory therapist, "I feel great! My grandson is graduating from high school next month, but he lives 500 miles away. Is there any way I could be there for that?" Mr. Continued shows the respiratory therapist a magazine article about a patient who had lung volume reduction surgery (LVRS). He asks the respiratory therapist, "Could Bea have this operation?"

Group Critical Thinking Exercise 1

TRADITIONAL AND EMERGING ROLES

After reviewing this chapter, the class should be divided into groups of 2 to 4 students. The faculty will provide a listing to the class of the various traditional and emerging roles for respiratory therapists and ask students to choose (randomly or deliberately) where they will work following graduation. Each group will prepare a written report on how to find and secure this type of position, providing specific names of individuals and organizations to contact. The report should also specify the job requirements, duties, salary, benefits, and other specific considerations. After submitting the written reports, each group should make a 10- to 15-minute oral report to the entire class. The oral and written reports should be part of the each student's earned grade for the respiratory therapy course.

KEY POINTS

- While the traditional role for the respiratory therapist has been in the acute care setting, recent changes in the delivery of health care, including changing government policies for reimbursement, the emergence of managed care, and an aging population have expanded the continuum of care.

- Respiratory therapists now enjoy careers in settings as varied as diagnostic laboratories and patients' homes.

- All levels of health care, from subacute and skilled nursing facilities, to wellness, disease prevention, and pulmonary rehabilitation, employ respiratory therapists.

- Respiratory therapists have expanded the services they provide to include diagnosis, case management, and education.

- Respiratory therapists are now frequently employed in areas that until a few years ago were not obvious choices, such as industry and research.

- The future for respiratory therapy in nontraditional settings looks bright.

ACKNOWLEDGMENTS

The author wishes to acknowledge the following people for their valuable contributions to this chapter:

Laura Beveridge, MEd, RRT
Respiratory Sales Specialist
US Human Health
Merck & Co., Inc.
Augusta, Georgia

Patty Joyner, RRT, CCM
Respiratory Disease Management Specialist
TLC Family Care Health Plan
Memphis, Tennessee

Kathy Owen, BS, RRT
Health Care Specialist
Lincare
Augusta, Georgia

Tony Patterson, BS, RRT
Pulmonary Case Manager
Piedmont Hospital
Atlanta, Georgia

Brenda Stafford, AS, RRT
Health Care Specialist
Lincare
Augusta, Georgia

REFERENCES

1. Ward JJ, Hemholz HF Jr. Roots of the respiratory care profession. In: Burton GG, Hodgkin JE, Ward JJ, eds. *Respiratory Care: A Guide to Clinical Practice.* 4th ed. Philadelphia: Lippincott; 1997: 21–23.

2. Mishoe SC, MacIntyre NR. Expanding professional roles for respiratory care practitioners. *Respir Care.* 1997;42:71.

3. Lewin Group Report. Respiratory care practitioners in an evolving health care environment. American Association for Respiratory Care, Dallas, Texas; 1999.

4. Sabo JS. Respiratory care in the 1990s. In: Burton GG, Hodgkin JE, Ward JJ, eds. *Respiratory Care: A Guide to Clinical Practice.* 4th ed. Philadelphia: Lippincott; 1997:33.

5. Health Care Financing Administration. Office of the Actuary. 1996.

6. Hafenschiel J. Home health reimbursement and the 1997 budget act. *Home Care Provider.* 1997;2(6): 279–281.

7. Health Care Financing Administration. Office of Managed Care. 1996

8. US Department of Commerce Bureau of Census. *Statistical Abstract of the United States.* 11th ed. 1991.

9. US General Accounting Office: *Long Term Care— Projected Needs of Baby Boom Generation.* GAO/HRD: 91: 86. Washington: US Government Accounting Office; June 1991.

10. Centers for Disease Control. National Center for Health Statistics. Chronic Obstructive Pulmonary Disease. http://www.cdc.gov/nchs/fastats/copd.htm

11. Centers for Disease Control. National Center for Health Statistics. Asthma. http://www.cdc.gov/nchs/fastats/asthma.htm

12. American Lung Association. Trends in chronic bronchitis and emphysema: morbidity and mortality. http://www.lungusa.org/data/copd/copd1.pdf Epidemiology & Statistics Unit, February 2000.

13. Scott F. The downside of downsizing. *Adv Respir Care Pract.* 1996;2:45–46.

14. Hanania NA, Wittman R, Keston S, et al. Medical personnel's knowledge and ability to use inhaling devices. *Chest* 1994;105(1):111–116.

15. Guidyt GG, Brown WD, Stogner SW, et al. Incorrect use of metered dose inhalers by medical personnel. *Chest* 1992;101:31–33.

16. Kollef MH, Shapiro SD, Clinkscale D, et al. The effects of respiratory therapist-initiated treatment protocols on patient outcomes and resource utilization. *Chest* 2000;117(2):467–475.

17. Heidegger R, Walton J. Subacute care. In: Fink JB, Hunt GE, eds. *Clinical Practice in Respiratory Care.* Philadelphia: Lippincott; 1999:465.

18. American Health Care Association. Consumer Information: Subacute Care. http://www.ahca.org/info/subacute.htm Washington, DC.

19. National Subacute Care Association. General information about subacute care & the industry. http://www.nsca.net/info/index.htm Washington, DC.

20. Council of Scientific Affairs. Home care in the 1990s. *JAMA* 1990;263(9):1241–1244.

21. Dunne PJ: Demographics and financial impact of home respiratory care. Respir Care. 1994;39(4):310.

22. Bunch D. Home care comes of age as health care moves outside hospitals. *AARC Times*. 1996:18–20, 23–24, 26–27.

23. Tingdale M. Case management of the geriatric patient. *AARC Times*. 1997;21(11):64–69.

24. Mullahy CM. A potent alliance. *RT J Respir Care Pract*. 1994;7(6):100–102.

25. Heiden D. Charting a new course. *RT J Respir Care Pract*. 1996;9(2):46–48.

26. Sheldon RL. RCPs can play an important role as physician extenders in pulmonary outpatient clinics. *AARC Times*. 1996;20(11):52–56.

27. Bunch D. Eligibility criteria for taking the case manager certification exam revisited. *AARC Times*. 1996;20(4):64–66.

28. Cornish K. Subacute care offers opportunities for respiratory therapists. *AARC Times*. 1995;19(2):22–27.

29. National Subacute Care Association. NSCA & the industry it serves. http://www.nsca.net/info/industry.htm Washington, DC.

30. Bunch D: Muse study shows respiratory therapists' positive impact. *AARC Times*. 1999;23(8):20–27.

31. Muse and Associates. *A Comparison of Medicare Nursing Home Residents Who Received Services from a Respiratory Therapist with Those Who Did Not*. Executive Summary. Dallas, TX: American Association for Respiratory Care; August 1999:1–3.

32. Ries AL, Carlin BW, Carrieri-Kohlman V, et al. Pulmonary rehabilitation: Joint ACCP/AACVPR evidence-based guidelines. *Chest* 1997;112(5): 1363–1396.

33. Arand DL, Bonnet MH. Sleep disordered breathing. In: Burton GG, Hodgkin JE, Ward JJ, eds. *Respiratory Care: A Guide to Clinical Practice*. 4th ed. Philadelphia: Lippincott; 1997:296.

34. http://www.nhtsa.dot.gov/people/perform/ human/ drwosy.html#NCSDR/NHTA

35. US Food & Drug Administration. FDA Consumer Magazine. Sleepless Society. Rockville, MD: July–August 1998. http://www.fda.gov/fdac/features/1998/sleepsoc.html

36. National Heart Lung & Blood Institute. National Center on Sleep Disorders Research. http://www.nhblisupport.com/sleep/about/about.htm

37. American Association for Respiratory Care. http://www.aarc.org. AARC clinical practice guidelines. Dallas, TX

38. American Association for Respiratory Care. Year 2001: Delineating the educational direction for the future respiratory care practitioner—Proceedings of a national education consensus conference on respiratory care education. Dallas, TX; October 2–4, 1992.

39. Smith R: Faces of the future. *RT J Respir Care Pract*. 1995;8(2):53–60.

6

USING AND DEVELOPING CLINICAL PRACTICE GUIDELINES, RESPIRATORY CARE PROTOCOLS, AND CRITICAL PATHWAYS

Lynda Thomas Goodfellow

For every problem under the sun, there is a solution
or there is none. If there be one, seek till you find it.
If there be none, then never mind it.
—MOTHER GOOSE

LEARNING OBJECTIVES

1. Define and describe clinical practice guidelines, respiratory care protocols, critical pathways, and the other key words for this chapter.

2. Discuss the advantages and disadvantages of clinical practice guidelines, respiratory care protocols, and critical pathways.

3. Describe the role of the respiratory therapist in the use of clinical practice guidelines, respiratory care protocols, and critical pathways.

4. Discuss the design and implementation of clinical practice guidelines, respiratory care protocols, and critical pathways.

5. Develop a strategy or strategies for successful implementation incorporating the critical thinking skills of respiratory care practitioners, with recommendations for the health care team, time lines, and patient care.

6. Describe outcomes evaluation and why it is necessary.

7. Describe the different types of outcomes that are monitored.

8. Define variances and the different types of variances that are tracked.

9. Discuss the link between critical thinking and clinical practice guidelines, respiratory care protocols, and critical pathways.

10. Generate a respiratory care protocol and/or critical pathway for an asthmatic patient.

11. Practice your communicating and negotiating skills in an attempt to gain acceptance of your proposed protocol or pathway.

12. Discuss the value of critical thinking in the use of clinical practice guidelines, respiratory care protocols, and critical pathways

CHAPTER DESCRIPTION

This chapter provides an overview of clinical practice guidelines (CPGs), respiratory care protocols, and critical pathways, defines some common terms, and discusses the advantages and disadvantages of each. It also elaborates upon the role of respiratory therapists in the use of CPGs, protocols, and pathways in health care. This chapter deviates slightly from other chapters in this text because case examples are not included. Here, critical thinking questions and exercises are utilized to help the student attain a deeper understanding of the applications, and ways to analyze these important topics. The questions and exercises are designed to provide students with opportunities for realistic application of the principles described here. For example, the chapter asks the student to develop a respiratory care protocol or pathway for a patient with asthma. In addition, students are given the opportunity to practice their communicating and negotiating skills to gain acceptance for the proposed pathway or protocol they develop.

INTRODUCTION TO GUIDELINES, PROTOCOLS, AND PATHWAYS

The health care system no longer consists merely of physicians' offices and hospitals. Today, the health care continuum also consists of ambulatory care clinics, surgi-centers, outpatient rehabilitation, subacute care centers, long-term care facilities, and home care services. The US health care industry reinvented itself during the 1990s, and a wealth of information exists in the medical literature about how to control costs throughout this continuum in many ways, such as with critical pathways, protocols, or algorithms, and with clinical practice guidelines. All of these methods claim to decrease length of stay (LOS) by employing more effective and efficient standards of care. Many of these claims have been substantiated, but many have not. It is important for practitioners to consider the alternatives so that the best possible clinical decisions are made, which in turn will lead to improved patient care.

Defining the Terms

The concepts of managed care, capitation, and case management are relatively unfamiliar terms to students and many staff practitioners. Effective resource utilization is a major concern and goal for everyone working in the health care industry. The following is a review of the definitions and a brief history of the methods used by health care facilities to control the cost of health care, while maintaining or improving the quality of care rendered.

Clinical Practice Guidelines. Clinical practice guidelines (CPGs) are systematically-developed statements to assist clinicians with appropriate respiratory care under specific clinical circumstances.[1] CPGs address the appropriateness of care by specifying indications for tests, procedures, and treatments. In other words, CPGs describe how specific disciplines should treat certain conditions, diseases, or modalities. The first 5 clinical practice guidelines for respiratory care practitioners were published in December 1991 in the journal *Respiratory Care*. The process of formally developing CPGs was initiated by the American Association for Respiratory Care (AARC) in 1990 to address the variability in clinical practice from one hospital to another and from one geographic region to another.[2] Differences were evident in patient outcomes, hospital LOS, and cost of care, which led to concerns among third-party payers and governmental agencies. The AARC has taken a leadership role not only for the respiratory care profession, but also in the eyes of other allied health organizations in the development of CPGs to improve the efficacy and reduce the costs of respiratory care practice throughout the country.

By 1999, there were almost 50 clinical practice guidelines published in *Respiratory Care*. Updates to existing CPGs and new guidelines are written and implemented regularly. These guidelines helped to establish respiratory care protocols, and have found their way into respiratory care services departmental policy and procedure manuals, provided clinical indicators for continuous quality improvement (CQI), and supported the enhanced role of the respiratory care practitioner.[3]

Respiratory Care Protocols. Respiratory care protocols, also known as therapist-driven protocols (TDPs) or patient-driven protocols (PDPs), were first described in the respiratory care literature in 1981.[4] Since then, respiratory care protocols have emerged as an integral part of many services provided by respiratory therapists. Respiratory care protocols are patient care plans initiated and implemented by credentialed respiratory therapists. Much-needed flexibility is provided by the use of respiratory care protocols and their use has led to an improvement in patient care, because therapy is more easily and efficiently modified according to the needs of the patient. Each protocol has a title, a purpose or objective, a description of the type of patient the protocol covers (eg, pediatric, postoperative), indications and contraindications, projected outcomes, and guidelines for reduction or discontinuation of therapy. In short, the respiratory care practitioner is allowed to initiate, adjust, discontinue, and restart respiratory care procedures once a protocol is ordered. Respiratory care protocols are developed by respiratory therapists with physician input, and must be approved by the medical staff and hospital administration prior to their implementation.

Respiratory care protocols can take several forms—algorithms, narratives, or worksheets. One of the main purposes of these protocols is to standardize decision making, and they may be patient-specific, diagnosis-specific, or symptom-

specific. Patient-specific protocols are usually based on an assessment of a patient's condition and treatment needs. Diagnosis-specific protocols are part of a patient's critical path of care (ie, CPT for cystic fibrosis). Symptom-specific protocols are implemented based on a particular problem, such as wheezing or atelectasis. Respiratory care protocols are typically generated by designating clinical practice guidelines that provide profession-oriented procedures to incorporate into the institution-oriented protocol.

Once the physician writes the order protocol, the respiratory therapist has the authority to evaluate and initiate care, and to adjust, discontinue, or restart respiratory care procedures on a shift-by-shift or hour-to-hour basis.[5] For respiratory care protocols to be successful, each respiratory therapist must have a strong knowledge base about cardiopulmonary care disorders and competence in the actual assessment process, including gathering clinical data, formulating a correct assessment, and treating the patient appropriately. Assessment skills are very important, as are communication skills, because more time is spent assessing and treating the patient, more time is spent communicating with other professionals, and more time is spent documenting what was done and what was observed.[6] Refer to Chapter 7 for a more detailed discussion of patient assessment.

Critical Pathways. Critical pathways (CPs) define the optimal sequence or timing of the key interventions done by all disciplines involved in patient care for a particular diagnosis, procedure, or symptom.[7] Interpreted informally, a CP is the sequence of events in a process that takes the greatest length of time.[8] This sequence of events outlines all the tests, procedures, treatments, and teaching services that patients utilize during their length of stay.[9] An example of a CP is provided in Fig. 6-1. CPs are also known by many other names throughout the medical literature (Table 6-1). Some institutions are reluctant to use the term "critical" pathway because of the implications it may have for the patients when they learn they are on a "critical" pathway. Others are bothered by the

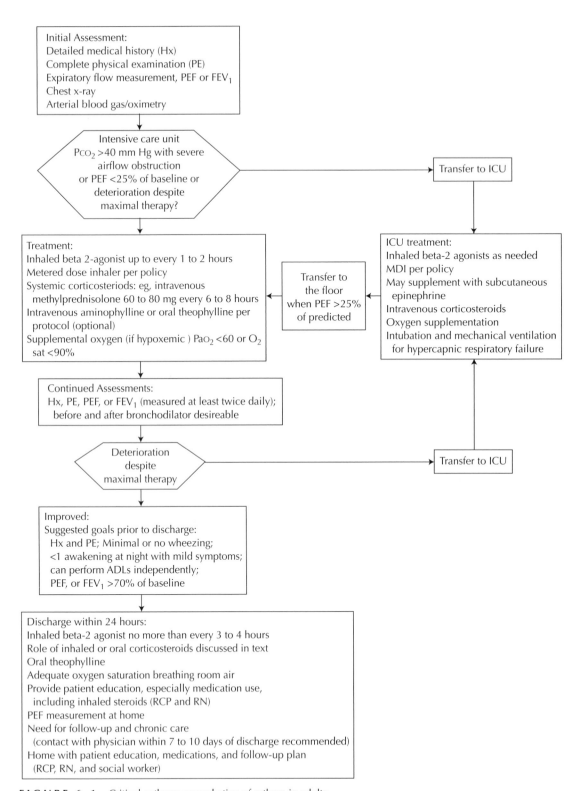

FIGURE 6-1 Critical pathway exacerbation of asthma in adults.

TABLE 6-1 CRITICAL PATHWAYS PSEUDONYMS

Critical pathways are also known as:
- Anticipated recovery paths
- Clinical paths
- Critical paths
- Clinical algorithms
- Care maps
- Collaborative plans of care
- Care paths
- Multidisciplinary action plans (MAPS)
- Practice parameters
- Practice protocols
- Practice standards
- Practice options

term "pathway" because it implies that there is one **best** way to deliver care and all others should be considered substandard. Regardless of the terminology used, much of the documented success comes from the use of CPs in the acute care setting. CPs can be utilized in any setting and currently many health care organizations outside of acute care are developing CPs to meet the needs of patients in other settings.

CPs have their roots in the construction and manufacturing industries as tools to identify and manage rate-limiting steps in production processes.[8] The purpose in these settings has been to maximize the efficiency of production given multiple contractors and limited resources. Using techniques like the critical path method (CPM), program evaluation review technique (PERT), and Gantt charts, all activities to be accomplished during a production process are identified and timed. Activities are then sequenced according to projected times of completion for each activity. By definition, a critical path is the key sequence of events that drives the timeline of the overall project. In other words, the critical path is the sequence of events that takes the most time to complete.

Coffey and colleagues have described the basics of CPs as they are applied in health care: "A critical pathway is an optimal sequencing and timing of interventions by physicians, nurses, and other disciplines for a particular diagnosis or procedure, designed to minimize delays and resource utilization and to maximize the quality of care."[7] CPs are strongly rooted in nursing as a blend of traditional nursing care plans, a need to provide care within the structured framework of a hospital setting, and a means to establish a standard of care for all patients.[10] Of all the diagnostic, therapeutic, social, and organizational interventions that are to be accomplished during an episode of care, the critical path is the sequence of milestone events that will have the greatest impact on clinical outcome, LOS, and resource consumption.

Clinical care or "case management" then becomes organized around these milestone events as activities supporting their accomplishment. Case management is known as the collaborative process that assesses, plans, implements, coordinates, monitors, and evaluates the options and services required to meet an individual's health care needs.[9] This is accomplished by the use of communication between practitioners and by utilizing available resources to promote quality, cost-effective outcomes.

There are instances where you may find that significant overlap exists with the use of all three of the concepts: clinical practice guidelines, respiratory care protocols, and critical pathways. All three of the tools described above are appropriate to use in certain situations and at certain times. For example, a respiratory care protocol may have been developed by using a specific CPG. Further, the respiratory care protocol may be incorporated into a CP and used for a specific disease or condition. In the literature, respiratory care protocols are straightforward in their description and use. However, some have found CPs and CPGs to be confusing. Table 6-2 compares and contrasts CPGs, respiratory care protocols, and CPs.

Overview of Design and Implementation. The general principles of design and implementation hold true across settings for all three of the tools you may need: CPGs, respiratory care protocols, and CPs. Whichever tool is chosen, your team must first identify desirable outcomes and then map out interventions intended to achieve those outcomes.

Critical Thinking Exercise 1

a. Discuss the ways in which clinical practice guidelines, respiratory care protocols, and critical pathways differ. Use your own words, and create examples within respiratory care to clarify your meaning.

b. Make an assumption about when it is appropriate to recommend the development and implementation of these three concepts in patient care and explain the anticipated or expected outcome.

c. Construct an argument that would convince someone with an opposing viewpoint that respiratory therapists have a valid role in the development and application of clinical practice guidelines, respiratory care protocols, and critical pathways.

This section provides an overview of the design and implementation process for CPGs, respiratory care protocols, and CPs.

Design and Implementation of Clinical Practice Guidelines

Fortunately there is no need for each institution to design and tailor-make its own CPGs. CPGs should provide the basis for appropriate respiratory care while maintaining flexibility to individualize for specific patients. The AARC's initiative to develop CPGs formally began in 1990. By 1999, there were approximately 50 practice guidelines published in *Respiratory Care*. The CPGs are brief but practical documents that address specific respiratory care modalities with the intent of standardizing care and improving the quality of respiratory care administered to our patients. For an overview of the design project for clinical practice guidelines, refer to editorials outlined by Hess[11,12] in *Respiratory Care*. All CPGs listed in *Respiratory Care* follow the same format and seek to answer similar questions (Table 6-3).

A CPG is initially developed from a thorough review of the literature, surveys of current practice, and the expertise of the members of the

TABLE 6-2   DISTINCTIONS BETWEEN CLINICAL PRACTICE GUIDELINES, RESPIRATORY CARE PROTOCOLS, AND CRITICAL PATHWAYS

Clinical Practice Guidelines:
- address appropriateness of care by specifying indications for tests, procedures, and/or treatments
- specify treatment plans, protocols, and algorithms for patient care
- describe how to perform procedures
- are developed by each discipline to guide practice
- are voluntary and evolve as the profession changes

Respiratory Care Protocols:
- are patient care plans
- are not standing orders
- each has a title, purpose, description of patients affected, indications and contraindications, outcome objectives, and guidelines regarding when it is appropriate to reduce or discontinue therapy
- must be approved by the medical staff and hospital administration prior to implementation

Critical Pathways:
- focus on efficiency and effectiveness after decisions regarding direction of treatment have been made
- are the completion of the protocol or guideline that results in the accomplishment of critical pathway events
- are affected by any delays or complications in treatment plans because the flow (timeline) of the critical pathway is altered
- are multidisciplinary in their development and execution
- employ health care practitioners with domain-specific or discipline-specific critical thinking skills earlier in the patient care process
- delineate specific timelines for the accomplishment of events
- describe when to perform procedures
- frequently become a permanent part of the medical record because of the comprehensive nature of their design

TABLE 6-3   FORMAT USED IN CLINICAL PRACTICE GUIDELINES

Procedure	Common names by which the procedure is known
Description or definition	Describes or defines the procedure in the context of the guideline
Setting	Describes places where the procedure can be appropriately performed
Indications	Recognized objectives or indications for the procedure
Contraindications	Relative and absolute conditions when it is not safe to use or employ the procedure
Hazards/complications	Those that are associated with the procedure
Limitations	Limitations of which the practitioner should be aware
Need	Determination that a procedure is indicated
Outcomes	Benefit (or lack thereof) derived from the procedure
Resources	Equipment and personnel required to perform the procedure
Monitoring	Issues related to specific monitoring needed
Frequency	Statements related to determination of how often a procedure should be performed
Infection control	Issues related to specific infection control
References	Studies that support the recommendations

SOURCE: From Hess.[2] Reprinted with permission from Daedalus Enterprises.

working groups.[2] The group then makes multiple revisions and edits. When the working group is satisfied, the guideline is reviewed by a steering committee and distributed for peer review by over 500 respiratory therapists, physicians, and others. The comments made by every reviewer are considered by the working group and the steering committee. Following this process, the CPGs are published in *Respiratory Care* and are widely distributed as reprints.[2]

There are several reasons why it is beneficial for institutions to take advantage of these published guidelines. Practice guidelines make an excellent tool for incorporation into respiratory care protocols that are institution-specific because they define and justify clinical practice. Respiratory care departments have incorporated CPGs into their consulting services and respiratory care protocol programs.[13–16] CPGs should provide a basis for therapist-physician interactions by helping the respiratory therapist to meet the expectations of the physician and vice versa. Thus CPGs should improve the consistency and appropriateness of care. The CPG can provide assistance to respira-

tory care departments in developing triage systems so that patient care is allocated most appropriately. In addition, CPGs can also serve as a guide for education and research as they become accepted as standards of care.[16] The role of CPGs in respiratory care remains to be researched, but in some professions (eg, anesthesiology) the adoption of clinical guidelines has resulted in lower malpractice premiums[17] and significant cost savings.[18]

CRITICAL CONTENT

PROPOSED ADVANTAGES OF CPGS

- Facilitate the development of respiratory care patient protocols
- Form a basis for respiratory therapist-physician interactions
- Contribute to consistency and appropriateness of care
- Assist in the triage of care
- Serve as a guide for education and research

Critical Thinking Exercise 2

How can a clinical practice guideline be used to standardize care?

Design and Implementation of Respiratory Care Protocols

Several studies are available for review in the literature regarding the clinical effects of allocation of respiratory care services using respiratory care protocols. The consensus is that there is less misallocation of respiratory care resources when respiratory care protocols are utilized, and no concomitant increase in adverse respiratory events.[13–15,19–25] For example, Brougher and colleagues[19] and Small and associates[22] investigated the misuse of oxygen therapy; Browning and co-workers[21] and Kester and Stoller[23] studied the misuse of arterial blood gases; and Shapiro and colleagues[20] reported on the misallocation of bronchial hygiene procedures. All of these studies demonstrate the need to investigate allocation of respiratory therapy procedures and treatments. Misallocation—overordering and underordering—of respiratory care procedures under the traditional physician-order system of allocating respiratory care was the major reason for the growing acceptance of respiratory care protocols in the 1980s and 1990s.[6] Misallocation may be further defined as providing treatment to patients who do not need it and may not benefit, or not providing therapy for those who do need it and would benefit.

An involved medical director and department manager committed to the respiratory care protocol program are essential for its success.[6] The medical director for the respiratory care department presents the structure and purpose of the program and teaches other physicians about the protocols. He or she is a key person in the implementation process. The medical director may be hesitant to implement respiratory care protocols if the educational level of the respiratory care staff is low, the political climate at the institution is not favorable, or the organization is uncomfortable with the concept. The department manager is also a key team player.

If the manager favors the status quo and is forced to cut costs by reducing staff, he or she may feel as if the resources are lacking to successfully implement a respiratory care protocol program. Finally, efforts to move forward may be hampered by unmotivated respiratory therapists. It is best that department managers be aware of their department's strengths and limitations before embarking on a program of respiratory care protocols.

Steps Toward Success. The first step is to establish indications for therapy by using the AARC's CPGs, an exhaustive review of the literature, and institutional preferences. With the respiratory care protocol system, indications for therapy (criteria) are developed by the respiratory care staff, the medical director(s), and the respiratory care department manager.[26] By generating various tools, such as algorithms, flowcharts, or protocol sheets, respiratory therapists can determine which treatments are indicated after a patient assessment and chart review are performed. Several institutions have designed their own triage system to be used for determining the frequency of respiratory care procedures. A scoring system of 1 to 3 or 1 to 5 is used to rank the severity of patient illness after each evaluation. As the patient progresses, the score given by a respiratory therapist on a particular shift can change hour to hour, shift to shift, or day to day.

Once the physician's order is written for the respiratory care protocol, the respiratory therapist does all the evaluations and reevaluations. A protocol for that particular patient, based on the diagnosis, is placed in the medical record for all caregivers to review. The patient's symptoms and indications for therapy are noted, as well as the respiratory therapist's adjustments and requests for medical consultation. All subsequent documentation is made on the protocol form. The assessment skills of the respiratory therapist are very important, and if the respiratory care staff has low self-confidence in its assessment abilities, then the program will not be successful. Please refer to Chapter 7 to review or develop your patient assessment skills and ability to develop an individualized care plan.

The assessment consists of evaluating information in the chart (progress notes), laboratory reports (radiographs, ABG, etc.), and from the patient. People who think in concrete terms may not be capable of thinking analytically, and will therefore have difficulty with making critical decisions.[6] Therefore patient assessment and decision making skills are fundamental to the success of respiratory care protocols. Experience and practice greatly enhance the effectiveness of respiratory care protocols. Practitioners who can think critically and analytically and are not limited by goal-oriented, objective-directed assessments are better prepared to deal with guidelines, protocols, and pathways. See Chapter 3 for additional information and exercises that enhance problem solving skills needed for effective decision making.

Education and Training Strategies. Good communication skills are essential because respiratory therapists report daily to each other regarding the patient's status, the reason the protocol was ordered, and the therapy currently being administered. As the patient's condition changes, an evaluation of appropriateness is needed to ensure the best possible care is provided. Examples include changing the type of equipment needed for aerosol therapy delivery from hand-held nebulizer to metered dose inhaler and adjusting ventilator settings. The respiratory care staff is constantly reassessing the therapy being given and makes any changes it feels are necessary for the delivery of quality care. By consulting with other respiratory care staff members who have treated the patient on other days, the therapist ensures that the changes suggested are effective and that any new changes are appropriate. Critical thinking skills are enhanced by the use of respiratory care protocols.

Education and orientation of the medical, nursing, and respiratory care staff are major components of the success of the program. Case studies and various forms of problem-based learning exercises are useful for training the respiratory care staff. Negative outcomes may be used to improve departmental quality by discussing prevention strategies that can be incorporated into future prac-tice. Having respiratory therapists develop a respiratory care protocol during an orientation session can be a great teaching tool for describing the process, as well as identifying the differences between the information gathering and decision making stages. All respiratory care staff should be involved in educating the other hospital staff. Handbooks are helpful, particularly for medical residents. These handbooks may include a set of the approved algorithms and outlines, as well as the method used to initiate the respiratory care protocol process.

Today, managers are using performance standards as process evaluations. Respiratory care protocols are incorporated into the employee evaluation process. For instance, one goal of the protocol program is ensuring that practitioners make patient evaluations correctly. If an incorrect evaluation is made too frequently, pulmonary physicians could lose trust in the protocol system. Consequently, physicians may revert to writing their own medical orders, disregarding the protocol system. Because of this concern, performance standards are set high. Practitioners are expected to make the correct assessment 95% to 100% of the time. Thus the protocol allows managers to assess each therapist's performance in relation to these standards.[26] If a therapist is not performing as required, more training and education are needed.

Advantages resulting from the implementation of respiratory care protocols include recruitment of better therapists because of the challenging work environment, and increased job satisfaction.[6] Cost containment is a major asset for managers whose departments use protocols, because patients are getting the most appropriate care, therefore the total charges against the diagnostic-related groups (DRG) are low.[26] For instance, if a patient is very ill, almost continuous therapy can be ordered and changed as appropriate to every 2 hours or every 4 hours as the patient's condition improves. Another example of how protocols assist in cost containment is discontinuing therapy when it is no longer needed. As the respiratory therapy profession changes, the protocols can and should be updated to reflect the latest in technology or research with little change or disruption in the overall program. AARC's web site (www.aarc.org) has a link to guidelines for preparing a respiratory care protocol.

CRITICAL CONTENT

ADVANTAGES OF IMPLEMENTATION OF RESPIRATORY CARE PROTOCOLS

- Recruitment of better respiratory therapists
- Increased job satisfaction
- Cost containment
- Increased appropriateness of care provided

Critical Thinking Exercise 3

a. How does the medical director play a vital role in the success of a respiratory care protocol program?

b. How do normal and unusual findings affect the triage system of respiratory care protocols in patient care?

c. Consider the advantages and disadvantages of using the performance evaluation system to determine the effectiveness of a respiratory therapist using respiratory care protocols. How can the respiratory care manager effectively implement these criteria?

Group Critical Thinking Exercise 1

COMMUNICATING AND NEGOTIATING RESPIRATORY CARE PROTOCOLS

Demonstrate how you would communicate and negotiate with other members of the health care team regarding the rationale and implementation of a respiratory care protocol program. Role play with your classmates or invite the key personnel to your class or meeting. Who are the key personnel to inform? What forms of communication will work best and which forms of communication will not work well? Why? Develop and present an evaluation plan to monitor the success of the respiratory care protocol program you are recommending.

Critical Pathways and Multidisciplinary Design

In an era of increasing competition in health care, critical pathways are intended to reduce costs while maintaining or even improving the quality of care.[8] CPs are developed primarily for high-volume procedures or frequent hospital diagnoses and provide the ideal sequence and timing of staff actions for optimal efficiency. Despite the rapid dissemination of CPs in hospitals throughout the United States, many uncertainties remain about their development, implementation, and evaluation.[27]

Health care professionals may be instructed to develop CPs with little or no instruction. Very few continuing education activities relating to CP development and implementation have been offered outside of hospitals. The few that exist concentrate on the development of CPs. Most of the literature also centers around how to develop and implement CPs. Like other promising medical innovations and technologies, CPs are being used before controlled clinical trials have been done to evaluate their effectiveness. No one knows for sure if CPs are cost effective for the overall operation of the institution over the long haul. Preliminary studies have shown cost savings when CPs are used under specific circumstances.

So why advocate CPs? One reason is that the short-term benefits are evident. Developing multidisciplinary CPs is a major step toward coordinating and organizing health care, and therefore short-term benefits are realized. Most of the CPs in hospitals were developed by nurses for nursing care alone, but multidisciplinary teams soon began developing pathways to encompass all aspects of care for hospitalized patients.[28,29] A basic assumption behind pathway development is the "80/20 rule,"[9] which states that 80% of patients follow a predictable path, and that the remaining 20% stray from that path, with a portion of that 20% deviating far from the expected pathway.

For this reason, CPs should be developed by the professionals who will use them. A team of health care providers from a wide range of professions, offering a variety of views in the multidisciplinary meetings, is most effective. Chances are that the views held by committee members will be mirrored by other staff members outside the task force during implementation.

With increasing economic and consumer pressures on the health care industry for more effective outcome management, it is easy for institutions to jump on the critical pathway bandwagon. CPs are a change in philosophy for many institutions and should not be taken lightly. Without a firm commitment from the leadership, CPs will not achieve what they are intended to do, which is to reduce cost and LOS in the short-term while improving on quality and patient satisfaction. CPs are being used more and more as a part of a continuous quality improvement (CQI) plan. CQI monitoring and evaluation of appropriateness of patient care in a large hospital is a difficult task in terms of time and efficiency. Therefore, CPs outline "daily triggers" that can be used to help identify potential and actual variations in the health response to a planned intervention.[10] The daily triggers are a visual reminder to the care provider that anything out of the ordinary that occurs can have a negative impact on outcomes. For example, an asthmatic patient is audibly wheezing 2 days after a status asthmaticus attack. This event is a trigger to the care providers that an unexpected event has occurred. The wheezing noted by the respiratory therapist forces a deviation from the planned course of care on the asthma CP. Another example is the presence of atelectasis 3 days postoperatively on the chest radiograph of a patient who underwent abdominal surgery. The presence of atelectasis triggers a variance that requires immediate attention. Triggers can be used to assist practitioners to respond to changes in the clinical course of the illness. This model provides a means for providers to promote and document their excellence of care so they can remain competitive.

Getting Started.   Critical pathways are available in the literature for specific diagnoses or procedures,[30] and some organizations and agencies (ie, the AARC) provide critical pathways for a fee.[31] Although it may seem like a simple solution to pur-

chase a set of CPs and just implement them, this does not afford the health care practitioners the opportunity to learn about CPs, or give them the time they need to work through the problems or questions they may have. Although the internal development of CPs is a very time consuming, complex process, it is also beneficial to the institution. In working together to institutionalize CPs, team members gain valuable insight into their own unique contributions to patient care, as well as a greater understanding of the roles of other health care providers. It is customary for a physician or nurse to chair the group, which also includes representatives from hospital administration, quality management, pharmacy, and all appropriate ancillary support services. It is appropriate for a respiratory therapist to be responsible for the development of a CP on ventilator weaning or prolonged mechanical ventilation. This developmental process can help to diminish the perception that CPs offer a pre-formulated approach to care.

Practitioner input in the development and implementation are also important because the buy-in and success of the CP program are increased. It is wise to spend time at the beginning securing a "buy-in" within the institution. If the leadership is supportive, the next step is to get buy-in from the staff. To get all staff members committed to CPs is possibly the greatest challenge in any setting. An opportunity for the staff to express concerns and a forum to resolve them are effective steps to achieve buy-in. As with any change, there is bound to be dissension within the staff. Old ways of practice need to be let go and a grieving process with an adjustment phase must ensue. Therefore the CP team must be carefully chosen.

Choosing the Critical Pathway Team.   When choosing staff members for multidisciplinary teams, it is important to select staff members who are team players who are able to work as a group.[9] One to two members from the disciplines or areas affected by the CP are useful to the makeup of the committee. It is also useful to choose staff members who are not necessarily agents of change. It is useful and healthy to hear a variety of the views held by committee members that are mirrored by other staff members outside of the task force. The meetings may be the scenes of lively dialogue before all points of view are heard. Thorough discussion of pros and cons can prevent any new concepts or ideas from blindly being implemented without all disciples being firmly behind the CP. By addressing concerns openly, problem areas can be resolved before the CP is designed. The meetings may not always be pleasant; reaching consensus can be challenging and time consuming, but the effort is well worth it.

Once the administrative decision has been made to implement CPs and the multidisciplinary team has been chosen, the team must decide what diagnosis or procedure to address first. Critical pathways are most often developed for very specific high-volume modalities and treatments used in a predictable patient population, such as total hip procedures, pneumonia, and coronary artery bypass surgery. Generally, DRGs should be considered if they involve high cost, high volume, high risk, or a combination of these factors. It is also helpful to choose a diagnosis that is well documented in the literature and has associated, research-based practice standards or CPGs that can be utilized when mapping out the care elements and interventions. It may be best to choose a simple diagnosis for your institution because the care involved varies little among patients, and it can be used as a pilot study to design and implement the first CP. For example, if your facility is known as a regional heart center and many open heart surgeries are performed each day, then begin with coronary artery bypass graft surgery (CABG). This will provide a learning tool and minimize frustration in the initial stages of pathway development (see Table 6-4 for helpful hints in selecting a CP). One strategy in the formulation stage of CP development is to set down your best expert practices on paper. Once this is done, even the least experienced practitioner can follow the best practices.[32]

CPs are also designed along specific timelines, sometimes even in hour-by-hour detail. CPs not only spell out specific actions, but also enumerate expected intermediate patient outcomes that serve

---

TABLE 6-4   SELECTION OF A CRITICAL PATHWAY

- Choose a critical pathway that assures success for your institution
- Use a DRG that is high cost, high volume, and high risk
- Choose an uncomplicated and a complicated critical pathway for the same diagnosis (eg, uncomplicated acute myocardial infarction (AMI) and complicated myocardial infarction with congestive heart failure (CHF)

---

as checkpoints for the performance of both the patient and the pathway.[8] In other words, CPs begin on day 1 of admission and progress through all the steps that will be taken by all health care providers involved in the patient's treatment (see Fig. 6-1). General outcomes are described in Table 6-5.

TABLE 6-5   EXAMPLES OF PATIENT OUTCOMES

Positive Patient Outcomes:
- Achieve the desired end result of patient care
- Document improvements in the patient's condition
- Document reversal or resolution of a patient's medical problem
- Increase patient satisfaction
- Minimize complications
- Decrease costs
- Decrease length of stay
- Lower morbidity and mortality rates
- Improve quality of life
- Improve patient self-management
- Achieve patient compliance with care plans
- Document patient satisfaction

An example of a positive patient outcome is when a patient demonstrates the correct usage of the MDI.

CPs for medical diagnoses (eg, congestive heart failure) involve inherently more variability and are therefore more difficult to distill into CPs than those for specific procedures (eg, coronary artery bypass grafts). It is therefore crucial that each discipline be clear as to what it is trying to achieve before it maps out how it will achieve it. Subsets of CPs are currently being developed; for example, CPs for asthma in children in the emergency department or for the condition of failure to wean.

Before a CP is implemented, staff members from each discipline are educated on how to use CPs. The content and amount of education necessary varies and is done for each discipline (at least in part) by a representative from that discipline so the material is presented in a relevant way. Implementing a single pathway allows the staff to learn the concept and to adapt to associated changes in a more controlled and less stressful manner. Once the lessons from the pilot pathway are learned, other pathways are introduced. Having an individual in charge of overseeing implementation of the CP on the unit or clinic level helps with consistency and compliance. This may be the case manager or clinical specialist for that area or department, or any staff person who has a solid working knowledge of practice issues and of CPs. Please refer to Chapter 5 for a detailed discussion of the respiratory therapist's role as case manager. When the CP is not used the way it was designed to be used, it is seen as a liability and the benefits are not realized. Tremendous coordination and teaching efforts are required, as well as ongoing communication and contact between the health care providers and patients.

The rapid push for CP implementation comes from intense competitive pressures and the persistent evidence of unexplained variance in medical practice.[8] It is believed that because CPs are designed around patient outcomes, if all aspects of the CP are considered, the patient outcomes will improve. But as critical thinkers, we must ask, "Is the evidence there to support this notion?" Bailey and colleagues[33] found no significant reduction in LOS, but they conclude that the CP for acute exacerbations of bronchial asthma is associated with an increase in conversion from hand-held nebulizers to metered dose inhalers because of the respiratory care assessments, resulting in substantial cost savings. No studies have shown a CP to reduce the duration of hospital stay or to decrease resource use, nor has any study shown CPs to improve patient satisfaction or outcomes in the long term.[34,35] Perhaps the limitations of CPs have been underestimated and are magnified if CPs are used as policing or auditing mechanisms rather than processes to improve clinical outcome.[34] We do know that CPs have organized health care and facilitated recovery of patients through the CQI process.[27] This has resulted in specific outcomes being influenced by care coordination, and therefore substantial cost savings for the institution are realized.

Critical Thinking Exercise 4

a. How might you choose the key personnel to include on the task force when a CP on the neuromuscular disease myasthenia gravis is being formulated? An alternative exercise would be to formulate a multidisciplinary team of students to develop the CP as part of a course or clinical grade.

b. Choose one of the different timelines that CPs use and describe a situation in respiratory care in which this timeline would be used.

Group Critical Thinking Exercise 2

THE ROLE OF THE RESPIRATORY THERAPIST IN DEVELOPING A CRITICAL PATHWAY

You are the supervisor of a respiratory therapy department in a 250-bed nonprofit hospital. Your manager has asked you to join a new multidisciplinary team of health care providers being assembled to develop CPs in your institution. At the first meeting you attend, you are asked to explain to the other committee members how your service (respiratory therapy) should be incorporated into a new CP being developed on asthma. How would you respond?

Group Critical Thinking Exercise 3

THE ROLE OF CPGS, RESPIRATORY CARE PROTOCOLS, AND CPS IN HOME HEALTH CARE

You are part of a committee to make recommendations regarding which is the appropriate tool for your organization. Develop a strategy for the clinical practice guideline, respiratory care protocol, or critical pathway design and implementation. Describe the steps taken and the reasons used when making the decision of which tool to develop for a particular disease process or procedure. How will your committee's plan be communicated to physicians, respiratory therapists, nurses, and other relevant personnel? Explain and justify the role of the respiratory therapist in the implementation phase of the process.

OUTCOMES EVALUATIONS —THE ULTIMATE GOAL

Regardless of which tool you are using in your practice, clinical practice guidelines, respiratory care protocols, or critical pathways, various outcomes should be collected and analyzed (Table 6-5). These include patient outcomes, care provider outcomes, or institutional outcomes. Why? Because the process and structure of your practice lead to these outcomes, whether they are good or bad. It is helpful to consider the purpose the data will serve for the institution when determining which outcomes to collect. There are several uses of clinical outcomes documented in the literature.[36] These include but are not limited to compliance with regulatory agencies, benchmarking, research, patient compliance, patient education, marketing, and clinical operations management. Your outcomes have the potential to change practice over time. Until the use of CPs or respiratory care protocols, the relationship between providing care in a certain way and achievement of certain outcomes had never been looked at scientifically. The former fee-for-service health care reimbursement system con-

tributed greatly to the misuse, overuse, and lack of scientific evidence to back up the health care provided. The following section is intended for practitioners using CPGs, respiratory care protocols, or CPs to design and implement outcomes evaluation.

Patient Outcomes

Indicators of patient outcomes include mortality rate, complications, patient satisfaction, and improved quality of life as evidenced by increased longevity and improved functional capacity, (eg, self-care and health-promoting behaviors).[17] Morbidity and mortality rates are the most commonly measured indicators of patient outcomes. Patient satisfaction is gaining in importance with third-party payers and should be considered an outcome to measure. Questions to address when determining which outcomes to measure include the following: Is the patient better off as a result of this treatment? Is the quality of life improved, maintained, or has it declined? Is the patient able to care for himself or herself, manage his or her own disease, and demonstrate health-promoting behaviors?

Care Provider Outcomes

Care provider outcomes include increased satisfaction with the care delivered, autonomy in practice, participation in decision making, and reduced turnover rates. Studies have shown that positive care provider outcomes lead to better patient outcomes. In a study of 9 critical care units,[37] improved patient outcomes (as evidenced by reduced risk-adjusted mortality) were demonstrated in units with the following qualities: a patient-centered focus; strong leadership as evidenced by shared visions; supportive, visible leaders; a collaborative approach to problem solving by all members of the health care team; and effective communication. Managers, who are leaders, work to provide institutional climates that promote teamwork and effective problem solving to achieve improved patient outcomes. Managers, in turn, look for these attributes when recruiting new graduates.

CRITICAL CONTENT

FOOD FOR THOUGHT

Will you be the type of respiratory therapist who is an asset to the organization where you work because you possess the skills and traits of a critical thinker? How will you contribute to the scientific foundation of your discipline and the quality of respiratory care?

Institutional Outcomes

Outcomes related to the health care facility are primarily related to costs and quality of care. LOS is commonly correlated with cost, and some studies show that the majority of costs are incurred within the first few days of a patient's stay.[37] To decrease costs to the institution, the LOS should be as short as possible; therefore, LOS is the number one variable to manipulate when attempting to save money in a health care institution. Conversely, quantifying quality of care is a harder task. To this end, it is more important to document what the patient learned, as opposed to what content was taught. This is why the evaluation of progress of the CPs or protocols becomes a verification of outcomes.[38] For instance, patient education on a COPD CP may include the need to assess understanding of the indications and use of bronchodilators. The institutional outcome to evaluate is whether the patient understands when to contact their physician. The patient is then followed after discharge to document whether the physician's office was notified or not notified prior to the next emergency department visit. These data can be used to improve patient education at discharge.

Another example of the concept of measuring what was taught versus what was learned occurs in respiratory therapy education. Respiratory therapy schools are evaluated on student outcomes. The content taught is important to outside accreditation agencies, but what really matters is what the students learn. If students learn the content, applica-

tion, and analysis, they should do well on the national board examinations. If students have not mastered the content, they will likely not do well on the national board examinations. Therefore, student performance on these board exams is one example of an institutional outcome indicator for quality. Beyond mastering the content, an important goal of respiratory therapy education is to help students develop the critical thinking skills and traits that are important to effective practice. This book has been developed to help respiratory therapy students as well as practicing respiratory therapists to engage with the content in a meaningful and practical way.

Variance Tracking

A variance is defined as the difference between how patient care and outcomes were described in the CP, protocol, or guideline, and what actually happened. In other words, variance is the difference between what you expect (good outcomes) and what you find. Variances reflect patient or caregiver issues that can have an impact on patient outcomes (Table 6-6).[39] A variance occurs when a patient does not progress as anticipated or when an expected outcome is not achieved.[40] As one author put it, "Variances alert a caregiver to the need for action, and of equal importance, serves as a database retrospectively for continuous quality improvements."[41]

Monitoring for Variances.   Monitoring for variances is a key part of the process of creating and implementing successful CPGs, respiratory care protocols, and CPs. In fact, CQI, CPGs, CPs, and respiratory care protocols work well together. The guideline, pathway, or protocol helps the health care team engage the positive challenge of reducing variation as part of the general improvement process.[40] For example, achieving an outcome earlier than expected provides clues for more cost-effective care. Timely recognition and addressing of any deviations using a CQI format is the most important step that can be taken to assure the suc-

TABLE 6-6　VARIANCES

Variances may be positive or negative. Variances are the differences between what is expected and what actually happens.

Types and examples of variances:
- *Hospital or system*: Related to the hospital or health care system
  Example:　Unable to schedule a patient for a test due to a backlog of cases; CT unavailable due to equipment malfunction
- *Clinician or caregiver:* Related to the health care provider caring for the patient
  Example:　A delay in providing specific treatment needed to move along the expected plan of care; a delay in discharge teaching for a parent of an ill child
- *Patient or family:* related to patients or family
  Example:　Having a complication from a procedure (eg, an infection); patient refuses a test that is required prior to discharge
- *Community:* Related to care provided outside of the hospital
  Example:　Lack of respiratory therapists in the community to provide needed home care; lack of nursing home beds delays a patient's discharge

cess of CPGs, CPs, or protocols and assure delivery of quality patient care. Unless a review process is in place to detect variances, a CP or respiratory care protocol is only a CPG. Protocols can be developed from CPGs as stated earlier, by incorporation of an explicit review process to measure outcomes, including variances.

Respiratory therapists are already involved in variance tracking when working under CPGs, CPs, or respiratory care protocols. For example, as part of the CQI process, a record of the number of self-extubations, the number of reintubations within 24 hours, and the number of arterial blood gas punctures are documented for a specific patient or for a specific period of time. If the number recorded exceeds the standard of care, then a variance has occurred. Students and practitioners should be aware of the advantages and disadvantages of the CQI process for tracking variances. Its advantages are that it not only includes a mechanism for tracking variances, but it serves as an educational tool to guide changes that can save time and money, and enhance the quality of patient care. The disadvantage is that tracking variances constitutes an audit process that may make clinicians wary of changes in procedures (a necessary step in individ-

ualizing care) lest there be a variance.[34] After the data are collected, analysis and reporting are the next tasks. Case managers typically develop and implement a quality improvement process for any recurrent variances found under CPs.

Respiratory therapy students should be mindful that the principles of CQI (including variance monitoring and tracking) are included on the NBRC content outline matrix for the written, registry examination. For example, Content Area I—Clinical Data includes, "develop/implement quality improvement program," and under Content Area III—Therapeutic Procedures, "conduct patient education and disease management programs" are required knowledge.

Documentation.　Accurate recording of variances is extremely important to effectively determine trends and manage problems. By effectively orchestrating all of the care given by all of the caregivers involved in the patient's treatment, CPs and respiratory care protocols can increase the efficiency and timeliness of care. Documentation on the CP or respiratory care protocol serves as a way of recording variances. Because of the amount of interaction the respiratory therapist has with the patient, he or she is able to heavily influence patient outcomes over the course of a day. Variances require timely intervention if the desired outcome is to be accomplished. If variance collection is not addressed in a timely manner, outcome measurement will not help that particular patient—only future patients will be helped as problems are solved over time.

By keeping track of variance data, administrators are able to document effectiveness of the care provided, producing effective health care that can lead to reduced LOS and presumably fewer complications. The relationship between providing care in a certain way and achievement of outcomes has not been scrutinized scientifically through randomized controlled studies, so it is difficult to sort out speculation from fact. The data are lacking to promote any particular means for providing the most effective care with the best outcomes. The National Institute of Health (NIH) and Agency for Health Care Policy and Research (AHCPR), as well as other organizations including the AARC, have called for and funded proposals to study patient outcomes. More research in this area is needed, and respiratory therapists are ideal candidates to carry out these inquiries.

Categories of variances that affect patient progression include the following:

1. Patient/family variance—These variances include anything related to patients or families that result in variance from the path. For example, noncompliance resulting in wound infection belongs in this category. Family members being unavailable or other inadequate social support systems are included as well.
2. Caregiver/clinician variance—This category includes variances related to providers, such as a delay in treatments necessary to move along the expected treatment plan, resulting in a delay in the accomplishment of an event in the pathway or protocol. Examples include timed orders not being written, slow physician response time, lack of documentation, and treatments or procedures being omitted.
3. Hospital/system variance—Includes elements of the hospital health care delivery system that

cause variances, such as lack of bed availability, schedule conflicts, and consultants and other services not being available pending payer approval.
4. Community variances—These result from community health care delivery problems that have traditionally been considered out of the scope of influence of health care practitioners. Included here are the lack of extended care nursing beds and shortage of health care providers in rural settings or in certain geographic regions of the US.

There are many formats useful for collecting and analyzing variance. The literature provides a variety of examples of practical ways to collect data on variances (or outliers) but little in terms of how to analyze variances. Generally, statistical methods are used to evaluate quantitative (numerical) data. Qualitative methods may be used to analyze nonnumerical data such as descriptions of variances if a tool like the one presented in Table 6-7 is used.

Collection of variance data tends to fall into one of four categories: notations written directly on the CP or respiratory care protocol document itself; retrospective chart review; with a separate variance data collection sheet (Table 6-7); and with computerized systems. After identifying the outliers, variance analysis is undertaken to explain the clinical reason or reasons for the deviations. Cause-and-effect relationships can be established between medical condition, treatment variables, and resource utilization within the given pathway or protocol. Armed with this information, data from current care plans can be compared to these "standard" performance indicators and changes can be made to maximize patient benefit. Thus the treatment approach is altered in real time to prevent over- or underutilization of resources.

Another reason variances are analyzed is to compare statistics relating to the effectiveness of different medical treatment plans among health care providers.[9] This process of peer comparison, or benchmarking, is the foundation of the standardization of health care delivery, as well as the

TABLE 6-7   EXAMPLES OF A VARIANCE REPORT

VARATIONS TO EXPECTED PATIENT OUTCOMES

Date: _____
Patient: _____
Date of Admission: _____
Diagnosis of DRG: _____

Unmet patient outcomes must be explained. Circle each applicable reason/cause and action. Justify actions when necesssary. Specify results of action.

Expected outcome	Reason/cause outcome not met	Actions	Results of Action
Verbalizes symptom improvement	a. Meds/O_2 not started b. Inadequate respiratory effort c. Other (specify)	1. Meds/O_2 given 2. Ventilatory support 3. Other (specify)	i. SOB relieved ii Other
Verbalizes understanding to call for assistance	a. Instructions not given c. Unable to call d. Other (specify)	1. Instructions given 2. Easy press call bell is provided 3. Other (specify)	i. Verbalizes when to call for help ii. Other
Patient transferred out of ICU on post-op day 3	a. Fever b. Hemodynamically unstable c. Unable to extubate d. Other (specify)	1. Culture sputum 2. Begin vasoactive drips as needed 3. Wean as tolerated	i. Temp. <101°F ii. V/S stable iii. SpO_2 >92%

Signature: _____

Place in Variance Box upon Discharge

maximization of its benefits. The term **benchmarking** is a general one applied to all efforts to determine not the average *utilization* of a particular diagnosis, but the *most medically appropriate utilization* per diagnosis.[9] For example, consider a decision tree diagram from a portion of the critical pathway for acute asthma in the adult shown in Fig. 6-1. Let's construct a scenario in which monitoring LOS in this CP flags an outlier case for review because of increased LOS. Among the factors contributing to increased LOS could be noncompliance to guidelines, treatment errors resulting in corrections and rework, and severity and complications of the condition. Upon chart review we find that the patient also had increased costs per day for laboratory, radiology, and respiratory care. Further investigation revealed that the reasons for the increased costs were the performance of procedures that were not in the treatment guidelines for asthma. Reviewing the progress notes tells us that the additional procedures were necessary to diagnose and treat nosocomial pneumonia developed by the patient. Because the extra procedures ordered were flagged as being a variance from the CP, the laboratory, radiology, and respiratory care services were able to react faster to investigate changes necessitated by the patient's worsening condition. Efficiency indicators are elevated for the three services, but it can be concluded that the extra procedures were medically necessary for this patient. These necessary procedures are used to justify changing the DRG from uncomplicated asthma to asthma complicated with pneumonia for reimbursement from third-party payers. The CP is adjusted for the extra time and care required to return the patient to the expected pathway.

Critical Thinking Exercise 5

a. Explain why outcomes are important to measure in the process of CQI.

b. What is the rationale for tracking variances when using CPs or respiratory care protocols?

c. Describe specific outcomes that are monitored in outcomes evaluation.

d. When negotiating respiratory care for your patients using critical pathways or respiratory care protocols, what outcomes are you seeking?

e. Consider the following question to analyze your motives when negotiating respiratory care: When you make a recommendation for respiratory care in your workplace, is it a change in therapy you are seeking or are you teaching/informing when you negotiate changes? Or are you doing both when you negotiate respiratory care? Provide examples for each possibility.

WHAT IS THE LINK BETWEEN CRITICAL THINKING AND CPS, RESPIRATORY CARE PROTOCOLS, AND CPGS?

Critical thinking in respiratory care is essential. Respiratory therapists must possess excellent assessment, decision making, and communication skills which require critical thinking. Critical thinking skills and dispositions have been researched and described in the literature.[42–44] The development and implementation of CPGs, respiratory care protocols, and CPs has opened many opportunities for respiratory therapists. However, for CPs or respiratory care protocols to be successful, respiratory therapists must become more active members of the multidisciplinary health care team and understand very clearly the potentials and problems associated with their use. A clinician who can articulate the strengths and weaknesses and advantages and disadvantages of numerous approaches to managing patients is not only a more effective health care team member, but is an excellent candidate for a leadership role.

As respiratory therapists demonstrate their use of critical thinking skills, physicians and nurses will rely even more on the technical skills for which respiratory therapists are so well trained. Various opportunities are available for respiratory therapists to merge CPs, respiratory care protocols, and CPGs into an integrated health care approach. The role of the respiratory therapist can expand to include clinical pathway team leader, respiratory consultant/assessor, disease state case manager, patient educator, CQI coordinator, and collaborative care manager, to name a few. Please refer to Chapters 5 and 9 for further discussion of the opportunities for respiratory therapists in these roles.

As respiratory therapists reflect on their practice, it is important for them to take the lead in designing the information infrastructure needed to support value-added decisions regarding efficiency and effectiveness of respiratory care and other aspects of health care. Respiratory therapists who are critical thinkers will need to create algorithms for clinical assessment of patient outcomes, construct information networks among providers, and look toward establishing CPs, respiratory care protocols, and CPGs for wellness. Respiratory therapists should immediately begin to determine the clinical information needs of patients and endeavor to meet these needs with information and appropriate education wherever they find them. Table 6-8 lists a number of questions that need to be explored further. This list is certainly not exhaustive, but it may serve as a good starting point for discussion. Research and analysis of these questions are needed because the health care delivery system of the future will be increasingly consumer-driven, and the future is here.

In conclusion, complete the following exercises individually and as group activities to facilitate your understanding, application, and analysis of the principles outlined in this chapter.

TABLE 6-8   QUESTIONS FOR FURTHER INVESTIGATION

- What are the readmission rates using CPs or respiratory care protocols?
- Is this the best practice?
- Is the patient satisfied with the care received?
- Was the quality of care maintained or improved?
- Can pathways and protocols be merged?
- Are respiratory care protocols prepared to take a leadership role in this process?
- Are adequate evaluation and accountability processes incorporated into the program?
- Are the ethical considerations, concerns, and fears being evaluated?
- Is the case manager the answer?

 Critical Thinking Exercise 6

a. Describe the role of research in connecting clinical practice guidelines, respiratory care protocols, and critical pathways.

b. Explain collaborative care. Provide reasons to institute collaborative care in patient care.

c. Explain case management.

d. Describe some of the challenges and opportunities awaiting respiratory therapists in the future.

 Group Critical Thinking Exercise 4

CRITICAL THINKING AND THE USE OF CPGS, PROTOCOLS, AND PATHWAYS

a. Debate the role of critical thinking in the use of critical pathways, respiratory care protocols, and clinical practice guidelines.

b. Discuss the value gained by the use of CPGs, respiratory care protocols, and CPs in the practice of respiratory care.

c. How will the future practice of respiratory care be impacted by the use of critical thinking skills?

 **Group Critical Thinking Exercise 5
The Pro/Con Debate**

WHICH CONCEPT IS BEST: PATHWAYS, PROTOCOLS, OR CPGS?

Divide your class or discussion group into 3 separate groups. Each group is to take one of the concepts developed in this chapter, either critical pathways, respiratory care protocols, or clinical practice guidelines.

a. Debate which concept is best to use and when. Be sure to include advantages and disadvantages of each concept. Make your argument as informative and persuasive as possible.

 Group Critical Thinking Exercise 6

DEVELOP A PATHWAY OR PROTOCOL FOR ONE RESPIRATORY DISEASE

a. Develop a critical pathway or respiratory care protocol for one of the disease processes discussed in this book.

b. Outline the critical elements of the pathway or protocol that will provide the best and most efficient patient care possible.

 Group Critical Thinking Exercise 7

REFLECTION TO IMPROVE FUTURE CLINICAL DECISION MAKING

a. Propose questions to be asked (as in Table 6-8) and present ways to investigate these questions. For example, a patient is enrolled in a pulmonary rehabilitation program. Ask questions such as the following: Is your patient satisfied with care? Is it the best practice? Is the quality of life maintained or improved after a 6-week program? Are there any ethical considerations? How do ethics and costs affect the long-term management plan? Who should answer these questions?

b. Draw a conclusion about the level of participation required of a staff RT in answering your questions.

REFERENCES

1. Hess D. Clinical practice guidelines—Valuable resources. *NBRC Horizons.* 1997;23:1, 6.

2. Hess D. The AARC clinical practice guidelines. *Respir Care.* 1991;36:1398–1401.

3. Brougher P. CPGs 1994: Where are we? Where have we been? Where are we going? *Respir Care.* 1994;39:1146–1148.

4. Nielson-Tietsort J, Poole B, Creagh CE, et al.: Respiratory care protocol: An approach to in-hospital respiratory therapy. *Respir Care.* 1981;26:430–441.

5. Des Jardines T, Burton GG, Tietsort J. *Respiratory Care Case Studies: The Therapist-Driven Protocol Approach.* St. Louis: Mosby-Year Book; 1997.

6. Weber K, Milligan S. Conference Summary—Therapist-driven protocols: The state of the art. *Respir Care.* 1994;39:746–756.

7. Coffey R, Richard J, Remmert C, et al. An introduction to critical paths. *Quality Manage Health Care.* 1992;1:45–54.

8. Pearson SD, Goulart-Fisher D, Lee T. Critical pathways as a strategy for improving care: Problems and potentials. *Ann Int Med.* 1995;123:941–948.

9. Dykes PC. An introduction to critical pathways. In: Dykes PC, Wheeler K, eds. *Planning, Implementing and Evaluating Critical Pathways: A Guide for the 21st Century.* New York: Springer; 1997.

10. Birdsall C, Sperry S. *Clinical Paths in Medical-Surgical Practice.* St. Louis; Mosby-Year Book; 1997.

11. Hess D. The AARC clinical practice guidelines. *Respir Care.* 1991;36:1398–1401.

12. Hess D. Clinical practice guidelines: Why, whence, and whither? *Respir Care.* 1995;40:1264–1267.

13. Stoller JK, Haney D, Burkhart J, et al. Physician-ordered respiratory care vs. physician-ordered use of a respiratory therapy consult service: Early experience at the Cleveland Clinic Foundation. *Respir Care.* 1993;38:1143–1154.

14. Shrake KL, Scaggs JE, England BA, et al. Benefits associated with a respiratory care assessment-treatment program: Results of a pilot study. *Respir Care.* 1994;39:715–724.

15. Komara JJ Jr, Stoller JK. The impact of a post-operative oxygen therapy protocol on use of pulse oximetry and oxygen therapy. *Respir Care.* 1995; 40: 1125–1129.

16. Orens DK: A manager's perspective on respiratory therapy consult services. *Respir Care.* 1993;38:884–886.

17. McGinn P. Practice standards leading to premium reductions. *AMA News.* 1988 Dec;2:1, 28.

18. Thompson RS, Kirz HL, Gold RA. Changes in physician behavior and cost savings associated with organizational recommendations on the use of routine chest x-rays and multichannel blood tests. *Prevent Med.* 1983;12:385–396.

19. Brougher LI, Blackwelder AK, Grossman GD, et al. Effectiveness of medical necessity guidelines in reducing cost of oxygen therapy. *Chest.* 1986;90:646–648.

20. Shapiro BA, Cane RD, Peterson J, et al. Authoritative medical direction can assure cost-beneficial bronchial hygiene therapy. *Chest.* 1988;90:1038–1042.

21. Browning JA, Kaiser DL, Durbin CG Jr. The effect of guidelines on the appropriate use of arterial blood gas analysis in the intensive care unit. *Respir Care.* 1988;34:269–276.

22. Small D, Duha A, Wieskopf B, et al. Uses and misuses of oxygen in hospitalized patients. *Am J Med.* 1992;92:591–595.

23. Kester L, Stoller JK: Ordering respiratory care services for hospitalized patients: Practices for overuse and underuse. *Cleveland Clin J Med.* 1992;59:581–585.

24. Shrake KL, Scaggs JE, England KR, et al. A respiratory care assessment-treatment program: Results of a retrospective study. *Respir Care.* 1996;41:703–711.

25. Stoller JK, Skibinski CI, Giles DK, et al. Physician-ordered respiratory care vs. physician-ordered use of respiratory therapy consult service: Results of a prospective observational study. *Chest.* 1996;110:422–429.

26. Tietsort J. The respiratory care protocol: A management tool for the '90s. *AARC Times* 1991;15:55–62.

27. Berger JT, Rosner F. The ethics of practice guidelines. *Arch Intern Med.* 1996;156:2051–2056.

28. Gruiliano KK, Porrer CE: Nursing case management: Critical paths to desirable outcomes. *Nursing Manage.* 1991;22:52–55.

29. Hoffman PA. Critical path method. J Quality Improvement 1993;June:235–246.

30. Ignatavicius DD, Hausaman KA. Clinical *Pathways for Collaborative Practice*. Philadelphia: Saunders; 1995.

31. American Association for Respiratory Care, 11030 Ables Lane, Dallas, Texas 75229.

32. Benner, P. *From Novice to Expert: Excellence and Power in Clinical Nursing Practice*. Menlo Park, Calif: Addison-Wesley; 1984.

33. Bailey R, Weingarten S, Lewis M, et al. Impact of clinical pathways and practice guidelines on the management of acute exacerbations of bronchial asthma. *Chest*. 1998;113:28–33.

34. Zander K. Collaborative care: Two effective strategies for positive outcomes. In: Zander K, ed. *Managing Outcomes through Collaborative Care*. American Hospital Association, 1995.

35. Falconer JA, Roth EJ, Sutin JA, et al. The critical path method in stroke rehabilitation: Lessons from an experiment in cost containment and outcome improvement. *QRB Quality Rev Bull*. 1993;19:8–16.

36. Docherty J, Dewan N: Guide to outcomes management. Paper presented at the meeting of the National Association of Psychiatric Health Systems, Greater Bridgeport Mental Health Center, Bridgeport, Conn. In Dykes PC, Wheeler K, eds. *Planning, Implementing and Evaluating Critical Pathways: A Guide for the 21st Century*. New York: Springer; 1997.

37. Dykes CD, Slye DA. Data collection, outcomes measurement, and variance analysis. In: Dykes PC, Wheeler K, eds. *Planning, Implementing and Evaluating Critical Pathways: A Guide for the 21st Century*. New York: Springer; 1997.

38. Zimmerman JE, Shortwell SM, Rousseau UM. Improving intensive care: Observation based on organizational case studies in nine units: A prospective multicenter study. *Crit Care Med*. 1993;21: 1443–1451.

39. Schriefer J. Managing critical pathway variances. *Quality Manage Health Care*. 1995;3:30–42.

40. Aronson B, Maljanian R. Critical path education: Necessary components and effective strategies. *J Continuing Education Nursing*. 1996;27:215–219.

41. Zander K. Critical pathways. In: Melum M, Sinoris M, eds. *Total Quality Management: The Health Care Pioneers*. Chicago: American Hospital Association Publishing; 1992, 305.

42. Facione P. Critical thinking: A statement of expert consensus for purposes of educational assessment and instruction. The Delphi Report: Research findings and recommendations for the American Philosophical Association. ERIC Doc. No. 315–423; 1990.

43. Paul RW. *Critical Thinking: How to Prepare Students for a Rapidly Changing World*. Santa Rosa, Calif: The Foundation for Critical Thinking; 1993.

44. McPeck JE. Teaching critical thinking: Dialogue and didactic. New York: Routledge; 1990.

7

PATIENT ASSESSMENT AND RESPIRATORY CARE PLAN DEVELOPMENT

David C. Shelledy and Stephen P. Mikles

The pause—that impressive silence, that eloquent silence, that geometrically progressive silence, which often achieves a desired effect where no combination of words, however felicitous, could accomplish it.

MARK TWAIN
(1835–1910)

LEARNING OBJECTIVES

1. Discuss the significance of reviewing the patient history to include: demographic data, chief complaint (CC), history of present illness (HPI), past medical history (PMH), family history.

2. Describe the important aspects of the patient interview as performed by the respiratory therapist.

3. Summarize these aspects of physical assessment of the pulmonary patient: vital signs, inspection, palpation, percussion, auscultation.

4. Define the acronyms POMR and SOAP.

5. Distinguish key diagnostic data to include: arterial blood gases, chest radiography, pulmonary function studies, complete blood count.

6. Evaluate patient history, physical assessment, and diagnostic data for a pulmonary patient.

7. Write a SOAP note for a pulmonary patient using the information from history, physical assessment, and diagnostic data.

8. Explain how to assess a patient for respiratory care plan development, to include medical record review, patient interview, physical assessment, and bedside measures of pulmonary function.

9. Identify the key elements of a respiratory care plan.

10. Give examples of the types of respiratory care plans.

11. Describe the goals of a basic respiratory care plan, including appropriate outcome measures.

12. Outline the key steps in development and implementation of the respiratory care plan.

13. Identify techniques to consider for the respiratory care plan to improve oxygenation, provide for secretion management, treat bronchospasm and mucosal edema, and deliver lung expansion therapy.

14. Develop a respiratory care plan to maintain adequate tissue oxygenation.

15. Create a respiratory care plan for the treatment and/or prevention of bronchospasm and mucosal edema.

16. Design a respiratory care plan to mobilize secretions.

17. Propose a respiratory care plan for the treatment and/or prevention of atelectasis and pneumonia.

INTRODUCTION

The purpose of this chapter is to review the basic principles of assessment needed for the development and modification of a respiratory care plan. Patient history, physical assessment, and a review of important diagnostic data are included. Development of the respiratory care plan is described to include a review of the various respiratory care treatment options, patient assessment for care plan development, and key elements of a basic respiratory care plan. Sample care plans and protocols for typical patient conditions are also included with this chapter.

Rationale for Patient Assessment

There are several important reasons for the respiratory therapist to routinely use assessment skills on patients. Admitting history and physicals are often rushed. The respiratory therapist may find something significant that was overlooked. Change over a period of time in chest physical findings (for better or worse) is a key indicator of the patient's progress. Government and other third-party payers are insisting that objective, documented results of therapy be obtained; otherwise they may not pay. And last, an informal patient history can do no worse than simply improve the therapist's relationship with the patient.

In summary, the rationale for routine use of the basic principles of assessment by the respiratory therapist include:

- to augment admission history and physical
- to recommend therapy
- to monitor the patient's condition over time
- to modify or terminate therapy
- to provide documentation of results of therapy
- to develop, implement, and monitor the respiratory care plan

PATIENT ASSESSMENT FOR CARE PLAN DEVELOPMENT

In order to select the appropriate care for a specific patient, the respiratory therapist must complete a thorough patient assessment. Patient assessment for respiratory care plan development should include a review of the patient's medical record or chart, a patient interview, and physical assessment. The bedside measurement of parameters related to oxygenation and pulmonary function should be considered, where appropriate. SpO_2 may be measured to assess the patient's oxygenation status. Arterial blood gases should be obtained if there is a concern regarding ventilatory status, acid-base balance, or the reliability of pulse oximetry values. Inspiratory capacity and/or vital capacity should be measured in patients for whom lung expansion therapy is being considered. Peak expiratory flow (PEF) and/or FEV_1 may also be assessed, in order to determine the need for and effectiveness of bronchodilator therapy.

PATIENT HISTORY

The general medical history taken on the patient should include the collection of demographic data, chief complaint (CC), history of the present illness (HPI), past medical history (PMH), and family history.[1] The general patient history may be taken by the physician or nurse during an initial office or clinic visit, or by the physician, nurse, physician's assistant, respiratory therapist, or other health care worker upon admission to the acute care facility.[1] A brief overview of the general medical history follows, with an emphasis on findings related to the cardiopulmonary patient.

Demographic Data and Patient Profile

Demographic data and the patient profile provide the respiratory therapist with a snapshot of the patient in terms of name, address, age, gender, ethnicity, admitting diagnosis, and medical problems.

Other information to obtain includes the name(s) of the physician(s) caring for the patient and a brief description of why the patient sought medical care. The patient profile may include the what, where, how, why, and when of the patient's current condition. A personal history including place of birth, home environment, education, socioeconomic status, and marital status may also be useful.

Chief Complaint

The chief complaint is a succinct statement by the patient relating their reason for seeking medical attention.[1] Examples may include shortness of breath, cough, fever, or chest pain. It is their primary symptom described in their own terms. Breathlessness is perhaps the most common pulmonary complaint.[2] For example, the patient may say, "I can't get enough air when I walk to the mailbox." Wheezing may be related as, "my chest is tight." Cough is often considered the "watchdog" of the lung. In general, it should be considered abnormal to cough.[2] Development of a cough, or a change in a chronic cough, may be significant. For example, a nonproductive cough is an early finding in the development of chronic bronchitis due to cigarette smoking.[2] Sputum production is often a primary complaint whether the disease is acute or chronic in nature. The previously healthy person may refer to the recent expectoration of "rust-colored phlegm." The patient with chronic bronchitis may report an increase in volume of sputum expectorated with a concomitant change in color and consistency. The chief complaint provides a starting point from which to guide the patient history, physical exam, and laboratory work-up. Identifying the chief complaint is often the first step in determining the admitting or principal diagnosis.

History of Present Illness (HPI)

The history of the present illness is a detailed narrative by the patient.[1] The skilled interviewer uses effective questioning techniques to encourage an open exchange with the patient about their illness. Every symptom that the patient relates is fully described regarding such pertinent factors as onset, location, frequency, and severity. The importance of the HPI cannot be overstated because it directs the subsequent physical assessment and pertinent laboratory tests. When complete, a clear chronological account of the present illness should result. The principal symptoms should be described in terms of location, quality, quantity or severity, timing (onset, duration, frequency), the setting in which they occur, factors which aggravate or relieve them, and associated manifestations.[1] The key elements of the HPI are summarized in the critical content box.

CRITICAL CONTENT

ITEMS TO INCLUDE IN THE HISTORY OF THE PRESENT ILLNESS

- Onset (date, time, sudden, gradual)
- Nature of complaint (quality and quantity)
- Course of the complaint (progression over time)
- Location (Where is the pain, discomfort or other symptom? Does it spread?)
- Exacerbations (What is the cause? When has it gotten worse? What makes it better or worse?)
- Treatment (What has been done?)

Past Medical History (PMH)

The past medical history may range from brief to extensive. The PMH is primarily determined by the nature of the illness. For example, the past medical history for a 60-year-old patient with longstanding chronic bronchitis will greatly exceed in length that of a 20-year-old athlete with acute viral pneumonia. When taking the patient's history, the interviewer should assess the patient's ability to accurately answer specific questions. It may be prudent to interview family members and request past medical information on file if the patient is confused or disoriented. Medications, past reasons for hospitalization, and smoking history are critical components of a good past medical history.[1] For example, in the asthmatic patient a past medical history of intubation, prior admission to an intensive care unit, two or more hospitalizations or three or more ED visits in the past year, use of more than two canisters per month of short-acting bronchodilators, systemic steroid use, or an ER visit or hospitalization due to asthma in the last month may place the patient at risk for death from asthma.[3] Information that should be included in the general past medical history is summarized in the critical content box.

CRITICAL CONTENT

ITEMS TO INCLUDE IN THE PAST MEDICAL HISTORY

- General state of health (as the patient perceives it)
- Childhood illnesses (measles, rubella, mumps, whooping cough, rheumatic fever, scarlet fever, polio, cystic fibrosis, bronchiectasis, aspiration)
- Adult illnesses
- Psychiatric illnesses
- Accidents and injuries
- Operations
- Hospitalizations
- Thoracic trauma, surgery
- Respiratory care received (oxygen, history of intubation, history of mechanical ventilation, use of metered dose inhalers [MDIs] or aerosolized medication, other)
- Pulmonary disease-tuberculosis, bronchitis, emphysema, asthma, bronchiectasis, etc.
- Cardiac problems-congestive heart failure (CHF), myocardial infarction (MI), cor pulmonale, etc.
- Cancer—lung, other
- Testing—allergies, pulmonary function tests (PFTs), tuberculin (PPD), fungal skin tests, chest radiographs, etc.
- Exposure to respiratory infections, influenza, tuberculosis

Family History

The list of cardiopulmonary diseases with hereditary or infectious association is extensive. For infectious diseases, the nuclear family is typically the focus. The health status of relatives, including parents, siblings, and grandparents, often plays an important role in establishing a familial link with hereditary diseases. Asthma, cystic fibrosis, and panlobular emphysema are notable pulmonary diseases with a hereditary predisposition. Pneumonia and tuberculosis are infectious diseases that often spread via contact with immediate family members. A family history of cancer, heart disease, renal disease, or diabetes should be noted.

CHART REVIEW AND PATIENT INTERVIEW

Regardless of who obtains the patient's initial history, the respiratory therapist should always perform a chart review, and when possible a patient interview, in order to assess the patient's respiratory care. The purpose of the patient interview performed by the respiratory therapist is to determine the appropriateness of ordered respiratory care, to determine goals of therapy, and to monitor, evaluate, and modify or discontinue therapy based on the patient's response. A patient interview performed by the respiratory therapist is essential for respiratory care plan development, implementation, and evaluation.

Chart Review

The chart review should include patient age, gender, diagnosis, problem list, and current physician orders. Previous blood gas studies, chest x-ray, and pulmonary function testing reports should be reviewed, as well as the results of other diagnostic studies, including sputum, acid-fast bacillus (AFB) culture, sensitivity, cytology, and silver stain. Table 7-1 outlines the key elements of the review of the patient medical record.

TABLE 7-1   ITEMS IN THE MEDICAL RECORD TO BE REVIEWED WHEN DEVELOPING A RESPIRATORY CARE PLAN

Patient Data	Diagnostic tests ordered (ABGs, PFTs,
Name	sputum exam, CBC, electrolytes, etc.)
Age	Cardiac/cardiovascular medications
Gender	Antibiotics
Height	Anticoagulants
Weight	History and physical examination
Ideal body weight	Results of diagnostic testing
Physician	Arterial blood gases
Floor or unit	Chest x-ray reports
Room number of bed	Pulmonary function test results
Diagnosis	Sputum samples
Problem list	Other lab work (CBC, electrolytes, etc.)
Current physician orders	Respiratory care progress notes
Oxygen therapy	Therapy given
Aerosol bronchodilators	Patient response to therapy
Chest physiotherapy	Measured Parameters (SpO$_2$, IC, VC, MIP,
IPPB and/or incentive spirometry	MEP, PEFR, FEV$_{1.0}$, etc.)
Other current respiratory care orders	

SOURCE: Used with permission from the University of Texas Health Science Center at San Antonio, Department of Respiratory Care, Patient Assessment and Respiratory Care Plan.

Patient Interview

As noted above, the patient interview is an important part of patient assessment performed by respiratory therapists. The purpose of the patient interview is to collect subjective data from the patient and/or family members. During the interview the respiratory therapist asks a series of questions to get a clear idea of the patient's condition.

The respiratory therapist must have good communication skills, including effective listening, to conduct a successful patient interview.[4] Interviewing skills can improve with practice and experience. Communication skills are so important for effective respiratory care that an entire chapter is devoted to this topic. You should refer to Chapter 4 to gain a clear understanding of the importance of communications for numerous aspects of respiratory care practice. You are encouraged to complete the exercises in Chapter 4 to help you to gain experience and confidence in your communication skills. As you further develop and refine your communication skills, you will be able to conduct successful patient interviews. You will also be able to function more effectively as a member of the health care team.

The successful patient interview includes these components:

1. Establish patient rapport so you can obtain the most accurate description of the patient's condition.
2. Gather information about the patient's condition, including a chronology of events and the patient's impressions of his or her health.
3. Obtain feedback from the patient regarding your understanding of the patient's answers to your questions.
4. Involve the family, especially caregivers, in the patient interview whenever possible.
5. Demonstrate to the patient and the family that you understand the patient's problems and will work with them to obtain the appropriate care.

6. Build on initial rapport to enhance further assessment, evaluations, and treatment plans.
7. Provide additional assessment, evaluation, and treatment plan for chronic cardiopulmonary conditions to facilitate disease management.

The patient interview should include questions to assess cough, sputum production, hemoptysis, wheezing, whistling or chest tightness, dyspnea, past history of chest illness, smoking history, occupation, and where appropriate, hobby and leisure activities. The patient interview should also include questions regarding the patient's current medications, use of oxygen in the home, use of other respiratory care equipment, and history of previous episodes requiring intubation or mechanical ventilatory support. The patient interview should also include questions to assess the benefits of any respiratory care the patient is currently receiving, as well as any adverse effects of respiratory care the patient may have experienced. Table 7-2 outlines the key elements of the patient interview for care plan development.

Cough and Sputum Production. During the interview the respiratory therapist should ask questions to determine: 1) when the patient coughs (morning or other times?), 2) how often the patient coughs (most days?), and 3) if the cough is associated with a specific activity or location. A morning cough is common in smokers. A cough on most days for as many as 3 months of the year, which is productive of a tablespoonful or more of sputum in the absence of other pulmonary disease, is by definition chronic bronchitis. A cough associated with plants, pets, dusts, or other allergens may be treatable by avoidance of the allergen or irritant. A cough or shortness of breath that subsides over the weekend and recurs on Monday morning may be a sign of an occupationally-related disorder; a classic example is byssinosis. Cotton workers exposed to the dust of cotton will develop a COPD-like syndrome and complain of shortness of breath, chest tightness, or wheezing on Monday mornings when they return to work after the weekend.[5] A change in the nature of the cough may indicate a major change in the patient's condition. Remember, in any case a cough is not normal and its presence may indicate a problem.

Sputum production is also very important. Some sputologists go to great lengths to monitor the volume, consistency, color, odor, and even microscopic appearance of sputum. One method of monitoring sputum production is to simply place a clean sample container at the bedside for a 24-hour period. The able, cooperative patient is instructed to deposit all sputum produced into the container. Frequently, respiratory therapists only record sputum produced following a specific treatment or procedure. The use of a 24-hour collection and monitoring system helps ensure that the therapist is aware of sputum production that occurs when he or she is not present.

T A B L E 7 - 2   ITEMS TO INCLUDE IN THE PATIENT INTERVIEW FOR RESPIRATORY CARE PLAN DEVELOPMENT

Cough	Smoking
Sputum production	Occupational history
Hemoptysis	Hobby and leisure history
Wheezing, whistling, or chest tightness	Medications
Breathlessness	Home respiratory care
History of chest illness	History of intubation and/or mechanical
Previous hospitalizations and/or ICU	ventilation
admissions	Response to respiratory care received

SOURCE: Used with permission from The University of Texas Health Science Center at San Antonio, Department of Respiratory Care, Patient Assessment and Respiratory Care Plan.

Table 7-3 provides an introduction to sputology, the interpretation of sputum production, color, consistency, and other characteristics. The key factors to be considered when evaluating a patient's cough and sputum production are summarized in the critical content box.

Wheezing, Whistling, and Chest Pain or Tightness. The patient should be asked about their breathing using open-ended questions. Patients with cardiopulmonary disease may describe wheezing, whistling, and chest pain or tightness. For example, recurrent wheezing, chest tightness or difficulty in

---

TABLE 7-3   BASIC INTERPRETATION OF SPUTUM PRODUCTION: AN INTRODUCTION TO SPUTOLOGY

With respect to gross examination of sputum produced, the following items are important for assessment:

Change in sputum production. An increase or decrease in sputum production may mean the patient is getting better or it may mean he or she is getting worse. Sputum production should decrease gradually with improvement.
   1. Sudden increase: Rupture of abscess or release of blocked bronchi
   2. Sudden decrease: Obstruction, dehydration, poor humidity

Color. Green-colored sputum is associated with acute infection, sometimes from draining sinuses. White or yellow purulent sputum is also indicative of infection, such as in pneumonia or bronchitis. Brown or off-white brownish sputum is associated with a longstanding infection such as chronic bronchitis. A classic "currant jelly" appearance or brick-red color to the sputum is associated with a *Klebsiella* infection. Alcoholics and elderly diabetics often develop *Klebsiella* pneumonia. Frothy pink sputum may indicate pulmonary edema. Also, some inhaled medications turn sputum pink.

Hemoptysis. Blood tinged sputum is associated with a large number of pulmonary disorders. If the blood is bright red and in significant amounts, the origin is probably the upper airway or large lower airway.

Consistency. The viscosity of sputum is partly a function of the sputum's water content. It should be noted whether the sputum is tenacious (associated with dehydration), mucoid, or purulent.

Odor. Foul smelling sputum is associated with long-term infections such as those found with bronchiectasis, lung abscess, cystic fibrosis, or aspiration. *Pseudomonas* has a peculiar sweet smell.

Curschmann's spirals. These are mucus plugs that have been coughed out; they are associated with bronchial asthma.

With advanced cases of bronchiectasis, the sputum settles out into three layers:
   1. Top layer: Cloudy
   2. Middle layer: Clear saliva
   3. Bottom layer: Cloudy purulent

Obtaining a satisfactory sputum specimen for gram stain, culture, and sensitivity or cytology requires special care. Methods for obtaining a sputum specimen include the directed cough, use of ultrasonic nebulizers with sterile distilled water, or hypertonic (3% to 7% NaCl) heated aerosols. The latter must be used with caution. The high salt content of the inhaled aerosol may literally pull water out of the mucosa (osmolar transudation) to help provide a sputum specimen.

CRITICAL CONTENT

COUGH AND SPUTUM SUMMARY

1. Onset: sudden, gradual; duration
2. Nature of cough: dry, moist, wet, hacking, hoarse, barking, whooping, bubbling, productive, nonproductive
   a. Sputum production: duration, frequency, with activity, at certain times of day
   b. Sputum characteristics: amount, color (clear, mucoid, purulent, blood-tinged, mostly blood), foul odor
   c. Sputum volume (estimate in mL, teaspoons, or tablespoons)
3. Pattern: occasional, regular, paroxysmal; related to time of day, weather, activities, talking, deep breaths; change over time
4. Severity: severe enough to tire patient, disrupt sleep or conversation, cause chest pain
5. Associated symptoms: shortness of breath, chest pain or tightness with breathing, fever, upper respiratory signs, noisy respirations, hoarseness, gagging, choking, stress
6. Efforts to treat: prescription or nonprescription drugs, vaporizers, other

breathing, or a cough that is worse at night are associated with a diagnosis of asthma.[3] The interviewer should ask direct questions to determine any changes in the frequency, duration, and related circumstances. Remember that all that wheezes is not asthma. Once again, a major point of interest is a change in symptoms and what factors are associated with that change. For example, exercise-induced asthma is associated with breathing cold air while exercising.[6] Occupational or environmental irritants or allergens may be pinpointed by a careful patient interview. Some patients may experience shortness of breath at night, known as paroxysmal nocturnal dyspnea (PND). PND is associated with congestive heart failure, which can also cause wheezing, and therefore it is sometimes referred to as cardiac asthma.

Chest Pain. There are 3 basic types of chest pain a patient may describe:

1. Substernal: associated with angina pectoris and MI. The patient may complain that it feels as if someone is "standing on my chest." The pain may radiate down the arms or up to the jaw. Unexplained severe central chest pain lasting 2 minutes or longer in at-risk patients with no known cardiac disease may indicate an MI, and appropriate action should be taken immediately.
2. Pleuritic: sharp, localized pain, often at the periphery of the chest.
3. Musculoskeletal: associated with rib fractures and/or chest trauma. Musculoskeletal pain often varies as the patient breathes and moves about.

CRITICAL CONTENT

THREE BASIC TYPES OF CHEST PAIN

- Substernal
- Pleuritic
- Musculoskeletal

The onset and duration of chest pain, and whether the pain is associated with trauma, coughing, movement, or lower respiratory infection should be noted. Associated symptoms such as shallow breathing, fever, uneven chest expansion, coughing, anxiety about getting enough air, or radiation of the pain to the neck or arms should also be noted during the patient interview. Efforts to treat chest pain with heat, splinting, or pain medication should also be included.

Shortness of Breath. Dyspnea is defined as the conscious sensation of being short of breath. Shortness of breath is often the chief complaint in patients with cardiopulmonary disorders.[2] It is very helpful to quantify the degree of dyspnea a patient suffers. This can be done by asking the patient

TABLE 7-4   SEVERITY OF DYSPNEA IN THE EVALUATION OF PERMANENT IMPAIRMENT

Class I	Dyspnea only on severe exertion ("appropriate" dyspnea)
Class II	Can keep pace with person of same age and body build on a level surface without breathlessness, but not on hills or stairs
Class III	Can walk a mile at own pace without dyspnea, but cannot keep pace on a level surface with a normal person
Class IV	Dyspnea present after walking about 100 yards on a level surface, or upon climbing one flight of stairs
Class V	Dyspnea with even less activity, or even at rest

Source: Modified from Committee on Rating of Mental and Physical Impairment. Guides to the evaluation of permanent impairment—the respiratory system. *JAMA.* 1965:194;919.

about activity and any resulting breathlessness as illustrated in Table 7-4. Key factors to be considered when evaluating a patient's shortness of breath are summarized in the critical content box.

CRITICAL CONTENT

SHORTNESS OF BREATH SUMMARY

Factors to be considered when evaluating a patient for shortness of breath:

1. Onset: sudden or gradual; duration; gagging or choking event a few days before onset
2. Pattern:
   a. Position most comfortable, number of pillows used
   b. Related to extent of exercise, certain activities, time of day, eating
   c. Harder to inhale or exhale
3. Severity: extent of activity limitation, tiring or fatigue with breathing, anxiety about getting air
4. Associated symptoms: pain or discomfort (relationship to specific point in respiratory exertion, location), cough, diaphoresis, swelling of ankles

Chest Illness.   A past history of chest illness can be useful in assessing a patient's current cardiopulmonary status. The patient should be questioned as to the frequency of chest colds, bronchitis, or pneumonia. The patient should also be asked if he or she has ever been told that they had any type of lung disease or chest injury. Medications taken for breathing problems (current or past) should be noted. Exposure to tuberculosis or influenza should also be noted.

Smoking History.   Obviously, obtaining a smoking history is an important part of the patient interview. The patient should be questioned about the use of pipes, cigars, and cigarettes. The number of years smoked as well as the amount consumed per day should be noted. For cigarettes, 1 pack/day × 1 year = 1 pack year. Occasionally patients will be less than forthcoming in describing current tobacco use. Inspection of the fingers for nicotine stains can be helpful in identifying closet smokers. Measurement of carboxyhemoglobin (CoHb) levels as part of an arterial blood gas study can also be useful in identifying patients who continue to smoke, yet who deny that they are still smoking. Smoking causes chronic bronchitis and is strongly associated with the development of emphysema and lung cancer. Smokers also seem to be at risk for developing more severe disease in the presence of coal worker's pneumoconiosis (CWP) and asbestosis. Successful smoking cessation programs include an individualized patient evaluation, patient-specific education, addiction therapy, follow-up, and relapse prevention. A relatively recent and apparently widespread smoking problem in terms of lung disease is the use of marijuana. Marijuana smoking has been associated with the development of bronchitis. The smoking of crack cocaine has been associated with the development of cough, dyspnea, chest pain, hemoptysis, airway burns, and other acute respiratory symptoms. Therefore, a history of smoking marijuana or other drugs should be noted.

Occupational History and Environmental Data. There are a large number of lung diseases that are associated with specific occupations. Patients should be questioned regarding occupational exposure and environmental factors associated with the development of lung disease. A list of occupations associated with specific lung disease is found in Table 7-5.

In addition, some types of lung diseases are endemic to specific areas or activities. For example, histoplasmosis is endemic to the Ohio and Mississippi river valleys. Coccidioidomycosis is prevalent in the San Joaquin valley in California, as well as parts of New Mexico, Utah, and Texas. Cryptococcoses are associated with excreta from pigeons and other birds. Psittacosis is associated with bird fanciers. Finally, with respect to specific environmental data, one should question the patient about allergies, hobbies, and pets.

The following summarizes the elements of an abbreviated pulmonary history. One can quickly ask the patient about these major areas, with a positive response prompting a more in-depth interview.

CRITICAL CONTENT

ABBREVIATED PULMONARY HISTORY

- Cough and sputum production
- Wheezing, whistling, and chest tightness
- Breathlessness
- Past chest illness
- Smoking

PHYSICAL ASSESSMENT

Overview

Physical assessment of the patient provides additional important information needed to develop and assess the respiratory care plan. The physical assessment should include general appearance, level of consciousness, assessment of oxygenation and perfusion (skin color, nailbeds, skin characteristics, capillary refill), chest inspection including use of accessory muscles, chest excursion and respiratory pattern, and assessment of breath sounds.[2,7] Palpation techniques may be used to determine the presence of tactile rhonchi or vocal fremitus. Percussion of the chest may be helpful to assess hyperinflation or pneumothorax (hyperresonance), atelectasis, or pleural fluid (dullness on percussion). Bedside measurement of pulse and respiration should be performed to assess for tachycardia, bradycardia, or tachypnea. Blood pressure should be measured in patients who seem to be doing poorly. SpO_2 should also be assessed for most patients, as it is a simple and low-cost method of determining oxygenation status. Inspiratory capacity should be measured in patients at risk of developing atelectasis and in all patients being considered for or receiving lung expansion therapy. Patients receiving bronchodilator therapy should also have FEV_1 measured before and after therapy, or at minimum a peak expiratory flow rate (PEFR) measurement. Arterial blood gases may be obtained to confirm suspected hypoxemia, identify suspected hypoventilation, and assess acid-base status. Lastly, bedside measurement of vital capacity (VC) and maximum inspiratory force may be helpful in assessing ventilatory muscle strength and the ability to cough and breathe deeply. Table 7-6 summarizes the key elements of the physical assessment for care plan development.

Vital Signs

Temperature. Temperature is an important vital sign that can be obtained orally, rectally, axillary, or tympanically. The site used to obtain body tempera-

TABLE 7-5   OCCUPATIONS ASSOCIATED WITH SPECIFIC LUNG DISEASES

Aluminum pneumoconiosis
  Ammunition maker
  Fireworks maker
Asbestosis (associated with smoking)
  Asbestos weaver
  Brake manufacturer
  Clutch manufacturer
  Filter maker
  Floor tile maker
  Insulator
  Lagger
  Mill worker
  Miner or miller
  Roofer
  Shipbuilder
  Steam fitter

Beryllium disease
  Alloymaker
  Bronze maker
  Ceramics worker
  Demolition person
  Electronic tube maker
  Extraction worker
  Fettler
  Flame cutter
  Foundryman
  Grinder
  Metalworker
  Metalizer
  Polisher
  Scarfer

Bagassosis: Sugar cane worker

Byssinosis: Cotton flax or hemp mill worker

Baritosis (Barium)
  Barite miller and miner
  Ceramics worker
  Fluorescent lamp maker
  Glassmaker
  Metallurgist
  Missile worker
  Neon sign maker

  Nuclear energy worker
  Phosphor maker
  Propellant manufacturer
  Toxicologist
  X-ray tube maker

Coal worker's pneumoconiosis (CWP)[a]
(Black lung associated with smoking)
  Coal miner
  Motorman
  Roof bolter
  Tipple worker
  Trimmer

Interstitial Lung Disease (ILD)
  Farming (associated with moldy hay)

Kaolinosis (Clay)
  Brick maker
  Ceramics worker
  China maker
  Miner
  Potter

Occupational asthma
Animal-derived materials
  Laboratory workers (medical labs,
    veterinarians)
  Breeders (birds, rabbits, other)
  Food processors (poultry, seafood)
Plants and vegetable products
  Food processors
  Grain handlers
  Textile workers
  Bakers
  Printers
  Laxative manufacturers
Enzymes, chemicals, and drugs
  Detergent manufacturers
  Food processors
  Pharmaceutical workers
  Printers
  Chemical workers
  Foam manufacturers
  Plastic workers

Continued

TABLE 7-5   Continued

Dye workers	Fettler
Farmers	Filter Maker
Hairdressers	Foundryman
Hospital workers	Miner or miller
Food wrappers	Motorman
Wood dust (carpenters, woodworkers, etc.)	Paint maker
Metal workers (aluminum soldering, metal plating, etc.)	Polisher
	Quarry man
	Sandblaster
Siderosis (Iron)	Shotblaster
Ship breaker	Stonecutter
Welder	Stone driller
	Well driller
Silicosis	
Abrasives worker	*Talcosis* (certain talcs)
Bentonite mill worker	Ceramics worker
Brick maker	Cosmetics worker
Ceramics worker	Miner or miller
Coal miner	Papermaker
Diatomite worker	Plastics worker
Enameler	Rubber worker

a Most pneumoconiosis (disease caused by dust) results in scar tissue formation in the lung (fibrotic lung disease). Important exceptions are bagassosis, byssinosis, and farmer's lung. The latter disorders are thought to be related to an immune or allergic response to an irritant.

ture will affect the reading. Taking body temperature at the same site allows for easier tracking. A persistent fever typically indicates that infection is present in the body. Causes other than infection are numerous but are less common and may be ruled out during the course of the assessment. Tachypnea and tachycardia often accompany the febrile process because the metabolic rate is increased. Consequently, there can be increased oxygen consumption and increased carbon dioxide production. Hypothermia is rarely encountered, but it can be a significant diagnostic or prognostic sign. Hypothalamus involvement should be strongly suspected if a patient presents with hypothermia following a neurological incident. Hypothermia reduces the metabolic rate and tissue demand for oxygen. The prognosis for cold water near-drowning patients is therefore

more favorable than that of a patient with an equal period of submersion in warm water.

Heart Rate. Heart rate varies considerably with age. A rate of 150 BPM in the neonate is well within normal limits. The adult range is commonly thought to be between 60 and 100 BPM.[8] A heart rate over 100 BPM, tachycardia, is associated with myriad clinical conditions including hypoxemia, hypotension, and fever. A heart rate under 60 BPM, bradycardia, is associated with the administration of certain cardiac medications such as beta blockers, as well as severe hypoxia. Well-trained endurance athletes maintain resting heart rates in the thirties and forties. Patients with third degree heart block typically exhibit bradycardia. The respiratory therapist should be aware of significant deviations from

TABLE 7-6   KEY ELEMENTS TO INCLUDE IN THE PHYSICAL ASSESSMENT FOR RESPIRATORY CARE PLAN DEVELOPMENT

General appearance
Level of consciousness
Oxygenation and perfusion
   Skin color and characteristics
   Nailbeds and mucosa
   Capillary refill
Chest inspection
Pulse, respirations, and blood pressure
   (optional)
SpO_2
Inspiratory capacity and/or vital capacity
Peak expiratory flow rate (PEFR) and/or FEV_1
Assessment of the work of breathing
Breath sounds
Palpation (tactile, vocal fremitus, chest
   excursion, trachea position)
Percussion (dullness, resonance, hyper-
   resonance)

SOURCE: Used with permission of the University of Texas Health Science Center at San Antonio, Department of Respiratory Care, Patient Assessment and Respiratory Care Plan.

baseline heart rate due to a respiratory care procedure or medication. Generally, a change of ± 20 BPM warrants suspension of the therapy and careful assessment of the patient's condition.

Respiratory Rate.   Respiratory rate also varies with age as evidenced by the full-term neonatal respiratory rate range of 35 to 45/min.[8] The normal adult range is 12 to 20/min.[8,9] Tachypnea is defined as an adult respiratory rate of greater than 20/min.[9] Tachypnea may be triggered by physiologic stimuli such as acute hypoxemia or interstitial pulmonary edema. Bradypnea is defined as a respiratory rate of less than 12/min.[9] Bradypnea is often associated with a depression of the medullary center. Common causes include narcotic overdose and neurological insult from trauma or disease. A respiratory rate of greater than 30/min when combined with a spontaneous tidal volume of 300 mL or less is associated with impending ventilatory failure.[10]

Blood Pressure.   As with heart and respiratory rate, blood pressure (BP) is also age-related. BP values steadily climb from birth and reach the adult mean normal values of 120/80 at approximately 18 to 20 years of age.[8,9] Systemic hypertension is characterized by a sustained systolic pressure of greater than or equal to 140 mm Hg and a sustained diastolic pressure of greater than or equal to 90 mm Hg.[4] Contributing factors associated with primary hypertension include smoking, obesity, heredity, and type A personality profile. A sustained systolic pressure of less than 90 mm Hg and a sustained diastolic pressure of less than 60 mm Hg are evidence of hypotension.[4] Common causes of hypotension include circulatory shock and hypovolemia.

Inspection

Inspection of the cardiopulmonary patient should include general appearance, level of consciousness and sensorium, extremities, and inspection of the head, neck, and chest. Inspection of the patient should begin at the moment you first see the patient and continue throughout your assessment. The patient's general appearance should be noted, including overall condition, level of consciousness, condition of extremities, respiratory rate and pattern, retractions, color, diaphoresis, position, and ancillary equipment in use.

Color.   The presence of peripheral cyanosis indicates that the level of desaturated oxyhemoglobin within the capillaries of the hands and feet is significantly elevated. The nailbeds of the fingers and toes reveal a bluish hue when this condition is present. Patients with chronic hypoxemia and resultant polycythemia typically present with cyanosis. It should also be noted that a pale, cold, clammy appearance may be just as ominous as cyanosis, because it is strongly associated with shock.

Other conditions that may affect color include skin rash, allergic reactions, carbon monoxide poisoning, and elevated carbon dioxide levels. A skin rash combined with mucosal edema, nasal polyps, and aspirin intolerance are common in allergic asthma and is known as triad asthma. Carbon monoxide inhalation produces a bright cherry red skin color, while elevated carbon dioxide levels are sometimes associated with redness of the skin.

Diaphoresis.   Sweating is a sign of acute distress and is often associated with respiratory failure or cardiopulmonary distress. *Diaphoresis* is the term used to indicate excessive sweating and should be noted whenever present.

Sensorium and Levels of Consciousness.   The difference between an awake, relaxed, and oriented patient and a confused, anxious, disoriented patient could be a lack of adequate oxygenation. The respiratory therapist should always be alert to the physical signs of hypoxia and respiratory failure. Please refer to the critical content box for a list of terms often used to describe levels of consciousness.

CRITICAL CONTENT

LEVELS OF CONSCIOUSNESS

- *Oriented × 3*: the patient is aware of person, place, and time
- *Confused*: the patient may have difficulty in understanding directions or be confused regarding person, place, or time
- *Delirious*: hallucinations may be present
- *Lethargic*: patient is sleepy but can be aroused
- *Obtunded*: patient may be difficult to arouse, but responds appropriately
- *Stuporous*: patient does not completely awaken when attempts are made to arouse
- *Comatose*: patient is unconscious, does not respond

Position.   Positional dyspnea is common in CHF as well as chronic obstructive pulmonary disease (COPD). For example, the patient with severe COPD may have great difficulty breathing while in a supine position. These patients often sit up, using one or more pillows for support, even while sleeping. These patients have orthopnea.

Inspection of the Extremities.   Capillary refill, color, skin temperature and moistness or dryness, digital clubbing, and the presence of edema should be noted. Inspection of the fingers for the presence of nicotine stains should also be performed. Good capillary refill is an indication of adequate peripheral circulation and oxygenation. Peripheral cyanosis (as opposed to central cyanosis) may indicate poor peripheral circulation and oxygenation. Warm, moderately moist extremities indicate good peripheral perfusion and/or poor oxygenation. Cold, clammy extremities indicate poor perfusion and circulation. Edema, particularly in the ankles and feet (pedal edema), and in severe cases in the arms and legs, is associated with congestive heart failure and fluid overload. Edema of the feet, legs, and arms is common in patients with multisystem organ failure. Edema of the lower legs and particularly the ankles, pedal edema, is also commonly seen in patients with right heart failure due to chronic lung disease (cor pulmonale). The patient with left heart failure (CHF) also presents with pedal edema. A complete history and physical examination helps establish the differential diagnosis.

Clubbing.   Digital clubbing is associated with chronic pulmonary disease, and on occasion, lung cancer (CA).[11] Clubbing is characterized by a bulbous swelling of the distal phalanges of the fingers and toes. The etiology of this condition is unknown, but possible factors associated with the development of clubbing may include chronic infection, circulating vasodilators or unspecified toxins, and chronic hypoxemia.[12] Clubbing is sometimes seen with cystic fibrosis, bronchiectasis, interstitial lung disease, bronchogenic CA, lung abscess, or chronic cardiovascular disease.[12] Digital clubbing may be associated with decreased oxygen delivery to the tissues; however, clubbing may or may not be associated with cyanosis, and COPD alone does not lead to clubbing.[11,13] Normal, mild, and severe digital clubbing are pictured in Fig. 7-1.

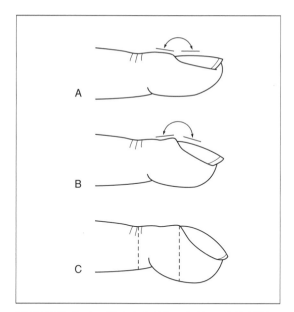

FIGURE 7-1 Digital clubbing. A. Normal. B. Mild digital clubbing. C. Severe digital clubbing. *(SOURCE: From Wilkins et al.)*

Ancillary Equipment in Use. Always note the presence or absence of IVs, respirators, cardiac monitors, urinary catheters (Foley bags), oxygen or aerosol equipment, isolation equipment, incentive spirometry equipment, chest drainage systems, sputum cups, restraints, and other equipment. The presence or absence of each of these items tells you something about the patient's condition.

Inspection of the Head and Neck. Observation of the mouth offers two signs associated with respiratory disease. The presence of central cyanosis indicates that the level of desaturated oxyhemoglobin within the capillaries of the oral mucosa is significantly elevated. The lips and adjacent oral tissues reveal the same bluish hue seen with peripheral cyanosis. Central cyanosis is associated with severe hypoxemia and warrants immediate intervention.

The patient who appears to be blowing out candles upon expiration is exhibiting a pursed lip breathing pattern. Patients with COPD who are prone to airway collapse upon expiration may intuitively incorporate this technique or, more frequently, are taught this exercise as part of their pulmonary rehabilitation program. The slight expiratory resistance afforded by this maneuver helps to "splint" the airways open and prevent their premature collapse and resultant air trapping.

Observation of the neck also offers two distinctive signs associated with respiratory disease. Inspection of the internal and external jugular veins for jugular venous distention (JVD) allows one to assess the degree of right heart failure in patients with pulmonary hypertension due to chronic hypoxemia. JVD is also associated with other clinical disorders, including left heart failure; however, cor pulmonale is the leading cause of this finding. Figure 7-2 illustrates the technique for jugular venous pressure estimation. This evaluation should be done at end-exhalation and is simply graded as normal, increased, or markedly increased.[7]

Use of Accessory Muscles of Inspiration. Use of the accessory muscles of inspiration often indicates an increased work of breathing (WOB) and difficulty in maintaining adequate ventilation. Accessory muscle use is commonly associated with an increased WOB due to decreases in compliance, obstruction, or increased airway resistance.

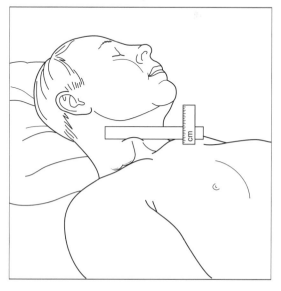

FIGURE 7-2 Jugular venous pressure estimation. *(SOURCE: From Wilkins et al.[1])*

During inspiration, visible contraction of the accessory muscles of the neck, notably the sternomastoid and scalenes, is also a common finding in patients with COPD. Hyperinflation of the lungs from gas trapping causes a depression of the diaphragm and thus limits normal abdominal excursion during inspiration, forcing a more apical adaptation to the breathing pattern and the incorporation of the accessory neck muscles. Patients with advanced obstructive lung disease develop a "clavicular lift" upon inspiration with intense contraction of the neck accessory muscles.

Inspection of the Chest. For inspection of the chest, the patient should be sitting upright to allow the examiner to adequately observe the anterior, lateral, and posterior aspects of the thorax. The transverse distance across the chest is normally measurably greater than the anteroposterior distance. This difference decreases with age and is significantly altered with the development of COPD. The term *barrel chest* refers to the dramatic in-

crease in the anteroposterior (AP) dimension of the chest in these patients. Figure 7-3 compares a patient with a normal chest to a patient with an increased AP diameter.

Flail chest occurs when there are multiple fractures of adjacent ribs with resulting instability of the chest wall. Flail chest leads to a paradoxical movement of the affected area: in upon inspiration and out upon expiration. Flail chest may be noted following the traumatic impact to the chest often incurred in motor vehicle accidents or other blunt trauma. Pneumothorax and lung contusions are typical sequelae and warrant immediate medical intervention.

An inward movement of the upper abdomen upon inspiration (rather than the normal outward movement) characterizes *abdominal paradox*, a phenomenon associated with paralysis or fatigue of the diaphragm. It is commonly noted in patients with COPD with the development of respiratory failure.

Paralysis of the hemidiaphragm can occur with phrenic nerve damage caused by trauma or surgery. This may result in a lack of chest motion on the affected side of the thorax.

Deformities of the bony thorax should also be assessed, because they are associated with restrictive pulmonary disease. Scoliosis, a lateral spine curvature, is noted upon inspection of the posterior aspect of the chest. Kyphosis, an anteroposterior spine curvature, is noted upon inspection of the lateral aspect of the chest. Scoliosis is often congenital in nature, while kyphosis is often associated with osteoporosis in the elderly population. Kyphoscoliosis is a combination of the two deformities that causes a more significant restrictive pattern. Key items to be reviewed during inspection of the chest are listed in Table 7-7.

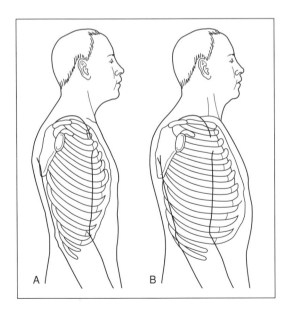

F I G U R E 7 - 3 Normal chest configuration (*A*) and a patient with increased anteroposterior (AP) diameter (*B*). (*Source: From Wilkins et al.*[1])

Respiratory Rate and Pattern. Respiratory rate and pattern should be assessed whenever the respiratory therapist interacts with the patient. As described above, tachypnea as well as an uneven respiratory pattern such as Cheyne-Stokes breathing should be noted, because their presence may indicate impending ventilatory failure. Bradypnea

TABLE 7-7   SUMMARY OF THE CHEST INSPECTION

The following key elements should be noted during chest inspection:

Increased anteroposterior diameter. An increase in anteroposterior (AP) diameter of the chest is associated with pulmonary overinflation. This is a common finding with COPD and is sometimes seen with cystic fibrosis patients and in acute asthma exacerbations.

Unilateral apparent hyperexpansion. A decrease in compliance on one side, a pneumothorax, or bronchial intubation can all result in this appearance. A severe unilateral pneumonia or pneumonectomy are possible causes of decreased or absent chest wall movement on one side. Types of pneumothorax include spontaneous, traumatic, and tension.

Chest wall or spinal deformity. Pectus excavatum, pectus caravatum, kyphosis, and other disorders may all affect the patient's thoracic compliance.

Flail chest. Flail chest is the instability of the chest wall due to multiple rib fractures (generally 2 to 3 consecutive ribs broken in 2 or more places each). The chest wall sinks in on inspiration with flail chest.

Obesity, pregnancy, or ascites. All of these conditions indirectly reduce compliance (extrapulmonary or thoracic compliance). Obesity is also associated with disorders of ventilatory control and obstructive sleep apnea.

Intercostal retractions. These are often caused by upper airway obstruction, increased resistance to air flow, or inadequate gas flows via closed systems such as mechanical ventilators.

Symmetry of respiration. By placing both hands parallel to one another on the chest wall (right and left) and observing chest expansion for symmetry, one can sometimes note changes associated with such things as major atelectasis, pneumothorax, or other unilateral disorders of lung or chest wall expansion. Other possible causes of asymmetrical movement of the chest include bronchial intubation, unilateral pneumonia, or pneumonectomy. Trauma and the associated presence of a flail chest may cause paradoxical chest wall movement.

Scars due to trauma or surgery and radiation markers. Surgical scars relating to pneumonectomy, lobectomy, or thoracotomy are of obvious interest, as is sternal scarring from open heart surgery. Radiation markers are also of obvious interest.

may be associated with CNS problems, sedatives, hypnotics, or impending respiratory arrest.

Synchronicity of Chest Wall and Diaphragm. The chest wall and abdomen should rise and fall together as the patient inhales and exhales. Asynchronous and/or spasmodic diaphragmatic contractions are strong indicators of acute ventilatory failure (excluding hiccups, of course) and respiratory muscle fatigue. Often this sign is a prelude to respiratory arrest.

Retractions. Retractions between the ribs (intercostal), above the clavicles (supraclavicular), or below the xiphoid process (xiphoid) are noted as the tissue in these areas moves inward with inspiration. They are associated with marked negative pleural pressure on inspiration. Retractions can be caused by upper airway obstruction (supraclavicular), decreased lung compliance (intercostal and/or xiphoid), or inadequate gas flow to the mechanically ventilated patient.

Palpation

Palpation involves touching the chest wall of a patient in order to determine chest expansion and the degree of tactile fremitus. Although palpation is not a routine part of every patient assessment, it may be of help in quantifying the degree of impairment involved in certain disease processes. Palpation techniques and findings with common problems are summarized in Table 7-8.

Chest Expansion.   The degree and symmetry of chest expansion are evaluated as the patient is instructed to take a deep breath from end exhalation. Chest expansion is most easily assessed by positioning the tips of the thumbs so they are touching at approximately the level of the eighth thoracic vertebra along the posterior chest wall.

The palmar surfaces of the hands and fingertips are spread out across the lower chest wall. The tips of the thumbs should move symmetrically away from one another approximately 3 to 5 cm at the end of an inspiratory vital capacity maneuver.[4] Limitations to chest expansion may be unilateral or bilateral. Bilateral limitation is noted with COPD and neuromuscular disease. Unilateral limitation may be present with unilateral disorders such as lobar atelectasis or lobar pneumonia.

Tactile Fremitus.   This technique involves placing the fingertips or ulnar surface of the hand or fist on the anterior and posterior surfaces of the chest wall in a systematic order as the patient repeats a number such as "99".[7] The tactile sensation felt by the examiner from the vibrations caused by the

TABLE 7-8   PALPATION TECHNIQUES AND CLINICAL IMPLICATIONS OF SPECIFIC FINDINGS

PALPATION TECHNIQUE	POSSIBLE IMPLICATIONS
Tactile vocal fremitus. To perform this exam, one simply places the lateral edge of one's hand against the patient's chest wall. The patient then repeatedly speaks the number "ninety-nine." The examiner shifts his or her hand from side to side noting the vibrations felt through the chest wall as the patient speaks.	A marked increase in vibration over a given area is indicative of consolidation.
Tactile rhonchi. These are vibrations or a rumbling or gurgling feeling when the examiner places his or her hands flat (palms down) over portions of the chest wall.	Rumbling or tactile rhonchi are associated with secretions in a larger airway. They may clear following a cough or suctioning.
Subcutaneous emphysema. This is air under the skin, usually of the neck and face. Upon palpation, the skin feels crackly, similar to what is felt when one balls up a sheet of waxed paper or plastic.	Subcutaneous emphysema is associated with pneumothorax (especially tension pneumothorax) and pneumomediastinum.
Tracheal deviation. This is movement or a shift in the trachea away from the midline. One can feel the position of the trachea by placing the index finger in the suprasternal notch.	A shift toward the affected side is caused by massive atelectasis, severe pneumonia, and spontaneous or traumatic pneumothorax (without tension). Bronchial intubation and tension pneumothorax may shift the trachea away from the affected site.

patient's phonation is referred to as *tactile fremitus*. Air is a poor transmitter of sound waves and vibrations, while solid substances tend to enhance transmission. Conditions that increase the air:lung tissue ratio such as pneumothorax and emphysema will decrease fremitus. Conditions that decrease the air:lung tissue ratio such as consolidation and atelectasis will increase fremitus.

Percussion. Percussion is also used to assess the air:lung tissue ratio by listening to the transmission quality of sound waves created by striking the patient's chest wall with one's fingertip. The examiner systematically taps the anterior and posterior aspects of the chest. The resonance that is evoked by percussion over normal lung tissue has been compared to the sound heard by tapping on a watermelon.[4] Conditions that increase the air:lung tissue ratio such as pneumothorax and emphysema will increase resonance. The transmission of sound in the presence of increased resonance can be compared to the sound heard when striking a hollow log. Conditions that decrease the air:lung tissue ratio such as consolidation and atelectasis will decrease resonance. Decreased resonance or dullness can be compared to the sound heard when striking a solid log.

There are two basic methods of percussion: mediate and intermediate.[7] With mediate percussion, one thumps directly on the chest wall. With intermediate percussion, one interposes the first and second finger of one hand between the chest wall and the hand used for percussion. Figure 7-4 illustrates the technique used for intermediate percussion of the chest. The box below compares the clinical implications of resonant, hyperresonant, and dull percussion sounds.

CRITICAL CONTENT

CLINICAL IMPLICATIONS OF PERCUSSION SOUNDS

Percussion Sound	Possible Implications
Resonant	Normal lung tissue underlying percussion point
Hyperresonant (tympanic)	Hyperinflation (asthma, emphysema) or pneumothorax
Dull	Pleural effusion, empyema, atelectasis, consolidation, percussion over liver, heart, or kidneys

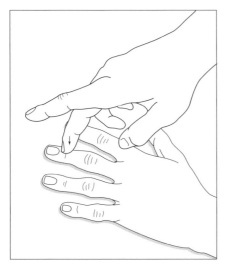

FIGURE 7-4 Intermediate percussion technique. (*Source: From Bates B*. A Guide to Physical Examination and History Taking. *5th ed. Philadelphia: Lippincott; 1991.*)

Auscultation

Auscultation is the process of using a stethoscope to listen for sounds produced by the body. Auscultation over the chest is performed to identify normal or abnormal lung (breath) sounds.

Chest auscultation provides the examiner with essential information regarding the status of the airways and the lung parenchyma. Auscultation is carried out in a systematic manner as the examiner positions the patient in an upright sitting position and proceeds to listen to the patient's breath sounds with his or her stethoscope. Sources differ as to whether one should progress from the apices to the bases or vice versa, but there is consensus that one should auscultate from side to side over both the anterior and posterior aspects of the chest.

Normal Breath Sounds.   Tracheal breath sounds are heard over the trachea and are loud and high in pitch. Bronchovesicular breath sounds are heard between the scapulae and around the sternum. These sounds are attenuated in intensity and lower in pitch than tracheal breath sounds. Vesicular breath sounds are heard over the remaining aspects of the chest and are soft in intensity and low in pitch. The differences in these breath sounds are explained by the role that healthy lung tissue plays in "filtering" or actually muffling the harsh sounds produced by turbulent flow in the trachea and large airways.

Adventitious Breath Sounds.   These breath sounds indicate that there is some underlying pathology in the parenchyma and/or the airways. Abnormal parenchymal sounds are classified as either bronchial or diminished. Bronchial breath sounds develop as alveolar surface area is lost due to disease processes that lead to atelectasis, fibrosis, or consolidation of the lung parenchyma. These conditions lead to a loss of the normal alveolar muffling of the tracheal breath sounds from the upper airways, and thus the sounds produced are louder and harsher than vesicular sounds. Diminished breath sounds are associated with hypopnea as seen in neuromuscular disease and drug overdose, or with an increase in the air:tissue ratio in the lung as seen with emphysema and pneumothorax.

Abnormal airway sounds are acoustically classified as continuous or discontinuous. The continuous sound maintains a uniform pattern for at least one tenth of a second, while the discontinuous sound does not hold such a pattern.[14] Wheezing and stridor are continuous sounds associated with narrowing of the airways. *Stridor* is a sign of upper airway obstruction that can be heard without the use of a stethoscope, as it is loud and high in pitch. Stridor is a classic finding in laryngotracheobronchitis or croup.

Wheezing indicates that the caliber of the lower airways has been reduced. Wheezes vary in pitch depending on the site and degree of narrowing. The severe bronchospasm that develops in the bronchioles of the asthmatic during an acute exacerbation produces a sound that is high in pitch. Obstruction of the bronchi that develops with chronic bronchitis as copious amounts of tenacious sputum narrow the airways leads to a wheeze that is low in pitch.

During an asthma attack, one would anticipate hearing wheezing on auscultation. Wheezes are generated by the vibration of the wall of a narrowed or compressed airway as air passes through at high velocity. During an asthma attack, the diameter of the airway can be reduced due to mucosal edema, secretions, and bronchospasm. When listening to breath sounds, you should note the pitch, intensity, and portion of the respiratory cycle occupied by the wheeze. For example, the patient may have a high-pitched wheeze throughout inspiration and expiration (the entire respiratory cycle). Following bronchodilator therapy, the wheezing may be heard only during the later part of exhalation and may also decrease in pitch and intensity. An increase in the patient's airway caliber can affect the pitch and intensity, as well as the portion of the respiratory cycle occupied by the wheeze. High-pitched wheezes at end expiration indicate less airflow obstruction than a lower pitched wheeze throughout inspiration and expiration. However, wheezing can be an unreliable indicator of obstruction because in extreme cases severe obstruction can result in silent chest. Serious reduction in airflow to the point where the clinician cannot hear any breath sounds, called *silent chest*, is a serious clinical finding.

Crackles are discontinuous sounds associated with the sudden expansion of closed bronchioles and alveoli upon inspiration, or the flow of gas through airway secretions. The type of crackles associated with expansion of bronchioles has been described as similar to the sound made when the two parts of Velcro are pulled apart, and these crackles are noted with pulmonary edema. The type of crackles associated with gas flow through secretions are very discor-

TABLE 7-9 TYPICAL BREATH SOUNDS NOTED UPON AUSCULTATION AND RELATED CLINICAL IMPLICATIONS

BREATH SOUNDS	POSSIBLE IMPLICATIONS
Vesicular	Normal over most of the chest *except* over major airways.
Tracheal or bronchial	Harsh, loud sounds. Normal if found over a large airway; indicative of consolidation if heard elsewhere.
Bronchovesicular	Normal over or near large airways. Associated with consolidation if heard elsewhere.
Diminished or absent	Associated with hypoventilation of that portion of the lung, severe COPD, pneumothorax, pleural effusion, atelectasis, bronchial intubation.
Wheezing (high pitched rhonchi)	Bronchospasm as in asthma. Sometimes heard with tumor, aspiration, or other irritation.
Rhonchi (low pitched rhonchi or gurgles)	Associated with secretions in a larger airway. May clear following cough.
Crackles (rales)	Associated with fluid in the alveoli as in pulmonary edema.
E-A egophony	An audible A sound when the patient says E. Associated with consolidation.
Pleural friction rub	Loud, dry, creaky, coarse, leathery sound associated with pleural irritation and inflammation.

dant in quality and may clear or improve following an effective cough.

With respect to normal and abnormal breath sounds, one should be cautious in the interpretation of findings. In one study of tape recorded breath sounds, there was very little agreement between physicians even as to the type of breath sounds being heard. However, in general, most would agree to the terms and possible implications of these sounds as described in Table 7-9.

DIAGNOSTIC STUDIES

Books and chapters have been published that provide comprehensive coverage of the principles involved in the review and analysis of arterial blood gases, chest radiography, pulmonary function testing, and hematology, as well as other laboratory studies. The following sections of this chapter offer a concise synopsis of relevant information commonly used in helping to quantify cardiopulmonary disease or dysfunction.

Arterial Blood Gases

The information from the results of an arterial blood gas (ABG) sample is critical for proper management of the patient with a cardiopulmonary disorder. The pH allows ready interpretation of the patient's acid-base status with a normal mean value of 7.40 and a normal range of 7.35 to 7.45.[15] The lungs and the kidneys are the primary organ systems that influence arterial pH. The lungs control the level of carbon dioxide (CO_2), which dictates the balance of carbonic acid (H_2CO_3) in the blood. The kidneys control the level of bicarbonate (HCO_3), the major base in the blood. Primary increases in blood bases (decreased acids) result in a condition called *metabolic alkalosis*, while primary decreases in blood base (increased acids) cause *metabolic acidosis.*

Acidemia occurs when the arterial blood pH falls below 7.35.[15] A gain in carbon dioxide will increase the level of carbonic acid in the blood and result in respiratory acidosis. Normal ventilation maintains arterial carbon dioxide partial pressure values between 35 and 45 mm Hg. *Hypoventilation* is documented when arterial carbon dioxide values climb above 45 mm Hg.[15] The resultant respiratory acidosis may be acute or chronic in nature and may be referred to as *acute* or *chronic ventilatory failure.* There are many exceptions in interpretation of ABGs, and you will find examples of ABG interpretations in Part II with many of the case chapters.

Alkalemia occurs when the pH rises above 7.45.[15] A loss of carbon dioxide will decrease the level of carbonic acid in the blood and result in respiratory alkalosis. Hyperventilation is documented when arterial carbon dioxide values fall below 35 mm Hg.[15] The resultant respiratory alkalosis is most commonly acute and transient in nature.

Chest Radiography

There are many pulmonary diseases that cause distinctive changes in chest radiographic findings. For example, the radiographic signs associated with emphysema are numerous and fit a very particular pattern that is unique to that disease. A number of disturbances can only be determined by evaluating the results of special procedures, such as a ventilation-perfusion scan for the detection of pulmonary emboli. The majority of cardiopulmonary disorders can be detected through careful inspection of an anteroposterior or a posteroanterior view chest film. The most common disturbances relate to changes in air volume (radiolucent/dark) or fluid volume (radiopaque/white). Keep in mind that the tissue

cells are all "fluid density" and thus are radiopaque/white on a radiograph.

Atelectasis is the loss of lung volume due to collapse of small airways and alveoli. Small areas of atelectasis are difficult to discern and may only be manifested on the radiograph as small, white streaks as the radiolucent alveoli are lost and tissue density is increased. Collapse of a lung segment or lobe will cause the following features: narrowing of the rib spaces on the affected side, shifting of fissure lines and hilar structures toward the affected area, and a rise in the hemidiaphragm on the affected side.

Hyperinflation is due to the trapping of air during exhalation noted in patients with asthma, chronic bronchitis, and emphysema. Features noted with hyperinflation include wide rib spaces; low, flat diaphragms; narrow heart shadow; and radiolucent/dark lung fields.

Pneumothorax is manifested when excessive air accumulates in the pleural space. The pleural cavity fills with air and the adjacent lung collapses towards the hilum. The chest radiograph shows a radiolucent/dark hemithorax on the affected side.

Fluid changes will translate into an increase in opacity or whiteness on the chest film. The type of fluid is determined by the underlying pathology. A plasma-like transudate will fill the parenchyma in congestive (left-sided) heart failure. A purulent exudate will fill the affected lung tissue with bacterial pneumonia. The pleural space may fill with a transudate or an exudate with the development of pleural effusion. Keep in mind, however, that no matter what type of fluid accumulates in the lung, it will be radiopaque on the radiograph.

Please refer to the cases in Part II of this textbook for examples, questions, and cases related to chest radiography.

Pulmonary Function Studies

The spectrum of complete pulmonary function testing encompasses very sophisticated and specialized testing equipment and techniques. The cornerstone of pulmonary function testing for the vast majority of patients, however, is basic spirometry.

Basic spirometry can be quickly accomplished at the patient's bedside with a variety of compact devices that meet American Thoracic Society standards and American Association for Respiratory Care guidelines.[16–18] The evaluation of spirometric lung volumes and expiratory flow rates allows ready classification of a patient's primary mechanical disturbance affecting their breathing.

Restrictive pulmonary disorders are characterized by a decrease in lung volumes.[19] The forced vital capacity (FVC) is the most commonly used pulmonary function test and is useful in assessing both restrictive and obstructive pulmonary disease. The maneuver requires that the patient take a maximal inspiration followed by a forceful maximal expiration that is recorded by a spirometric device. Patients with restrictive pulmonary diseases exhibit FVC values that are reduced below 80% of predicted normal values; however, patients with obstructive disease may also demonstrate a decrease in FVC.[19] Most restrictive disorders are parenchymal in nature, such as coal worker's pneumoconiosis (CWP), or thoracic in nature when the bony thorax is involved, such as kyphoscoliosis. Neuromuscular diseases also are classified as restrictive diseases.

Obstructive pulmonary disorders are characterized by a decrease in expiratory flow rates.[19] The forced expiratory volume in 1 second (FEV_1) to forced vital capacity (FVC) ratio is the most commonly used index used in assessing obstructive pulmonary disease. Healthy young subjects can exhale slightly more than 80% of their forced vital capacity in 1 second. This ratio falls with age as the airways lose elastic tissue support and become prone to premature narrowing and collapse upon expiration. A ratio of less than 70% is indicative of obstructive airways disease. Patients with asthma, chronic bronchitis, cystic fibrosis, and emphysema have dramatic declines in their FEV_1/FVC ratios.[19]

Figure 7-5 gives examples of normal, restrictive, and obstructive spirometry. Please see the critical content box for guidelines for interpretation of pulmonary function data.[20–22] In addition, increase your knowledge, application, and analysis of PFTs through completion of questions and exercises with the cases in Part II of this textbook.

CRITICAL CONTENT

BASIC PULMONARY FUNCTION STUDY INTERPRETATION

Obstructive Defects

FEV_1/FVC .70 to .75* AND

FEV_1/FVC .70 or	
FEV_1 80% of predicted	= mild obstruction
FEV_1/FVC .60 or	
FEV_1 60% of predicted	= moderate obstruction
FEV_1/FVC .40 or	
FEV_1 40% of predicted	= severe obstruction

Restrictive Defects

$FFEV_1$/FVC .70 to .75 AND

FVC 80% predicted	= mild restriction
FVC 60% predicted	= moderate restriction
FVC 50% predicted	= severe restriction

---

*In the presence of obstruction, measurement of total lung capacity (TLC) should be used to assess restriction, with TLC 80% predicted being mild, 70% predicted being moderate, and 60% predicted being severe restriction.[21]

Laboratory Tests

Hematology. The complete blood count (CBC) entails an analysis of the red and white blood cells. Red blood cell analysis involves red blood cell (RBC) count, hemoglobin (Hb), and hematocrit (Hct). Erythrocyte indices are also measured, but are of limited value in the evaluation of cardiopulmonary disorders. RBC count is the total number of erythrocytes, or mature RBCs. The normal adult value is approximately 5 million per microliter.[23] Hemoglobin is the portion of the RBC that carries oxygen, and it is reported in grams per deciliter.[23] Normal adult values range from 12 to 16 g/dL. Hematocrit is a percentage that relates RBC volume to total blood volume. Normal adult average values fall below 50%[23] and are approximately three times the hemoglobin value (Hb × 3).

Polycythemia is a disease of red blood cells that leads to an increase in all RBC analysis results.

FIGURE 7-5 Normal, restrictive, and obstructive spirometry. (*SOURCE: From Fishman AP et al.* Fishman's Pulmonary Diseases and Disorders. *New York: McGraw-Hill; 1998:546.*)

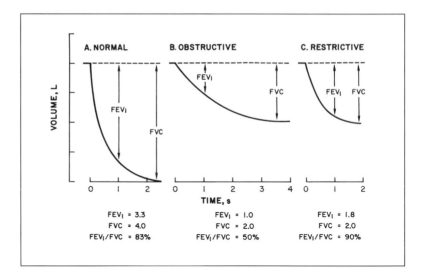

Polycythemia may be classified as either primary or secondary as determined by etiological factors: Secondary polycythemia is noted in patients with chronic hypoxemia. Chronic hypoxemia triggers the release of erythropoietin from the kidneys. Erythropoietin stimulates the bone marrow to produce more red blood cells to allow an adaptive increase in oxygen-carrying hemoglobin. Secondary polycythemia is a cardinal sign noted in patients with COPD.

White blood cell (WBC) analysis includes a measure of the total number of white blood cells, as well as differentiation of the cell types. These cells are integral components of the immune system and respond to infection. Normal WBC count is between 5000 and 10,000 cells per cubic millimeter of blood.[23] Leukocytosis denotes an elevated WBC count. A decrease in WBC count is termed leukopenia.

A more specific diagnostic evaluation of the white blood cells by exact cell type is performed during the differential count. There are five types of white blood cells, each reported as a percentage of total WBCs. The neutrophils are the most prevalent, about 40% to 70% of all WBCs.[23] An increase in numbers of these cells, neutrophilia, is most commonly associated with bacterial pneumonia. Lymphocytes number a distant second to the neutro-

phils, at about 20% to 45%.[23] Lymphocytosis is a sign associated with viral pneumonia. The notably paradoxical development of lymphocytopenia is seen with the progression of HIV infection. Monocytes normally represent 2% to 10% of the differential.[23] Monocytosis is seen with tuberculosis and some of the mycotic lung diseases. Eosinophils normally account for less than 6% of all WBCs. Eosinophilia may be noted in asthmatic patients. Basophils comprise 1% or less of WBCs and do not play a role in any pulmonary disorders.[23]

Chemistry. Numerous studies are classified under blood chemistry, including electrolyte, enzyme, glucose, tumor marker, and drug level monitoring. Electrolyte analysis of the major serum cations and anions is used to identify and monitor myriad metabolic disorders including acid-base disturbances. Kidney function can be assessed via analysis of serum levels of creatinine. The blood urea nitrogen (BUN) is used to assess protein metabolism, as well as liver and kidney function. Serum enzymes, such as aspartate aminotransferase (AST), alanine aminotransferase (ALT), alkaline phosphatase (ALP), lactate dehydrogenase (LDH), and creatine kinase (CK) are used in the diagnostic evaluation of liver and heart disease. Glucose monitoring is critical for both the diabetic patient and those receiving parenteral feedings. The monitoring of cholesterol and triglycerides is also important in cardiac profiling for coronary artery disease. Tumor marking involves analysis of the blood for hormones, enzymes, and certain antigens associated with various cancers. The monitoring of serum levels of various drugs is critical in order to ensure proper therapeutic benefit and to avoid toxicity. Commonly quantitated cardiac and pulmonary drugs include digoxin and theophylline, respectively.

Microbiology. The analysis of tissues and fluids for the presence and identification of microbes is of significant diagnostic value. The collection and examination of sputum is commonly used to identify pneumonias caused by bacteria, fungi, protozoa, and viruses. Histology, the study of tissue, involves a bronchoscopic or biopsy sample that is examined for microbes or cancerous lesions. Cytology, the study of cells, includes the analysis of sputum, bronchial brushings from a bronchoscopic procedure, lung mass cells from fine-needle aspiration (FNA), or pleural fluid for atypical or cancerous cells.

AGE-SPECIFIC CONSIDERATIONS

Infants and Children

There are a number of special considerations when assessing infants and children. Low birthweight is associated with prematurity, the development of hyaline membrane disease, and the need for surfactant replacement therapy and mechanical ventilation. Children requiring mechanical ventilation at birth may develop bronchopulmonary dysplasia, a chronic lung disease of infancy.

Recurrent spitting up and choking in infants may be a sign of gastroesophageal reflux which can result in recurrent pneumonia. Sudden infant death of a sibling is a danger sign for apnea and the need for an infant apnea monitor. Coughing or difficulty breathing that develops suddenly in infants or small children may be caused by aspiration of a small object, toy, or food. Young children are also

prone to ingestion of poisons or drugs if they are left within reach of the child.

Older Adults

When performing an assessment of an older adult, risk factors for respiratory disability should be considered. These include smoking, frequent respiratory infections, immobilization, marked sedentary habits, difficulty swallowing, or a history of chronic exposure to environmental pollutants or toxic inhalants. Older adults are at particular risk for chronic lung disease, lung cancer, and tuberculosis. Consequently, in older patients it is especially important to inquire about smoking history, cough, dyspnea on exertion, fatigue, significant weight changes, fever, and night sweats. Alteration of daily living habits or activities as a result of respiratory symptoms should also be noted. The elderly may also have physical or mental disabilities that may greatly affect the interview and assessment process. See Chapter 9 for more detailed descriptions and exercises on communicating with patients who have limitations due to disability and/or aging.

SOAP NOTES

Respiratory therapists must be able to systematically collect and document data in order to properly assess and treat the patient. Clinically, the problem-oriented medical record (POMR) may be used for these purposes. The POMR is used to collect and document data, assess the patient, and develop an appropriate treatment plan. The most common POMR is the SOAP note. The acronym *SOAP* refers to a type of clinical note that allows the practitioner to report their examination finding, assessment, and treatment plan. The four letters of the acronym distinguish the salient features of the SOAP note.

S: This is the patient's **subjective** expression of the symptoms that have brought him or her to medical attention. The chief complaint is the leading statement reported by the patient. The history of present illness and past medical history is also inherently subjective.

O: This part of the note includes all of the **objective** signs that are exhibited by the patient and discovered by the examiner. This includes all of the findings of physical assessment, including vital signs, inspection, palpation, percussion, and auscultation. Diagnostic data, such as the results of ABG analysis, chest radiography, pulmonary function, and other laboratory tests are also typically recorded.

A: Refers to the examiner's **assessment** of the findings noted in the S and O sections of the clinical note. This is commonly an assessment of various clinical signs and symptoms that is followed by a disease or disorder diagnosis. For example, the symptoms, physical findings, and diagnostic data uncovered during the examination of the asthmatic patient present a very characteristic disease pattern.

P: Involves the development of a care **plan** based on the assessment findings. The plan should address the treatment of particular symptoms or signs noted on examination, such as the administration of an adrenergic bronchodilator to alleviate acute bronchospasm in an acute asthmatic attack.

RESPIRATORY CARE PLANS

Introduction to Care Plans

The respiratory care plan is simply a written explanation of the respiratory care the patient is to receive. It can be viewed as an individualized care protocol for the specific patient. It is based on a careful patient assessment and a review of the respiratory care diagnostic and treatment modalities available to the respiratory therapist. The respiratory care plan may take the form of physician's orders, a detailed progress note in the medical record, an established protocol, completion of a standardized respiratory care form, or the use of POMRs using SOAP notes. The respiratory care plan may include the goal of the therapy, device, or procedure; medications given; method or appliance used; gas source and/or flow; and frequency

and duration of therapy. The care plan may also include a statement of how the intensity and/or duration of therapy will be adjusted and when the therapy will be discontinued. Assessment of the outcomes of therapy may also be included. In summary, the respiratory care plan may be defined as the written plan of treatment that the patient will receive. The respiratory care plan may include goals, rationale, and significance, and a description of how the care will be assessed. The key elements of a respiratory care plan are described in Table 7-10.

Common Conditions Requiring Respiratory Care Plan Development

Following a careful patient assessment, the respiratory care plan is developed. Conditions requiring respiratory care plan development can be categorized as either obstructive or restrictive pulmonary disease. Some patients present with combined obstructive and restrictive disease. The most common obstructive pulmonary diseases are asthma, chronic bronchitis, emphysema, and combined COPD. The most common restrictive pulmonary diseases are pneumonia, atelectasis, acute respiratory distress syndrome (ARDS), and pulmonary edema.

C R I T I C A L   C O N T E N T

THE MOST COMMON PROBLEMS REQUIRING RESPIRATORY CARE

Obstruction
Chronic bronchitis: secretion management
Emphysema: air trapping
Combined/COPD
Asthma: bronchospasm/mucosal edema

Restriction
Pneumonia: consolidation
Atelectasis: secretions and plugging, inadequate
   lung expansion
ARDS
Pulmonary edema (CHF)

TABLE 7-10   KEY ELEMENTS OF A BASIC RESPIRATORY CARE PLAN

Goal of therapy
  Maintain adequate tissue oxygenation
  Treat/prevent bronchospasm and/or mucosal edema
  Deliver antiinflammatory or antiasthmatic agents
  Secretion management
  Sputum induction
  Prevent or treat atelectasis

Device or procedure
  Oxygen therapy (nasal cannula, air-entrainment mask, other masks)
  Aerosol medication via small volume nebulizer
  MDI via holding chamber
  Incentive spirometry
  IPPB
  Chest physiotherapy (postural drainage and chest percussion)
  High volume bland aerosol with or without supplemental oxygen
  Directed cough
  Suctioning

Medications
  Bronchodilators
  Mucolytics (acetylcysteine, dornase alpha)
  Antiinflammatory agents and decongestants (steroids, racemic epinephrine, others)
  Antiasthmatic agents (cromolyn sodium, nedocromol sodium)
  Bland aerosol (normal saline, ½ normal saline, sterile distilled water)

Method or appliance
  Mask, mouthpiece, mouthseal, trach mask, nose clips, aerochamber, etc.

Gas source, flow and/or pressure
  Oxygen or compressed air
  Liter flow and/or FIO_2
  Pressure (IPPB)

Frequency and duration of therapy
  BID, TID, QID, q6 hours, q4 hours, q2 hours, q1 hour, PRN, etc.
  Duration of therapy in minutes or continuous

Volume goals
  Incentive spirometry minimum of one third of predicted IC (⅓ × IBW in kg × 50)
  IPPB minimum of one third predicted IC or at least 10 mL/kg

Assessment
  Improvement and/or reversal of clinical signs and symptoms
  Oxygenation and ventilation—reversal of the manifestations of hypoxia and/or hypoventilation
  Decreased work of breathing
  Decreased cardiac work
  Improved breath sounds (air movement, wheezing, rhonchi, crackles)
  Pulse oximetry and ABG
  Bedside pulmonary function (rate, volumes, inspiratory force, PEFR, IC, FVC, FEV_1)
  Chest x-ray

Developing and Implementing the Respiratory Care Plan

The process for respiratory care plan development generally includes the receipt of an order for a specific type of respiratory care or for a respiratory care consult. In some care settings, the respiratory therapist is responsible for determining the priority of care ordered for the patient. This is especially critical when the workload exceeds the available manpower. Following receipt of an order, the respiratory therapist performs a detailed patient assessment including chart review, patient interview, and physical assessment, which may include the bedside measurement of SpO_2 and basic pulmonary function parameters. Following this assessment, the respiratory therapist may then select the appropriate care based on the patient's condition. The goal is to optimize the match between the care needed and the treatment options that are available. These options may include techniques to improve oxygenation, or for secretion management, sputum induction, treatment for bronchospasm and mucosal edema, and lung expansion therapy. A typical respiratory care treatment menu is found in Table 7-11. Following selection of a respiratory care treatment regimen, the patient's physician should be notified and given the opportunity to review and/or modify the care plan. The care is then delivered. The patient is monitored and the care plan is reevaluated based on the patient's response to therapy. The critical content box summarizes the steps in respiratory care plan development and implementation.

GOALS OF THE RESPIRATORY CARE PLAN

The respiratory care plan may be aimed at management of secretions, treatment of bronchospasm and mucosal edema, or lung expansion therapy for the treatment and/or prevention of atelectasis and pneumonia. Supportive respiratory care may include techniques for improving oxygenation and providing ventilatory support. Diagnostic respiratory care procedures include techniques to assess oxygenation, ventilation, acid-base balance, and pulmonary function, as well as obtaining sputum

CRITICAL CONTENT

STEPS IN THE DEVELOPMENT AND IMPLEMENTATION OF AN INDIVIDUALIZED RESPIRATORY CARE PLAN

Order for respiratory care received
↓
Perform assessment
Chart review
Patient interview
Physical assessment
↓
Establish desired treatment goals, objectives, or outcomes
↓
Evaluate/select/modify treatment
↓
Physician notification and review
↓
Deliver respiratory care
↓
Chart in the medical record
↓
Monitor and reevaluate based on patient response

samples for Gram's stain, cultures, or cytologic examination. Table 7-12 provides the most common goals of a typical respiratory care plan and the associated outcomes assessment. We will now turn to the development of specific respiratory care plans based on an assessment of the patient's needs and the related goals of therapy.

Maintain Adequate Tissue Oxygenation

Oxygen therapy is indicated for documented or suspected hypoxemia, severe trauma, acute MI, and immediate postoperative recovery. It also may be indicated to support the patient with chronic lung disease during exercise and to prevent or treat right-side congestive heart failure (cor pulmonale) due to chronic pulmonary hypertension. A Pao_2 of less than 60 and/or a Spo_2 of less than 90% to 92% are considered clear indications for oxygen therapy in most patients.[24,25] Exceptions to this rule include patients with chronic CO_2

TABLE 7-11   RESPIRATORY CARE TREATMENT MENU

Basic care treatment menu
Oxygenation
   Nasal cannula
   Oxygen masks (simple/partial/nonrebreather)
   High flow systems (venturi masks, large volume
      entrainment nebulizers)
   CPAP by mask
Secretion management
   Directed cough and deep breathing instruction
   Suctioning [nasotracheal (NT), endotracheal (ET),
      trach suctioning]
   Chest physiotherapy (postural drainage, percus
      sion, vibration)
   High volume bland aerosol therapy (ultrasonic
      nebulizer, heated large volume nebulizer)
   Mucus-controlling agents (mucolytics)
Sputum induction
   Directed cough
   Hypertonic saline aerosol
   Suctioning (NT, ET, trach suctioning)
Bronchospasm and mucosal edema
   Bronchodilator therapy (small volume nebulizer,
      MDIs)
   Antiinflammatory agents (steroids)
   Antiasthmatic aerosol agents (cromolyn sodium,
      etc.)
Lung expansion
   Cough and deep breath
   Suctioning
   Incentive spirometry
   IPPB
Frequency of treatment options
   Continuous
   Q1 to 2 hours
   Q4 hours
   Q6 hours
   QID
   TID
   BID
   PRN

Critical care
Ventilator management
   Volume limited ventilation

   Pressure limited ventilation (pressure support,
      pressure control)
   Noninvasive ventilation (CPAP, BiPAP)
   Adults, children, infants
Physiologic monitoring
   Pulse oximetry
   ABG
   Capnography
   Arterial line insertion
   Metabolic studies and monitoring
   Cardiac monitoring and hemodynamics
   Mixed venous oxygen saturations (SvO_2)
   Compliance, resistance, and work of breathing
Mechanical circulatory assistance (IAPB,
   intraaortic balloon pump)
Airway care
Basic care

Diagnostic testing
Pulmonary function laboratory
   Pulmonary mechanics
   Lung volumes
   Diffusion
   Tests or reactive airways
   Pulmonary exercise testing
Sleep laboratory
Noninvasive cardiology (echocardiography)
Invasive cardiology (Cath lab)
Cardiac stress testing
Pulmonary stress testing

Other specialized procedures
Transport
Advanced cardiac life support
Intubation
Airway care
Patient education
Home care
Discharge planning
Disease management (asthma, COPD, CF)
Pulmonary rehabilitation
Smoking cessation
Patient assessment and respiratory care plan
   development, implementation, and
   monitoring

T A B L E 7 - 1 2   GOALS OF BASIC RESPIRATORY CARE AND RELATED OUTCOME MEASURES

Overall goal of therapy: Maintain adequate tissue oxygenation

Specific goals:

Treat suspected or documented hypoxemia

Decrease or eliminate the clinical manifestations (signs and symptoms) of hypoxia

Maintain SpO_2 between 92% and 98%

Maintain PaO_2 between 60 and 100 (50–60 in chronic CO_2 retainers and 50–70 in premature neonates)

Decrease work of breathing

Decrease cardiac work

Prevent hypoxemia (immediate postoperative recovery period, trauma, acute MI, and during exercise with chronic lung disease)

Treat/prevent pulmonary hypertension secondary to chronic hypoxemia [PaO_2 ≤55 or SaO_2 ≤85 with COPD or PaO_2 56–59 (SaO_2 <90) with existing pulmonary hypertension]

Outcome measures:

Clinical improvement (pulse, respirations, blood pressure, mental function/level of consciousness, cyanosis, work of breathing, cardiac work, exercise tolerance)

Measurement of SpO_2 and/or arterial blood gas values

Decreased pulmonary artery pressure

Treat and/or prevent bronchospasm and mucosal edema

Specific goals:

Treat asthma

Treat COPD

Treat wheezing

Treat increased airway resistance (ventilator patients)

Provide aerosolized antiinflammatory or antiasthmatic agents (steroids, cromolyn, nedocromol sodium)

Outcome measures:

Clinical improvement (breath sounds, accessory muscle use/work of breathing, improved expiratory gas flow, pulse, respirations, blood pressure, mental function/level of consciousness, cyanosis)

Improved PEF (good response is improvement to 70%–80% of predicted)

Improved FEV_1 (increase ≥15%) or FVC (increase ≥12%)

Improvement in SpO_2 and/or arterial blood gas values

Decreased airway resistance (decrease PIP → ventilator patients)

Improved control of asthma symptoms

    PEF (good response is improvement to 70%–80% of predicted)

    FEV_1 to ≥80% of predicted

    For steroids and antiasthmatic drugs (cromolyn, nedocromil) → decrease need for bronchodilators

    For cromolyn or nedocromil → decrease or eliminate need for corticosteroids

Improved quality of life

    Patient subjective improvement (patient believes therapy is of benefit)

    Absence of adverse side effects (tachycardia, dizziness, nausea, vomiting, headache, tremors, tingling, anxiety or nervousness, chest pain, increased wheezing, increased dyspnea)

TABLE 7-12   Continued

Mobilize/remove secretions

Specific goals:
Provide mucolytic therapy
Provide chest physiotherapy (for atelectasis caused or suspected to be due to mucus plugging)
    Postural drainage and chest percussion
Provide other methods for mobilizing secretions
    Flutter, vest, or PEP therapy
    IPV
    Directed cough
    Airway suctioning
Provide for sputum induction
    Bland aerosol or hypertonic saline via large volume nebulizer or ultrasonic

Treat upper airway edema (croup, subglottic edema, postextubation edema)

Provide humidification for a bypassed upper airway (tracheostomy or endotracheal tube)

Outcomes measures:
Clinical improvement (improved breath sounds, decreased accessory muscle use/work of breathing,
    improved pulse and respirations, decreased dyspnea)
Patient subjective improvement (patient believes therapy is of benefit)
Cough effectiveness
Production of sputum, secretion volume, and ease of expectoration
Improved SpO_2, blood gases
Absence of adverse side effects (tachycardia, dizziness, nausea, vomiting, headache, tremors, tingling,
    anxiety or nervousness, chest pain, increased wheezing, increased dyspnea)

Lung expansion therapy to treat and/or prevent atelectasis and pneumonia

Specific goals:
Provide incentive spirometry
Provide IPPB

Outcome measures:
Volumes achieved during therapy $\geq 1/3$ predicted IC
Clinical improvement (improved breath sounds, decreased accessory muscle use/work of breathing,
    improved pulse and respirations, decreased dyspnea)
Subjective improvement (patient feels that therapy is beneficial)
Cough effectiveness
Production of sputum, secretion volume, and ease of expectoration
Improved SpO_2, blood gases
Absence of adverse side effects (tachycardia, dizziness, nausea, vomiting, headache, tremors, tingling,
    anxiety or nervousness, chest pain, increased wheezing, increased dyspnea)

retention and the premature neonate. Critical values in the COPD patient may be a PaO_2 of ≤ 55 with a SpO_2 of $\leq 85\%$ at rest or a PaO_2 of 56 to 59 and SaO_2 90% in the presence of pulmonary hypertension.[25,26] A critical PaO_2 for the newborn may be a PaO_2 of less than 50 torr and/or an SpO_2 of less than 88%.[24]

Hypoxemia should be suspected whenever the patient is exhibiting the signs and symptoms of hypoxia. Initial signs of hypoxia may include tachycardia, increased blood pressure, tachypnea, hyperventilation, restlessness, disorientation, dizziness, excitement, headache, blurred vision, impaired judgment, and confusion. Clinical manifestations of severe hypoxia may include slowed, irregular respirations, bradycardia, hypotension, and loss of consciousness, somnolence, convulsions, and coma. Severe hypoxia may lead to cardiac and/or respiratory arrest. The respiratory therapist should obtain an SpO_2 or ABG in order to confirm the presence of hypoxemia. The indications for oxygen therapy in the acute care setting are summarized in the critical content box.

CRITICAL CONTENT

INDICATIONS FOR OXYGEN THERAPY

Documented hypoxemia (SpO_2 or ABG)
    Adults and children: PaO_2 <60; and/or SpO_2 <90
    Neonates (less than 28 days old): PaO_2 <50 and/or
        SpO_2 <88%
Suspected hypoxemia (follow with SpO_2 or ABG)
Severe trauma
Acute MI
Postoperative recovery
Treat or prevent pulmonary hypertension secondary
    to chronic hypoxia [PaO_2 <55 or SpO_2 ≤85 with
    COPD or PaO_2 56 to 59 (SpO_2 <90) and preexist
    ing hypertension]

(SOURCE: © The University of Texas Health Science Center at San Antonio, Department of Respiratory Care, Patient Assessment and Respiratory Care Plan.)

Once it is established that oxygen therapy is required, the respiratory therapist must decide on the appropriate equipment, oxygen flow or FIO_2, and assessment of therapy. In general, the lowest FIO_2 needed to ensure adequate tissue oxygenation should be chosen. Generally, this means a target PaO_2 of 60 to 100 with a SpO_2 of 92% to 98%.[24,25] You should avoid excessive oxygen levels in patients who are chronic CO_2 retainers and in newborn infants, espe-

cially premature infants. Oxygen therapy for the COPD patient with chronically elevated $PaCO_2$ may be targeted at maintaining a PaO_2 of 50 to 60 torr with a SaO_2 of 88% to 90% in order to avoid oxygen-induced hypoventilation.[25,26] The newborn should have a PaO_2 maintained in the range of 50 to 70, as these levels should not result in retinopathy of prematurity, a disorder caused by high arterial oxygen concentrations in the newborn.[27]

One should also avoid high oxygen levels (greater than 50% to 60%) for extended periods of time because of the threat of oxygen toxicity. If high levels of oxygen (>50%) are needed for more than a brief period of time, alternative methods to improve oxygenation should be considered. Other techniques that may improve the patient's oxygenation status include positive end-expiratory pressure (PEEP) or continuous positive airway pressure (CPAP), bronchial hygiene techniques to mobilize secretions, and bronchodilator therapy. Prone positioning has been shown to improve oxygenation in patients with ARDS,[28] although this suggestion is not without controversy. Attention to maintaining cardiac output and blood pressure may be required to ensure adequate oxygen delivery to the tissues in patients with cardiovascular instability. Replacement of blood in patients with severe anemia may also be helpful.

The selection of an oxygen delivery method should be based on the desired FIO_2, as well as patient-specific factors such as disease state or condition, ventilatory pattern, patient comfort, and patient acceptance of the oxygen appliance. Generally, patients with hypoxemia due to low ventilation/perfusion (V/Q) or hypoventilation respond well to low to moderate concentrations of oxygen. This group includes patients with asthma, emphysema, chronic bronchitis, bronchiectasis, and cystic fibrosis. Often, patients with CHF without acute pulmonary edema and patients with coronary artery disease also respond well to low to moderate concentrations of oxygen.

The device of choice for most patients requiring low to moderate concentrations of oxygen is the nasal cannula. When set at ½ to 6 L/min, the nasal cannula will deliver from approximately 22% to 40% oxygen.[24,25] The nasal cannula is well tolerated, easy to use, and effective for most patients. The only major problem associated with the cannula is that the delivered FIO_2 will vary with the patient's ventilatory pattern. An air-entrainment mask should be considered as an alternative in patients with a variable ventilatory pattern or those with rapid, shallow breathing. Air-entrainment ("venturi") masks will deliver a stable FIO_2 for most patients and are available to deliver 24%, 28%, 30%, 35%, and 40% oxygen.[25] A sample respiratory care plan for providing oxygen therapy by nasal cannula using the SOAP note format is provided in the critical content box. Figure 7-6 contains a simple oxygen therapy protocol.

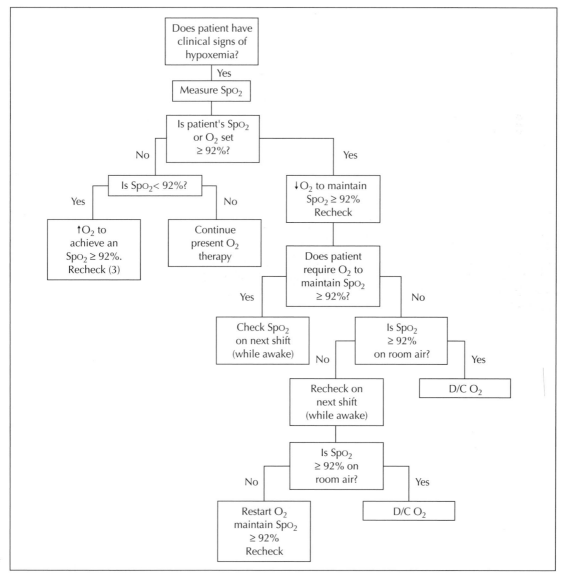

FIGURE 7-6 An oxygen therapy protocol. (*SOURCE: From Scanlon CL, Wilkins RL, Stoller JK (eds):* Egan's Fundamentals of Respiratory Care, *7th ed. St. Louis: Mosby; 1999:762.*)

CRITICAL CONTENT

A RESPIRATORY CARE PLAN FOR OXYGEN THERAPY

Admitting History and Physical Examination
A 61-year old man with a history of COPD is under scrutiny. He has a 60 pack-year history of smoking. He came to the emergency room acutely short of breath. He was admitted to the hospital 6 months ago due to acute exacerbation of COPD with documented CO_2 retention. Physical assessment revealed accessory muscle use and tachypnea with an increased pulse and blood pressure. Oximetry on room air reveals a SpO_2 of 80%. The patient has a weak, nonproductive cough, and breath sounds are diminished on auscultation.

Respiratory Assessment and Plan (SOAP Note)
S: "I'm real bad this time. I can hardly get my breath."
O: Respiratory rate, 32; pulse, 110; BP, 138/90; accessory muscle use; SpO_2, 80% on room air; diminished breath sounds bilaterally
A: Patient in acute distress secondary to exacerbation of chronic lung disease with documented hypoxemia
P: • Administer oxygen via nasal cannula at 1 to 4 L/min per protocol
   • Titrate O_2 based on oximetry and blood gases to maintain PaO_2 of 50 to 60 torr and an SpO_2 of 88% to 90%
   • Obtain ABGs on oxygen to access ventilatory status
   • Begin albuterol and atrovent bronchodilator administration per protocol
   • Continue to monitor patient

Patients with hypoxemia due to pulmonary shunting and patients suffering from acute MI or trauma may require moderate to high concentrations of oxygen therapy. Short-term oxygen therapy for patients needing moderate to high concentrations of oxygen may be provided using a simple mask (35% to 50% O_2 at 5 to 12 L/min),[24,25]

a partial rebreathing mask (35% to 60% at 6 to 10 L/min),[25] or a nonrebreathing mask (55% to 70% at 6 to 10 L/min).[25] Air-entrainment nebulizers via aerosol mask, trach mask, or T piece can be very useful in providing a stable oxygen concentration from 28% to 50%. Above 50% oxygen, typical air-entrainment nebulizers do not have an adequate total gas flow to deliver a dependable FIO_2. In recent years, a newer generation of nebulizers has been developed that can achieve high FIO_2s while maintaining high flows. For example, The Misty-ox High FIO_2-High Flow nebulizers will deliver 60% to 96% oxygen with total gas flows of 42 to 80 L/min.[29]

To summarize, for selection of oxygen delivery method, if the patient requires a low to moderate concentration of oxygen, the nasal cannula is the device of choice. In patients with unstable ventilatory patterns or rapid, shallow breathing, an air-entrainment (venturi) mask may be considered. For moderate to high concentrations of oxygen therapy for short-term use, consider a simple partial rebreathing or nonrebreathing mask. For a stable oxygen concentration via aerosol mask, trach mask, or T piece, consider a standard air-entrainment nebulizer for an FIO_2 of .28 to .50 and a high flow-high FIO_2 entrainment nebulizer for 60% to 96% oxygen.

Treat and/or Prevent Bronchospasm and Mucosal Edema

Bronchodilator Therapy. The primary indication for bronchodilator therapy is to treat or prevent bronchospasm.[27,30] Bronchodilator therapy is indicated in the treatment of asthma, COPD (including chronic bronchitis and cystic fibrosis), and whenever wheezing is due to reversible bronchoconstriction. A documented response to bronchodilator therapy may be demonstrated by an improvement in PEF, FEV_1, or FVC following therapy.[31] An improvement in clinical findings such as decreased wheezing, improved aeration, or a subjective improvement as judged by the patient are also important indicators of bronchodilator effectiveness.[31] With mechanically ventilated patients, bronchodilator therapy may be helpful to decrease airway resistance. An improvement in peak inspiratory pressures or expiratory gas flow curves may be useful in documenting the effectiveness of the therapy in these patients. The critical content box summarizes the indications for bronchodilator therapy.

CRITICAL CONTENT

INDICATIONS FOR BRONCHODILATOR THERAPY

Asthma

COPD (emphysema, chronic bronchitis, cystic fibrosis)

Wheezing

Documented response to a bronchodilator:

  Increase in FEV_1 of >15% following therapy, or

  Increase in FVC of >12% following therapy, or

  Increase in PEF

  Increase in PEFR to >70% to 90% of baseline with good response

  Increase in PEFR to 50% to 70% of baseline with incomplete response

  Increased airway resistance in patients receiving mechanical ventilation

(SOURCE: © The University of Texas Health Science Center at San Antonio, Department of Respiratory Care, Patient Assessment and Respiratory Care Plan.)

For bronchodilator therapy based on a specific protocol, the respiratory therapist must first assess the appropriateness of the therapy. Once the respiratory therapist has determined that a bronchodilator is appropriate, the specific medication, method of delivery, and frequency of administration must be determined using a specific patient protocol. Excellent clinical practice guidelines for the management of asthma have been developed by the National Institutes of Health.[3] A protocol for management of acute asthma exacerbation is found in Fig. 11-2. Generally, for adult asthmatics in the ED, 2.5 to 5 mg of albuterol is administered via small volume nebulizer every 20 minutes × 3. Following the initial bronchodilator administration, 2.5 to 10

mg of albuterol is administered by small volume nebulizer every 1 to 4 hours as needed, or 10 to 15 mg/hr continuously. Ipratropium bromide may be added, initially beginning with 0.5 mg every 30 minutes × 3, then every 2 to 4 hours as needed. These medications may be given with equal effectiveness via MDI and holding chamber if the patient is able to coordinate the use of the MDI. The frequency of administration is then reduced based on the patient's response and measurement of PEF or FEV^1. Figure 7-7 lists the medication dosages for treatment of asthma exacerbations.

Bronchodilator therapy is also indicated in the treatment of COPD as described in the American Thoracic Society standards.[32] Generally, intermittent symptoms are treated with 1 to 2 puffs of a $beta_2$ agonist via MDI every 2 to 6 hours. Regular or daily symptoms are treated with ipratropium MDI 2 to 6 puffs every 6 to 8 hours. A severe exacerbation of COPD may require a $beta_2$ bronchodilator via MDI or small volume nebulizer every ½ to 2 hours and/or increasing the dose of ipratropium. Figure 7-8 describes the use of bronchodilator therapy in the management of patients with COPD. See Chapter 12 for a more thorough discussion of the treatment of patients with COPD.

For other disease states or conditions where bronchospasm is suspected, the frequency of administration of a bronchodilator is generally every 4 hours to 4 times a day, depending on the patient's response and the duration of effect of the medication. For example, the recommended dosage of albuterol by small volume nebulizer is 2.5 mg three or four times a day, with onset of action occurring in about 15 minutes, a peak effect in 30 to 60 minutes, and a duration of action of 3 to 8 hours.[30] Salmeterol, on the other hand, has an onset within 20 minutes, a peak effect in 180 to 300 minutes, and duration of action of 12 hours.[30] The normal dose for salmeterol via MDI is two puffs every 12 hours.

Antiinflammatory Agents and Antiasthmatic Medications.

Antiinflammatory aerosol agents and antiasthmatic drugs include inhaled steroids, cromolyn sodium, nedocromol sodium, afirlukast, and ileuton, the latter two medications being

	Dosages		
Medications	**Adult dose**	**Child dose**	**Comments**
Inhaled short-acting beta$_2$ agonists			
Albuterol Nebulizer solution (5 mg/mL)	2.5–5 mg every 20 minutes for 3 doses, then 2.5–10 mg every 1–4 hours as needed, or 10–15 mg/hour continuously	0.15 mg/kg (minimum dose 2.5 mg) every 20 minutes for 3 doses, then 0.15–0.3 mg/kg up to 10 mg every 1–4 hours as needed, or 0.5 mg/kg/hour by continuous nebulization	Only selective beta$_2$ agonists are recommended. For optimal delivery, dilute aerosols to minimum of 4mL at gas flow of 6–8 L/min
MDI (90 µg/puff)	4–8 puffs every 20 minutes up to 4 hours, then every 1–4 hours as needed	4–8 puffs every 20 minutes for 3 doses, then every 1–4 hours inhalation maneuver. Use spacer/holding chamber	As effective as nebulized therapy if patient is able to coordinate
Bitolterol Nebulizer solution (2 mg/mL)	See albuterol dose.	See albuterol dose. Thought to be half as potent as albuterol on a mg basis	Has not been studied in severe asthma exacerbations. Do not mix with other drugs.
MDI (370 µg/puff)	See albuterol dose.	See albuterol dose.	Has not been studied in severe asthma exacerbations.
Pirbuterol MDI (200 µg/puff)	See albuterol dose.	See albuterol dose. Thought to be half as potent as albuterol on a mg basis	Has not been studied in severe asthma exacerbations.
Systemic (injected) beta$_2$ agonists			
Epinephrine 1:1000 (1 mg/mL)	0.3–0.5 mg every 20 minutes for 3 doses SQ	0.01 mg/kg up to 0.3–0.5 mg every 20 minutes for 3 doses SQ	No proven advantage of systemic therapy over aerosol
Terbutaline (1 mg/mL)	0.25 mg every 20 minutes for 3 doses SQ	0.01 mg/kg every 20 minutes for 3 doses then every 2–6 hours as needed SQ	No proven advantage of systemic therapy over aerosol

Medication			Comments
Anticholinergics			
Ipratropium bromide nebulizer solution (0.25 mg/mL)	0.5 mg every 30 minutes for 3 doses then every 2–4 hours as needed	0.25 mg every 20 minutes for 3 doses, then every 2 to 4 hours as needed	May mix in same nebulizer with albuterol. Should not be used as first-line therapy; should be added to beta$_2$ agonist therapy
MDI (18 µg/puff)	4–8 puffs as needed	4–8 puffs as needed	Dose delivered from MDI is low and has not been studied in asthma exacerbations
Corticosteroids			
Prednisone Methylprednisolone Prednisolone	120–180 mg/day in 3 or 4 divided doses for 48 hours, then 60–80 mg/day until PEFR reaches 70% of predicted or personal best	1 mg/kg every 6 hours for 48 hours then 1–2 mg/kg/day (maximum = 60 mg/day) in 2 divided doses until PEFR 70% of predicted or personal best	For outpatient "burst" use 40–60 mg in single or 2 divided doses for adults (children: 1–2 mg/kg/day, maximum 60 mg/day) for 3–10 days

Note: No advantage has been found for higher dose corticosteroids in severe asthma exacerbations, nor is there any advantage for intravenous administration over oral therapy, provided gastrointestinal transit time or absorption is not impaired. The usual regimen is to continue the frequent multiple daily dosing until the patient achieves an FEV$_1$ or PEFR of 50% of predicted or personal best and then lower the dose to twice daily. This usually occurs within 48 hours. Therapy following a hospitalization or ED visit may last from 3 to 10 days. If patients are then started on inhaled corticosteroids, studies indicate there is no need to taper the systemic corticosteroid dose. If the follow-up systemic corticosteroid therapy is to be given once daily, one study indicates that it may be more clinically effective to give the dose in the afternoon at 3 PM, with no increase in adrenal suppression.

F I G U R E   7 - 7   Medication dosages for treatment of asthma exacerbations. (*SOURCE: From National Institutes of Health.*[3])

Intermittent Symptoms* **MILD**	Regular/Daily Symptoms* **MILD TO MODERATE**	Exacerbation* **SEVERE**
Beta$_2$ agonist MDI 1–2 puffs every 2–6 h not to exceed 8–12 puffs every 24 h	**Ipratropium MDI** 2–6 puffs every 6–8 h; not to be used more frequently	**Increase beta$_2$ agonist dose** 6–8 puffs every ½–2 h, or nebulized solution, every ½–2 h, or subcutaneous epinephrine or terbutaline
	plus ↓	**and/or** ↓
	Beta$_2$ agonist 1–4 puffs as required 4 times daily PRN or regular supplement	**Increase ipratropium dose** MDI with spacer 6–8 puffs every 3–4 h or nebulized ipratropium 0.5 mg every 4–8 h
	UNSATISFACTORY RESPONSE OR INCREASE IN SYMPTOMS	↓
	Theophylline sustained release, 200–400 mg twice daily, or 400–800 mg at bedtime for nocturnal bronchospasm and/or consider **Sustained release albuterol** 4–8 mg twice daily or at night only and/or consider using **Mucokinetic agent**	**Theophylline IV** serum level 10–12 µg/mL and **Methylprednisolone IV** 50–100 mg immediately, then every 6–8 h, taper as soon as possible and add **Antibiotic** if indicated and add **Mucokinetic agent** if sputum is very viscous
	CONTROL OF SYMPTOMS SUBOPTIMAL ↓	
	Oral steroids eg, prednisone, up to 40 mg/d for 10–14 days. If improvement occurs, wean to low daily dose or alternate day use (eg, 7.5 µg) or consider inhaled steroids. If no improvement occurs, stop abruptly.	

F I G U R E 7 - 8   Bronchodilator therapy in the COPD patient. *Includes addition of steroids and mucokinetic agents, as needed. [*Source: Adapted from* Am J Respir Crit Care Med. *1995;152(5 Suppl):S78.]*

administered in tablet form. The indications for antiinflammatory aerosol agents and antiasthmatic agents are shown in the critical content box.

CRITICAL CONTENT

INDICATIONS FOR ANTIINFLAMMATORY AND ANTIASTHMATIC AGENTS

Antiinflammatory Aerosol Agents (Inhaled steroids)
- Asthma
- COPD (emphysema, chronic bronchitis, cystic fibrosis)
- Upper airway edema (postextubation, croup)

Antiasthmatic Aerosol Agents (Cromolyn, Nedocromol)
- Asthma

(SOURCE: © The University of Texas Health Science Center at San Antonio, Department of Respiratory Care, Patient Assessment and Respiratory Care Plan.)

The appropriate use of corticosteroids for the treatment of asthma is well described in the NIH guidelines.[3] Cromolyn or nedocromil may be added to the asthma patient's care regimen for the long-term management of asthma.[3] See Chapter 11 for a comprehensive discussion and case studies for asthma management.

With respect to upper airway edema following extubation, the use of a cool aerosol with supplemental oxygen has been recommended.[10] Racemic epinephrine (0.5 mL of 2.25% in 3 mL of diluent) or dexamethasone (1 mg in 4 mL of diluent) by nebulizer have also been recommended.[10] Helium-oxygen mixtures (60% He and 40% O_2) by nonrebreathing mask may be helpful in decreasing the severity of stridor and reducing the need for reintubation.[10] Helium-oxygen therapy may also be of value in treatment of acute severe asthma exacerbation and has been used in an attempt to reduce the need for intubation and mechanical ventilation in these patients.[3]

For pediatric patients suffering from croup (laryngotracheobronchitis), treatment typically consists of cool mist therapy. Aerosolized racemic epinephrine, dexamethasone, and budesonide may be effective in reducing severity of symptoms in patients suffering from croup.[33] See Chapter 14 for examples, exercises, and a comprehensive discussion of croup management.

Mobilize and Remove Secretions

Techniques to mobilize or remove secretions include mucolytic therapy (acetylcysteine, dornase alpha), directed cough, suctioning, and chest physiotherapy. In addition, high-volume bland aerosol may be of value in the presence of a secretion clearance problem. Specific indications for each of these therapies are listed in Table 7-13.

The least expensive method that is effective for mobilization of secretions should be selected. For example, a patient with chronic bronchitis who is able to easily remove secretions using a directed cough probably has no need for mucolytic therapy, chest physiotherapy, or use of a high-volume bland aerosol. Thick, viscous, retained secretions in the same patient might require aerosolized acetylcysteine given with a bronchodilator followed by vigorous chest physiotherapy.

Frequency of therapy will vary with the respiratory care modality selected and the patient's condition. For example, 3 to 5 mL of a 10% to 20% solution of acetylcysteine with a bronchodilator is generally administered by aerosol three or four times a day.[30] (Acetylcysteine given by aerosol should always be accompanied by a bronchodilator to avoid inducing bronchospasm.) Aerosolized dornase alpha is specifically indicated in cystic fibrosis patients, in a dose of 2.5 mg four times a day.[30]

Directed cough or huff coughing (especially with COPD patients) should follow any therapy used to mobilize secretions and may be useful for obtaining a sputum specimen. Suctioning should be applied to patients with artificial airways on an as-needed basis. Routine schedules (every 2 hours, four times a day, etc.) for suctioning should be avoided.

TABLE 7-13   INDICATIONS FOR THERAPY TO MOBILIZE AND REMOVE SECRETIONS

Mucolytic therapy
Evidence of viscous/retained secretions which are not easily removed via other therapy
Chronic bronchitis, cystic fibrosis, bronchiectasis

Directed cough
Retained secretions
Atelectasis
At risk for postoperative pulmonary complications
Cystic fibrosis, bronchiectasis, chronic bronchitis, necrotizing pulmonary infection, or spinal cord
    injury
During/following other bronchial hygiene therapies
To obtain sputum specimens
Presence of endotracheal or tracheostomy tube

Suctioning
Inability to clear secretions in spite of best cough effort (secretions audible in large/central airways)
Need to remove accumulated pulmonary secretions in presence of an artificial airway
    Coarse or noisy breath sounds (rhonchi, gurgles)
    Increased PIP during mechanical ventilation or decreased VT during pressure controlled ventilation
    Ineffective spontaneous cough
    Visible secretions in airway
    Suspected aspiration
    Increased WOB
    Deterioration of ABGs
    CXR changes consistent with retained secretions
    To obtain sputum specimen
    To maintain artificial airway patency
    To stimulate cough
    Presence of atelectasis or consolidation presumed to be associated with secretion retention

Chest physiotherapy
  Postural drainage and percussion
  Suggestion/evidence of problems with secretion clearance
    Difficulty clearing secretions with volume >25–30 mL/day (adult)
    Retained secretions in presence of an artificial airway
    Atelectasis caused or suspected to be due to mucus plugging
    Cystic fibrosis, bronchiectasis, cavitating lung disease
    Presence of a foreign body in airway

High volume bland aerosol
  Cool large volume nebulizer
    Postextubation
    Upper airway edema
    Delivery of precise FIO_2 via aerosol mask and high humidity
  Heated large volume nebulizer
    Evidence or potential for secretion clearance problem
    Deliver precise FIO_2 via aerosol mask and high humidity

SOURCE: Used with permission of the University of Texas Health Science Center at San Antonio, Department of Respiratory
Care, Patient Assessment and Respiratory Care Plan.

Chest physiotherapy may include postural drainage, percussion, and vibration. Postural drainage positions are generally applied for 3 to 15 minutes per position for a total treatment time of 20 to 45 minutes or more, as tolerated by the patient.[34] Chest percussion or vibration may be applied for each postural drainage position for 3 to 5 minutes per position.[34] Frequency of performance of chest physiotherapy should be based on the patient's ability to tolerate the procedure and its effectiveness in mobilizing secretions. Generally, postural drainage and chest percussion in the acute care setting is applied four times a day every 4 to 6 hours.

The use of high-volume bland aerosol (normal saline, ½ normal saline, and sterile distilled water) for the mobilization of secretions remains controversial. It would seem to be clear that most pneumatic cool mist aerosol generators are unable to deliver enough water to the airway to mobilize secretions. Heated pneumatic nebulizers, babbington nebulizers, and ultrasonic nebulizers may be used to deliver large volumes of bland aerosol to assist in mobilizing secretions; however, the value of bland aerosols in secretion mobilization remains a matter of opinion. Generally, heated aerosols and ultrasonic nebulizers are reserved for use in sputum induction, either using sterile distilled water or a hypertonic saline solution of 3% to 7% NaCl.[34-36] Heated bland aerosols are also used routinely to provide humidification in patients with artificial airways for which there is evidence or potential for secretion problems.[36]

Other techniques sometimes used to aid in mobilizing secretions include the use of the huff cough (forced expiratory technique, or FET), active cycle breathing, autogenic drainage, mechanical insufflation-exsufflation, positive expiratory pressure (PEP), and high frequency compression/oscillation (high frequency chest wall compression, flutter valve, and intrapulmonary percussive ventilation).[34] An example of a respiratory care plan designed to assist in mobilizing secretions in a patient with chronic bronchitis is found in Table 7-14.

Provide Lung Expansion Therapy

Indications for lung expansion therapy include the treatment and/or prevention of atelectasis. Incentive spirometry should be considered in patients who are able to perform the maneuver every 1 to 2 hours while awake and are able to achieve an inspired volume of at least one third of predicted inspiratory capacity.[37] Inspiratory capacity may be predicted by multiplying the patient's estimated ideal body weight (IBW) in kilograms by 50 mL/kg:

$$\text{Minimum volume for incentive spirometry} = \text{IBW} \times 50 \text{ mL/kg} \times .33$$

The formula for ideal body weight for men and women in kilograms:

$$\text{IBW for men} = [106 + 6(\text{H} - 60)]/2.2$$
$$\text{IBW for women} = [105 + 5(\text{H} - 60)]/2.2$$

where H is the person's height in centimeters.

TABLE 7-14   SAMPLE RESPIRATORY CARE PLAN FOR SECRETION MOBILIZATION AND BRONCHODILATOR THERAPY IN A PATIENT WITH ACUTE EXACERBATION OF COPD (CHRONIC BRONCHITIS)

4 mL of 10% acetylcysteine with 2.5 mg of albuterol QID by small volume nebulizer powered by compressed air

Follow aerosol therapy with postural drainage and chest percussion to RLL, LLL, anterior, posterior, and lateral segments

Directed cough following each of the above, or may try huff cough

Ipratropium 6–8 puffs via MDI with spacer q4 h while awake and PRN at night

Continue nasal cannula at 1–4 L/m to maintain SpO_2 ≥92%; monitor SpO_2 during chest physiotherapy

Note: Severe acute exacerbations of COPD may also require the administration of theophylline, corticosteroids, and antibiotics, if indicated. An SpO_2 of 88%–90% with a PaO_2 of 50–60 torr may be appropriate for the COPD patient who is also a chronic CO_2 retainer in order to prevent oxygen-induced hypoventilation.

Intermittent positive-pressure breathing (IPPB) should generally be reserved for patients who have clinically important atelectasis, in whom other therapy has been unsuccessful.[38] When used as a form of lung expansion therapy, minimum delivered tidal volumes during IPPB therapy should probably be at least one third of predicted inspiratory capacity (IC). Another common sense approach is that the volume delivered with IPPB should exceed the patient's maximum spontaneous volume, preferably by more than 25%.[39] There is little logic to using IPPB for lung expansion therapy unless it actually exceeds spontaneous efforts at lung expansion.

IPPB may also be considered for patients at risk of developing atelectasis who cannot or will not take a deep breath on their own. IPPB may also be useful in a few patients for delivery of bronchodilators or other medication where patient coordination and the ability to take a deep breath are compromised.

Recommended frequency and duration of an incentive spirometry session is once every hour while awake times 10 to 15 breaths of at least one third predicted IC (or >10 mL/kg). IPPB as a form of lung expansion therapy usually includes the administration of an aerosolized bronchodilator, and therapy is usually given three or four times a day or every 2 to 4 hours for approximately 10 to 20 minutes. The indications for lung expansion therapy are outlined in the critical content box. A sample protocol for delivery of lung expansion therapy is found in Fig. 7-9.

CHART REVIEW

Patient name: _____   Age: _____

Physician(s): _____   Height: _____

Hospital ID No.: _____   Weight: _____

Floor/Unit: _____   Sex: _____

Admitting diagnosis: _____

Other problems from problem list or patient history and physical:

1. _____   4. _____

2. _____   5. _____

3. _____   6. _____

Current physician orders for respiratory care: _____

_____

Most recent ABGs and/or Spo_2: _____

_____

Most recent chest x-ray reports: _____

_____

Most recent pulmonary function testing: _____

PATIENT INTERVIEW

Cough: _____   Sputum production: _____

Hemoptysis: _____   Wheezing, whistling,

                                            or chest tightness: _____

Breathlessness: _____

FIGURE 7-9 A protocol for lung expansion therapy.

PATIENT INTERVIEW (*continued*)

Chest illness: _____

Smoking: _____

Occupational history: _____

Hobby and leisure history: _____

Medicines or respiratory care used: _____

Response to current respiratory care: _____

PHYSICAL ASSESSMENT

General appearance: _____

Pulse: _____   Respirations: _____   Blood pressure: _____

Level of consciousness: _____

Chest inspection: _____

Auscultation: _____

Percussion: _____

Palpation: _____

Bedside spirometry: IC: _____   PEFR: _____   VC: _____ FEV_1 _____

ASSESSMENT FOR THERAPY

Evaluate whether or not each specific therapy listed would be indicated and/or appropriate for this patient based on your chart review, patient interview, and physical assessment data. NOTE: Check all indications present REGARDLESS of whether the patient is currently receiving a particular therapy or not.

Assessment for oxygen therapy (check all indications present for oxygen therapy)

Yes No

☐ ☐ documented hypoxemia (SpO_2 or ABG)

  adults and children — PaO_2 <60 and/or SpO_2 <90

  neonates (less than 28 days) — PaO_2 <50 and/or SpO_2 <88%

☐ ☐ corrected hypoxemia — a PaO_2 of less than 90–100 torr while receiving oxygen therapy would be consistent with corrected hypoxemia

☐ ☐ suspected hypoxemia based on chart review and/or physical assessment (follow with SpO_2 or ABG)

☐ ☐ severe trauma

☐ ☐ acute MI

☐ ☐ immediate post-op recovery (recovery room or ICU)

Continued

FIGURE 7-9   *Continued*

Assessment for bronchodilator therapy (check all indications present for bronchodilator therapy)

Yes   No

☐   ☐   asthma
☐   ☐   COPD or chronic obstructive lung disease (emphysema/chronic bronchitis/cystic fibrosis/bronchiectasis
☐   ☐   wheezing
☐   ☐   documenting response to a bronchodilator
    – increase in FEV_1 of ≥15% or increase in FVC of ≥12%
      or
    – increase in PEFR
      ↑ PEFR to >70–90% base line → good response
      ↑ PEFR to 50–70% base line → incomplete response

Assessment for anti-inflammatory aerosol agents (inhaled steroids) (check all of the indications present)

Yes   No

☐   ☐   asthma
☐   ☐   COPD (emphysema/chronic bronchitis/cystic fibrosis/bronchiectasis)
☐   ☐   upper airway edema (postextubation, croup)

Assessment for antiasthmatic aerosol agents (cromolyn, etc.) (check all of the indications present)

Yes   No

☐   ☐   asthma

Assessment for mucolytic therapy (check the indications present for this patient)

Yes   No

☐   ☐   evidence of viscous/retained secretions which are not easily removed via other therapy
☐   ☐   chronic bronchitis, cystic fibrosis, bronchiectasis

Assessment for lung expansion therapy

Incentive Spirometry (check the indications present for this patient)

Yes   No

☐   ☐   Patient is able to perform the maneuver q1–2 hours while awake and is able to achieve an inspired volume of at least ⅓ of predicted inspiratory capacity (or VC ≥ 10 mL/kg) AND:

FIGURE 7-9   A protocol for lung expansion therapy.   *Continued*

Assessment for lung expansion therapy (*continued*)

Check as many as apply:

☐	☐	patient predisposed to development of atelectasis
☐	☐	upper abdominal surgery
☐	☐	thoracic surgery
☐	☐	surgery in patients with COPD
☐	☐	patient debilitated/bedridden
☐	☐	presence of atelectasis
☐	☐	quadriplegic and/or dysfunctional disphragm

Intermittent positive-pressure breathing (check the indications present for this patient)

Yes   No

☐	☐	presence of clinically important atelectasis AND other therapy and has been unsuccessful
☐	☐	inability to spontaneously deep breathe (inspired volumes less than ⅓ predicted IC or VC <10 mL/kg) in patients with inadequate cough and/or secretion clearance AND other therapy has been unsuccessful
☐	☐	to provide short-term ventilatory support in an attempt to avoid intubation and continuous mechanical ventilation
☐	☐	to deliver aerosol medication in patients who are unable to adequately deep breathe and/or coordinate the use of other aerosol devices

Assessment for chest physiotherapy (check all of the indications present for this patient)

Postural drainage and percussion

Yes   No

☐	☐	suggestion/evidence of problems with secretion clearance
☐	☐	difficulty clearing secretions with volume > 25–30 mL/day (adult)
☐	☐	retained secretions in presence of an artificial airway
☐	☐	atelectasis caused/suspected to be due to mucus plugging
☐	☐	cystic fibrosis, bronchiectasis, cavitating lung disease
☐	☐	presence of a foreign body in airway

FIGURE 7-9   *Continued*

Assessment for high-volume bland aerosol (check all of the indications present for this patient)

Cool large-volume nebulizer

Yes	No	
☐	☐	postextubation
☐	☐	upper airway edema
☐	☐	delivery of precise F_{IO_2} via aerosol mask, trach mask, or T-piece and high humidity

Heated large-volume nebulizer or USN

Yes	No	
☐	☐	evidence/potential for secretion clearance problem
☐	☐	deliver precise F_{IO_2} via aerosol mask, trach mask, or T-piece and high humidity

Assessment for directed cough (check all of the indications present)

Yes	No	
☐	☐	retained secretions
☐	☐	atelectasis
☐	☐	at risk for postoperative pulmonary complications
☐	☐	cystic fibrosis, bronchiectasis, chronic bronchitis, necrotizing pulmonary infection, or spinal cord injury
☐	☐	during/following other bronchial hygiene therapies
☐	☐	to obtain sputum specimens
☐	☐	presence of endotracheal or tracheostomy tube

Assessment for suctioning (check all of the indications present for this patient)

Yes	No	
☐	☐	inability to clear secretions in spite of best cough effort (secretions audible in large/central airways
☐	☐	need to remove accumulated pulmonary secretions in presence of an artificial airway
☐	☐	coarse or noisy breath sounds (rhonchi, gurgles)
☐	☐	increased PIP during mechanical ventilation or decreased VTduring pressure controlled ventilation
☐	☐	ineffective spontaneous cough
☐	☐	visible secretions in airway
☐	☐	suspected aspiration
☐	☐	increased WOB
☐	☐	deterioration of ABGs
☐	☐	chest x-ray changes consistent with retained secretions
☐	☐	to obtain sputum specimen
☐	☐	to maintain artificial airway patency
☐	☐	to stimulate cough
☐	☐	presence of atelectasis or consolidating presumed to be associated with secretion retention

FIGURE 7-9 (*Continued*) A protocol for lung expansion therapy.

CRITICAL CONTENT

LUNG EXPANSION THERAPY

Incentive Spirometry

Patient must be able to perform the maneuver every 1 to 2 hours while awake and be able to achieve an inspired volume of at least one third of predicted inspiratory capacity (or VC >10 mL/kg) AND one or more of the following:

Patient predisposed to development of atelectasis:
    Upper abdominal surgery
    Thoracic surgery
    Surgery in patients with COPD
    Patient debilitated/bedridden
Presence of atelectasis
Quadriplegic and/or dysfunctional diaphragm

IPPB

Patient should have one or more of the following indications:

    Presence of clinically important atelectasis
        AND other therapy has been unsuccessful
    Inability to spontaneously deep breathe)inspired
        volumes less than one third predicted IC or
        VC <10 mL/kg) in patients with inadequate
        cough and/or secretion clearance AND
        other therapy has been unsuccessful
    To provide short-term ventilatory support in
        an attempt to avoid intubation and
        continuous mechanical ventilation
    To deliver aerosol medication in patients who
        are unable to adequately deep breathe and/or
        coordinate the use of other aerosol devices

(*SOURCE:* © *The University of Texas Health Science Center at San Antonio, Department of Respiratory Care, Patient Assessment and Respiratory Care Plan.*)

RESPIRATORY CARE PLAN FORMAT

Many institutions have developed various forms and formats for use in writing and organizing the respiratory care plan. One common format uses problem-oriented charting including the use of a SOAP note as described earlier. Figure 7-10 contains a suggested format for organizing a respiratory care plan using the SOAP technique.

Another format includes problems or complaints, possible sources of problems or complaints, actions taken to relieve problems or complaints, short- and long-term goals, evaluation, and documentation.

A third possible format for the respiratory care plan is found in Fig. 7-11. This format includes patient demographic data, indications for specific respiratory care and a care plan oriented toward maintaining oxygenation, treatment and prevention of bronchospasm and/or mucosal edema, delivering antiinflammatory and antiasthmatic medications, therapy to mobilize and remove secretions, and lung expansion therapy.

SUMMARY OF RESPIRATORY CARE PLAN

The respiratory care plan is simply a written explanation of the respiratory care that the patient is to receive. The respiratory care plan may take the form of physician's orders, a detailed progress note in the medical record, an established protocol, completion of a standardized respiratory care form or the use of problem-oriented medical records using SOAP notes. In the clinical setting, respiratory care plan development requires an initial physician's order, a well-designed protocol or policy, and careful patient assessment. The physician's order may be specific or may simply state "respiratory care per protocol." Developing and implementing the respiratory care plan requires a careful patient assessment. Following the patient assessment, the respiratory therapist selects the appropriate care based on the patient's condition and the indications for each type of therapy, as described above. The respiratory care plan may include the goal of the therapy, device, or procedure; medications given; method or appliance used; gas source and/or flow; volume goals; and frequency and duration of therapy. The care plan may also include a statement of how the intensity

Patient name: _____   Age: _____

Physician(s): _____   Height: _____

Hospital ID no.: _____   Weight: _____

_____   Sex: _____

Admitting diagnosis: _____

Problems or complaints:

1. _____   4. _____

2. _____   5. _____

3. _____   6. _____

Subjective findings: _____

_____

_____

_____

Objective findings: _____

_____

_____

Assessment: _____

_____

_____

_____

Plan: _____

_____

_____

_____

F I G U R E 7 - 1 0   Sample respiratory care plan using SOAP.

Oxygen therapy

    Goals: _____

    Device: _____

    Liter flow and/or F_{IO_2}: _____

    Frequency and duration of therapy (cont., PRN, etc.): _____

    Assessment: _____

Bronchodilator therapy

    Goals: _____

    Device or procedure (MDI, SVN, etc:) _____

    Medications: _____

    Method or appliance (mask, mouthpiece, aerochamber, etc.): _____

    Gas source and flow: _____

    Frequency and duration of therapy: _____

    Assessment: _____

F I G U R E 7 - 1 1   Patient assessment and respiratory care plan. (*SOURCE: Used with permission of the University of Texas Health Science Center at San Antonio, Department of Respiratory Care, Patient Assessment and Respiratory Care Plan.*)

Antiinflammatory aerosol (inhaled steroids)

    Goals: _____

    Device or procedure (MDI, SVN, etc.): _____

    Medications: _____

    Method or appliance (mask, mouthpiece, aerochamber, etc.): _____

    Gas source and flow: _____

    Frequency and duration of therapy: _____

    Assessment: _____

Mucolytic therapy

    Goals: _____

    Device or procedure (MDI, SVN, etc.): _____

    Medications: _____

    Method or appliance (mask, mouthpiece, aerochamber, etc.): _____

    Gas source and flow: _____

    Frequency and duration of therapy: _____

    Assessment: _____

Lung expansion therapy

    Goals: _____

    Device or procedure: _____

    Medications: _____

    Method or appliance (mask, mouthpiece, etc.): _____

    Gas source, flow and pressure: _____

    Frequency and duration of therapy: _____

    Volume goals: _____

    Assessment: _____

Chest physiotherapy

    Goals: _____

    Procedure: _____

    Method or appliance (percussor, etc.): _____

    Frequency and duration of therapy: _____

    Assessment: _____

Directed cough

    Goals: _____

    Procedure: _____

    Frequency and duration of therapy: _____

    Assessment: _____

Continued

FIGURE 7-11 *Continued*

Suctioning

    Goals: _____

    Procedure: _____

    Method: _____

    Frequency and duration of therapy: _____

    Assessment: _____

Comments:

FIGURE 7-11   Patient assessment and respiratory care plan.   *Continued*

and/or duration of therapy will be adjusted and when the therapy will be discontinued. Assessment of the outcomes of therapy may also be included. These may include evidence of clinical improvement, measurement of bedside pulmonary function data such as PEF or FEV_1, improvement in oxygenation or SpO_2, improved quality of life, patient subjective improvement, and the absence of adverse side effects. In summary, the respiratory care plan may be defined as the written plan of treatment that the patient will receive. The respiratory care plan may include goals, rationale, and significance, and a description of how that care will be assessed.

CASE STUDY 1

CARL CHILLS

Case Scenario

A 39-year-old computer programmer is admitted to your hospital via the ED. He is divorced and maintains custody of his two teenaged sons. Mr. Chills has health insurance through his company's PPO. His neighbor drove him to the ED because he felt too ill to drive. He states, "I feel tired, have bouts of chills and sweats, and keep coughing up brown-colored phlegm." Initially the cough was dry and nonproductive, but has become more persistent and productive during the last 24 hours.

Onset of fever was noticed approximately 3 days prior to admission. Past medical and family history are not contributory to the current condition.

 Critical Thinking Exercise 1

PRIORITIZING PATIENT CARE

Explain how you would prioritize your assessment of this patient based on his admitting data.

CASE STUDY 1 *(continued)*

PHYSICAL ASSESSMENT

Vital signs	Temperature: 39°C; Pulse: 110/minute; Blood pressure: 125/85; Respiratory rate; 25/min.
Inspection	No central cyanosis. Normal chest/abdominal excursion.
Palpation	Asymmetry noted during thoracic expansion with a right-sided limitation. Increased tactile fremitus noted over the lower posterior right chest wall.
Percussion	Dull/flat noted upon percussion of the lower posterior right chest wall.
Auscultation	Bronchial breath sounds heard over the lower posterior right chest wall with discordant crackles.

LABORATORY DATA

ABG, room air sample	pH: 7.48; $Paco_2$: 30 mm Hg; Pao_2: 58 mm Hg; HCO_3^-: 20mEq/L.
Chest radiograph	Increased opacity noted throughout the right lower lobe.
PFT	None ordered.
CBC	RBC, hemoglobin, and hematocrit all within normal limits. WBC: 20,000/mm^3 with neutrophils at 85% of the differential.

Critical Thinking Exercise 2

MAKING INFERENCES BY CLUSTERING DATA

a. What inference can you make about the possible diagnosis?

b. Practice clustering the data that lead you to this inference and describe how each piece of data contributed to your hypothesis.

Critical Thinking Exercise 3

ANTICIPATING FINDINGS

a. What laboratory and diagnostic data would be of further assistance in assessing this patient?

b. What specific findings do you anticipate and how would they guide your management of this patient?

Critical Thinking Exercise 4

PROBLEM SOLVING USING CLINICAL DATA

a. What does the laboratory and diagnostic data suggest about this patient's diagnosis? Explain the rationale for your interpretation.

b. What additional data would you request to assist in making your diagnosis? Explain the rationale for each procedure or test.

Critical Thinking Exercise 5

ANTICIPATING PROBLEMS AND SOLUTIONS

a. How would you track this patient's clinical progress?

b. What pulmonary complication may develop during this patient's clinical course?

CASE STUDY 1 *(continued)*

SOAP Note and Care Plan

S: "I feel tired, have bouts of chills and sweats, and I keep coughing up brown-colored phlegm."

O: Temperature: 39°C; HR: 110/min; BP: 125/85; RR: 25/min. Inspection findings are normal. Palpation reveals right-sided limitation upon expansion and increased tactile fremitus in right lower posterior chest wall. Flat percussion note in right lower posterior chest wall. Bronchial breath sounds in right lower posterior chest wall with discordant crackles. ABG results: pH: 7.48; $Paco_2$: 30 mm Hg; Pao_2: 58 mm Hg; HCO_3^-: 20 mEq/L. CXR results: RLL opacity. CBC results WBC: 20,000/mm^3, 85% neutrophils.

A: The patient is febrile (39°C) and tachypneic (25/min).

The limited right-sided expansion and increased tactile fremitus indicate consolidation. The percussion and auscultation findings are also indicative of consolidation with airway secretions, as evidenced by the bronchial breath sounds and presence of crackles.

ABG results reveal a partially compensated respiratory alkalemia (alveolar hyperventilation) with moderate hypoxemia.

CXR results indicate a RLL infiltrate.
CBC results denote leukocytosis with neutrophilia.
These findings are consistent with bacterial pneumonia.

P: Begin oxygen via nasal cannula at 4 L/min per protocol to maintain SpO_2 ≥92%. Follow-up with ABG on oxygen. May monitor with pulse oximeter. Institute bronchial hygiene per protocol.

Critical Thinking Exercise 6

DECISION MAKING AND REFLECTION

---

a. Discuss the average length of stay (LOS) you would expect for this patient, Mr. Chills.

b. Estimate the direct and indirect costs for acute care based on your care plan and your understanding of the treatment for bacterial pneumonia.

c. Finally, estimate if your hospital can make a profit in this case if the PPO-negotiated payment is based on the DRG.

KEY POINTS

- The primary goals for patient assessment by respiratory therapist are to augment admission history and physical exam, recommend therapy, monitor the patient's condition over time, modify or terminate therapy, provide documentation of the outcomes of therapy, and to develop, implement, and monitor the respiratory care plan.

- Additional goals of patient assessment and development of a respiratory care plan include collection of data to assess cost/benefit and other cost analyses of effective patient care.

- Before the patient interview and assessment, it is important to review the patient history to include: demographic data chief complaint (CC), history of present illness (HPI), past medical history (PMH), and family history.

- The respiratory therapist must have effective communication skills, including active listening to conduct a successful patient interview. Interviewing skills can improve with practice and experience.

- Important aspects of physical assessment of the pulmonary patient include vital signs, inspection, palpation, percussion, and auscultation (IPPA).

- Clinicians use the problem-oriented medical record (POMR) to collect and document data, assess the patient, and develop an appropriate treatment plan. The most common POMR is the SOAP note. The acronym SOAP refers to a type of clinical note that allows the practitioner to report their examination finding, assessment and treatment plan to include *S*ubjective, *O*bjective, *A*ssessment, and *P*lan.

- In the clinical setting, respiratory care plan development requires an initial physician's order, a well-designed protocol or policy, and careful patient assessment. The physician's order may be specific or may simply state "respiratory care per protocol."

- The respiratory care plan can be defined as the written plan of treatment for a specific patient to include goals, rationale, significance, and a description of how that care will be assessed, including the outcomes to be measured.

- The respiratory care plan is an individual protocol for the care of a specific patient.

- The respiratory care plan may take the form of physician's orders, a detailed progress note in the medical record, an established protocol, completion of a standardized respiratory care form or SOAP notes.

- The respiratory therapist determines the respiratory care plan based on careful patient assessment and a review of the available respiratory care diagnostic and treatment modalities available.

REFERENCES

1. Krider SJ. Interviewing and respiratory history. In: Wilkins R, Krider S, Sheldon R, eds. *Clinical Assessment in Respiratory Care.* 3rd ed. St. Louis: Mosby-Year Book; 1995:9–34.

2. Andreoli TE, Bennett JC, Carpenter CCJ, et al. *Cecil's Essentials of Medicine.* 4th ed. Philadelphia: Saunders; 1997:113.

3. National Institutes of Health, National Heart Lung and Blood Institute Guidelines for the Diagnosis and Management of Asthma: Expert Panel 2 Report. (NIH Publication No. 98-4051). Bethesda, Md: US Department of Health and Human Services; 1998.

4. Des Jardins T, Tietsort JA. Assessment skills core to practitioner success. In: Burton GG, Hodgkin JE, Ward JJ, eds. *Respiratory Care—A Guide to Clinical Practice.* 4th ed. Philadelphia: Lippincott; 1997:153–183.

5. Redlich CA, Balmes J. Occupational and environmental lung disease. In: George RB, Light RW, Matthay MA, et al, eds. *Chest Medicine.* 3rd ed. Baltimore: Williams & Wilkins; 1995:365.

6. Des Jardins T, Burton GG. Asthma. In: Des Jardins T, Burton GG. *Clinical Manifestations and Assessment of Respiratory Disease.* 3rd ed. St. Louis: Mosby; 1995:195–207.

7. Wilkins RL. Physical examination of the patient with cardiopulmonary disease. In: Wilkins R, Krider S, Sheldon R, eds. *Clinical Assessment in Respiratory Care.* 3rd ed. St. Louis: Mosby-Year Book; 1995:47–77.

8. Krider SJ. Vital signs. In: Wilkins R, Krider S, Sheldon R, eds. *Clinical Assessment in Respiratory Care.* 3rd ed. St. Louis: Mosby-Year Book; 1995: 35–46.

9. Mathews PJ, Gregg BL. Monitoring and management of the patient in the ICU. In: Scanlan C, Wilkins RL, Stoller J, eds. *Egan's Fundamentals of Respiratory Care.* 7th ed. St. Louis: Mosby-Year Book; 1999: 921–965.

10. Shelledy DC. Discontinuing ventilatory support. In: Scanlan CL, Wilkins RL, Stoller JK, eds. *Egan's Fundamentals of Respiratory Care.* 7th ed. St. Louis: Mosby; 1999:967–991.

11. Wilkins RL, Stoller J. Bedside assessment of the patient. In: Scanlan CL, Wilkins RL, Stoller JK, eds. *Egan's Fundamentals of Respiratory Care.* 7th ed. St. Louis: Mosby; 1999:295–319.

12. Des Jardins T, Burton GG. Patient assessment. In: Des Jardins T, Burton GG, eds. *Clinical Manifestations and Assessment of Respiratory Disease.* 3rd ed. St. Louis: Mosby; 1995:3–118.

13. George RB. History and physical examination. In: George RB, Light RW, Matthay MA, et al, eds. *Chest Medicine.* 3rd ed. Baltimore: Williams & Wilkins; 1995:81–91.

14. Wilkins R, Dexter J. *Respiratory Disease: A Case Study Approach to Patient Care.* 2nd ed. Philadelphia: F.A. Davis; 1993.

15. Shapiro BA, Peruzzi WT, Templin R. *Clinical Application of Blood Gases.* 5th ed. St. Louis: Mosby; 1994.

16. American Thoracic Society. Standardization of spirometry. *Am Rev Respir Dis.* 1979;119:831.

17. American Thoracic Society. Standardization of spirometry-1994 update. *Am J Respir Crit Care Med.* 1995;152:1107–1136.

18. American Association for Respiratory Care Clinical Practice Guideline. Spirometry, 1996 Update. *Respir Care.* 1996;41:629–636.

19. Ruppel GL. *Manual of Pulmonary Function Testing.* 7th ed. St. Louis: Mosby; 1998.

20. Enright PL, Hodgkin JE. Pulmonary function tests. In: Burton GG, Hodgkin JE, Ward JJ, eds. *Respiratory Care—A Guide to Clinical Practice.* 4th ed. Philadelphia: Lippincott; 1997:225–248.

21. Ries AL, Clausen JL. Lung volumes. In: Wilson AF, ed. *Pulmonary Function Testing—Indications and Interpretations.* Orlando, Fla: Grune & Stratton; 1985:69–85.

22. Light RW. Clinical pulmonary function testing, exercise testing, and disability evaluation. In: George RB, Light RW, Matthay MA, et al, eds. *Chest Medicine.* 3rd ed. Baltimore: Williams & Wilkins; 1995:132–159.

23. Brown B. *Hematology: Principles & Procedures.* 6th ed. Philadelphia: Lea & Febiger; 1993:83–102.

24. American Association for Respiratory Care Clinical Practice Guidelines. Oxygen therapy in the acute care hospital. *Respir Care.* 1991;36:1410–1413.

25. Scanlan CL, Heuer A: Medical gas therapy. In: Scanlan CL, Wilkins RL, Stoller JK, eds. *Egan's Fundamentals of Respiratory Care.* 7th ed. St. Louis: Mosby; 1999:737–770.

26. American Association for Respiratory Care Clinical Practice Guideline. Oxygen therapy in the home or extended care facility. Respir Care. 1992;37:918–922.

27. Kacmarek RM, Mack CW, Dimas S. *The Essentials of Respiratory Care.* 3rd ed. St. Louis: Mosby; 1990.

28. Crouser ED, Dorinsky PM. Acute lung injury, pulmonary edema and multiple system organ failure. In: Scanlan CL, Wilkins RL, Stoller JK, eds. *Egan's Fundamentals of Respiratory Care.* 7th ed. St. Louis: Mosby; 1999:507–523.

29. Higgins JT, Hernandez JA, Peters JI, et al. The effectiveness of the Misty-ox High FIO_2-High Flow nebulizer in delivering high oxygen concentrations. Respir Care. 1998;43:870.

30. Rau JL. *Respiratory Care Pharmacology.* 5th ed. St. Louis: Mosby; 1998.

31. American Association for Respiratory Care Clinical Practice Guideline. Assessing response to bronchodilator therapy at point of care. *Respir Care.* 1995;40:1300–1307.

32. American Thoracic Society. Standards for the diagnosis and care of patients with chronic obstructive pulmonary disease. *Respir Crit Care Med.* 1995; 152:577–620.

33. Malinowski C, Wilson B. Neonatal and pediatric. In: Scanlan CL, Wilkins RL, Stoller JK, eds. *Egan's Fundamentals of Respiratory Care.* 7th ed. St. Louis: Mosby; 1999:993–1045.

34. Scanlan C, Myslinski MJ. Bronchial hygiene therapy. In: Scanlan CL, Wilkins RL, Stoller JK, eds. *Egan's Fundamentals of Respiratory Care.* 7th ed. St. Louis: Mosby; 1999:791–816.

35. American Association for Respiratory Care Clinical Practice Guideline. Bland aerosol administration. *Respir Care.* 1993;38:1196–1200.

36. Fink J, Scanlan CL. Humidity and bland aerosol therapy. In: Scanlan CL, Wilkins RL, Stoller JK, eds. *Egan's Fundamentals of Respiratory Care.* 7th ed. St. Louis: Mosby; 1999:661–681.

37. Fink JB. Volume expansion therapy. In: Burton GG, Hodgkin JE, Ward JJ, eds. *Respiratory Care—A Guide to Clinical Practice.* 4th ed. Philadelphia: Lippincott; 1997:525–553.

38. American Association for Respiratory Care Clinical Practice Guideline. Intermittent positive pressure breathing. *Respir Care.* 1993;38:1189–1195.

39. Respiratory Care Committee of the American Thoracic Society. Guidelines for the use of intermittent positive pressure breathing (IPPB). *Respir Care.* 1980;25:365–370.

ETHICAL AND COST CONSIDERATIONS

James B. Fink and Shelley C. Mishoe

*Ethics and law guide each other, but a major dilemma
is that ethical behavior is not always legal and that
following the law sometimes does not seem ethical.*
—SHELLEY C. MISHOE, SEMINARS IN RESPIRATORY CARE, 1996

LEARNING OBJECTIVES

1. Identify and describe key guidelines in ethical decision making.
2. Discuss the history of health care and factors that have increased costs for providing care.
3. Differentiate costs from charges and compare the implications of both fee-for-service and managed care.
4. Identify factors that require an organization to reduce costs of providing health care.
5. Apply specific formulas and theory to assist in clinical decision making with consideration of limited health care resources.
6. Differentiate and discuss management strategies to reduce expenditure of resources and both the positive and negative effects on patient care.
7. Develop a management plan to reduce expenditure of resources and improve quality of care.
8. Interpret data from case examples.
9. Apply the critical thinking skills of prioritizing, anticipating, negotiating, communicating, decision making, and reflection by completing exercises and case examples, including the effects of cost reduction in various clinical environments.
10. Communicate facts, evidence, and arguments to support evaluations and recommendations for care plans to reduce costs and improve care.
11. Practice the skill of negotiating in an attempt to persuade acceptance of your proposed plan.
12. Evaluate treatment and outcomes of interventions to determine need to modify plans.
13. Describe the role of the respiratory care practitioner in providing ethical, cost-effective respiratory care.

KEY WORDS

Advanced Directive	Confidentiality	Fixed Costs	Misrepresentation
Allocation	Conflict	Futility	Resources
Autonomy	Cost Containment	Insurers	Self-Determination
Beneficence	Efficacy	Justice	Third Parties
Benefit	Ethics	Maleficence	Variable Costs
Charges	Fee-for-Service	Managed Care	Veracity

INTRODUCTION

Overview

It is truly a marvelous age in which we live. It is estimated that medical science knowledge doubles every 3 years. Many conditions considered to be a death sentence at the turn of the last century can now be cured or controlled with common medical interventions. As we learn more through research and practice, we translate that knowledge into development of new and improved drugs, devices, and techniques that further alleviate suffering, reduce morbidity and mortality, improve quality of life, and prolong expected life spans. All of these innovations, from basic science research to marketing new products, requires tremendous investment of resources (both time and money). The costs of development drives the price as these innovations become commercially available to the health care provider. The new and improved medications or devices often cost considerably more than older (and presumably less effective) therapies previously used to treat the same illnesses. In short, the proliferation of knowledge directly correlates with increased costs of drugs and devices.

Increased consumption of more expensive treatments explains in large part why costs for health care have consistently escalated at a rate that exceeds the inflation rate for other goods and services. In addition to costing more, these breakthrough innovations reduce morbidity and mortality. Consequently, with access to better health care the general population lives longer and requires more health care resources than did previous generations. More expensive drugs and devices, a longer life span, and increased consumption have exponentially increased health care costs. From a public policy viewpoint, health care costs are soaring out of control and must be contained within a defined and affordable set of resources.

On a more personal level, when you or your loved one is ill, you expect and demand the best medical care available. Whether it is the latest drug to control hypertension or the transplantation of organs, there seems to be no limit to expecta-

tions placed on the health care system to meet the needs of the individual. The difference between what we expect (the sky's the limit) and the limited resources that society (ie, government, employers, insurers, and individuals) is willing to pay for health care has become a source of tension and conflict. These transformations within the health care industry are the source of the ethical issues that are the focus of this chapter.

The respiratory care profession has an important role in either squandering resources or providing cost-effective care. While resource allocation issues may be best decided by the government and the courts, the realities of day-to-day operations places much of the allocation of resources within the scope of the clinician and clinical service operations. Our approach to care and the way policies and procedures are disseminated at the bedside have a tremendous impact on departmental and institutional costs. As new technology emerges we try to embrace it, and add it to our clinical armamentarium, often expanding the costs of providing care. Respiratory care practitioners have an ethical obligation to apply new technologies in their practice while keeping an eye on streamlining and optimizing care and reducing or eliminating ineffective care. In this chapter we will discuss the need to control costs, define key ethical concepts, and provide examples of effective and ineffective cost control management.

CRITICAL CONTENT

FACTORS CONTRIBUTING TO INCREASED HEALTH CARE COSTS

- Proliferation of knowledge correlates with increased costs of drugs and devices
- A longer life span for the general population means increased consumption of health care resources
- Increased public expectations increase the demand for new technology

Our Biases

In the spirit of the ethical principles espoused in this chapter, we feel compelled as clinicians, managers, and administrators, to divulge to the reader stated biases and potential conflicts of interest. Everyone has biases that affect how we think, interact, feel, and behave. Our biases can lead to potential conflicts of interest, which can interfere with our thinking and decision making. Therefore we must examine our biases on a regular basis. Critical thinking is enhanced whenever we examine our biases. Critical thinking can be further enhanced when we consider the biases of others, including clinicians, authors, researchers, teachers, students, patients, and other health care professionals. Here are our biases for your discussion, reflection, and consideration.

Bias #1: Most respiratory care services are not so efficiently managed that they cannot make major changes in how they operate, largely in accordance with evidence-based clinical information and guidelines, that not only will reduce costs, but substantially improve the quality of care provided to their patients. We believe that there is no service that could not further reduce costs and improve quality with appropriate technology, analysis, coordination, support, and negotiation.

Bias #2: Administrators (and managers) who respond to the need to reduce costs for the organization by across-the-board cuts, personnel freezes, and management by attrition (those who leave the organization are not replaced, no matter what their role), are lower in the moral food chain than used car salesmen (with apologies to used car salesmen). These "leaders" abdicate their obligation to manage, waiting to see where the chips fall, and taking a minimum of personal risks by avoiding making the tough, data-driven decisions that their organization needs to survive and flourish. These managers place their organization, care providers, and patients at tremendous risk, and exacerbate the financial crisis facing heath care.

Whether you are a staff practitioner, supervisor, manager, or administrator, you have a legal and ethical obligation to participate in the process of providing your patients the best possible care with the resources available. We will explore the use of critical thinking skills and ethical principles to facilitate that goal.

CRITICAL CONTENT

CHALLENGES FACING HEALTH CARE RESPIRATORY THERAPISTS

- Optimize the health care provided
- Reduce or eliminate ineffective care
- Measure outcomes to assess efficacy of care
- Allocate resources based on sound ethical and legal decisions

COST CONSIDERATIONS

The amount of money spent on health care in the United States exceeded $1.6 trillion in the year 2000.[1] That's more than $4000 for every man, woman, and child in the US, and our health care costs consume a larger percentage of the gross domestic product than in any other developed country. Health care costs are growing far faster than the gross national product or rate of inflation. Even with all the resources expended, the United States is still not the leader in indices such as infant mortality, raising the question of whether we are efficiently expending these health care dollars. In other words, are we getting enough "bang for our buck"? As health care expenditures continue to increase at a rate faster than inflation, government agencies, third-party payers, and employers, who pay many of these health care costs, have expressed increasing concerns that costs are escalating out of control. Consequently, we have seen mandated measures to curb these costs.

Managed Care

Managed care, patient-focused care, preferred provider organizations (PPOs), and health maintenance organizations (HMOs) have all evolved as attempts to more effectively manage the nation's health care dollars. No matter what you call it, the bottom line is that the clinician at the bedside is increasingly being called upon to do more with less. When that is not enough, the organization may feel that it must reduce or eliminate services. Therefore, services that the patient and public may have benefited from, and may even be entitled to, can be discontinued because no one can pay for the costs of care.

Managed care is not a recent fad, having its roots in the early 1900s. The first managed care organizations were established to meet the needs of employees of large industries (such as the railroads). In the 1920s, escalating health care costs meant that patients in the hospital could generate bills that surpassed their ability to pay. Ultimately, this could burden the resources of the institution such that the financial foundation of the hospital could be at risk. Consequently, the argument was raised that hospitals exist to serve the community, and the financial risks of providing care should be shared or spread throughout the community. The ensuing discussions led to the development of Blue Cross insurance. At the same time, physicians developed the Blue Shield plan to protect physicians and patients from allowing employers to select providers for their work force that excluded other providers in the community. In the 1930s and 1940s, the larger business community began exploring prepaid health plans, leading to the precursors to modern health maintenance organizations (HMOs) such as Kaiser Permanente. After World War II, employers, in an attempt to provide a relatively inexpensive competitive fringe benefit in lieu of higher wages, became the major source of health insurance for the American work force.

In 1965, the US Congress legislated Medicare and Medicaid to provide comprehensive health care coverage for the elderly and poor. At that time, most physician and hospital charges were on a fee-for-service basis. The more services provided to the patient, the higher the total fees charged under the fee-for-service system. Charges were equated with revenue. As more patients were eligible for comprehensive health care coverage, the total number of

dollars spent on health care soared. The fee-for-service system was thought to create incentives that encouraged physicians and hospitals to treat disease, with no financial incentives to provide preventative health care. This led to the passage of the Health Maintenance Organization Act in 1973. By 1980, HMO and PPO enrollment in the US had increased to 55 million. Faced with soaring costs of traditional health insurance plans, employers developed strategies to make these alternative systems more accessible and less expensive to their employees.

Ironically, these organizations, created to improve access to health care with financial incentives to prevent disease and promote health, developed "gatekeeper systems" to reduce operating costs by limiting patient access to subspecialists and expensive interventions. This gatekeeping function restricts access to care for individuals with some of the greatest medical needs, with the insurer claiming the need to fairly allocate limited resources for the benefit of all of the plan's members.

Meanwhile, government and insurers began to discount fee-for-service charges, and developed contractual relationships that reduced reimbursement to the hospital to as little as 50% of the bill. The incentive to keep patients in the hospital longer, while providing extensive testing and therapies, was rapidly disappearing. This shifting of payment meant that hospitals had to find methods to treat patients in less time, with fewer resources expended.

It was predicted that health care reform would result in closure of up to 16% of the hospitals in the US, but less than 3% actually folded. This is a testament to the many communities that feel their local hospitals are essential to their economic viability and stability. Nevertheless, all institutions were faced with the very real requirement to evaluate and reorganize their operations to reduce costs and improve efficiency. The need to downsize was irrefutable.

Respiratory Care Providers

Respiratory medicine represents approximately 7% of total health care costs and 10% of total prescription costs in the United States. This correlates with the 5% to 10% of the total population with asthma, and another 6% with chronic obstructive pulmonary disease (COPD). Over the last 40 years, respiratory medicine evolved from a base of physicians who treated tuberculosis to the pulmonary/critical care specialist. At about the same time, respiratory care emerged as an allied health specialty. Respiratory care services accounted for more than 10% of the institutional costs. Therefore, respiratory care sometimes became the first place an administrator would look when making cuts in services. This is not evil, immoral, or unethical. In fact, the institution would be remiss in not carefully assessing the role of all of the major players expending major resources. Our goal is to apply critical thinking and the technical tools of our profession to meet the needs of both our institutions and our patients in a cost-effective and ethical manner.

The effective application of critical thinking can make the difference between removing resources that undermine fundamental services, placing patients and the institution at peril, or investing resources in programs that reduce operational overhead, eliminating unnecessary services, and improving the quality of patient care.

CRITICAL CONTENT

MEASURES TO CONTROL SPIRALING HEALTH CARE COSTS

- Managed care, HMOs, PPOs
- Gatekeeping to limit access to expensive care
- Shift to prospective payment systems or capitated payment
- Hospitals downsize, use patient-focused care and alternate sites
- Greater focus on wellness, health promotion, disease management

IS ALL MEDICAL CARE NECESSARY?

This seems to be a reasonable starting point in our analysis of cost containment. While we understand factors that drive up costs of new innovations, we have not dealt with resources required to provide care that is not necessary. There are at least three categories of unnecessary medical care: 1) small ticket items (laboratory tests and x-rays), which can represent 25% of costs for hospital and ambulatory care; 2) big ticket items (expensive operations and procedures that are used in circumstances in which they are known to be of no value); and 3) aggressive care for terminally ill patients when palliative care is more appropriate.

In a New York teaching hospital, 10% of the hospital budget was spent on the final admissions of 4% of patients who died in the hospital. About 40% of these patients had diagnoses such as cancer that would suggest a terminal status at the time of admission.

It is crucial to differentiate medical care in the hospital that is useful and expensive from that which is just expensive. There is a world of difference between a 75-year-old cancer patient with terminal COPD on a ventilator for 3 months and a 12-year-old child who receives a liver transplant. Unfortunately, much of the expensive care provided is lacking cost and benefit analyses. For example, there is limited evidence that the benefits justify the costs for coronary bypass surgery, neonatal and adult intensive care, invasive monitoring, new imaging techniques, as well as older, more established techniques such as mastectomy, hysterectomy, tonsillectomy, chemotherapy, and radiation therapy. The evidence for the benefits and risks of these procedures is simply inadequate.

In 1979, the Health Care Financing Administration set up the National Center for Technology Assessment to try to develop accurate information on the risks and benefits of new technologies. With a budget of only $4 million dollars, it managed to determine the lack of value in intermittent positive-pressure breathing (IPPB) prior to being abolished at the beginning of the Regan era. Today the Agency for Health Care Policy and Research (AHCPR) has taken an active role in developing evidence to support medical practice issues.

Is Preventive Medicine the Answer?

It has been argued that rather than investing in more technology, we should turn towards preventive measures. It is no doubt true that if the population had proper nutrition, adequate exercise, and did not smoke or abuse drugs or alcohol, health care demands would be considerably lower. However, these changes are far beyond the range of influence of the health care system. The means to influence our habits, including health promotion, are largely educational, social, economic, and political. Preventive care is important, but is not a panacea for reducing health care costs to the exclusion of technical innovation and development.

What can respiratory therapists do to contain costs, both as individuals and as a profession? As individuals, we must do the best we can for each patient. We must not provide unnecessary tests and procedures. Even when the patient requests a procedure that he or she believes will be of value, the respiratory therapist should take time to explain why the procedure would not be worth the costs or risks. As a profession we need to support the revision of fee schedules and charges that rewards the judicious use of tests and procedures. We also need to press for and participate in adequate technology assessment. We need to work to base our practice on available evidence that supports cost-effective care.

Product Costing in Hospitals

The health care industry has been slow in enabling its accounting systems to make accurate cost determinations for specific treatments or illnesses. Historically, hospitals have divided patients into two classes of payers: those who will pay and those unable to pay. Those who could pay were charged enough to produce revenue to defray the costs of the charity patients. As third-party payers, insurance companies and Medicare and Medicaid came to represent a larger piece of the financial pie, the gap increased between standard charges made by the hospital and the amount of money that hospitals received in payment, and pressure increased to further shift costs to privately paying patients.

One of the avenues that hospital management has taken to respond to the shift from promoting charges to minimizing costs has been to make an effort to assign actual costs to products and ser-

vices, and to make decisions based on these costs. Managers now need to ask questions like, "What does it actually cost to give another 10 chest physiotherapy treatments a day?"

Cost Centers and Revenue Centers   Hospitals used to distinguish between revenue centers and cost centers. Cost centers were departments that accumulated costs without the ability to charge for individual services. Revenue centers had individual charges and were expected to carry the load of the cost centers. Charges had to cover the costs of providing the service, the overhead of a portion of nonreimbursable services, and whatever margin of profit the institution wished to generate. This resulted in hospital bills in which the patient might be charged $2.00/tablet for aspirin. In this example, the charge ($2.00) has little apparent direct correlation to the cost of providing the particular service ($0.02/tablet). However, if the hospital reduced the charge for the aspirin, it would have to increase other charges to maintain its operating margin.

Traditionally, respiratory care has been a revenue center, while nursing would be considered a cost center. Respiratory charges not only had to cover the direct costs of providing respiratory care services, but also the costs of services provided by cost centers. It was common practice for hospitals to allocate all overhead costs to revenue-producing centers. A typical revenue center would have "indirect" costs (reflecting a percentage of environmental services, central supply, hospital administration, etc.), and "direct" costs, those actually incurred for providing the service. Indirect allocations were based on the revenue center's "ability to bear" or pay the cost.

With the introduction of diagnosis-related groups (DRGs) from Medicare, reimbursements for health care services are not based on costs or charges, but for specific disease and treatment groups. Revenue is no longer received from charges for the treatments administered to a COPD patient. With DRGs and prospective payment, a bulk payment is based on mean number of days and projected costs of providing care for that diagnosis. While hospitals still need to establish charges, there are increasing proportions of patients for which payment is based on per diem (daily) rates, capitation, or percentage of charges.

The hospital needs to collect a certain amount of money in order to pay all its bills and keep operating. The problem comes in deciding the proper mix of services to maximize revenue and minimize costs. It could be crucial to the management process to be able to assign a realistic cost to a specific procedure. For instance, does it make more sense to increase the staff to handle the workload of increased treatments, or should the hospital reduce services and not admit patients who require the increased service? The pricing of services and establishing the cost of providing care is essential to address this problem.

Fixed and Variable Costs In order to price prospective services properly according to the real cost, it is necessary to differentiate between variable and fixed costs. Total cost is the sum of the total fixed cost and the total variable cost. Fixed costs are the factors of production that do not vary in the short run. For example, once the decision has been made to staff a respiratory care service on a 24-hour basis, there are certain fixed costs incurred, whether or not any treatments are performed. Fixed costs might include allocating the space, electricity, basic equipment, and staff members required to provide baseline coverage. Whether that staff is busy or idle, the costs are the same. Fixed costs are those required to keep a certain level of service in operation.

Any costs above that level are variable costs since they vary with the amount of work performed. Total variable cost varies with the output and increases directly once the limits of output exceed the allocated fixed costs. Marginal cost is the addition (or subtraction) to total cost of producing one more (or one less) unit of output. For example, if one respiratory care practitioner (RT) is always on the night shift and can handle up to 4 ventilators, then 1 to 4 ventilators are covered within the fixed costs. When there are more than 4 ventilators running, the extra staff member added to the shift to cover the extra ventilators would represent a variable cost.

HEALTH CARE COST CONTAINMENT ISSUES

- Reduce or eliminate all unnecessary care, such as questionable clinical procedures, tests, and surgical procedures, and overly aggressive terminal patient care
- Preventive care is important, but it is not a panacea
- Actual costs are hard to determine due to the past practice of cost-shifting

Critical Thinking Exercise 1

**PROBLEM SOLVING—
CALCULATING COSTS AND CHARGES**

Calculate costs and complete the table using this information: The staffing standard is that no RT will be assigned more than 4 ventilators, an RT costs $200 per shift, and the hospital charges $150/ventilator/shift. How would the cost per ventilator and cost/charge ratio change as the numbers of ventilated patients increase?

	Cost/Ventilator	Total Cost	Total Charge	Cost/Charge Ratio
1 ventilator				
2 ventilators				
3 ventilators				
4 ventilators				
5 ventilators				
6 ventilators				
7 ventilators				
8 ventilators				

ETHICAL GUIDELINES

Medical ethics is a set of moral principles that govern the behavior of health professionals. These principles have evolved over time, heavily influenced by religious teachings and legal conventions, as health care practitioners struggle to embrace changes in technology and economics.[2,3] Ethical standards have certain maxims that help guide clinicians in decision making and conflict resolution, but they are not written in stone. Legal and ethical considerations are irrevocably intertwined with clinical practice.[4]

In clinical medicine, ethical problems arise because there are sound reasons for conflicting courses of action. A systematic approach to sorting out and responding to ethical problems helps to ensure that no important considerations are overlooked and that similar cases are consistently resolved. It is important that every respiratory therapist has a basic understanding of ethical decision making and the legal implications attendant to ethical issues. In resolving ethical dilemmas, practitioners should be able to refer to the following maxims to help select and justify actions and choices.

Respect Patient Autonomy

Autonomy is the right and the ability to govern one's self. Autonomy (or self-rule) means that individuals are free from interference and control by others. Patients have a right to self-determination, independence, and freedom, and people should not infringe on these rights or try to control their actions. In health care, autonomy means that the patient has the right to choose actions that are consistent with their goals, values, and life plan.[5,6] Patient autonomy should be respected even when some choices made by the patient conflict with the wishes of family members or recommendations of the physician or health care team.

In modern medicine, respecting patient autonomy begins with the process of informed consent. Table 8-1 shows the elements of informed consent. Table 8-2 provides information on ways to determine a patient's ability to provide informed consent. Every patient needs to be properly informed of his or her options in order to make decisions about their health care. Patients have a right to decline interventions prescribed by their physician. On the other hand, no patient is free to violate the autonomy of others, harm others, or impose unfair claims on society's resources. Table 8-3 provides exceptions to the need for obtaining informed consent for health care. Respecting patient autonomy is

related to other ethical guidelines such as avoiding misrepresentation, maintaining confidentiality, and keeping promises.[7] Concern for patient autonomy resulted in the Patient Self-Determination Act, which mandated that health care facilities and agencies provide patients with written information about their rights under law when making decisions concerning their medical care. Advanced directives, living wills, and medical powers of attorney specify what treatments patients desire or wish to refuse.[8]

Patients can express decisions concerning their care in the form of advance directives that are placed in their medical records. The health care team should be familiar with each patient's

TABLE 8-1   ELEMENTS OF INFORMED CONSENT

- Present a clear, concise statement of the patient's condition, disease, disorder, or problem.
- State the nature and purpose of the proposed treatment (or course of therapy) in language that is specific enough to be commonly understood.
- Describe the risks and consequences of the proposed treatment.
- Describe and discuss any feasible alternatives to treatment.
- Tell the patient his or her prognosis if the proposed treatment is or is not given.

TABLE 8-2   PSYCHOPATHOLOGY AND INFORMED CONSENT

Check the patient for:
    Primary thought disturbance
    Hallucinations or delusions
    Disturbing or aggressive behavior
    Difficulties in communication
    Affective disorders
    Disturbances of memory, orientation, and
       cognition
    Severe mental retardation
    Suicidal or homicidal ideation

TABLE 8-3 EXCEPTIONS TO THE DOCTRINE OF INFORMED CONSENT

> **Waiver:** The patient insists that he does not want to know the details of treatment.
> **Emergency:** In a life-or-death crisis with a serious and imminent threat, the practitioner may assume that the patient would want intervention. Once the crisis has passed, the requirement for informed consent is restored.
> **Implied agreement:** Commonly encountered procedures with little or minimal risk (eg, routine blood work) can be performed without specific consent.
> **Therapeutic privilege:** If informing the patient will cause her or him serious and identifiable harm, the informed consent need not proceed. Fear of producing anxiety or depression is not adequate to abridge the consent process.

advance directives, and should review any advance directives in the medical records. Failure to adhere to stipulated advanced directives is a violation of both ethical and legal principles.[8] When a patient is

Group Critical Thinking Exercise 1

ETHICAL DECISION MAKING AND NEGOTIATING WHEN DEALING WITH PATIENT ADVANCED DIRECTIVES

A patient in the coronary care unit who was admitted with massive myocardial infarction begins to show signs of increased cardiac failure. The patient and family have signed an advanced directive to make it clear to the staff that the patient wants no extraordinary life-saving efforts if complications should arise. The patient stops breathing and the resident begins to intubate and asks the respiratory therapist for a ventilator.

Class discussion:

a. What should the respiratory therapist do?

b. Should the respiratory therapist follow orders?

c. Should he or she attempt to convince the resident to reconsider and call the attending physician should the resident refuse to consider the advanced directive?

incapable of making informed decisions, respect for autonomy may take a backseat to acting in his or her best interests.

Avoid Misrepresentation (Veracity)

Avoiding misrepresentation means that you cannot lie to your patient. Applying the ethical principle of veracity means telling the truth. This principle implies that the practitioner should tell the patient the truth at all times. It is based on the belief that health care is best served in a relationship of trust where the practitioner and the patient are bound by truth.[9]

Sounds simple, doesn't it? We know it is important to tell the truth, and that lying is dishonest. However, in medicine, withholding information about proposed interventions or the patient's condition, or providing information that is true but misleading, are all serious forms of misrepresentation. While patients should not be forced to receive information against their will, most patients want to know their diagnosis and prognosis, even if they are terminally ill. Truthful and complete information is fundamental for the patient to be able to make informed decisions.

Practitioners may be tempted to misrepresent information to third parties. Patients may ask their care provider to misrepresent their condition to third parties to obtain benefits such as insurance and disability payments. This can be particularly difficult, because while we want to help our patients, we are obligated by law to provide accurate information to government agencies, employers, and insurers. Misrepresentation of this type can be unfair to other patients, who may ultimately pay higher insurance premiums or taxes, and undermine the public's trust in the health care profession. In dealing with third-party payers, misrepresenting a patient's condition to help them obtain insurance coverage or disability is both illegal and unethical.

Maintain Confidentiality

Maintaining confidentiality of medical information is fundamental to respecting the patient's privacy. In addition, maintaining confidentiality encourages patients to seek medical care, fosters trust in the provider-patient relationship, and prevents discrimination based on illness. Confidentiality protects the patient from harm that might occur if information about their condition, illness, personal habits, sexual preferences, and other personal activities were widely known. Patients and the public expect health care providers to keep medical information confidential.

The obligation to maintain patient confidentiality is not absolute. Overriding patient confidentiality may be warranted under certain circumstances, such as when 1) there is potential for serious harm to third parties or a high likelihood of harm; 2) there is no alternative means to warn or protect those at risk; and 3) the harm that results from the breach of confidentiality is minimized and acceptable. However, failure to maintain confidentiality due to careless or unthinking behavior is not acceptable. Breaches of confidentiality are often caused by practitioner indiscretions, ranging from leaving the patient's medical record exposed to casual view, to discussing patients by name in hospital elevators or cafeterias.

Patients may waive their right to confidentiality and give permission to disclose information about their condition to others (eg, allowing staff to discuss their condition with family and friends, or releasing information to insurance companies). An ethical dilemma arises when a patient is too sick to authorize such disclosures.

Act in the Patient's Best Interest (Beneficence)

Health care providers have a responsibility to work in the best interest of their patients. Beneficence means charitable or merciful, and the exercise of beneficence requires practitioners to take active steps to benefit patients. In other words, it is the respiratory therapist's duty to act in the patient's best interest. Health care practitioners generally have medical expertise that their patients do not, and patients may be vulnerable because of their illness. Therefore, patients rely on health care professionals to provide sound advice and competent care to promote the patients' well being.

 Group Critical Thinking Exercise 2

DECISION MAKING: "WHAT WOULD YOU DO?"

Debate the pros and cons of maintaining patient confidentiality in the situation described below. This exercise can be performed by an individual who would identify the arguments on both sides of the issue, or the assignment can be done as a group CT exercise: Students can be divided into two groups, and one group should be assigned the position of supporting Mr. Folk's request, and the other presenting the arguments for reporting this situation to the proper authorities.

Mr. Folk is a 55-year-old truck driver with 30 years' driving experience. He is a union member in good standing and spends as long as 3 weeks away from home during long distance hauls. Every 5 years, his employer and union contract require a physical examination. Mr. Folk went to his family physician, who in the course of the examination and thorough history, suspected a sleep-disordered breathing problem. The patient denied ever falling asleep at the wheel, but was scheduled for a sleep study, and the sleep study found evidence of obstructive sleep apnea. He was prescribed nasal continuous positive airway pressure (CPAP). The respiratory therapist instructed Mr. Folk in use of the CPAP, and informed Mr. Folk that he should not drive the truck until the repeat sleep study showed that the CPAP was effective. The patient became very upset, and said that if he told his boss that he couldn't drive for a few weeks, his boss would know something is wrong, and Mr. Folk would lose his job. The RT explained that his sleep apnea was severe enough to place him and others at risk, and asked him to consider the potential danger to others on the road. Mr. Folk said, "I can handle it. I am only a few years from retirement, and don't want to lose my pension. I'll be careful. Don't worry."

The respiratory therapist is aware of relevant state law mandating a report to the Department of Health if the patient "has ever experienced a lapse of consciousness or is likely to do so while driving." Reporting Mr. Folk could result in revocation of his driver's license. Mr. Folk tells the RT, "This is between you and me. I can deal with this. I just want to work a couple more years."

a. What are the ethical implications for the RT?

Serving the health interests of patients should take priority over the interests of practitioners themselves or the interests of third parties, such as hospitals or insurers. Clinicians should act in a manner that maximizes the benefits of treatment and minimizes the potential harm. This is facilitated in part by fundamental training, development of clinical competencies, and continuing education that keeps the practitioner aware of evolving technology. In accord with this maxim, prior to performing ordered therapy, the respiratory therapist should ask, "Will my actions benefit the patient?" and "Do I possess the knowledge and skills required to safely perform this procedure so that it will benefit the patient?"

Does the exercise of beneficence justify the practitioner overriding unreasonable refusals of care by competent patients? Acting in what we believe to be the patient's best interests, even when they contradict the patient's own choices, is termed

Critical Thinking Exercise 2

REFLECTION AND DECISION MAKING

a. Describe a situation in which treating a patient against his or her wishes might be appropriate.

b. Describe how beneficence and medical paternalism affect the situation in your clinical example, the process of reflection used to make your decision, and the ultimate decision.

Critical Thinking Exercise 3

DECISION MAKING AND COMMUNICATION—"YOU DECIDE!"

A patient with an acute exacerbation of COPD has borderline respiratory failure. The doctor orders noninvasive ventilation. As you begin to apply the mask, the patient pushes it away and says, "I don't want that." The patient's intent may range from, "I don't want that mask on my face while I am having so much trouble breathing" to "I don't want this therapy at all".

a. What can you do to differentiate whether the refusal for treatment is a response to discomfort or whether the patient is refusing lifesaving treatment?

medical paternalism. The problem with paternalism is that clinicians do not have the expertise to make value judgments for their patients, no matter how obvious they presume their clinical choices to be.

Nonmaleficence is the ethical principle of "do no harm," which prevents clinicians from knowingly providing ineffective therapies, acting selfishly or maliciously.[10] Nonmaleficence is not as simple as it appears, since many beneficial interventions, including common medications, may have serious side effects. The principle of double effects occurs when the benefits of a treatment are accompanied by undesired side effects that could cause harm.

Forego Ineffective or Futile Interventions

Physicians and practitioners should forego ineffective intervention because these measures do not offer any possibility of benefit to the patient. This is certainly the case for a patient who has died, at which time the benefits of all interventions become futile. But in most cases, the judgment that intervention is ineffective or futile reflects greater or lesser probability of benefit. For the respiratory therapist, using resources to provide therapy when there is strong evidence that it will not meet the clinical goals may pose an ethical dilemma.

Conflicts of interest may explain why ineffective or futile interventions occur in health care. Conflicts of interest occur when the practitioner is influenced by motivations other than the best interest of the patient. In such a situation, the practitioner may abuse the trust of the patient for personal gain. Even the appearance of conflict of interest can adversely affect the trust in the individual practitioner, the respiratory care profession, and the entire health care system. Clinicians need to consider how the patient, public, or profession would react if they witnessed or knew the details of the situation.

Allocate Resources Fairly

Health care practitioners should allocate the amount of health care resources needed by each patient for proper treatment. This is a form of justice. *Justice* is the principle that deals with fairness and equity in the distribution of scarce resources such as time, services, equipment, and money.[8] While this concept may seem simple, in reality it is a major challenge for our health care system. Resources should be allocated fairly and consistently. People in comparable situations should be treated similarly, and patients in different ethical situations should be treated differently. Health care resources are limited, so allocation decisions are necessitated by these resource limitations.

How should limited health care resources be distributed? There are several theories that deal with that question. The egalitarian theory states that there should be equal access to goods and services, but in reality this is not always possible. The health care resources available in rural or inner-city areas of the US are not the same as the health care available in more affluent suburban areas.

The utilitarian theory of justice states that the distribution of resources should be such that it achieves the greatest good for the largest number of persons. The libertarian theory emphasizes the personal rights to social and economic liberty. Another theory of justice is the maximum view of justice, in which one maximizes the minimum, even if doing so does not maximize the total amount of good done. In other words, the person needing the resources the most is helped, even if others are not helped. Another way to look at this theory is that the maximum amount of health care goes to a minimum number of patients (ie, the most critical patients).

With health care resources stretched thin these days, health care justice has become an important topic. Determining who gets the resources is never an easy decision. This question has stimulated discussion everywhere from Congress to homes across the country. Ideally, decisions of allocation of health care resources should be made as part of public policy and determined by government officials or judges, because rationing at the bedside tends to be inconsistent, discriminatory, and inefficient. Care providers should be advocates for their patients, securing resources required to optimize care, within limits determined by society and good practice. Conflicts arise when two or more patients compete for the same limited resources, such as an intensive care bed, an organ for transplant, or a practi-

CRITICAL CONTENT

THEORIES OF JUSTICE TO GUIDE ALLOCATION OF RESOURCES

- *The egalitarian theory:* equal access to goods and services for all
- *The utilitarian theory:* distribution of resources to achieve the greatest good for the greatest number of persons
- *The libertarian theory:* emphasizes the personal rights to social and economic liberty
- *The maximum theory:* provide resources to those with the greatest need (maximize the minimum)

tioner's time. Limited resources need to be rationed and distributed according to the medical needs of the patient and the probability of benefit.

Fidelity to Colleagues

Fidelity exists among colleagues and is an important ethical principle guiding clinical practice. *Fidelity* means faithfulness and loyalty. There is an obligation of loyalty to co-workers and the profession. There may be times when this loyalty is in conflict with loyalty to the patient. The principle of loyalty to colleagues does have exceptions. Most professional organizations have ethical codes that require members to report incompetent or dishonest practices and/or impaired colleagues. In such cases, the fidelity to the patient would outweigh the loyalty to the colleague. The American Association of Respiratory Care (AARC) code states that the respiratory care practitioner "shall refuse to conceal illegal, unethical, or incompetent acts of others."[11]

Avoid Nonabandonment

A final ethical consideration is the principle of nonabandonment. Nonabandonment is the total commitment by the practitioner to seek solutions to problems throughout the course of illness of the patient, particularly toward the end of life, no matter what the anticipated outcome. Dying patients should receive palliative care to ease pain and suffering, even after it becomes clear that critical care interventions may be futile. Physical and psychological supports are crucial for the dying patient and family.

Please refer to Table 8-4 and review the AARC Code of Ethics for Respiratory Therapists.[11] Respiratory therapists should have a broad understanding and deep appreciation for ethics as a basis for clinical decision making. However, all of health care ethics can be reduced down to its four guiding principles: autonomy, beneficence, nonmaleficence, and justice.[12] Please keep these major ethical principles at the forefront of your thoughts and discussions as you work your way through the exercises in this chapter and throughout the entire textbook.

CRITICAL CONTENT

MAXIMS TO HELP RESOLVE OR AVOID ETHICAL DILEMMAS

- Respect patient autonomy
- Act in the patient's best interest (beneficence and nonmaleficence)
- Allocate resources fairly (justice)
- Avoid misrepresentations
- Maintain confidentiality
- Forego ineffective or futile interventions
- Balance role fidelity (loyalty)
- Avoid nonabandonment

TABLE 8-4   AARC STATEMENT OF ETHICS AND PROFESSIONAL CONDUCT

In the conduct of professional activities, the respiratory care practitioner shall be bound by the following ethical and professional principles. Respiratory care practitioners shall:

- Demonstrate behavior that reflects integrity, supports objectivity, and fosters trust in the profession and its professionals.
- Actively maintain and continually improve their professional competence, and represent it accurately.
- Perform only those procedures or functions in which they are individually competent and which are within the scope of accepted and responsible practice.
- Respect and protect the legal and personal rights of patients they treat, including the right to informed consent and refusal of treatment.
- Divulge no confidential information regarding any patient or family unless disclosure is required for responsible performance of duty or required by law.
- Provide care without discrimination on any basis, with respect for the rights and dignity of all individuals.
- Promote disease prevention and wellness.
- Refuse to participate in illegal or unethical acts, and shall refuse to conceal illegal, unethical, or incompetent acts of others.
- Follow sound scientific procedures and ethical principles in research.
- Comply with state or federal laws which govern and relate to their practice.
- Avoid any form of conduct that creates a conflict of interest, and shall follow the principles of ethical business behavior.
- Promote the positive evolution of the profession, and health care in general, through improvement of the access, efficacy, and cost of patient care.
- Refrain from indiscriminate and unnecessary use of resources, both economic and natural, in their practice.

SOURCE: AARC.[11]

LIFE SUPPORT ISSUES

Over the past two decades, much of the debate in medical ethics has focused on where to draw the line on providing or discontinuing life support. The decision to administer, withhold, or withdraw life support arises daily in intensive care units. Life support is offered to most acute care patients unless it conflicts with advance directives or the patient has no reasonable chance of survival. Unfortunately, four common factors contribute to care providers intervening beyond the point of ensuring the best interest of the patient. These factors include:

1. Technological imperative, or the perceived need to do everything possible, regardless of the potential adverse effects or costs for the patient. This is most commonly applied when the patient will die without aggressive management, and cannot make his or her own decision concerning care. A sign of this problem is reflected in the statement "Well, we haven't tried _____ yet."

2. Specialists who become focused on supporting a specific organ or system, without taking a holistic view of the patient's overall situation and viability.

3. Fee-for-service and procedure-oriented reimbursement, which persist in providing financial incentives to the physicians for prolonging and intensifying care.

4. Concerns about legal repercussions resulting in the practice of "defensive medicine." Clinicians may perform tests or procedures to cover all possibilities in a misguided attempt to defend against litigation for malpractice.

In the ICU, critical care medical professionals tend to value making decisions based on patient quality of life, likelihood of surviving hospitalization, chronic disorders, reversibility of acute illness, patient advance directives, and premorbid cognitive function.[13] In Canada, 1361 intensivists, house staff, and ICU nurses in 37 ICUs were asked to rate 18 determinants of withdrawing life support.[14] More than 50% agreed that surviving the current illness, advanced directives, premorbid cognitive function, and the likelihood of long-term survival were extremely important. However, when the participants were asked to respond to 12 clinical scenarios, the results were widely varied. The results suggest that previously unidentified and unmeasured patient and professional factors were more influential in making such decisions.[14]

Care providers often form opinions about a patient's attitude toward life support or resuscitation, although these opinions may only weakly correlate with the preference expressed by the patient or family. Surveys have found that physicians tend to vary discussions about intubation for end-stage chronic obstructive lung disease patients to influence patient choice. The way a physician approaches the patient can influence whether the patient will want intubation and mechanical ventilation for the inevitable respiratory failure with end-stage COPD. The physician's approach will influence some patients to prepare advanced directives refusing intubation or the patient's decision to "do everything possible" (meaning intubation). Surveys also indicate that care providers consider quality of life of the elderly to be worse than do the patients. These misconceptions are substantial barriers to effective communication between the health care provider and patient.

Virtually all patients want some control over health care decisions, and many patients are concerned that they may receive interventions without being consulted. Patient and family decisions about life support expressed long before the onset of illness are of limited use. Both care provider and patient preference often change with new information. Patients should be informed of the utility of a living will in specifying their health care wishes. Health care professionals, especially respiratory therapists who manage life support technologies, should discuss living wills with patients, families, co-workers, and friends. Even when patients make end-of-life decisions, such as do not resuscitate (DNR) orders, health care personnel may ignore these decisions or may be unaware of the patient's intentions.

How we discuss information influences patient decisions. When patients and health care professionals are from different backgrounds (religious, racial, cultural), the values and ethnocultural identities that influence many of their decisions may be in conflict. Even decisions based on the best available evidence are colored by a health care worker's ethical, social, and religious values. Consequently, end-of-life treatment options and life support issues should be discussed in culturally sensitive and meaningful ways.

The critical care environment may be conducive and supportive of ethical thinking and decision making or it may erect barriers to the process. The ethical framework of an organization provides guidelines for problem solving and for determining what behavior is acceptable under certain circumstances. Some organizations espouse patient-centered care in marketing the institution's services, but when they actually deal with patients and family, a paternalistic philosophy predominates. Discussions with patients and surrogates too often are reduced to notifying them of the treatment plan and meeting legal requirements rather than engaging in meaningful dialogue. Economic and political pressures guide most organizations.

Utilitarian principles are aimed at maximizing outcome for the greatest number of patients. Focus on outcomes that reflect values such as efficiency, objectivity, cost containment, and economic stability may be in opposition to providing quality care, respecting patient choice, and free expression of one's own values. For example, resources expended to provide quality end-of-life care, including psychosocial programs, pastoral care, or bereavement programs might not be viewed by the organization as cost-effective.

Policies may be developed to limit admission of critically ill patients to the intensive care units when a DNR order has been written for them. Similar policies may dictate moving dying patients out of the ICU, making room for patients who are more likely to survive. A systematic ethical analysis can differentiate whether these decisions are made to promote the well being of patients and family members, or are simply a mandate created with an eye on the financial bottom line.

CRITICAL CONTENT

FACTORS CONTRIBUTING TO INTERVENTION BEYOND THE PATIENT'S BEST INTERESTS

- Technological imperative: "We've got the technology—we have to use it!"
- Not taking a holistic view of each patient
- Specialists too focused on their specialty
- Reimbursement incentives: "Provide the care now and send the bill later!"
- Defensive medical practices
- Substantial barriers to effective communication leading to interventions not desired by patients

Group Critical Thinking Exercise 3

DEBATE THE ETHICS OF THIS COST REDUCTION STRATEGY

This exercise may be done individually, or the instructor may assign two groups to debate this issue, with one group taking the "pro" policy stance, and the other taking the "con" stand.

You are working in a hospital where the administration has recently announced a policy that any patient with a DNR order will not be admitted to ICU or remain in the ICU.

a. Identify several ethically-based arguments in support of and in opposition to this policy.

ETHICS AND MANAGED CARE ORGANIZATIONS

Managed care organizations (MCOs) include group and staff model health maintenance organizations, preferred provider organizations, and independent provider associations. All MCOs share some common characteristics, including those shown in Table 8-5.

TABLE 8-5   CHARACTERISTICS OF MANAGED CARE ORGANIZATIONS (MCOs)

Organized delivery—centering on a primary care provider who acts as a gatekeeper controlling utilization of services.

Team care—a collaborative effort between primary care providers and specialists in managing clinical decisions and financial resources.

At-risk financing—The primary care provider's treatment choices and referral behavior are influenced by being financially at risk for the choices made (as well as being subject to practice guidelines and retrospective review of practice patterns).

Risk pooling—financing on a capitated basis (receiving a fixed number of dollars per insured patient) requires a large enough pool of patients that cost of treating high-cost patients can be distributed (and subsidized) from savings generated by healthy patients whose care costs less.

Demographic determinants of care—The MCO provides care for an entire population, so that it becomes aware of demographic determinants of illness, promoting a focus on efforts that maintain the health of the population through screening and prospective treatment.

Payer demands—The large portion of business expenses that have been allocated to health insurance have led employers to realize that health expenditures might be viewed as an investment. Self-insured employers have become interested not only in controlling costs by direct contracting with providers, cost-sharing with employees, and utilization review, but with efforts to promote improved health status of employees. Managed care has begun to include cost-effectiveness analysis. To improve health outcomes of the entire employee or insured population, it is necessary to reduce individual practice variations so that predictable medical outcomes can be identified and measured.

Focus on outcomes and practice guidelines—MCOs have become interested in development and use of practice guidelines to decrease practice variation and improve patient outcomes.

Dual agency of provider—The MCO creates some specific and predictable categories of dual moral agency for the physician. At-risk financing can lead to two conflicting incentives: the well being of the patient versus the financial well being of the provider.

The ethical responsibilities of the health care provider, in or out of the managed care organization, are threefold: 1) they have a duty to maintain and provide a level of skill; 2) a duty to make that skill maximally available to the patient and explain limits of availability; and 3) a duty to patient advocacy. The ethical responsibilities of health care providers have been challenged throughout history. However, the introduction of managed care has created unique challenges.

Managed care organizations attempt to provide their members with the highest quality of health care benefits at the lowest cost to the payer (eg, employer, government). Health care payers include the government (Medicare and Medicaid), employers (health insurance fringe benefits), and individuals. Lowest prices are often achieved through volume purchasing and minimizing unnec-

essary and inappropriate treatment. Lowest prices can also be achieved by offering financial incentives to members to use the plan's facilities and providers. Incentives to the physician are to reduce utilization of services. This alters the traditional physician relationship. An emphasis on limiting unnecessary care may benefit the patient with an emphasis on quality over quantity; however, it may also be perceived as a threat to quality, reducing necessary procedures. This fear that cost containment considerations may override the provision of quality care is pervasive among patients and in society in general.

Care providers are obligated to provide or recommend care when it will benefit the patient, and not withhold care to benefit the plan to the detriment of the patient. Care providers should not engage in bedside rationing if at all possible. This is accomplished by establishing treatment guidelines. Keep in mind that even with guidelines it is important to recommend treatment for a particular patient against the guidelines when indicated. However, decisions made at the bedside can extend beyond the limitations of established guidelines. Exceptions to guidelines are unavoidable, although guidelines are generally useful. Conditions must exist that allow ethics to play a role in resource allocation, including universal access to a basic minimum level of care.

Practitioner or physician level of income must not be directly related to treatment choices. In addition, an ethically acceptable framework for decision making must balance resource allocation with patient needs and consideration of practitioner income. Unethical decisions occur when income of practitioners or companies is the major priority.

With national failures to legislate universal insurance coverage, physicians in general are left with an inadequate framework for making ethical decisions. Practitioners must attempt to offer treatments to patients who are most likely to benefit and discourage or withhold treatments from patients whose chance of benefit is very limited. If care providers fail to make these decisions, the decisions become administrative functions, further limiting fair and just allocation to meet unique needs of individual patients.

Within the managed care organization, the care providers are dealing with a population that universally has coverage. It can be argued that clinicians, as patient advocates, can apply their own resources and skills to the patient unstintingly (utilizing resources within their control). In contrast, resources that are not directly within their command are constrained by the administrative guidelines of the MCO, and cannot be offered on an unrestricted basis. In reality, administrative scheduling policies and productivity standards place constraints on the amount of time clinicians can spend with their patients, limiting that resource as well. Consequently, the just allocation of resources remains an issue, for clinicians because of limitations on the time available for them to meet the needs of patients, and also because of limitations imposed on referrals for other specialists, procedures, or treatments.

To minimize the negative implications of these resource limitations, practitioners should participate in the development of guidelines that they will utilize in providing care. Practice guidelines affect the relationships of health professionals with patients, ranging from productivity standards to policies for withdrawing life support. Evidence-based clinical practice guidelines (CPGs) allow the clinical staff the opportunity to incorporate practices supported by sound empirical evidence.[14] Unfortunately, many clinical practices have not had the benefit of expensive, rigorous, and time-consuming randomized controlled trials. Therefore, practitioners are often required to reach consensus on integrating their best guess with available science to form workable guidelines. At their best, clinical practice guidelines represent a culmination of graded empirical evidence and expert opinion that summarizes what is known about the efficacy of various management strategies for specific conditions.

Critical Thinking Exercise 4

USING CPGS FOR CLINICAL DECISION MAKING

a. When do guidelines best benefit the provider, patient, and organization?

b. When do guidelines undermine care? Choose specific respiratory care CPGs to provide examples and support your arguments.

Once guidelines are established, the next major problem is implementation. A major difficulty in evidence-based medicine is the practical problem of how to encourage practitioners to incorporate new guidelines into their current practice. This appears to be a major problem for virtually every discipline-related organization that has produced or monitored use of its CPGs. Even with the well-publicized National Heart Lung Blood Institute guidelines for asthma education in 1991 and the revision in 1997, a majority of internal medicine and family practice physicians have not effectively incorporated the guidelines into their practice.[15] This is a case in which application of the guidelines appears to improve quality of care and reduce health care costs, meeting the objectives of the institution, physicians, and patient. However, we still do not know how to effectively integrate asthma guidelines into daily clinical practice. One strategy of interest to respiratory therapists is developing protocols based on guidelines that are invoked by the practitioners in lieu of specific orders. We will explore some examples of this later in the chapter.

Patients also have a role in the MCO. To support autonomy, patients should be well informed of plan benefits at the time they subscribe to the plan. Once subscribed, they have the responsibility to recognize that allocation decisions may limit their benefits. If patients feel these limitations are unfair, they must be free to appeal without penalty or prejudice to their future care. Under managed care, patients seek care from individual providers but they contract with organizations. MCOs have an ethical obligation to make ethically sound contracts, and to assure that the individual providers behave ethically on a consistent basis. Plans should allow care providers to explain all treatment options to patients, even if they are not offered by the plan. MCOs should not compromise patient well being to profit plan investors.

The corporate goal for MCOs of generating profits inherently conflicts with providing costly care. Health care did not originate as a business and was not designed to be for-profit. However, escalat-ing costs of health care due to overutilization, lack of foresight, and fraud and abuse required implementation of cost containment measures. MCOs evolved as means to limit costs of health care in the United States, and they have to constantly balance reinvestment of profits into expanded services and distribution of profit to stockholders. Nonprofit MCOs may have less potential for conflict in these areas.

There are highly publicized debates about end-of-life decisions often seen in the public media. These discussions are motivated by a desire to limit costs for ineffective or futile care. Open communication about differential access to health care resources appears to be virtually ignored. Limited debate on fair allocation of resources results in unfair decisions being made at the bedside. All too often, these decisions are unduly influenced by racial, cultural, social, and age-related factors.

ETHICAL AND COST CONSIDERATIONS: CASE STUDIES

Thus far we have reviewed the maxims of ethical medical behavior, as well as the economic forces at work in determining health care allocation, that have brought about major changes in health care delivery. You may have completed some of the chapter questions. Now apply this information to a few cases.

CASE STUDY 1

THE VIRTUAL DEPARTMENT—RESPIRATORY CARE IN ACUTE CARE

You are a respiratory care practitioner in a 300-bed urban community hospital with 30 critical care beds. There are 21 respiratory care practitioners providing 24-hour coverage, with an average of 2 full-time equivalents (FTE) in overtime. Typical workload in the ICU: 10 ventilators in the medical-surgical ICU (average 12 vent days/patient), with an additional 2 postoperative heart patients recovering on ventilators (average 1 to 2 days on ventilator) Monday through Friday. Ventilators are checked every 2 hours; standard circuits with heated water humidifiers and closed suction catheters are changed daily.

There is an active emergency room that treats approximately 10 moderate to severe asthmatic patients each day, with >60% of those patients admitted to the hospital after an average of 3 hours of treatment in the ED, often with around-the-clock albuterol nebulizer treatments every 1 hour. The ordered workload for respiratory care on the

---

---

acute care floors averages 120 nebulizer treatments per day, 30 MDIs, 20 CPT treatments, and 20 IPPB treatments, with 30 patients receiving oxygen, typically 40 O_2 saturation spot checks (often ordered every 4 hours), and 10 patients on continuous Sao_2 monitoring. Even with the overtime, 30% of ordered therapies are routinely not being accomplished due to lack of staff.

The annual department budget is $1,150,000. Personnel costs for staff with benefits is $840,000, with $90,000 in overtime. Supply costs are $220,000. One full-time equivalent employee is 2080 hours costing $30,000 in direct salary, and $8000 to $15,000 per year in benefits. One FTE of overtime at time and a half is $45,000.

Hospital administration has just announced that due to a financial crisis, all budgets will be cut by 10%, and a hiring freeze imposed on all departments. The department manager is told to stop all overtime, and reduce costs by 10% immediately. He is also told that this appears to be the first of many cuts. The manager states that he is already missing 30% of ordered therapy, and the overtime is required to provide safe coverage

of sick calls that would reduce shift staffing to dangerously low levels.

The manager complains that the doctors order the therapy and he has to give the ordered therapy by law. He says that if he has to cut staff by 10%, patients will suffer. He believes the increased liability to the hospital will be much greater than the few dollars saved. The administrator tells the manager it is his job to manage the doctors, the service, and the patients, and that if he cannot manage the situation, the hospital will find someone else who can.

 Group Critical Thinking Exercise 4

REFLECTION AND ANTICIPATION

a. Debate the pros and cons of the position of the administrator, including discussion of across-the-board cuts, the hiring freeze, and no overtime. Include in your debate the ways the manager should communicate each cost-reduction strategy.

b. In addition, what are the ethical implications of the manager's actions?

THE SUBACUTE VENTILATOR UNIT AND THE CASE OF MRS. SNOOZER

The hospital has been told that reimbursement for all Medicare patients will be based on the national average length of stay for the diagnosis-related group (DRG). The hospital has determined that patients requiring mechanical ventilation beyond 12 days cannot remain in acute care because the costs are prohibitive. It is financially desirable for these patients to be transferred as soon as feasible to a subacute long-term ventilator center. These centers receive reimbursement for

long-term ventilator management on a different basis than the acute care hospital, allowing an additional 30 days of cost coverage.

Lydia Snoozer is a 74-year-old woman who was admitted to the hospital from a nursing home for the treatment of pneumonia. Prior to admission, the patient was in poor health and limited to bed and chair, requiring total nursing support. During her hospitalization, Ms. Snoozer had a cardiac arrest, resulting in her being intubated

CASE STUDY 2 *(continued)*

and placed on a ventilator. Although the patient regained consciousness, attempts to wean the patient from mechanical ventilation did not meet with success. After 12 days the ICU team reviewed her situation and recommended that she be transferred to a long-term subacute ventilator management facility. The patient agreed that she wanted to be maintained on the ventilator as long as necessary.

Group Critical Thinking Exercise 5

REFLECTION AND DEBATE OF ETHICAL ISSUES

a. What are the ethical considerations of transferring this patient to a subacute ventilator unit?

b. Debate the pros and cons of patient autonomy and allocation of resources.

CASE STUDY 3

THE EMERGENCY DEPARTMENT AND MS. WHEEZE

You are called to the ED to treat Ms. Wheeze, a 24-year-old asthmatic who has been having progressive difficulty breathing over the past 34 hours. She claims to have used frequently her MDI albuterol without effect. She has previously been diagnosed with asthma, and has visited the ED on 2 prior occasions in the past year. Ms. Wheeze stopped taking her prescribed inhaled steroids because she could not afford them on her minimum-wage salary, which pays her just enough to keep her from qualifying for Medicaid. She is apprehensive that she cannot afford this ED visit. She is extremely short of breath, with audible wheezing in all lung fields, and her peak expiratory flow rate is <40% of predicted.

Critical Thinking Exercise 5

PRIORITIZATION AND ETHICS OF CARE

What is the first priority in the management of this patient?

Ms. Wheeze is given a small volume nebulizer with 2.5 mg of albuterol in 3 mL of normal saline. The treatment lasts 10 minutes. The patient does not appear to have any relief of symptoms.

The doctor has ordered the same dose be given in treatments every 20 minutes over the next 3 hours. You are one of 3 therapists covering the entire hospital, working with 2 less than your normal staffing on the shift, and with an assignment including care of 3 ventilated patients in one critical care unit, and 12 treatments to patients on two acute care floors during the next 3 hours.

Critical Thinking Exercise 6

PRIORITIZING YOUR WORK

a. How would you set your priorities?

b. List the options for providing optimal care to Ms. Wheeze that would not keep you occupied in the ED for the next 3 hours.

c. What are the pros and cons, as well as relative costs, for each of these options?

d. What are the minimum requirements of a treatment option for Ms. Wheeze?

e. Anticipate which options would meet your patient's needs, reduce the time you might be required at the bedside, and be most acceptable to the attending physician and nursing staff.

CASE STUDY 3 *(continued)*

Group Critical Thinking Exercise 6

COMMUNICATIONS AND NEGOTIATIONS WITH OTHER HEALTH PROFESSIONALS

a. Role play how you would communicate your resource (time) limitations, and negotiate your preferred treatment option.

b. What would you say to the physician, the nurse, and the patient?

In the case of Ms. Wheeze, suppose that you have communicated your need to be in several places at once, and that you cannot spend the next 3 hours in the ED taking care of just one patient. When you attempt to negotiate a treatment strategy that would be as good or better for the patient and require less of your time at the bedside, the physician responds that he is not comfortable with your proposed strategy. The physician insists that his order be followed.

Critical Thinking Exercise 7

NEGOTIATIONS—THE DOCTOR DOESN'T CHANGE THE ORDER

a. Describe the ethical issues facing you.

b. What are your options for action?

CASE STUDY 4

YOU CANNOT STAY IF YOU CANNOT PAY!

A patient presents to the ED via ambulance with no evidence of health insurance. The hospital administrator on call says that if the patient cannot pay, he cannot stay, and directs the ED staff to transfer the patient to the local county hospital. The ED physician insists on examining the patient prior to making any decision to transfer the patient, stating that transferring the patient before assuring the patient was stable would be unethical. The administrator cites hospital policy that states, "patients without proof of insurance will not be seen." The administrator notes that the ED is already gravely over budget, and threatens the physician with disciplinary action unless she immediately transfers the patient to the county facility.

Critical Thinking Exercise 8

ETHICAL DECISION MAKING

a. If you were the physician, what would you do?

b. What are the ethical and legal issues?

KEY POINTS

- Ethics is the study of how societies and individuals make decisions about what is right or wrong.

- Many factors affect respiratory therapists' decisions as to what is right or wrong, including culture, religion, morals, and the mores of their society.

- Seven important ethical principles to guide health care are veracity, autonomy, confidentiality, beneficence, nonmaleficence, justice, and fidelity.

- Veracity is the principle guiding the health care practitioner to tell the patient the truth.

- In health care, autonomy means that the patient has the right to choose actions that are consistent with his or her goals, values, and life plan.

- Confidentiality ensures that information revealed to the health care practitioner will not be revealed to others except when necessary to carry out their duty.

- Beneficence is the principle that dictates that the health care practitioner has the responsibility to seek good for the patient.

- Nonmaleficence is the principle that dictates that the health care practitioner refrain from harming the patient.

- Justice is the principle that deals with the fair and equitable distribution of health care resources, a major controversy today.

- Fidelity is the principle that says that one should be faithful to their duty.

- Managed care, patient-focused care, preferred provider organizations (PPOs), and health maintenance organizations (HMOs) have evolved to effectively manage the nation's health care dollars, provoking numerous ethical and legal issues.

- Hospitals and other health care organizations have established ethics committees to deal with ethical issues in patient care and to educate health care professionals.

- Each respiratory therapist has a duty and responsibility to provide quality health care guided by legal and ethical principles.

- The AARC code of ethics describes the ethical behaviors for respiratory therapists that should guide professional practice.

REFERENCES

1. Kuttner R. The American Health Care System: Employer-sponsored health coverage. *N Engl J Med.* 1999;340:248–252.

2. Perlin TM. *Clinical Medical Ethics:* Cases in Practice. Boston: Little, Brown and Company; 1992.

3. Beauchamp TL, Childress JF. *Principles of Biomedical Ethics.* 4th ed. New York: Oxford University Press; 1994.

4. Levine C. *Taking Sides: Clashing Views on Controversial Bioethical Issues.* 6th ed. Guilford, Conn: Dushkin Publishing Group; 1995.

5. Mappes TA, DeGrazia D. *Biomedical Ethics.* 4th ed. New York: McGraw-Hill; 1996.

6. Jonsen R, Siegler M, Winslade WJ. *Clinical Ethics.* 3rd ed. New York: McGraw-Hill; 1992.

7. Lo B. *Resolving Ethical Dilemmas.* Baltimore: Williams & Wilkins; 1995.

8. Mahlmeister M, Bigler J. Legal and ethical considerations. In: Fink JB, Hunt G, eds. *Clinical Practice of Respiratory Care.* Philadelphia: Lippincott; 1998.

9. Cowdrey ML, Drew M. *Basic Law for the Allied Health Professions.* 2nd ed. London: Jones and Barlett International Publishers; 1995.

10. Jonsen AR. Do no harm. *Ann Intern Med.* 1978; 88:827–832.

11. American Association for Respiratory Care: Statement of Ethics and Professional Conduct. *Respir Care* 41(9):835, 1996.

12. Idziak JM. *Ethical Dilemmas in Allied Health.* Dubuque, Iowa: Simon & Koltz Publishing; 1999.

13. Cook DJ. Health professional decision-making in the ICU: a review of the evidence. *New Horiz.* 1997;5:15–19.

14. Cook DJ, Guyatt GH, Jaeschke R. Canadian Critical Care Trials Groups: Determinants in Canadian Health care workers for the decision to withdraw life support from the critically ill. *JAMA.* 1995; 273:703–708.

15. Doerschug KC, Peterson MW, Dayton CS, Kline JN. Asthma guidelines: An assessment of physician understanding and practice. *Am J Respir Crit Care Med.* 1999;159:1735–1741.

9

PATIENT EDUCATION

Amy Travis and Shelley C. Mishoe

Education is what remains
after the facts are forgotten.
ANONYMOUS

LEARNING OBJECTIVES

1. Discuss the importance of patient education, including health promotion and quality-of-life issues.
2. Describe the differences and similarities between the patients' goals and the health care providers' goals for patient education.
3. Discuss the types of communication as well as the importance of communication for effective patient education.
4. Identify the strategies to improve patient communication to achieve the desired outcomes of patient education for pediatric, adult, and geriatric patients.
5. Describe the process of education from the planning stages through assessment.
6. Apply the critical thinking skills of prioritizing, anticipating, negotiating, communicating, decision making, and reflecting by completing exercises and case examples for providing patient/caregiver education.
7. Using the chapter case, develop, implement, and assess a plan for providing caregiver education, including recommendations for therapy and disease management, with consideration of the cost, and ethical and quality-of-life issues.
8. Describe the role of respiratory therapists in patient and caregiver education for management of acute and chronic cardiopulmonary diseases.

KEY WORDS

Affective
Caregiver
Cognitive
Disease Management
Chronic
    Cardiopulmonary
    Disease

Health Care Professional
Health Education Provider
Learning Objectives
Patient Compliance
Patient Rapport
Psychomotor
Pulmonary Rehabilitation

INTRODUCTION

Background

Educating the public on health issues is not a modern idea. In 1842, Horace Mann proposed to provide health education in schools,[1] but it was not until 33 years later the idea became widespread. In the last century, English leaders recognized that school was not the only place for health education.[1] At that time families were the ones caring for the sick, therefore a campaign was begun to educate families on health issues.[1] The goal of health education was and continues to be to enable individuals to make informed decisions and take responsible action regarding their health.

Patient education was reborn in the 1970s.[2] In the past, patient education was relatively simple. There was a sufficient number of staff to plan and provide education, and patients were in the hospital longer. By the early 1980s, patient education had become more challenging.[2] Reimbursement services diminished, hospital stays shortened, and there was an increase in the number of outpatient procedures done.[2] Patients now are rarely hospitalized after surgery or only stay in the hospital for 24 to 48 hours postoperatively. Education is usually conducted preoperatively in the physician's office and during follow-up visits. Consequently, when patients are discharged from the hospital, they and their families perform technical and monitoring procedures that once were performed solely by health care providers.[2]

Patient education has become a crucial component of health care. Four of the major causes of death in the United States are heart disease, cancer, cerebrovascular disease, and chronic obstructive pulmonary disease (COPD).[1] Primary causes of these diseases include high-fat diet, excessive alcohol use, use of tobacco, and inactivity. All of the causes of these major diseases are preventable. Three percent of the $750 billion spent on health care in the US has been allotted to patient education.[2] Recently, standard medical practice has shifted from physicians diagnosing and treating disease to a greater emphasis on illness prevention.[3] Massive education campaigns have spread to provide information to the public. There are widely publicized campaigns on the hazards of drinking and driving, smoking, and eating foods high in fat and cholesterol. Patient education has become a key part of health care. Health care providers must effectively transfer knowledge, skills, and attitudes to patients.[1] Patients must be well informed and self-sufficient.

AARC Description

The recognition that health professionals played a vital role in health education caused many professional organizations to develop policy statements. For example, the American Association of Respiratory Care (AARC) developed guidelines for clinical practice for respiratory therapists to use when providing patient education. In the clinical practice guideline (CPG) providing patient and caregiver training, the AARC defines patient education as the procedure of providing patient training, initiated by a health care provider, to facilitate the patient's knowledge and skills related to his or her medical condition and participation in its management.[4] The guideline goes on to address the need for the training process to occur with every visit and to include family and/or caregivers as shown in Table 9-1.[4]

Importance of Patient Education

Today's patients need to assume a greater degree of responsibility for their health behaviors. Why? The answer is simple. Today, most physicians need to see more patients in the same amount of time, spending less time per patient, in order to maintain past income levels. As patient volumes increase, physicians have less time for educating their patients. Consequently, patients and their families must take the responsibility to achieve better health outcomes. In the past, health care providers were considered experts and the ones solely involved in making decisions on the patient's behalf.[5] The relationship of the patient and the physician was similar to that of a parent and child.[5] The physician was perceived to be on a level above the patient because of extensive training and medical knowledge. However, the emphasis has shifted and the issues of patient education have become more complex than ever before.

At present, one major emphasis of health care is making the patient well informed, knowledgeable, and self-sufficient. The physician and patient are considered equal partners who share the goal of improving health. The physician serves as the facilitator who assists in the patient's decision making.[5]

TABLE 9-1 PROVIDING PATIENT AND CAREGIVER TRAINING

Description/Definition
- Patient and caregiver education provides the patient and family with a means of participating in the patient's health care management to the extent feasible, depending on physical condition and awareness.
- The training process should occur with every encounter between the health care provider (HCP) and the patient.
- The goal of the HCP should be to elicit a positive change in the patient's behavior through the use of verbal, written, and visual communication, in the affective, cognitive, and psychomotor domains.
- A final goal of the HCP is to provide the patient and family with the means to reap the economic benefits of improved utilization of the health care system.

Indications
The presence of a patient population with the need to:
- increase knowledge and understanding of health status and therapy
- improve necessary skills for safe and effective health care
- foster a positive attitude, strengthen motivation, and increase compliance with therapeutic modalities

Contraindications
- There are no contraindications to patient and caregiver training when the need exists.

SOURCE: AARC.[4]

Studies have shown that patient compliance has improved when patients are given the opportunity to participate in their treatment decisions.[6] One author summarizes the point thusly: "Effective health care is an equal partnership. Help your clients to make health care choices, but let them lead the way."[6] Patient education is important for three reasons: better self-management, cutting health care costs, and reduction in morbidity.

CRITICAL CONTENT

ADVANTAGES OF PATIENT EDUCATION
- Greater self-management
- More efficient health care
- Reduction in morbidity

The principle of self-management fosters patient autonomy. Autonomy is the right of the patient to make his or her own decisions regarding health care.[7]

For example, a patient may be prescribed an inhaled bronchodilator, ipratropium, to be taken regularly for COPD. The patient may decide that the medication is not working or that the drug has undesirable side effects. With patient education, the patient would consult the physician to report the side effects and discuss alternate therapies. This example illustrates the importance of open communication between the physician and the patient, because this can help the patient make a better treatment choice.

Research has shown that health care education can be cost effective.[8–12] The AARC states that one of the goals of patient education is to supply the patient with the knowledge needed to utilize the health care system more advantageously.[4] It has become clear that the present health care system is driven by economic incentives to cut costs and reduce a health care budget that has become out of control.[2] Recently health care expenditures have reached the trillion dollar mark.[2] The government is trying to control the problem by shifting responsibility from the health care provider to the patient. As the baby boom generation approaches its retirement years, it is presenting with chronic, debilitating diseases. This places considerable economic pressure on a health care system that is already strained. A better-informed patient will go a long way toward improving the effectiveness and efficiency of health care in the United States.[2] Ultimately, the cost of health care can be reduced.

Research has also shown that patient education can reduce morbidity.[8–12] By promoting open communication with the patient, the provider can ensure that the patient understands and adheres to the regimen necessary to live a healthier life. A review of studies reveals that only 25% to 50% of patients are compliant with treatment regimens, and this low compliance with prescribed therapy continues to be a challenge.[8–12] By continuing to integrate education into the health care system, patients have a better chance of preventing serious illness.

GOALS OF PATIENT EDUCATION

The AARC states that the ultimate goal of patient education is to provide the knowledge, skills, and attitudes needed so that patients may better understand their conditions and actively participate in their health care.[13] This goal can be met by identifying two components: the patient's goals in education and the health care provider's goals.

The Patient's Goals

The patient hopes to obtain factual information about their health condition.[1,14] When first diagnosed, most patients know very little about their disease. The information they receive from health professionals should be discussed and understood. When equipped with the appropriate information, patients should be able to make well-informed decisions about their health care.

Second, the patient hopes to have the opportunity to learn skills that encourage self-care and allow them to continue activities of daily living.[1,14] The patient should also be aware of health services available to them that enhance self-care. For example, pulmonary rehabilitation programs may bene-

fit patients by giving them the skills and knowledge to maintain the highest quality of life possible, even with COPD.

Another goal of patient education is to help the patient feel less anxious about his or her disease.[1,14] When a patient is first diagnosed with a condition, it is common for the patient to feel anxiety.[15] The professional team can be essential in providing emotional support to the patient and the patient's family. Many times, when patients understand the disease process, the feeling of distress is relieved.[15]

CRITICAL CONTENT

THE PATIENT'S GOALS FOR PATIENT EDUCATION

- To obtain accurate information about their disease
- To have the opportunity to learn skills useful in treating their disease
- To reduce anxiety about their disease process

The Health Care Professional's Goals

The health care professional has a different set of goals from those of the patient. The professional's primary goal is to increase the effectiveness and efficiency of health care.[11] The approach recently gaining the most attention is to manage a patient's overall health rather than solely treating disease.[15,16] Prevention and early detection of cardiopulmonary disease is the key. Managing the disease involves identifying a specific population at high risk for undesirable outcomes and intervening to modify that risk.[3] For example, approximately 25% of US residents smoke cigarettes, greatly increasing their chance of developing congestive heart failure (CHF) or COPD.[16] By providing information through a smoking cessation class, many may become enlightened and choose to stop smoking to reduce health hazards.

Respiratory therapists strive to make hospital admissions efficient. Research has shown that practicing disease management leads to fewer exacerbations overall and fewer severe exacerbations that require a patient to return to the hospital.[3] By providing patient education, health care professionals can reduce the number of patient hospitalizations, thus the hospital and physicians can achieve a reduction in health care delivery costs.

The health care professional also provides patient education in the hope of improving patient compliance. Noncompliance is costly.[14] When patients do not comply with treatment plans, it wastes valuable medical expertise and finite health care resources. In addition, failure to comply with treatment plans can be hazardous to patients. The

foundation of patient compliance is a trusting relationship with the caregiver. Respiratory therapists need to support patients' decisions if they expect them to comply with medical advice.

Patient education is a professional responsibility. In recent years, patient education has gained considerable credibility and acceptance. This has led to professional organizations developing guidelines to follow to accomplish patient education. The guidelines for patient education developed by the AARC are shown in Table 9-2.[13] While providing patient education, respiratory therapists must also meet their professional practice requirements.[14]

TABLE 9-2 TRAINING THE HEALTH CARE PROFESSIONAL (HCP) FOR THE ROLE OF PATIENT AND CAREGIVER EDUCATOR

Description/Definition

The process of training the HCP as patient and/or caregiver educator includes addressing and assuring adequate knowledge, skills, and attitude mastery for patient rapport and effective teaching.

The ultimate goal of the process is to provide education to the patient and/or caregiver that will equip him or her with the knowledge, skills, and attitudes to better understand the patient's condition and to more fully participate in their health care.

Assessment of Need

All HCPs who have patient care contact and the opportunity to provide patient and/or caregiver education should be assessed for training as education providers by:
1. Observation of the HCP in a patient education setting to determine if the needed skills are present.
2. Verbal questioning by a specialist as to knowledge of the topics being taught.

Assessment of Outcome

1. Evidence from HCP evaluations that the training has met the goals and objectives for preparing patient and/or caregiver educators through:
   a. Verbal or written evaluation; and
   b. Observation of the HCP in a teaching setting.
2. Evidence that the HCP educator can assist patients and/or caregivers to meet the goals of their patient education through:
   a. Knowledge gained by the patient or patient care provider;
   b. Skills mastered by the patient or the patient care provider;
   c. Positive change in patient outlook and/or attitude; and
   d. Compliance of patient or caregiver in following the care plan.
3. Long-term assessment through departmental or institutional continuous quality improvement indicators or other quality monitoring system.

SOURCE: AARC.[13]

THE HEALTH CARE PROFESSIONAL'S GOALS FOR PATIENT EDUCATION

- To increase the effectiveness and efficiency of health care
- To improve patient compliance with care plans
- To meet professional practice requirements

ROLE OF THE RESPIRATORY THERAPIST

In light of the changes accompanying managed care and the growing interest in disease management, respiratory therapists have expanded into the role of patient educator.[17] Besides physicians, respiratory therapists are considered experts in cardiorespiratory care. To be experts, respiratory therapists must ensure they stay up to date and have the most accurate information to relay to patients. The AARC recognizes that respiratory therapists are in a unique position to provide leadership in patient education.[18] For example, it is respiratory therapists that lead pulmonary rehabilitation programs, smoking cessation classes, and asthma management discussions, as well as initiatives to limit the costs and improve the care of patients with chronic pulmonary disease.

Building a good rapport with the patient is a start to being a competent instructor, one who is often admired by patients, families, and other health care professionals.[19] A good relationship between the patient and the respiratory therapist leads the way to an improved alliance in the fight for better health. With the patient's trust, the respiratory therapist is able to assist in diagnosing a disease by helping the patient understand the importance of disclosing pertinent medical history.[19]

One of the best ways to illustrate desired behaviors is by role modeling.[1] Unless health care professionals model healthy behaviors, successful health outcomes cannot be expected from the public.[1] For example, the media stress the dangers of smoking. However, a patient might see a respiratory therapist smoking and ask, "How can smoking be harmful when I see respiratory therapists doing it?" The trust of the relationship is also jeopardized if the therapist says one thing but does another. The most effective respiratory therapist facilitates patient compliance by modeling the actions they desire. Remember the saying, "Actions speak louder than words."

Respiratory therapists must be flexible and prepared to educate in any setting. It could be at a patient's bedside before discharge, in a group setting like a pulmonary rehabilitation, or in a patient's home. The respiratory therapist involved in educating home health patients can instruct on infection control, troubleshooting, backup equipment, and plans for emergencies.[20] It is crucial to be alert for "teachable moments," because at any time a patient may pop up with a question or concern about their illness.[1] What a great opportunity to teach! Ideal educators and communicators are aware of teachable moments and utilize them to full advantage.

Another essential skill needed to become an exceptional educator is the ability to organize teaching strategies in a way that is best suited to the patient.[3,6,18] Respiratory therapists should identify patient needs and work with the entire caregiver team—nurses, physicians, and family—to implement plans to take care of those needs. Respiratory therapists should also take an active role in the development of educational materials to aid in training.[1] For instance, Peak Performance USA is a project sponsored by the AARC and developed by respiratory therapists to improve the delivery of asthma care to children.[21]

Modern medicine has offered and will continue to offer a lot for people with a chronic or life-threatening disease.[17] In the future, respiratory therapists will be at the center of patient education. As health promotion and disease management gain more visibility, the respiratory therapist will find opportunities to educate not only in hospital settings, but also in home care and public health facilities.[1]

ROLES OF RESPIRATORY THERAPISTS IN PATIENT EDUCATION

- Build rapport with patients
- Be a role model
- Be flexible in educating patients
- Organize tasks
- Take advantage of opportunities to educate patients

TEACHING AND LEARNING

Frequently, patients have no previous knowledge of the issues to be dealt with. They depend on health care workers to be resources, offering encouragement and assistance. The teacher must recognize patient education as a continuing process. Education is not simply telling the patient about a disease. Effective education can only exist when learning has occurred. Learning is defined as knowledge and skills gained that change behavior.[1] There are three categories of human learning: cognitive, psychomotor, and affective.[14]

CLASSIFICATION OF LEARNING

- Cognitive
- Psychomotor
- Affective

The cognitive domain refers to the actual knowledge and understanding an individual has about a certain subject.[14] For example, if a patient has COPD and is prescribed to wear oxygen, the patient should understand the anatomy and physiology of COPD and why it is beneficial to wear oxygen. Any factual information that the educator expects the patient to recall or recognize falls under the cognitive domain.[14]

If the educator hopes to enable the patient to perform certain procedures, providing facts is not enough; the patient must be taught the physical skills. The psychomotor domain includes these skills. For instance, in the previous example in which the patient was prescribed oxygen therapy, the patient would be taught how to operate an E cylinder, how to properly place a nasal cannula, and how to replace the equipment. If the patient only reads about or listens to a description of the procedure, it may not be fully understood. When the patient has gained the skill and demonstrates the procedure, the educator can be sure that learning has occurred. Patients, like most learners, will remember only 10% of what they hear, but over 59% of what they do.[22]

The affective domain refers to the patient's attitude.[14] The patient may be reluctant or unmotivated about utilizing the knowledge and skills they have learned because of an earlier negative reaction to a condition or treatment they received. For example, a patient may not wear oxygen in public because they may be anxious about how people will react. It is important for a patient in that situation that the health care professionals, especially respiratory therapists, give the patient many ideas and strategies for making him or her feel less self-conscious. A support group for patients dealing with long-term oxygen use may be the solution to help the patient and family comply with the care plan. For many patients, it is important to identify their concerns and fears so that the professional can develop strategies to help them cope.

The effective patient educator realizes that the most important part of their role is to improve patient compliance. Patient compliance is one outcome used to determine effectiveness of education. Only about 50% of patients comply with their treatment plans. This means that the other half do not follow through on implementation of their care plans. It is important for the patient educator to address all of the cognitive, psychomotor, and affective needs of each patient.[14] If the health professional can achieve over 50% compliance over an extended period, this is one indicator that the education is effective. Research shows that when patient compliance rates are initially high, they tend to drop off within 3 months to 1 year. Therefore education must be a continuing part of the health care process for health promotion and disease management.

Respiratory therapists must be adaptable in the methods of instruction used to accomplish patient education. Respiratory therapists recognize that all patients do not learn in the same manner. A RT's students can be anyone from young children to elderly adults. The task of the teacher is to identify the needs of each patient and provide information in a way that meets those needs.

Teaching the Adult Learner

A developmental approach to patient education helps the respiratory therapist identify with the patient at a particular point in the individual's life. Life stages are apparent in children, but occur in adulthood as well. Adults have three stages: young adult, middle aged, and later years.[14]

Young adults are at a point in their lives where they are getting married, beginning careers, or starting a family. Knowledge of the different aspects of an individual's life helps the therapist determine patient responsibility and potential barriers to carrying out treatment recommendations.[14] The main concern for young adults is stress. Stress is an unpleasant fact of life, and individuals need to understand the consequences and learn to minimize the damage of stress-related overwork and the other health hazards associated with chronic stress. The cartoon in Fig. 9-1 pokes fun at the way many adults operate today, feeling the need to stay on the cutting edge, which often works against stress management and deprives them of the relaxation they need. Helping patients learn to cope with stress is important; however, all aspects of health promotion are important. Encouraging health promotion is important for everyone and is another major role of education. The best road to good health (excluding genetic factors) is adoption of a healthy lifestyle. Proper diet and exercise, sufficient sleep, and avoidance of risk factors are important determinants of health. Risk factors to avoid include unprotected sex, drinking and driving, failure to wear a seatbelt, illegal drug use, and other reckless behaviors. Health practices established in youth often determine an individual's long-term health.

Mid-life is the transition between young adulthood and the elder years. During mid-life, individuals begin to reexamine their lives. For many of them their roles have shifted, children have left home and no longer need supervision, but older parents now require their attention and care. Middle aged adults become keenly aware of death.[14] This realization may motivate the individual to follow recommendations more closely or may cause the individual to deny illness and abandon health promotion almost entirely.[14] The best approach to middle aged adults is nonjudgmental interactions and a sincere attitude.

Patient education for older adults is no longer health promotion. Patient education for the elderly revolves around coping with chronic ailments, especially when chronic diseases become apparent. Other issues involved are nutrition, aging, disease prevention, and enhancement of quality of life. The educator should teach the patient how to make optimum use of his or her skills and functions.[5] Respiratory therapists are aware of potential compliance problems during this phase. Elderly adults often misinter-

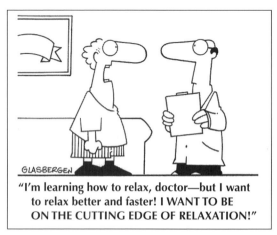

"I'm learning how to relax, doctor—but I want to relax better and faster! I WANT TO BE ON THE CUTTING EDGE OF RELAXATION!"

FIGURE 9-1   (*SOURCE: Cartoon by Randy Glasbergen © 1997.*)

pret information. They may also have physical limitations or lack financial resources that further limit adherence to treatment recommendations.

The Pediatric Learner

Children differ from adults in their reaction to illness.[14] It is important to encourage parents to foster the child's normal development despite illness limitations.[14] Children, too, go through developmental stages and each stage requires a different approach. As the child grows and develops, they should be included as much as possible in the teaching process whenever they are patients. Greater compliance occurs when children are accountable for their learning and are taught how to take responsibility for their health.[1] Nevertheless, it is the parent's responsibility to supervise the child and ensure that the health care plan is followed.

Teaching children is a unique opportunity to use a variety of teaching skills. The key for respiratory therapists in training children is to use humor, to be creative, and to have lots of patience. It is crucial to use language that includes words that children can relate to and understand. Short stories like fairy tales or sports-related events are useful in conveying information. In addition to games, children love to receive rewards when they accomplish set goals. Something as simple as candies or a small prize can be a powerful motivator for children. Educators should help caregivers establish a reward system to help children stay motivated when they have chronic illness. The right motivators can help most patients, including children, to set health goals and achieve care plans over the long term. Sessions should be brief so educators do not overload patients with information.

Each patient brings a diverse background that directly affects their ability to learn. Although the respiratory therapist should always approach each patient as an individual, an understanding of general human characteristics at various life stages can be practical.[9] Understanding age-specific learning needs and developmental issues helps define strategies for helping patients at various stages and makes patient education more meaningful and effective.

COMMUNICATION

A key element of patient education is communication. It is clear that satisfaction, compliance, and clinical outcomes depend on how health care professionals interact with patients. The basic purposes for communication in health care are to establish rapport with the patient and family, to obtain or relay information, to give instructions, and to persuade patients to change their behaviors.[23] Numerous factors affect communication. Attitudes, values, and cultural backgrounds sway opinions and thoughts. Feelings of fear, anxiety, or pain can hinder effective learning. Also, the environment where the interaction takes place can affect communication.[24] If lighting, noise level, or temperature is inappropriate, it may be more difficult to successfully teach the patient. There are two types of communication: nonverbal and verbal.

Nonverbal Communication

Nonverbal communication is the use of gestures, posture, facial expressions, manipulation of personal space, and other inaudible expressions to convey a message.[24] For example, a person might nod their head to indicate they understand. No words were spoken, but the gesture acknowledges that the person is listening and believes they understand the message. Nonverbal communication makes up 55% percent of communication.[25]

CRITICAL CONTENT

NONVERBAL COMMUNICATION

Nonverbal communication is conveying a message using facial expressions, gestures, or other means without using words.

Awareness of nonverbal cues can help make communication between the patient and health care worker more effective so the intended messages will be effectively exchanged.[24] Nonverbal behavior helps the health professional to determine the most appropriate way of responding to a patient at a given time. For example, a patient who frowns would require a different response than a person who looks puzzled. By observing nonverbal cues, the health care professional can obtain a more accurate picture of the progress being made by linking the patient's behavior to the words they speak.[14]

Not only is it important for health professionals to be aware of nonverbal cues from patients, but we also need to be aware of the meaning of their behavior.[14] For example, a health care worker obtaining a history from a patient, but who is shuffling papers at the same time, might convey the message to the patient that they are really too busy to listen. If patients react badly to nonverbal cues it can hinder the teaching interaction. If material is presented in a disinterested or hurried manner by the health care professional, patients may interrupt the communication because they may feel that the professional is not taking them seriously or not concerned about their needs. Patients can also incorrectly conclude that the information relayed is not important, because if it were, the health professional would take more time. Health care professionals should approach patients, as well as their families and visitors, in a warm, friendly manner that is accepting and considerate of their needs.[24]

Verbal Communication

The tone of voice and the actual words spoken comprise the remaining 45% of communication. Verbal communication, the actual spoken words, makes up only 7% of communication. The response to verbal statements can facilitate or hinder the degree to which teaching goals are reached. The important points in verbal communication are to be brief, clear, and simple.[26] If a patient is anxious or in pain, they may have difficulty comprehending detailed instructions.[24]

CRITICAL CONTENT

Verbal communication is using spoken words to express ideas.

It is important to remember that once a message is sent, it may be impossible to retrieve. Therefore, careful thought should go into all messages you communicate to others, especially to your patients. The verbal message may be changed by the tone of voice used.[26] Even greater are the effects of body language, the nonverbal message carried along with the verbal one. By emphasizing different words in a sentence the entire meaning can change.

Although verbal exchanges take place during any discussion with the patient, most often they are transmitted during interviews. The ideal interview, whether a 5-minute assessment or a 50-minute session, is one in which the patient feels secure and free to talk.[24] The interview should establish a trusting relationship between the patient and the professional. The interviewer must make a conscious effort to send signals of compassion, empathy, and professionalism.

When appropriate, probing questions are useful when interviewing the patient and his or her caregivers.[14] Patient feedback is used by the health professional to obtain additional information about the patient's understanding and ability to manage their disease. Instead of asking yes/no questions, open-ended questions are more helpful.[26] An example of a probing question is, "Tell me your understanding of your condition." This type of question is much better than, "Do you understand your condition?" This alternative can easily be answered, "yes," even when the patient does not understand. The worst alternative is asking a leading question such as, "You do understand your health condition, right?" This third alternative is most likely to be answered with, "Yes, I understand," when in fact they do not. It is important for the health care professional to know how much the patient understands about their health status. Whenever possible, ask the patient, caregiver, or other person you are teaching, to describe or demonstrate what they learned from the patient education session. Continuous feedback and updates are necessary throughout the course of treatment, especially for chronic conditions.

Improving Communication

Communication between patients and health care professionals has changed drastically over the years for many reasons. Computer technology has allowed the medical professions to improve the ways they communicate with patients.[22] A relatively new breakthrough communication tool is the Internet. Computers, and especially the Internet, provide an enormous amount of information to demanding patients. A recent survey revealed that 49% of information that patients receive comes from the Internet.[22] The fact is that all information on the Internet is not accurate. In some cases, obtaining certain information can be inappropriate and even detrimental to patient care and health. Effective communication must occur between patients and their providers to help patients evaluate the information they obtain so they are not misinformed.

Health care professionals have the ability to improve their communication with their patients. Studies have shown that during most patient interactions, health care professionals dominate the conversation.[15] To be effective in patient education as well as patient assessment, health professionals should listen more often! Being an active listener requires maintaining eye contact, clarifying by asking questions, and reinforcing by nodding or paraphrasing.[1] Patients should feel that they can participate and exercise choice in their health care. Skillful communicators know that people all have differing opinions, learning styles, and communication strategies. The effective patient educator allows others to express themselves freely.[15] Accepting input from others promotes growth and cooperation, not only for the patient but for the health professional as well.

CRITICAL CONTENT

WAYS TO ENHANCE PATIENT EDUCATION

- Health care providers should be active listeners.
- Patients should feel free to openly express their opinions.
- Heath care providers should be taught communication skills to enhance patient education and compliance.

The most promising improvements in communication are coming from the changes in medical education.[27] The increasing awareness of the need for patient education has led to formal training of health care practitioners on the most effective ways to communicate with patients and families. In the future, medical training will continue to give growing attention to the knowledge and skills necessary for effective communication with patients, their families, and other health care professionals.

Communication is such an important aspect of patient education and clinical practice that an entire chapter is devoted to this topic. Chapter 4 provides further discussion of communication, including the role of negotiation. Students should carefully read Chapter 4 and complete the questions and exercises to improve the communication and negotiation skills needed for respiratory care practice.

THE PROCESS OF PATIENT EDUCATION

Patient education is a systematic learning experience. The process consists of four major components. First, assessment requires the collection of information that will help implement teaching activities. Next, planning involves developing an individualized patient education program. The third step of the process is implementation, or the actual process of teaching using a variety of teaching methods and tools. Last, evaluation enables the instructor to determine whether learning has occurred. The completion of each component is critical to effective, successful patient education.

FOUR STEPS TO SUCCESSFUL PATIENT EDUCATION

- Assessment
- Planning
- Implementation
- Evaluation

Assessment

Effective assessment for patient education requires extensive data collection. Data can be collected from many sources. Simple observations can be a great source, but the most valuable source of information is the patient. The clinician should assess the learner's readiness to learn, ability to learn, previous knowledge of the subject, what the patient wants to know, and the educational needs of the patient and caregivers.[28]

CRITICAL CONTENT

Assessment is information gathering that assists the health care provider in planning teaching strategies.

Finding the right time to teach is essential. The learner's eagerness and ability to learn can be ascertained through the interview.[14] Asking questions gives the respiratory therapist a reasonable idea of the situation. With verbal and nonverbal communication, the therapist can determine the emotional state of the patient.[28] Emotions such as anger, anxiety, and sadness may be revealed in the patient's tone of voice. If a patient has just been informed of a diagnosis of a serious disease, he or she will probably not be able to retain information presented to them.[22] After the

patient has gotten over the initial shock is a better time to teach them about their condition.

All patients differ in their ability to learn. The intellectual level of the patient affects his or her ability to comprehend their illness, and also helps determine the teaching approach that should be employed by the educator. Some patients go to great lengths to mask their inability to understand.[14] Often, patients are given written materials without consideration of whether the patient can read or if the patient understands what he or she reads. Many patients feel inadequate or embarrassed about asking questions to clarify points of information. If a patient is given a handout without explanation, it is unlikely to benefit the patient. However, if the professional takes the time to explain and emphasize the risks of heart disease related to obesity, the communication is more likely to be effective. If the professional does not show that a point is important enough to discuss thoroughly, then the patient will feel it is not important.

It is advantageous for the health professional to know what previous knowledge or experience the patient has with their disease or condition.[14] The best way to assess this is to ask, "What have you been told about your illness?" If a patient diagnosed with emphysema simply states, "There is something wrong with my lungs," the educator can be sure the patient does not fully comprehend the extent of their condition. The patient's ability to understand health information is a prerequisite to patient compliance.[6]

Previous experiences of patients are likely to impact how they deal with their condition. For example, if a patient had a family member who had a similar problem, the patient will recall the experiences with the family member. The family member may have been unable to work, had frequent hospital visits, and had activities of daily living severely limited. These experiences will affect the patient's reactions and concerns for their own disease process.

The content of patient education depends on the needs and interests of the patient.[29] Adequately informed patients comply with instructions better than poorly informed ones.[22] Informed patients also seem to have faster recovery times and improved clinical outcomes.[22] Health professionals may feel that patients should be informed about all areas of their health care. However, it is important for the professional to establish realistic goals and to assess the likelihood of actually meeting those goals.[14] A 40-year-old patient smoking a pack of cigarettes a day and experiencing no respiratory or cardiac problems would probably be unwilling to simply quit smoking. A more realistic goal for the smoker would be to ensure the patient is well informed of the health hazards related to smoking.

CRITICAL CONTENT

During the assessment the health care provider can obtain information about the patient's:

- readiness to learn;
- ability to retain information;
- emotional state;
- past experiences; and
- educational needs and interests.

Planning

The second phase of the patient education process is planning. Planning necessitates the establishment of specific learning objectives and ways to accomplish those objectives.[14] The approach to patient teaching should reflect the patient's individual needs as well as his or her strengths.[14] Part of effective patient education is to set goals with the patients that are realistic and achievable.[1]

CRITICAL CONTENT

Planning is defining learning objectives for the patient to master. Ideal patient education involves the patient as much as possible in planning and every phase of patient education.

The purpose of planning in patient education is to help the health professional to develop clear, concise descriptions of teaching actions. The design is based on information gathered during the assessment process. No matter how comprehensive the teaching plan, patient education cannot be effective if the specified goals are impossible to attain. In some instances, the health professional is better off setting small, easy attainable goals.[14] In teaching a patient about prescribed medication, some short-term goals for the patient might be to first have the prescription filled; and second, to take the medication as recommended.

In setting goals for patient education, the health professional should establish priorities for the sequence of information being taught.[14] Information that is necessary to enable the patient to function safely and adequately should be covered first. Goals that are dependent on the accomplishment of prior goals can be included at a later time. It is important to realize that some goals take days, weeks, or months of teaching before they can be reached.[14]

Often the planning phase is skipped by the health practitioner.[14] Overenthusiastic educators forget the importance of planning and organizing and begin the teaching process without clear direction. Consequently, the educator can easily become frustrated and discouraged when obstacles pop up. Other planning considerations are financial limitations and time constraints.[22] Most departments do not have extra funds to spend on educational materials and the personnel required for effective education. Time is a scarce commodity for health care workers. The health professional's time has become more limited today because of the amount of reporting required by insurance companies.[22] A planned approach and the use of effective communication can help solve many of the problems regarding money and time spent teaching patients. Assessment of patient outcomes, including changes in the costs of care, must be documented and evaluated on a continual basis. The cost for patient education can be offset by decreased costs for acute and emergency care, but departments and organizations must document these results.

CRITICAL CONTENT

COMMON PROBLEMS IDENTIFIED DURING THE PLANNING PHASE

• Educator not prepared
• Resource limitations
• Time constraints

Implementation

Humans have a natural potential for learning, and learning will occur if the student perceives the subject as important.[29] Once the respiratory therapist has developed a plan, the teaching can begin. There are a variety of ways to provide information to patients. One of the most common ways to inform the patient is by lecturing.[14] The respiratory therapist talks to the patient and presents material to be taught. Lecturing can stimulate questions from the patients to help them better understand their condition. Respiratory therapists must remember that patients can suffer from information overload if they receive too much information at one time.[1] During lecturing, one way to ensure that patients understand is through repetition. Important instructions should be repeated several times in slightly different ways to increase retention.[29] After the lecture, printed material should be given to reinforce the material covered. Figure 9-2 shows an example of a printed handout that may be given to patients after explanation of coronary risk factors. Patients can refer to the printed materials at home to refresh their memory. The reading level of the patient determines the usefulness of any handout materials. Generally, illustrated handouts with bulleted key points work best. Some patients require specific literature or materials designed to accommodate special needs. For example, a geriatric patient might require a handout or brochure with large print, while a child or an illiterate person may require a handout with lots of pictures. Young school-age children might require handouts with both pictures and words to enhance understanding. Although lecturing is efficient and commonly used for patient education, it is not ideal. Patients can become disinterested and passive when lecturing is the primary teaching method used. Therefore patient educators should utilize a variety of teaching methods, especially those that allow greater learner participation in the process.

Demonstration is another valuable teaching strategy that requires the patient to actively participate in learning.[14] It allows the patient to hear and demonstrate comprehension of the information. Repeated demonstration will lead to a higher degree of competency. Videotapes can be useful in allowing the patient to observe the procedure and then illustrate competency of the task step-by-step.

Adults like to plan their own learning experiences. Facilitation and group discussions allow the student to become self-directed and accept the fact that the instructor will not guide each step.[29] Discussion groups can be powerful motivators that reinforce learning, encourage desirable behaviors, and develop positive personal values.[29]

Computers and computer software provide a newer approach to health education.[22] Increasingly, computer programs are being developed to facilitate patient education. Current computer programs can offer patients the most recent materials available. Computer programs for patient education cover a variety of topics, including health promotion and disease management strategies for a variety of chronic diseases, as well as medical, surgical, and pharmaceutical aspects of health care. Many computer programs allow patient interaction, including the ability to test the patient on their knowledge, assess their quality of life, and answer questions about their treatments or other aspects of their health care. For example, a multimedia game is now available that helps children to enhance asthma management skills.[30] Also available is an automated telephone-based smoking cessation system, with counseling available over the phone.[31] The telephone-linked care is designed to assist smokers in quitting and preventing relapse.[31] The system is convenient and inexpensive.

Patient Education: Coronary Risk Factors

The problem of coronary heart disease

The number one cause of death in modern Western society is coronary heart disease (CHD), whether it be from sudden fatal heart attacks or blocked coronary arteries causing angina and heart failure. CHD is responsible for 1 in 3 deaths in Austria. However, there has been a very pleasing reduction in deaths from coronary heart disease and stroke in the past 20 years because people have made an effort to reduce their risk factors. In spite of this, it is still a major cause of preventable death and we still need to work hard at reducing the risk.

What are the risk factors?

- Hypertension (high blood pressure)
- Smoking
- High cholesterol
- Diabetes
- Obesity
- Lack of exercise
- Stress
- Alcohol excess
- Family history

These risk factors increase the likelihood of development of hardening of the arteries (or *atherosclerosis*); the benefit of reducing them is obvious. The factors are interrelated; for example, excessive intake of alcohol will lead to hypertension.

Hypertension

The higher the blood pressure, the greater the risk. Regular checks, say yearly for people over 40 years, are advisable. Doctors recommend that you have the *diastolic level* (lower level) of blood pressure kept at 90 mm Hg or below.

Smoking

Cigarette smoking has been clearly shown to increase the risk of heart disease. The death rate from coronary heart disease is about 70% higher for smokers than for non-smokers and for very heavy smokers the risk is almost 200% higher. The more one smokes, the greater the risk. It has also been proved that the incidence of heart disease falls in those who have given up smoking.

High cholesterol

It has been proven that high blood cholesterol is related to heart attacks. High cholesterol is caused by a diet high in *saturated* fats, as compared with *polyunsaturated* fats. It is recommended that every effort should be made to keep the blood cholesterol level as low as possible and preferably below 5.5 mmol/L in adults. This acceptable level can usually be achieved through dieting. Saturated fats are found in regular milk and its products (e.g., cream, butter, cheese); fatty meats; pies and pastries, cakes, biscuits, and croissants; cooking fats; most fast foods and potato crisps.

Stress and heart attack

The stress of our modern lifestyle is regarded as a risk factor. Evidence for this is supported by the increase in incidence of heart attacks in Asians (who have a low incidence) when they move into Western societies or become business executives in their own environment. Consider ways to modify your stress factors and seek relaxation programs such as meditation.

The significance of risk factors

Most of the risk factors are interdependent, and if two or more are present they have a cumulative effect. If only one risk factor is present, the patient does not have as much cause for concern. Your doctor is the best person to assess the combined risk.

Rules for Living

- Do not smoke.
- Drink alcohol in only very small amounts or not at all.
- Keep to an ideal weight.
- Avoid saturated fats.
- Practice relaxation.

Note: The risk factors for coronary heart disease apply also to other cardiovascular disease, such as cerebral artery disease and hardening of the arteries of the legs.

FIGURE 9-2 Handout for patient education about coronary risk factors. (*Source: Murtagh J. Patient Education. 2nd ed. New York: McGraw-Hill;1999:76.*)

WAYS TO PROVIDE INFORMATION TO PATIENTS

- Lectures
- Handouts and other written materials
- Demonstrations
- Peer group discussions
- Computer programs and the Internet
- Telephone services
- Distance learning and telecommunications

Evaluation

The critical question after a teaching session is "Did the patient learn anything?" The cartoon in Fig. 9-1 depicts how the patient apparently did not grasp the meaning of the educational session, approaching even relaxation techniques from a position of stress and competition! Evaluation is the last step when conducting patient education. Evaluation is the measuring and documentation of patient education. Evaluation is an ongoing process and should be performed during every stage of patient education.[14] Throughout the evaluation process, patients provide positive and negative feedback. Based on this feedback, the respiratory therapist can reinforce desired behavior or adjust the education plan.[14] Learning can also be evaluated by having the patient complete a questionnaire or test that includes key points to be learned. The test or questionnaire enables the health professional to identify areas where the patient is lacking knowledge. Evaluation can also assist in identifying problems that may have prevented the patient from following the regimen.

If the outcome assessment shows that the teaching plan failed, the patient educator must initiate new strategies followed by additional assessment and evaluation. Demonstrations are effective ways to evaluate how well the patient understands.[29] If the patient cannot properly demonstrate a procedure

with the health professional, he or she cannot be expected to carry out the procedure at home alone.[29] Additional teaching may be necessary to reach long-term goals and effect desired behavior changes.

For example, the computer game used to enhance children's self-management skills showed that after using the game for an average of 7.6 months, children had fewer hospitalizations, better symptom scores, greater asthma knowledge, and increased functional status.[30] Figure 9-3 shows a checklist used by a hospital to evaluate asthma education. Each caregiver, as well as the patient, receives a score based on knowledge and demonstration. Another example is the use of a scale by pulmonary rehabilitation staff to rate the patient's perceived dyspnea. If the staff uses a dyspnea scale before the pulmonary rehabilitation session and then again at the end, it can help to evaluate the session's success by determining how effective it was in relieving dyspnea. Noncompliance with providers' instructions exacts a tremendous cost both on the patients and the clinics.[6]

Evaluation is the process of determining the success or failure of patient education.

DOCUMENTATION

Each health care professional should document patient education in the patient's chart, addressing each step of the education process as previously described. Documentation provides a means of communication between health professionals about what patient teaching has been delivered.[31] Documentation of patient education and comprehension helps other health professionals to reinforce the learning, answer questions, and provide encouragement.

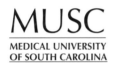

PATIENT EDUCATION RECORD
Asthma Education

Problem: **Physician/Clinic:**

Purpose: To provide the patient and caregiver with an educated understanding of asthma and methods to control the disease.

Plan:

Instructed	Scoring
1) Mother	0= No Understanding
2) Father	1= Can list item
3) Patient	2= Can demonstrate task
4) Other	NA= Not Applicable

Learning Objective/Skill	Date	Initials	Instr.	Score	Date	Initials	Instr.	Score	Comments
Pathophysiology									
Describe normal lung function									
What is asthma?									
Environmental									
Identify triggers									
Avoidance and control measure									
Medications									
Identify medication classes									
List patient's medications and purpose									
Demonstrates correct delivery technique									
Verbalize correct cleaning method									
Peak Flow Measurement									
Demonstrate correct technique									
Identify personal best									
Review recording sheets									
Verbalize correct cleaning/care									
Signs and Symptoms									
Verbalize early warning signs									
Verbalize peak flow zones									
Home Management									
Identify primary care physician									
Know medications and schedule									
Discuss asthma triggers									
Verbalize environmental control measures									
When to call physician									
Reviews school/daycare plan									

List persons taught (name): _____   List persons teaching and discipline:

FIGURE 9-3 Patient education record for asthma education. (*SOURCE: Medical University of Sourth Carolina, Charleston, SC.*)

In addition, documentation satisfies the needs of legal and regulatory agencies. Table 9-3 shows the 1998 Joint Commission on Accreditation of Healthcare Organizations (JCAHO) patient and family education standards.[32] The evidence that patient teaching was provided must reflect the patient's learning needs, teaching opportunities rendered, and patient's response to the teaching.[32] Documentation does not have to be elaborate or take a lot of time. It can be a simple checklist placed in the

TABLE 9-3   1998 JCAHO PATIENT AND FAMILY EDUCATION STANDARDS

PF.1 The patient's learning needs, abilities, preferences, and readiness to learn are assessed.

    PF.1.1   The assessment considers cultural and religious practices, emotional barriers, desire and motivation to learn, physical and cognitive limitations, language barriers, and the financial implications of care choices.

    PF.1.2   When called for by the age of the patient and the length of stay, the hospital assesses and provides for patients' academic education needs.

    PF.1.3   Patients are educated about the safe and effective use of medication, according to law and their needs.

    PF.1.4   Patients are educated about the safe and effective use of medical equipment.

    PF.1.5   Patients are educated about potential drug-food interactions, and provided counseling on nutrition and modified diets.

    PF.1.6   Patients are educated about rehabilitation techniques to help them adapt or function more independently in their environment.

    PF.1.7   Patients are informed about access to additional resources in the community.

    PF.1.8   Patients are informed about when and how to obtain any further treatment the patient may need.

    PF.1.9   The hospital makes clear to patients and families what their responsibilities are regarding the patient's ongoing health care needs, and gives them the knowledge and skills they need to carry out their responsibilities.

    PF.1.10 With due regard for privacy, the hospital teaches and helps patients maintain good standards for personal hygiene and grooming, including bathing, brushing teeth, caring for hair and nails, and using the toilet.

PF.2 Patient education is interactive.

PF.3 When the hospital gives discharge instructions to the patient or family, it also provides these instructions to the organization or individual responsible for the patient's continuing care.

PF.4 The hospital identifies and provides the educational resources required to achieve its educational objectives.

    PF.4.1   The patient and family educational process is collaborative and interdisciplinary, as appropriate to the plan of care.

SOURCE: Engelke Z, Trimborn S. Meeting the JCAHO standards for patient and family education. *Orthopedic Nursing* 1999;18(1):58.

chart with individual patient comments or a small written note in the patient's medical record.[14] Documentation can guide the educator in determining the best approach to use in devising a specific educational plan for a particular patient.[14]

Documentation includes informed consent.[32] Informed consent requires that patients have the capacity to understand the choices presented and the consequences of their decisions.[5] Once a patient has reached an informed decision, physicians have the responsibility to act upon these decisions.[5]

FUTURE TRENDS IN PATIENT EDUCATION

As the new millennium approached, the roles of health care professionals vastly changed. Managed care and other aspects of health care reform have been the driving force behind many of these changes.[27] The concept of patient education has grown and developed over the last decade. Although patient education has gained considerable credibility and acceptance, patient education remains one of the weakest links in health care delivery systems.[14]

Patient education continues to face challenges. Increasing pressure is felt by health care professionals to prove the cost effectiveness of patient education. Questions such as "Does patient education improve overall health status?" "Should patient education be supported because it reduces the chance of litigation?" or "How should patient education be reimbursed?" arise. Other challenges are determining who is the best qualified and most effective in providing patient education.

Medical schools, nursing programs, and programs in allied health sciences, including respiratory therapy, are adapting to the changing health care environment.[27] Health professions and medical curricula are integrating patient education into the students' education. As illustrated in Table 9-4, the respiratory therapists' list for scope of practice ranked patient education highly, at number 12.[27] The emphasis in health care today and into the future will continue to focus on interdisciplinary team building along with health promotion and disease management.[27] For patient education to conquer the challenges it faces in contributing to effective health care, it will depend on the commitment and leadership of all health professionals.

TABLE 9-4   RANKING OF RESPIRATORY THERAPISTS' SCOPE OF PRACTICE

1. Mechanical ventilation management/life support systems	19. Discharge planning
2. Invasive and noninvasive cardiodiagnostics and cardiopulmonary monitoring/cardiac monitoring/arterial-line/indwelling catheter	20. Sleep studies
	21. Research
	22. Medication administration
3. Traditional basic therapies (oxygen therapy, aerosol therapy, humidity therapy, incentive spirometry, etc.)	23. Stress/exercise testing
	24. Alternate site care delivery
	25. Bronchoscopy
	26. Infection control
4. Management	27. Electrolyte analysis
5. Pulmonary function testing	28. Geriatrics
6. Treatment assessment/outcome assessment	29. Quality/performance assessment
7. Home care	30. Case management
8. CPR/resuscitation	31. EEG/neurodiagnostics
9. Respiratory care of neonatal and pediatric patients	32. Computerization/information management
	33. Transport/trauma in-flight specialist
10. Arterial blood gases	34. Metabolics
11. Rehabilitation/cardiopulmonary rehabilitation	35. ACLS/NALS/PALS
12. Patient/family education	36. Mechanical cardiac support
13. Protocols	37. Ethics
14. Health promotion/disease prevention	38. Teaching/team management with other health professions
15. Smoking cessation/nicotine intervention	39. Patient-focused care
16. Hyperbaric oxygenation	40. Technology assessment
17. ECMO/other life support techniques	41. Charting and recordkeeping
18. Management	

INTRODUCTION TO THE CASE STUDY

The following case is included here so that learners can apply their understanding of education for caregivers of pediatric patients. The case presents exercises and asks specific questions to assess the learner's understanding of the assessment, planning, implementation, and evaluation of patient/caregiver education. The case challenges the learner to evaluate the age-specific considerations, patient education needs, caregiver needs, health care costs, and ethical concerns. Whenever possible, the case prompts more than one strategy for patient education to allow comparisons of the advantages, disadvantages, and limitations of various approaches.

Now you proceed with the most exciting part of this chapter: working through a hypothetical case. Your instructors will assign you to work on specific critical thinking exercises and group critical thinking exercises, depending on the available time, types of patients you are likely to encounter in your clinical rotation, and resources available. Your instructors may ask you to develop the learning issues as part of your problem-based learning (PBL) process, or you may be assigned specific predetermined learning issues that have been developed for this chapter. Please check with your program faculty before proceeding with the following case.

CASE STUDY 1

CAROL GIVER

You are the patient educator for the respiratory therapy department. You receive a call from a physician in the pediatric cardiothoracic intensive care unit. She would like you to consult with the parents of her patient on home care of their child. When you arrive in the ICU, you find a nurse and doctor at the patient's bedside performing a procedure. You obtain the medical record to review the patient's history and familiarize yourself with the case history.

 Critical Thinking Exercise 1

PRIORITIZING AND ANTICIPATING

a. What information would you look for in the medical record to assist with prioritizing the questions you will ask?

b. How would you use the information in the chart to anticipate potential problems?

Case History

The patient is a 3-month-old infant urgently traced at birth due to choanal atresia. She is being ventilated with a Servo 300. The infant has a hyperplastic left ventricle, which causes mixing of oxygenated and nonoxygenated blood. As a result, the normal pulse oximeter reading for this infant is 60% to 75%. Currently, the patient is awaiting heart surgery to repair the ventricle. The physician feels that after surgery the infant will easily wean from the ventilator and be able to go home on a trach collar. In order to allow sufficient time for the parents to learn trach care and tracheal suctioning, the parents are to be educated now. The parents should have the knowledge and skills to care for the infant after surgery. After reading the medical record, you return to the room to talk with the parents.

Upon arrival to the room, you find the mother sitting in a rocking chair. You begin talking to her while pulling up a chair and asking her if now is a good time to talk. She informs you that she has very little knowledge of the medical field since she is an accountant. However, she excitedly says, "But I've learned a great deal in the last 3 months since my baby has been in the intensive care unit!" She has two other children at home who are both under the

CASE STUDY 1 *(continued)*

age of 10. Her husband is in the Air Force, stationed about 2 hours from the hospital. He is taking care of the other children while she is staying at the hospital. He has returned to work and will come back to the hospital on the weekend. The mother appears to be composed and eager to learn. However, Mrs. Giver informs you as she looks down that she has a weak stomach and it is hard for her to look at the "hole in the baby's neck," though she understands why it was necessary to have the trach. After assessing the mother's needs and ability to learn, you both agree to scheduling an educational session for later that afternoon.

Critical Thinking Exercise 2

COMMUNICATION

a. How do you reconcile the nonverbal cues (appears composed and eager to learn) with the verbal information that she "has a weak stomach and it is hard to look at the hole in the baby's neck?"

b. What hidden messages does Carol reveal when she says the "hole in the baby's neck" rather than the "hole in my baby's neck"?

c. How can you use this information to establish rapport and provide effective education?

After talking to Mrs. Giver, you decide that she is ready to learn and has no real limitations, except she is a little hesitant about touching the trach. During the assessment, Mrs. Giver informs you that she learns best by doing one task at a time. She prefers to learn trach care before moving on to suctioning. Since the baby will have a few weeks of recovery time, you decide this will be acceptable. You and Mrs. Giver decide that the task she needs to know first is how to perform trach care, and then how to perform tracheal suction. You make a list of objectives to accomplish that day. The first objective is to reinforce why the baby requires the trach and to explain the impor-

tance of keeping it and the surrounding area clean. Second, the task of trach care will be demonstrated to Mrs. Giver and each step carefully explained. Third, an important objective is to answer any questions she has and build her understanding and confidence.

Critical Thinking Exercise 3

REFLECTION AND ANTICIPATION

a. Reflect on the information you have to plan how you will proceed with teaching trach care to Mrs. Giver

b. Anticipate how she will react and what you will do during each part of the training.

c. Reflect on what it may mean if Mrs. Giver does not ask you any questions.

d. Reflect on what it may mean if Mrs. Giver continually interrupts you with numerous questions.

That afternoon, you return to the room to find Mrs. Giver anxiously waiting to begin. You give her the material you have prepared as shown in Table 9-5. First, you read the handout with her. Then you tell her that you are going to demonstrate the procedure. You begin your demonstration, explaining each step slowly and inviting questions. Soon after beginning, Mrs. Giver grabs her stomach and tells you she feels very sick as she pulls up a chair to sit down. She watches you complete the procedure from a distance. The baby tolerates the trach care without complications. Mrs. Giver shakes her head and says "I am so sorry and will try again tomorrow" as you walk out of the room.

You document the trach care and the unsuccessful attempt to teach trach care to the baby's mother. The hospital also requires a checklist to be completed by the parents during each educational session demonstrating competence in caring for the infant.

CASE STUDY 1 *(continued)*

Critical Thinking Exercise 4

DECISION MAKING

a. What should you do and say when Mrs. Giver says she feels sick and sits down? Why?

b. What should you do and say when Mrs. Giver says she is sorry and will try again tomorrow?

The next afternoon you find Mrs. Giver waiting for you. She seems more confident today and says she is ready to begin. She listens carefully and nods understandingly as you explain the first step. As you begin cleaning the stoma, she is willing to hold the trach in place. You see that she is more receptive than yesterday to the patient education. Carol Giver is excited she made it through the entire process. She smiles encouragingly, saying she is ready to try it again next time as long as you are coaching.

As the days go on, Carol Giver gets more proficient at trach care. She is confident that she can complete the task at home without a respiratory therapist. She has completed all of the items on her checklist and is ready to move on to suctioning.

The baby has thick secretions and requires suctioning frequently. Carol has watched the procedure many times and is willing to try it. Before beginning, you explain to her the importance of sterile procedure. As she pulls the catheter back, it is loaded with thick yellow secretions. Carol is exhilarated; she did suction! Secretions extracted from the trachea are a way to evaluate suctioning. Ms. Giver has many opportunities to suction and she becomes a pro at it. The checklist for suctioning is complete and documentation of the teaching session is placed in the medical record.

Critical Thinking Exercise 5

TROUBLESHOOTING AND DECISION MAKING

a. What would you do if the suction did not work while Mrs. Giver was advancing the catheter into the baby's trach tube?

b. What would you do if Mrs. Giver broke sterile procedure while suctioning?

c. What would you do if Mrs. Giver was using a suction catheter that she says was provided in the room, and you find it is too large based on the size of the trach tube?

TABLE 9-5   TRACHEOSTOMY CARE: CAREGIVER EDUCATIONAL MATERIALS

Importance:
Rubbing of the trach tube and secretions can irritate the skin around the stoma. Daily care is needed to prevent obstruction, infection, and skin breakdown, especially under the tracheostomy tube and ties. Care should be done at least once a day, more often if needed. Children with new trachs or children on ventilators may need trach care more often. Tracheostomy dressings are used if there is drainage from the tracheostomy site or irritation from the tube rubbing on the skin.

Equipment needed:
- Sterile cotton-tipped applicators (Q-tips)
- Trach gauze and "unfilled" gauze
- Sterile water
- Hydrogen peroxide (half-strength, diluted with sterile water)
- Trach ties and scissors
- Two sterile cups or clean disposable paper cups

CASE STUDY 1 *(continued)*

TABLE 9-5 Continued

Procedure:
1. Open Q-tips, trach gauze, and regular gauze.
2. Cut trach ties to appropriate length.
3. Pour half-strength hydrogen peroxide into one cup and sterile water into the other.
4. Clean skin around the trach tube with Q-tip soaked in half-strength hydrogen peroxide. Work from the center outward using four swabs, one for each quarter around the stoma. Do not allow any liquid to get into trach tube or stoma area under the tube.
5. Rinse area with Q-tip soaked in sterile water.
6. Pat dry with gauze pad or dry Q-tip.
7. Check skin under ties, especially on back of neck.
8. Monitor skin for signs of infection. If the stoma area becomes red, swollen, inflamed, warm to the touch, or has a foul odor, call your doctor.

SOURCE: Adapted from *http://www.twinenterprises.com/trach/care.htm*

KEY POINTS

- Respiratory therapists should assume a primary role in patient education, especially for management of acute and chronic cardiopulmonary diseases.

- Although patient education has gained considerable credibility and acceptance, it remains one of the weakest links in health care delivery systems.

- Patient education is critical to foster patience, understanding, and adherence to treatment plans.

- Health promotion, wellness, and disease management programs require effective and continual patient education.

- Respiratory therapists and other health care specialists must tailor patient education programs to the individual, with consideration of specific criteria, including age, gender, race, ethnicity, and special needs.

- The emphasis in health care today and into the future will continue to focus on interdisciplinary team building along with health promotion and disease management.

REFERENCES

1. Scanlan C, Wilkins RL, Stoller JK. *Egan's Fundamentals of Respiratory Care*. St. Louis: Mosby; 1999.

2. Spencer K. Patient education: Then and now. *Plast Surg Nurs*. 1999;19:88.

3. Durbin C Jr. The role of the respiratory care practitioner in the continuum of disease management. *Respir Care*. 1997;42:159–165.

4. American Association for Respiratory Care. AARC clinical practice guideline: Providing patient and caregiver training. *Respir Care*. 1996;41:658–663.

5. Make B. Collaborative self-management strategies for patients with respiratory disease. *Respir Care*. 1994;39:566–583.

6. Capenito LJ. When clients teach me noncompliance. *Nurs Forum*. 1998;33:3–4.

7. Partridge M. Self-management in adults with asthma. *Patient Educ Counseling*. 1997;32:S1–S4.

8. Trautner C, Richter B, Berger M. Cost-effectiveness of a structured treatment and teaching program on asthma. *Eur Respir J*. 1993;6:1485–1491.

9. Bolton MB, Titley BC, Kudler J, et al. The cost and effectiveness of an education program for adults

who have asthma. *J Gen Intern Med.* 1991;6: 401–407.

10. Hindi-Alexander MC, Cropp GJA. Evaluation of a family asthma program. *J Allergy Immunol.* 1984; 74:505–510.

11. Lewis CE, Rachelefsky G, Lewis MA, et al. A randomized trial of A.C.T. (Asthma Care Training) for kids. *Pediatrics* 1984;74:478–486.

12. Clark NM, Nethwahr F, Gong M, et al. Physician-patient partnership on managing chronic illness. *Acad Med.* 1995;70:957–959.

13. American Association for Respiratory Care. AARC clinical practice guideline: Training the health-care professional for the role of patient and caregiver educator. *Respir Care.* 1996;41: 654–657.

14. Falvo DR. *Effective Patient Education.* Gaithersburg, Md: Aspen Publications; 1994.

15. Verhaak P. Editorial: Communication in medicine. *Patient Educ Counseling.* 1999;38:1–2.

16. Lawrence G. Respiratory care practitioners in ambulatory care. *Respir Care.* 1997;42:92–111.

17. Mishoe SC, MacIntyre NR. Expanding professional roles for respiratory care practitioners, *Respir Care* 1997; 42:71.

18. Cornish K. The respiratory care practitioner in extended care facilities. *Respir Care.* 1997;42: 127–130.

19. Shrake KL. The role of the respiratory care practitioner in the diagnosis of cardiopulmonary disease. *Respir Care.* 1997;42:148–156.

20. Dunne PJ. Respiratory care for the homebound patient. *Respir Care.* 1997;42:133–139.

21. Bunch D. AARC launches nationwide "Peak Performance USA" project. *AARC Times.* 1993;17: 39–41.

22. Gottesman J, Baum N. Patient education in the managed care era. *Contemp Urol.* 1999;11:42–56.

23. Visser A. Health care by head, heart, and soul. *Patient Educ Counseling.* 1999;36:2–6.

24. Wilkins R, Krider S, Sheldon R. *Clinical Assessment in Respiratory Care.* St. Louis: Mosby; 1995.

25. Drafke M. *Working in Health Care: What You Need to Succeed.* Philadelphia: F.A. Davis Company; 1994.

26. Redmond M. The importance of good communication in patient-family teaching. *J Post Anesth Nurs.* 1993;18:109–111.

27. American Association for Respiratory Care. Year 2001: Delineating the educational direction for the future respiratory practitioner. Proceedings of a National Consensus Conference on Respiratory Care Education. Dallas, Tex. October 2–4, 1992.

28. Lubkin IM. *Chronic Illness: Impact and Interventions.* Boston: Jones and Bartlett Publishers; 1990.

29. Knowles M. *The Adult Learner: A Neglected Species.* Houston: Gulf Publishing; 1990.

30. Bartholomew LK, Gold RS, Parcel GS, et al. Watch, discover, think, and act: evaluation of computer-assisted instruction to improve asthma self-management in inner-city children. *Patient Educ Counseling.* 2000;39:269–280.

31. Ramelson H, Friedman R, Ockene J. An automated telephone-based smoking cessation education and counseling system. *Patient Educ Counseling.* 2000; 39:269–280.

32. Engelke Z, Trimborn S. Meeting the JCAHO Standards for Patient and Family Education. *Orthoped Nurs.* 1999;18(1):58–62.

TIME AND RESOURCE MANAGEMENT

John Wright

In a valley dark a thousand years, one needs only one
candlelight to destroy the thousand years of darkness.[1]

LIAO FAN
(circa 1451)

LEARNING OBJECTIVES

1. Define and discuss time management, resource management, and critical thinking deficit (CTD), as well as how and why a respiratory therapy department or provider should implement a new time management system.
2. Outline the structured methods for patient assessment, establishing indications, and writing care plans.
3. Describe the ideal department environment for collective critical thinking. Discuss the
quality-productivity hybrid and the vicious cycle.
4. Define the productivity and quality perspectives when implementing a new time management system.
5. Describe methods for optimizing efficiency in health care and respiratory care practice.
6. Describe the relationships between critical thinking and time and resource management.

KEY WORDS

Added Value
Buffer
Critical Thinking
Critical Thinking Deficit (CTD)
Optimization
Prioritization

Resource Management
Synergy
Time Management
Time-Motion Study
Utilization Control
Vicious Cycle

INTRODUCTION

Reflecting—that is, the ability to examine your assumptions, opinions, and biases—is a crucial critical thinking skill for time and resource management, the focus of this chapter. To facilitate sig-
nificant changes at both the department level and within each individual respiratory therapist, the respiratory therapy department as a whole must adjust its thinking to adopt time and resource management strategies. As new strategies are implemented, your workday becomes more manageable **and** you can do more for your patients.

CRITICAL CONTENT

TIME MANAGEMENT

• A method used to prioritize scheduled activities and to improve efficiency

---

What is Time Management?

All activities can be grouped into one of three categories: critical activities that **must** be performed, important activities that **should** be performed, and optional activities that can be delegated or postponed. Time management skills assist respiratory therapists in focusing on the most critical procedures and allow them to delegate when appropriate.

CRITICAL CONTENT

PRIORITIZATION OF RESPIRATORY CARE ACTIVITIES

- Critical activities that **must** be performed
- Important activities that **should** be performed
- Optional activities that can be delegated or postponed

What Is Resource Management?

Closely related to time management, resource management is a method of allocating, in the most efficient way, material, informational, human, and financial resources.[2] In the best circumstances it involves staff respiratory therapists, the director of the department, hospital administration, and many others.

In terms of dollars spent, human resources are the most costly, followed by informational, material, and financial resources. *Human resources* refer to the employees who carry out various duties and tasks. *Informational resources* include computers and other forms of technology that store and manipulate vast amounts of data. *Material resources* are the supplies needed and the physical plant (ie, the building itself), as well as space within the building. *Financial resources* refer to budgets or money allocated to a specific department.

CRITICAL CONTENT

Resource management is a method of appropriately allocating four types of resources:
- Material (supplies, physical plant, space)
- Financial (money and budgets)
- Informational (computers, data storage, and manipulation)
- Human (personnel)

The Respiratory Therapist as a Time and Resource Manager

The drive to provide greater access to health care at a decreased cost has precipitated many changes in health care delivery. Prospective payment has changed how health care providers plan, manage, deliver, and assess care. As a result, the roles, skills, and traits expected of health care professionals, including respiratory therapists, have also changed. Practitioners of every discipline must work within managed care systems. Consequently, there is an unprecedented need to enhance the role of respiratory therapists as time and resource managers.

It is no longer sufficient to have health care personnel such as respiratory therapists who have only limited specialized knowledge and skills. There is an increased need for health care practitioners who have professional competence over and above mere technical training or clinical skills. The pressures to change old models, paradigms, and traditions of practice are not unique to respiratory care, but are experienced in all the health care professions, including nursing and medicine.

Respiratory therapists must have not only medical knowledge and technical skills, but also professional competencies and characteristics. To become effective time and resource managers, respiratory therapists must rely on basic critical thinking skills, be willing and able to break away from traditional mindsets, and try new approaches in the clinical setting. For example, if you focus mainly on your regular tasks, you may find it difficult to make time to develop a weaning plan with a physician because it would take time away from time spent doing the procedures you need to complete during your shift. Of course, the time invested in developing a weaning plan could benefit the patients, the respiratory care department, and increase productivity (eg, a faster weaning time could result in fewer ventilator checks overall). Furthermore, you should incorporate the

changed to titrated metered-dose inhaler (MDI). She consults with the physician (a second-year resident), who agrees with the suggestion. During morning rounds, the resident discusses the patient with the other physicians on his team and they concur that the change was appropriate.

A few hours later, the day shift respiratory therapist assesses the patient during a treatment and finds the patient can only obtain an inspiratory capacity measurement of 400 mL. This therapist then approaches the physician on duty, suggesting a change to intermittent positive-pressure breathing (IPPB). The moral of this story is that the physicians could be confused when two therapists suggest completely different respiratory care plans. More importantly, the physician team may begin to doubt the merit of any suggestions from respiratory therapists due to their inconsistency.

The lack of a standardized method for patient assessment can work against a respiratory therapy department. Such a method does not impede critical thinking skills or time and resource management techniques. Critical thinking skills should be built into the standardized method, so that change can be accommodated as needs arise.

A standardized approach to patient assessment can provide added value to the department as a whole by improving quality while effectively managing resources. Patient assessment is most visible with basic procedures: ones that have high volume and therefore high exposure. These procedures are vulnerable to restructuring agents who may think that some other department can do these simple tasks cheaper. However, such a maneuver can risk overall quality of care.

Patient assessments should be as objective as possible in prioritizing therapy. A standardized prioritization system should be established and enforced. Table 10-1 is a general structure with which to begin developing such a system.

Protocols. Protocols support the efforts of utilization control and financial management and they use the assessment skills and judgments of respiratory care staff, within physician-approved guidelines. Chapter 6 provides detailed descriptions and

TABLE 10-1   CATEGORIZING AND PRIORITIZING RESPIRATORY THERAPY

Category 1: Therapy that must be performed
- Cause or effect marker for immediately life-threatening condition
- Specific and immediate therapeutic action is needed
- A quick response is crucial

Category 2: Therapy that should be performed
- Necessary for diagnosis, triage, and follow-up therapy (eg, a generic assessment)
- Timeliness is a key factor but not as crucial as for Category 1 therapy

Category 3: Therapy or activities that can be delegated or postponed
- Routine patient care management (eg, maintenance dose for patients with COPD, prophylactic medications such as cromolyn sodium, pentamidine)
- Resource utilization/cost of treatment versus no treatment/total costs

exercises for using and developing protocols. There are many reasons why health care institutions should implement respiratory care protocols. A major advantage is that protocols are institution-specific guidelines for clinical decision making within specific clinical settings, taking into consideration the competencies of its staff, the needs of its patients, and numerous other contextual variables that influence health care. Many advantages of respiratory care protocols have been documented, such as improvements in allocation of respiratory care services, improvements in triage of care, objective criteria for initiation of respiratory care, discontinuation of therapy when no longer needed, decreased cost of care without adverse effects, and improvements in patient care outcomes.[9–19]

Another advantage that resulted from the implementation of respiratory care protocols is recruitment of better therapists because of the increased job satisfaction within a challenging work environment.[20] Cost containment is a major asset for managers whose departments use protocols, because patients are getting the most appropriate care. Therefore, the total charges against the diagnosis-related groups (DRG) are low. For instance, if a patient is very ill, a protocol order can achieve continuous therapy with assessment determining that treatments can be tapered, decreasing to every 2 hours, then every 4 hours, then twice a day, as the patient's condition improves. Tremendous cost savings can be realized when respiratory therapists are able to discontinue therapy the patient no longer needs. Because implementing protocols cuts the need for respiratory services, the costs associated with providing the treatments decrease. For this reason, protocol designs usually incorporate utilization control.

For example, a respiratory therapist could initiate chest physical therapy if the patient has the required indications. The protocol may allow the therapist to change the frequency of treatments according to sputum production and consistency, or stop them altogether if the patient is no longer in distress. The therapist would contact the physician if the patient complains of severe pain, if the need for treatments rapidly increases, or if the patient regresses.

Health care organizations should regularly update their protocols as the respiratory care profession changes and the organizational needs change to reflect the latest in technology or research. Regular updates to protocols should be part of the process; therefore there should be few or no deleterious effects on the overall program.

Information Resource Management

Efficiency can be improved with information management systems because tedious tasks become more automated. Examples of information resources include readily-available computerized x-rays, on-line laboratory results, computerized charting, and alpha-paging.

A computerized x-ray system allows clinicians to view the results in a matter of minutes without leaving the patient care setting (no more waiting for the x-ray to be developed and hand-delivered to the ICU). On-line laboratory results eliminate the need for results on paper. Once the blood gas analyzer produces a report, the results can be quickly disseminated by the computer network. Since results are available sooner, changes in patient care can be applied more readily.

Computerized charting systems allow several people to access the same file simultaneously. These systems are also designed to prompt clinicians as they update the charts, minimizing the omission of required information.

Computerized charting systems and respiratory care information systems can significantly improve quality assurance monitoring. A query can be developed which searches the extensive database for all relevant information. For example, if a cuff pressure assessment must be performed and documented at last once per shift, the supervisor would create a query, asking for any information on cuff pressure. All cuff pressure measurements would be displayed. She would then filter the data by providing limitations (eg, specific time frame, specific patient, etc.).

Finally, an alpha-paging system sends a message to individual pagers in the form of written text. Instead of waiting by a phone for a response, a therapist can receive clinical suggestions by alphapage. A "mass mailing" feature could allow a supervisor to inform all therapists on duty that the scheduled in-service is about to begin.

CRITICAL CONTENT

INFORMATION RESOURCE MANAGEMENT

- Information management systems improve efficiency by automating tedious tasks.
- Computerized charting systems and respiratory care information systems can significantly improve quality assurance monitoring.

Human Resource Management

Human resource management is closely related to financial resource management. It is the most costly expenditure for any organization or business. In essence, human resource management involves regulating the number of respiratory therapists according to clinical need, as well as providing methods to access the productivity, efficiency, and quality of products and/or services provided. The next section describes methods used for human resource management within the framework of time management.

TIME MANAGEMENT: METHODS FOR MEASURING EFFICIENCY AND QUALITY

This section describes time management as well as human resource management methods for measuring productivity, efficiency, and quality. Prior to implementing time and resource management strategies, it is important to know the current status of the respiratory care department and the staff therapists. Techniques for assessing the status of the work environment are discussed.

Measuring Productivity

One of the primary goals of time and resource management is to optimize the productive use of resources. Productivity can be defined as the relationship between output (ie, the therapy administered) and input (ie, human, financial, informational, and material resources).

Time-Motion Studies. Because they are responsible for efficiently operating their departments, respiratory care managers can measure that efficiency by performing time-motion studies. A time-motion study measures the actual productivity and efficiency of individual respiratory therapists and of the department as a whole. Management science personnel—efficiency experts—observe workers such as respiratory therapists in their natural work environment. They use stopwatches to time every activity of each therapist and make note of everything that occurs during a workday, from bathroom breaks to delays waiting for patients, elevators, and physicians. Because the time taken for every proce-

dure, such as a ventilator check, can vary, many samples are obtained. An average time is calculated and used as the standard.

Table 10-2 describes how to do a time-motion study. At the conclusion of such a time-motion study, you or the management science personnel assigned can provide a breakdown of the average time allotted to each procedure. Work assignments and productivity measurements are then based on these procedure times. Staffing needs can be adjusted to meet the requirements of the overall workload. The department can also compare its results with the results from other organizations (eg, relative value units [RVUs] and other measures of procedure times provided by the American Association of Respiratory Care).[21] When done in this fashion, the other organizations' results can be used as the benchmark for comparison purposes.

CRITICAL CONTENT

A TIME-MOTION STUDY

- Actual productivity of individual respiratory therapists and the department as a whole can be analyzed.
- A breakdown of the average time needed for each procedure is determined.
- Work assignments and productivity measurements are based on these procedure times.

Accounting for Emergencies. All patient care institutions, especially acute care facilities, must account for unexpected events. During the time-motion study, pay attention to unpredictable procedures (eg, stat ABGs, codes, high-risk deliveries, etc.). An average amount of time for each procedure should be calculated and then allotted to each shift for appropriate coverage. Also account for factors that increase the probability of unpredictable procedures (eg, Friday nights may be associated with an above average number of traumas. An increased number of ventilators in use may relate to an increased number of stat ABGs).

TABLE 10-2   PERFORMING A TIME-MOTION STUDY

1. With a stopwatch, measure each component (in minutes) for each procedure performed by the respiratory care department:

	HOURS	PERCENT
Direct Patient Care		
Perform procedure (patient assessment, wash hands, brief review of chart, brief communication with patient and family, position patient, preparing and returning equipment, actual procedure, monitoring, routine troubleshooting, adjusting settings, checking alarms, charting, equipment changes, suctioning, discontinuing therapy, cleaning up)	_____	_____
Delay (searching for chart, clarifying physician order, waiting for return call, collaboration with other caregivers, waiting for patient, rescheduling, waiting for escort [RN, MD, etc.], searching for equipment, waiting for elevator)	_____	_____
Personal (breaks, apparel changes, restroom break)	_____	_____
Fatigue (industry standard)	_____	_____
Direct Patient Care Subtotal	_____ hr	_____ %
Indirect Patient Care		
Report	_____	_____
Travel	_____	_____
Indirect Patient Care Subtotal	_____ hr	_____ %

2. Try to obtain about 20 timed measurements for each type of procedure. For seasonal or rarely performed procedures, obtain as many measurements as possible.

3. Multiply the Direct Patient Care Subtotal by 60 min/hr to obtain the number of minutes each respiratory therapist should complete per shift. This becomes the "Efficient workload/respiratory therapist/shift." For example, a direct patient care subtotal of 9½ hr × 60 min/hr = 570 min. This is the efficient workload/respiratory therapist/shift.

Source: Malinowski et al.[3]

Using Buffers to Fill Gaps in Staffing Levels.

Most time or resource measurement management systems are based on an average length of time per procedure. There are inherent problems with such a system: partial shifts that may be difficult to staff and periods of inactivity wedged between periods of predicted higher activity. Part-time or per diem staff can work partial shifts for coverage during peak times. Therefore, such staff may start working several hours after the shift has begun. Conversely, if the workload declines significantly in the middle of a shift, per diem staff should be dismissed immediately. To fill those periods of inactivity (and perhaps to supplement the workload of a per diem therapist assigned to a partial shift) use a buffer.

Critical Thinking Exercise 3

PRIORITIZING AND DECISION MAKING

Consider all of the procedures performed by a respiratory care department.

a. What procedures could be delayed with little or no risk to the patient?

b. What respiratory care procedure could be dispensed the longest without adverse results?

Examples of buffers include oxygen rounds, brief diagnostic procedures such as vital capacity measurements, and other procedures that are usually performed once per shift. Let's say there is a gap in one respiratory therapist's workload between 1:00 PM and 3:30 PM. If oxygen rounds are held in reserve as a buffer, the therapist could be kept busy for that 2.5-hour period. Done appropriately (ie, patient assessment and optimization of therapy are involved), the patient benefits from the procedure, the department maintains its productivity level, and the therapist enhances his or her efficiency.

Total Productivity Potential. Productivity measurements are a key component of financial management and can play a key role in determining a department's efficiency. However, productivity measurements may underrepresent the actual workload demand placed on a department. If staffing is not sufficient to perform all therapy ordered (ie, some therapy is missed), the total potential capacity of the department has not been achieved (ie, more patient care could be provided with additional staffing). The total productivity potential should be measured and reported.

Prioritization of the Workload. The standardized approach to patient assessment should help the respiratory therapist triage the workload, guiding the resources of the respiratory care department toward those patients who need our expertise and abilities the most. It should also guide prioritization of therapy. Table 10-3 provides an example of prioritization using the assessment of a patient's need for bronchodilator therapy. Priority 1 indicates the

---

TABLE 10-3   STANDARDIZED ASSESSMENT OF PATIENT'S NEED FOR BRONCHODILATOR THERAPY

Priority 1: Aerosolized bronchodilator therapy (regardless of modality used)

1. **Indications (any one of the following)**
   - Wheezing
   - Peak flow measurements that are <80% predicted
   - Peak flow measurements that do not improve by 15% or more after treatment

2. **Rationale for prioritization**
   The strongest indication for bronchodilator therapy is reversible bronchospasm. Effectiveness can be objectively evaluated through peak flow measurements. Breath sounds can also be used to determine effectiveness.

3. **Therapeutic strategy**
   Since patients receiving priority 1 treatments respond well to the therapy, these treatments should not be missed. Respiratory assessment skills are essential for properly caring for patients in this category.

4. **Restructuring strategy**
   Because assessment skills are essential for proper acute care of patients in this category, only clinicians who can 1) properly evaluate the effectiveness of the therapy, and 2) recommend the optimal modality to deliver the bronchodilator should give these treatments. Departments should ensure that all of their respiratory therapists have such competency—or require that they be obtained as soon as possible. If not, their value to their medical center is severely limited.

Priority 2: Aerosolized bronchodilator therapy (regardless of modality used)

1. **Indications (any one of the following)**
   - Documentation of wheezing in the last 12 hours (none currently present)
   - Patient was receiving a maintenance dose prior to hospitalization

2. **Rationale for prioritization**
   If the patient is currently not symptomatic (ie, wheezing; peak flows are within 20% of normal), the lack of current symptoms lowers the prioritization level. Indications are appropriate but not as strong as for priority 1 therapy.

Continued

TABLE 10-3   **Continued**

3. **Therapeutic strategy**

Priority 2 treatments could be missed or delayed for the sake of delivering higher-priority care. Respiratory assessment skills are essential for monitoring appropriateness of the therapy and for the development of symptoms.

4. **Restructuring strategy**

Again, assessment skills must be used to determine appropriateness of the physician order and to monitor the patient for symptoms. If an RC department is forced to relinquish a portion of its procedures, the priority 2 treatments would be a wiser choice than those needing priority 1 therapy. Priority 2 treatments could be delivered by a non-respiratory therapist if regular supervision and assessment is performed by a competent respiratory therapist. It is more difficult to justify why respiratory therapists should do priority 2 therapy than priority 1 therapy.

Priority 3: Aerosolized bronchodilator therapy (regardless of modality used)

1. **Indications (any one of the following)**
   - Tenacious secretions
   - A respiratory condition (eg, pneumonia)
   - Other symptoms

2. **Rationale for prioritization**

Indications for bronchodilator therapy are weak or nonexistent. While it is not contraindicated, other forms of therapy are more cost and clinically effective (eg, cool aerosol mask for tenacious secretions, incentive spirometer for postoperative prevention of atelectasis, etc.). The lack of any signs of bronchoconstriction lowers the prioritization level even further than for priority 2.

3. **Therapeutic strategy**

These treatments provide minimal benefit for the labor involved. By eliminating priority 3 procedures (or converting them to the optimal choice of therapy), RC departments can provide cost savings for their medical centers and focus their resources on higher-priority procedures.

4. **Restructuring strategy**

RC departments can increase their value by eliminating priority 3 bronchodilator therapy. A consistent approach to prioritization is equally important.

---

highest severity, and treatments for a patient in this category should not be missed. Priority 2 items could be delayed if needed, and priority 3 items should not be done at all. Respiratory therapists can use patient assessment and a similar priority system to triage all workloads.

The standardized approach should not be seen as a set of hard and fast rules. Rather, it represents a strategy and a goal to provide common direction. It does not prevent or inhibit the use of critical thinking skills, but it can lead to the kind of cohesive care that inspires confidence in the whole respiratory care department.

If respiratory care departments find that they do not have sufficient personnel to complete all therapy ordered, a prioritization system should be

constructed and presented to the medical staff executive committee (MSEC) for approval. Once the MSEC approves the system, it can be implemented.

CRITICAL CONTENT

STANDARDIZED APPROACH TO PATIENT ASSESSMENT

- Patient assessment and prioritization guidelines are not hard and fast rules.
- Assessment represents a strategy and a goal to provide common direction.
- Standardized patient assessments do not prevent or inhibit the use of critical thinking skills.

The goal is to direct respiratory care personnel to the patients who need our services the most, not only during times of insufficient staffing, but all day every day. Appropriate allocation of respiratory care services can optimize efficiency and effectiveness of respiratory therapists, a vital organizational resource.

Measuring Quality

Measuring quality of care is much more difficult than quantifying costs of care. Traditional measurements of quality tend to focus on objective data: the number of times a respiratory therapist did not wash his or her hands between patients, the number of self-extubations, and so forth. Objective quality measurements should be performed to monitor the effect of implementing time and resource management strategies. Variance tracking and outcome measurements can assess the quality of care. Health care outcomes include patient care outcomes, institutional outcomes, and care provider outcomes. Morbidity and mortality rates are the most common indicators of patient outcomes. In addition, indicators of patient outcomes include complications, patient satisfaction, and improved quality of life. Increased longevity, improved functionality, and emotional health are additional examples of desirable patient outcomes. Patient satisfaction is gaining in its importance, especially with third-party payers. In addition, each respiratory therapist should be evaluated to ensure that he or she is providing quality care.

For more on quality measurement, see the section later in the chapter, Follow-Up Measurements of Quality.

Competency Testing. One technique for ensuring that each respiratory therapist is providing quality care is competency testing. Establishing standards of quality is complicated by the increasing complexity of respiratory care technology that has created a need for lifelong learning and an escalating knowledge base. **Competency** can be defined as follows: the skills, knowledge, and ability to safely perform a specific task. To properly evaluate the level of performance of individual respiratory therapists before and after the imple-

TABLE 10-4   HOW TO IMPLEMENT COMPETENCY TESTING

1. Determine which procedures/areas need competency testing.
2. Establish a minimum safety level.
3. Select an expert who:
   - has the necessary clinical skills, knowledge, and abilities
   - can test staff in a fair, standardized manner
   - can develop tests
   - can train those who do not initially pass the competency test
   - can promote staff to others (ie, physicians, nurses, etc.) as experts
4. Obtain support from:
   - Staff: Explain rationale (ie, patient safety, overall evaluation of department competency, etc.)
   - Medical director
5. Perform competency testing on staff most likely to pass.
6. Expand competency testing to less experienced staff.

mentation of a new time and resource management system, a competency testing system must be in place. Table 10-4 describes the process for implementing a competency testing program.

Let's look at the process in more detail. Determine what areas and procedures need competency tests. Your initial reaction may be to create competency tests for high-tech procedures like inverse ratio ventilation (IRV), high-frequency ventilation (HFV), nitric oxide, or other complex modes of mechanical ventilation. However, one approach has greater potential for elevating the status of your department: focus on basic high-volume, high-exposure procedures. These are the very procedures that restructuring agents often want to hand over to some other department that could do these seemingly simple tasks cheaper. It is imperative that every respiratory care department develop competency standards for patient assessment skills. After that, test high-risk and high-tech procedures.

CRITICAL CONTENT

COMPETENCY TESTING

- It evaluates each respiratory therapist's basic level of performance against standard protocols
- It is the first crucial step to ensure consistently high quality
- Other goals are to optimize care and standardize clinical care
- Experienced respiratory therapists should not be exempt from the process

Establish Minimum Safety Levels. A minimum safety level essentially certifies that the therapist can perform all of the routine clinical activities in a specified area (or can perform a specific procedure) without placing the patient at unnecessary risk. You don't have to be an expert respiratory therapist in any specific ICU to safely work in the unit, but you should be able to competently perform all procedures commonly done in the unit.

Select Experts as Trainers. Expert therapists design the competency tests, and they clearly understand that a lot is riding on their approval. Their endorsement says a respiratory therapist is competent to perform his or her duties without supervision. Setting standards too low adds no value to the department, and setting standards too high limits flexibility. Standards should be relatively high, but obtainable. The staff should be required to achieve the standards. Some respiratory therapists may initially fail the test, but they can be schooled on their problem areas and retested.

Staff Acceptance. The medical director, the medical staff, and the respiratory therapists must all embrace the competency testing, or it will be worthless. Staff acceptance is essential to change the culture. As you can imagine, changing the culture requires strong leadership. Therefore, the technical director and the supervisors must be determined to enforce the rules, making competency testing part of the new culture. The benefits of a more flexible respiratory therapist staff need to be explained to new medical staff and other health care providers as they rotate into the unit.

Test All the Staff Members. Testing all the staff members adds flexibility and value to the department. Competency testing is expanded to include the less-experienced staff, old timers, and new graduates. Competency testing of staff most likely to pass the exam establishes a core group of staff respiratory therapists. This step provides a baseline level of performance in the unit. Once everyone is evaluated, the individual respiratory therapist's level of performance can be taken into account and the best performance ensured. A respiratory therapist's experience, including intuition, should be taken into consideration when level of performance is being evaluated. Experienced respiratory therapists should not be excluded from testing. In fact, they may be more mired in traditional mindsets and most in need of learning the new standardized approach.

Consider the following: As a new graduate, you have just been offered a job at a university teaching hospital. The hospital is a tertiary care center involved in numerous transplant programs and other high-tech procedures. As a student, you did a rotation at this hospital. Many of the staff showed you the ropes, and now you will be working with them. The department has just purchased several new, slightly different ventilators. The director of the department announces that every respiratory therapist must pass a competency test specifically designed for the new ventilator. One veteran tells you that the competency test is "a bunch of bureaucratic nonsense." He insists that he knows how to use the new ventilator without taking a competency test. Unsure of how difficult the test will be, you review the operator's manual and spend time with other therapists working with the ventilator connected to an artificial lung. You pass the competency exam, realizing that you did not really understand how the ventilator worked until you studied the material. The veteran therapist fails the exam.

To ensure that the highest quality care is provided, you also need commitment, compassion, and communication.

Commitment.　Commitment means that you are determined to do the job right. It starts within you, an attitude that cannot be taught, but can be enhanced. Competency tests, time and resource management, and all of the other factors involved with implementing the critical thinking process become second nature once the right attitude is in place.

Compassion.　Compassion means taking time to show the patient and family that you really do care. Our profession traditionally has had a high-tech image. Inability to display compassion deprives us of a certain level of communication and understanding that is not only humane, but is also important to critical thinking.

Communication.　Communication includes taking the time to contact the physician and/or supervisor. An extremely knowledgeable, intelligent respiratory therapist may recognize the best solution to a problem, but if it's not communicated, it isn't worth much.

One-on-One Observations.　Competency testing and training alone are unlikely to change a longstanding culture. To effectively alter behavior, quality assurance monitoring is required. However, traditional spot checks will not work. Instead the supervisor or quality assurance (QA) person should observe each individual's time and resource management as well as other critical thinking skills. These include prioritization (best noted at the beginning of the shift), communication, negotiation, implementation of suggestions, and troubleshooting skills. Areas that need improvement and successful transitions to new methods can be seen and later discussed with the respiratory therapist. With this approach, there is no chance for a staff respiratory therapist to say, "You don't know what my day was like."

Obviously, this method is more involved than the traditional spot check. However, it can be performed less often since it is more effective. As word about the new QA monitoring technique spreads among the staff, a new atmosphere and new expectations are created. This form of culture change is far more effective than traditional QA monitoring and in-service.

Education about time and resource management strategies and assurance of management backup can be informative and helpful, but alone they have very limited effect. One-on-one monitoring and mentoring not only supports these techniques, but also addresses the fact that respiratory therapists usually function as nomads. Often with minimal direct contact with other respiratory therapists and with limited direct supervision, they operate on a far more independent basis than many nurses (who are often trained by means of a preceptor). Therefore, individual training of therapists by a preceptor or mentor would be very rewarding.

Implementing critical thinking in a department may strike fear into respiratory care managers. Perhaps the one-on-one quality monitoring method could give the impression that staff members still have a free hand in their work. Also, if the respiratory care manager's only method of monitoring staff has traditionally been by productivity measurements, this new method might make his or her numbers look worse.

CRITICAL CONTENT

ASSESSING DEPARTMENTAL CRITICAL THINKING

- Traditional spot checks are *not* the optimal method for monitoring the implementation of critical thinking processes.
- One-on-one monitoring allows a supervisor to observe time and resource management as well as other critical thinking skills.
- Since respiratory therapists often work independently, training with a preceptor or mentor can yield better results.

Cross-Training.　*Cross-training* can be defined as educating therapists to be competent in many procedures and in many parts of the health care facility. For example, if a respiratory therapist has exclusively worked with adult patients, cross-training might involve teaching the respiratory therapist to work in pediatric and neonatal areas. Cross-training also pertains to the expansion of a skill base within the same patient population. For example, a respiratory therapist might have the experience to care for pediatric patients but may not have the skills, knowledge, or ability to work in the pediatric ICU or with certain pediatric equipment such as a high-frequency oscillator.

A lack of cross-training can significantly affect productivity, efficiency, and quality. If a respiratory care department has minimal cross training and the therapists can only work in limited areas, the supervisor can only hope that the workload in a particular area matches the number of qualified staff. With less than a full workload, the respiratory therapist assigned to that area cannot be very productive. If the skills and competency of the respiratory therapists on duty do not closely match the types of procedures done, the quality of care is at risk.

Training should not be limited by the personal desires of the staff therapists. The department needs respiratory therapists with multiple skills and competencies. To ensure flexibility, cross-training should be ongoing with an emphasis on training staff to work in all areas of the medical center and with *all* procedures. Competency testing can then be used for validation.

CRITICAL CONTENT

CROSS-TRAINING

- Provides flexibility
- Expands the number of therapists who can do many kinds of procedures
- Enhances the critical thinking skills and traits of staff
- Makes more staffing available to work in different areas
- Personal desires of the staff therapists should not strictly determine training needs

Subjective Measures of Quality.   Since many of the attributes associated with quality care (eg, commitment, compassion, and communication) are difficult to measure, a subjective measure of quality is required. Monitoring informal (verbal) and formal (written) feedback from co-workers, patients, and family members is important.

Feedback on quality can affect the image of the department. For example, if a medical director of an ICU states that the respiratory therapists are assessing more and informing physicians and nurses about clinical findings more often, the image of the department is enhanced and the chances of successfully implementing a new time and resource management system are improved.

Favorable comments from family members, patients, or visitors about a respiratory therapist's compassion, communication, or commitment certainly imply that the individual and the entire respiratory care department have a positive image. All significant subjective feedback should be compiled and reviewed along with the objective measures of quality.

CRITICAL CONTENT

QUALITY ASSESSMENTS

- Attributes associated with quality care are difficult to measure
- Quantitative and qualitative methods are needed to assess quality
- Subjective measures of quality are required
- Feedback regarding quality can affect the image of the department

ASSESSMENT OF THE WORK ENVIRONMENT

In addition to measuring productivity and quality, an assessment of the work environment should be performed to determine if any significant critical thinking deficits (CTDs) exist. If a CTD does exist, a strategy is developed to correct it. Otherwise, the underlying culture will continue to reinforce CTDs and the prevailing attitude, and this can significantly limit critical thinking.

In an effective work environment, information flows freely, facilitating the problem-solving process, critical thinking, and time and resource management. Although formal, well-defined systems for assessing the work environment have not yet been established, areas that should be reviewed are shown in Table 10-5.

Signs and Symptoms of a Critical Thinking Deficit

A serious lack of critical thinking is often revealed by a CTD. A CTD is characteristic behavior that is often based on tradition as opposed to efficiency or quality care. Improving time and resource management and increasing critical thinking need open-mindeness and an atmosphere conducive to brainstorming to flourish. Now you might be thinking, "The respiratory therapy department has some pretty sharp people working in it and I think they're doing the best they can." And in fact, most respiratory care departments have spent a great deal of time improving their clinical skills and adopting new techniques. However, a true assessment of the critical thinking status in a department is well worth the effort. Use of primarily one type of treatment is a strong indication that a department's time and resource management system needs revision.

TABLE 10-5   ASSESSING THE WORK ENVIRONMENT

Assess communication systems:
- Among staff respiratory therapists
- Between respiratory therapists and patients
- Between staff respiratory therapists and supervisors
- Between respiratory care managers and hospital administration
- Between respiratory therapists and nurses
- Between respiratory therapists and physicians

Systems for addressing complaints and new ideas:
- How well does respiratory care management receive a complaint from staff respiratory therapists?
- Does the department accept new ideas?
- How are new ideas conveyed from staff respiratory therapists to the respiratory care manager?

Department problem-solving process:
- How does the respiratory care manager approach staff respiratory therapists with:
  - A problem with their overall performance?
  - A problem for the department to solve?
  - Follow-up results?

Methods for assessing the environment:
- Surveys
- Interviews
- Observations

CRITICAL CONTENT

POSSIBLE INDICATORS OF CRITICAL THINKING DEFICITS

- Characteristic staff behaviors that become habitual
- Operations and decisions based on tradition rather than efficiency or quality care
- Use of primarily one type of treatment
- Similar ventilator settings for various patients
- Performing unnecessary procedures
- Expenditure of personnel and supply resources in a suboptimal manner
- Delays in high-priority work

Consider this illustration of a CTD. Patient A, who is being weaned after a craniotomy, has spontaneous tidal volumes of 13 mL/kg with a pressure support of 10 cm H_2O, and is breathing 16 times per minute on a synchronized intermittent mandatory ventilation (SIMV) of 10. Extubation is a possibility for this patient if other factors are also favorable. On the other hand, patient B, another postcraniotomy patient, has spontaneous tidal volumes of 5 mL/kg, and is breathing 30 times per minute on the same ventilator setting. ABGs for both patients are identical: pH, 7.42; Pco_2, 37; Po_2, 95.

Clinicians tend to treat blood gas results and not the patient. Normal blood gas results are obtained for both patients, but there is an important difference in respiratory status of the two patients. What is the major clinical difference?

Some of the reasons for overusing a particular mode or settings include:

- Habit or tradition: A comfort level with a familiar mode and weaning sequence
- Lack of information: A surgeon in the OR may only hear about a patient's ABG results and not know the rest of the clinical situation
- Lack of understanding or experience: A clinician may base decisions on the ABG results and not consider other pertinent information

Therefore the preponderance of any one particular ventilator order indicates that many patients have very similar clinical situations or a CTD is present that discourages variation.

If ventilator settings are not customized for each patient, the respiratory therapist will spend unnecessary time performing a procedure that does not provide optimal patient care. This also prevents the respiratory therapist from providing optimal therapy elsewhere. One study demonstrated that respiratory care services are overutilized by 32% and underutilized by 8% of respiratory care departments.[4] Both under- and overutilization present problems.

CRITICAL CONTENT

ROUTINE VENTILATOR SETTINGS AND MANAGEMENT

- The preponderance of any one particular ventilator order might indicate that many patients have similar clinical status.
- More than likely, routine settings indicate that a CTD is present, and it is discouraging variation.
- Time and resource management requires customized ventilator management for each patient.
- Both under- and overutilization present problems for both time and resource management.

These are some effects of the suboptimization of patient care: 1) Physical resources are wasted (ie, the ventilator may be used longer than necessary if a weaning plan is not well-developed); 2) human resources are wasted (a respiratory therapist stays with the patient with the less-than-optimal weaning plan instead of doing a more urgent procedure on another patient); 3) financial resources are wasted (unnecessary labor expense due to poor planning); and 4) information resources are wasted (eg, extra computer time is needed for the more complicated ventilator charting, additional use of computerized x-ray equipment, extra alpha-pages, etc.).

Limited Variation in Use of Ventilator Modes, Treatment Modalities, and Weaning Techniques

As in the previous CTD example, routine use of any mode, therapy, or technique warrants review. For example, if a respiratory care department exclusively uses volume ventilation (even on noncritical, weanable patients) the respiratory care staff will not have the opportunity to learn pressure ventilation. Or if a respiratory care department only delivers bronchodilator by means of a hand-held nebulizer (HHN), the therapists will be unfamiliar with other modalities, such as titrated MDI and continuous nebulizer therapy. The same concept holds true when only one weaning technique is used; it will be more difficult for the respiratory therapists to be open-minded about the available options.

Group Critical Thinking Exercise 1

DECISION-MAKING

a. Ask the students to form groups of six. Each group of six is subdivided into two groups of three students. Set A1 (three students from each group of six) are to determine which treatment modalities are capable of delivering large doses of bronchodilator in a short period of time during an acute case of bronchospasm. Set A2 (the second set of three students) is to answer the following questions: 1) what treatment modalities can minimize labor while providing the larger dose of bronchodilator? and 2) what modalities require repeated reloading of medication, thereby increasing the use of time and resources?

b. Once each set has discussed and answered its assigned questions, ask everyone to work together on the following problem. If the physician order is not questioned or challenged, three or four consecutive HHN treatments may be needed to relieve the patient's bronchospasm. The severity of the patient's condition may require another three or four consecutive treatments 2 hours later. Although HHN can provide effective bronchodilation, is it the optimal method in this situation? Cite evidence and state reasons to support your opinions.

Performing Unnecessary Procedures. Unless a respiratory therapy department has a *strong* protocol (or other strategy) to avoid performing unnecessary procedures, personnel and supply costs will be spent unwisely. In addition, higher-priority work might be delayed. Ideally, respiratory care practitioners should formally assess patients and physician orders prior to administering the therapy. The formal assessment should include a review of indications for therapy that have been approved on a hospital-wide basis by a high-level medical staff committee (eg, medical staff executive committee). If the patient does not present with any of the predetermined indications for therapy, it should not be initiated. This will avoid unnecessary consumption of valuable human and physical resources.

Obtaining hospital-wide approval for formal respiratory assessment is not necessarily difficult to accomplish. After developing a simple outline of priorities, seek approval from the committees concerned with the utilization of respiratory care human resources. The prioritization system should justify the need to eliminate unnecessary procedures so that staff therapists are available to help patients who can significantly benefit from respiratory care interventions. After obtaining committee approval, the proposal is presented to a medical staff executive committee for hospital-wide application.

Once such a mechanism is in place, the culture can change as physicians (and others) recognize that therapy will be not be started without appropriate indications. For example, a respiratory therapist receives physician orders for a new patient to start therapy. Department policy requires the therapist to complete a formal written assessment of the patient prior to initiating any therapy. The written assessment questions can only be answered with "yes" or "no" to minimize ambiguity. The answers to the questions guide the therapist with respect to prioritizing the therapy. Symptomatic patients with a higher acuity level will be treated before patients who are asymptomatic and more likely to be able to tolerate delays in therapy. If all answers are "no," respiratory therapy is not indicated.

A respiratory care department without a formal prioritization system or written assessments is less able to prioritize and coherently standardize therapy. Unnecessary treatments are administered, resources are mismanaged, and critical thinking is minimized. It is critically important that a respiratory care department have physician support for implementing policies and protocols that reinforce prioritization and resource management.

Implementation of New Procedures and Techniques. Although new procedures and techniques are usually associated with capital equipment or supply costs, new procedures and/or techniques can yield labor savings. For example, the incremental increase in supply cost for a continuous aerosol nebulizer set-up (compared to the cost of a hand-held nebulizer) may be offset by the decrease in labor cost[22] and is a useful alternative in the management of severe asthma in adults.[23]

More importantly, a new procedure tends to challenge traditional ways of thinking. It gives all staff respiratory therapists an equal opportunity to excel at a particular clinical skill or technique. As new procedures are introduced to the department, respect for seniority in its purest form (ie, years of service, *not* level of clinical expertise) is minimized, creating a work environment where *all* therapists recognize that the respiratory care profession is very dynamic. The pressure associated with the introduction of a new procedure allows staff therapists to break out of traditional mindsets and sets the stage for critical thinking.

Staff Members Taking Breaks at the Same Time. When staff therapists take breaks at the same time on a routine basis, a CTD and suboptimal staffing deficiency are indicated. A patient's clinical status can quickly change radically. Therefore, the probability that patients will need assistance at the same time (ie, during the synchronized break) on a routine basis is very high. Of course, the overall acuity level of the patients at an institution is a key factor. For example, a synchronized break at a skilled nursing facility (SNF) is more reasonable than such a break at a tertiary care hospital.

If staffing is heavy or the workload suddenly decreases, a synchronized break is feasible without sacrificing the quality of care. However, if such a situation occurs routinely, staffing efficiency is suboptimal, indicating that therapists have more time to perform procedures and care for patients than is actually needed. Therefore, the supervisor or manager should periodically review and intervene as necessary.

This inefficiency could also be explained by the lack of a management sciences study. Synchronized breaks can also occur when the staff is cutting corners. This could have serious implications because the staff is sacrificing quality care and other benefits provided by critical thinking. This type of CTD is often well established. The staff may feel that it is their only way to socialize, and is part of the department's culture. Staff therapists may provide suboptimal care by cutting corners to attend such synchronized breaks.

CRITICAL CONTENT

The probability that patients requiring respiratory services do not need assistance at the same time (ie, during the synchronized break) on a routine basis is very small. Of course, the overall acuity level of the patients at an institution is a key factor.

Typically, a staff respiratory therapist's workload covers a larger geographical area and allows for contact with a larger pool of patients and health care workers. More often, contact with fellow therapists is minimal. The amount of the time spent with any individual patient and/or co-worker is often much less than for nurses. As a result, respiratory therapists may feel a need to establish a sense of belonging in the departmental group.[24,25] This need for togetherness can be fulfilled by therapists planning a synchronized break for mutual support and emotional reinforcement.

Synchronized breaks should be monitored by supervisors and managers, who should intervene if the breaks are too long or if the habit becomes too deeply entrenched. If the supervisor finds that quality of work has been sacrificed for the sake of such a break, he or she must speak with the individuals involved to ensure that critical thinking is used and that patient care is not undercut.

The aforementioned rationale and intervention can be applied to three other CTDs: the times when staff linger in the department after report, when staff go to the cafeteria after report, and when lunches and breaks last longer than scheduled. Staff who linger in the department instead of going to the clinical setting show little regard for the importance of critical thinking skills (at least at the beginning of the shift after a half-hour report). Trips to the cafeteria immediately after report validate the priorities of some respiratory therapists. Extended lunches and breaks can indicate that the supervisor has overstaffed (because the respiratory therapist is not actually needed at the bedside), the time-motion study is inaccurate, or the therapist values the extra time at lunch more than being at the patient's bedside. An effective manager, supervisor, or clinical instructor can easily spot and correct these problems.

 Group Critical Thinking Exercise 2

REFLECTING, PROBLEM SOLVING, AND COMMUNICATING

Group discussion:

Imagine that you are the manager of a large respiratory therapy department. The hospital administrator tells you that you need to cut costs. You guess that at least 3 hours per day (above and beyond the allotted time for breaks and lunches) are not productive because staff members take extended lunches and synchronized breaks. Three hours per day equals 1095 hours per year, roughly half of the time that a full-time employee works in a year.

a. How has the culture been shaped to accept these practices?

b. How might you change such behavior?

c. What would you do?

d. How can a department break out of a vicious cycle?

e. Who do you think the key players are in this process?

f. Do you think that staff therapists will support the move to break free?

Workload Completion Rates are Very Consistent or Very High. Consistent workload levels are an unrealistic expectation in an acute care setting where the unexpected occurs on a regular basis. Therefore, variations in time and resources expended at the bedside should also be noticed occasionally at the department level. For example, one emergency patient can require the attention of one or more therapists for a disproportionately long time. Since time-motion standards are based on average time per procedure, productivity for the shift would decrease (unless offset by less time taken by other procedures). Consistent workload levels, therefore, can indicate a focus on productivity instead of assessment and critical thinking, which might require the occasional disproportionately longer procedure and more resources. Very high workload levels are often an indicator of cutting corners. Longer-than-average procedures are partially or completely offset by shorter-than-average procedure times, causing slight to moderate variations in time-motion workload completion rates.

"That's Just How We Do Things Around Here!" If you have ever heard this phrase in the work setting, you have definitely discovered a CTD. The phrase indicates both a rigid way of thinking and it reveals that the department culture accepts the behavior, either directly or indirectly. Quite often, the culture is based on certain mindsets that have become deeply entrenched in the behavior of staff respiratory therapists. Changing this type of rationale will require strong leadership from the manager and supervisors. Altering traditional mindsets will generally occur slowly. Implemen-

tation of time and resource management strategies can take place afterwards.

Attitudes that Foster CTDs

"My Supervisor Wants Me to Complete My Assignment." Management and supervisors can sometimes be part of the problem. This comment endorses the concept of productivity over quality. Staff respiratory therapists *do* sense what is important to managers and supervisors. Although productivity is critical to the success of any respiratory care department, leadership must understand the value of time and resource management and communicate their endorsement of such values to staff.

"The More Patients I Treat, the More Good I Am Doing for More People." Most if not all people who enter the health care professions want to help those in need. Developing a mindset based on this concept is easy to do. Seeing and treating more patients may seem superficially to be a more positive result than spending more time in fewer patient visits in order to perform critical thinking and provide optimal care.

Consider the following example. Three staff respiratory therapists (15 were assigned to work the shift) call in sick and cannot be replaced. The remaining 12 respiratory therapists divide the workload equally but there is more to do than they can complete. Some therapists will think that they are doing more for patients if they cut corners to avoid missing any procedures. The outcome is poor quality of care and no critical thinking. Critical thinking therapists will prioritize and provide quality care to those patients who need it most.

"If I Discontinue a Physician's Order, I'm Decreasing the Need for Staffing." Many therapists believe that the more work there is, the better off they are. Decreasing the workload for any reason seems counterproductive. A more appropriate attitude places the focus on obtaining more work because added value is being provided.

Sacrificing quality for the sake of completing the entire assigned workload is the antithesis of "demand management"—staffing is adjusted depending on the number of procedures there are to perform. In today's health care setting where capitated care (ie, insurance companies pay a predetermined amount for a specific diagnosis) prevails, performing unnecessary therapy creates an unnecessary cost to the hospital.

For example, a per diem respiratory therapist has a workload of 9.5 hours (570 minutes). According to the time-motion study conducted by the department, this is an optimal workload. During the first round of treatments, the respiratory therapist determines, through patient assessment, that two of his patients do not need the prescribed therapy. If he obtains a physician order to discontinue the unnecessary therapy, the overall workload (and specifically his personal workload) will decrease significantly and he may be sent home in the middle of the shift. To avoid being sent home early, he does not ask the physician to discontinue the orders. He has missed an opportunity to show others (ie, patients, physicians, nurses, and other respiratory therapists) the added value that is unique to respiratory therapists. In addition, the unnecessary therapy increases resource and time expenditures. As new work comes into the department, the staff is now forced to perform the unnecessary therapy along with therapy that is truly indicated.

CRITICAL CONTENT

DEMAND MANAGEMENT

- Staffing is adjusted depending on the therapies needed
- The antithesis is to sacrifice quality for the sake of completing the entire workload

Managers can promote problem solving by monitoring these clinical decisions and reviewing them with the respiratory therapist responsible. Repeated offenses should lead to disciplinary action. Some medical centers may allow downtime, in which the respiratory therapist can find other tasks to complete. Downtime tasks can include writing and developing protocols, consulting with physicians, and developing in-service education. If downtime is allowed, the respiratory therapist would work on these tasks instead of going home when the workload decreases. However, many medical centers do not permit nonproductive time, including downtime, regardless of the tasks that are performed during this period.

Q2 Ventilator Checks. If respiratory therapists have the mindset to get all of their work done on time with less focus on the quality of care delivered, Q2 ventilator checks are usually performed every 2 hours. There is nothing wrong with doing the check every 2 hours, especially in a setting where little clinical change takes place (eg, a long-term care facility with chronic patients). However, in an acute care setting, the time allocated to ventilator checks should vary in a manner consistent with the dynamic environment of an ICU, the ER, or an observation unit.

Let's say that during CTD determination you found that most staff respiratory therapists were very committed to performing ventilator checks every 2 hours (as outlined in the department policy). During a 12-hour day shift, the first ventilator check is initiated at 7:30 AM and repeated every 2 hours. This typical work pattern accounts for variations in procedure time due to retaping, suctioning, changing a setting, etc. Although unexpected crises (eg, code blues, emergency intubations, etc.) may occur to disrupt the repeated sequence of ventilator checks, this picture represents the underlying mindset of many respiratory therapy departments. This traditional behavior is neither realistic nor efficient in most acute care settings today. The clinical status of such patients is usually more fluid and requires more flexibility in treatment.

Although the clinical practice guideline for a patient ventilator check includes time for patient assessment, use of critical thinking skills can significantly increase the amount of patient assessment time.[26] Limited patient assessments allocate time for changes in care plans and shift-to-shift monitoring. Comprehensive patient assessments allocate time for new starts and a detailed review of the medical history, and implementation of critical thinking would definitely require the use of such procedures.

Other factors in the patient's acuity level (eg, hemodynamic instability, difficulty in obtaining optimal or stable ventilator settings, in-house transports, etc.) can create a need for a change in time and resource management. Implementation of critical thinking skills could also increase time allocated to observing the patient, communicating and negotiating with physicians, and consulting with nurses and other health care professionals.

As critical thinking skills are applied to the ventilator check procedure, the time management model should change considerably, as seen in Fig. 10-1. Note the following important points:

1. The time allocated for each ventilator check varies drastically between patients (compare the limited amount of time spent with patient Jones versus patient Johnson) as well as for any one patient (there's a difference between the first and second ventilator checks for patient Johnson).
2. The sequence does not always flow in order from patient 1 through 6 (eg, the last few hours of the shift), even though that pattern can be defaulted to when the overall situation is running smoothly (eg, the fourth round of vent checks).

Applying critical thinking skills can increase variations in ventilator checks. The first round of ventilator checks should intentionally be short to allow the clinician to prioritize once data on all patients have been reviewed and assessed. For example, for the first patient at the beginning of the shift, respiratory therapists often find reasons to spend an extensive amount of time at the bedside.

The first patient may need her endotracheal tube retaped. Quite often, the respiratory therapist addresses this clinical issue immediately. However, the respiratory therapist is unaware that another more serious situation exists with the fourth patient, and care is significantly delayed. To properly apply time management from the start of the shift, the respiratory therapist must quickly assess *all* the patients to determine prioritization of the workload.

In Fig. 10-1, patient Johnson had the highest priority, since a larger amount of time was spent with him after the first round of ventilator checks. Through assessment and prioritization, the critically thinking respiratory therapist found that patient Jones required less attention overall compared to the other patients (as evidenced by five small ventilator checks and a relatively large gap between the last two ventilator checks). The respiratory therapist focused on higher-priority work, knowing that Jones would most likely remain stable. However, the respiratory therapist did make one last check on Jones before the end of the shift.

Strong time and resource management skills can assist respiratory therapists in adapting to a more dynamic and flexible system.

Strategies to Minimize CTDs

Before critical thinking skills and time and resource management strategies are implemented, CTDs discovered during assessment of the work environment need to be addressed. It can be difficult for staff to adopt new systems if they won't let go of their traditional mindsets. The technical and medical directors of a respiratory care department

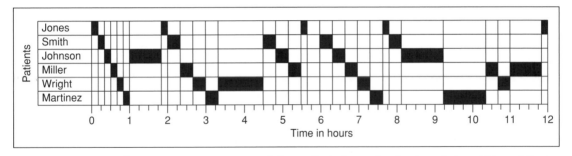

FIGURE 10-1 Differences in respiratory care needs for mechanically ventilated patients during a 12-hour shift.

play a key role in the overall implementation of new strategies. Staff usually follows their examples, therefore it is important that they model the desired behavior and offer positive reinforcement to facilitate changes.

Listen to Staff Ideas. The best source for time and resource management ideas is brainstorming—the open communication of ideas and concepts. Each individual has a different perspective and therefore something different to contribute. If anyone feels that the work environment is hostile or that management is merely paying lip service to the need for communication, he or she will refrain from contributing, the source of new ideas will dry up, and the culture will remain unchanged. When staff meetings are held on a frequent basis, therapists know they have a forum to hear the latest updates from the director and to voice their concerns and ideas about using time and resources wisely.

Accommodate Two-Way Communication. Not only should managers be open to staff ideas about time and resource management, they must actively encourage them. The manager may have experience in dealing with presentation of ideas to superiors, but staff therapists may not be familiar with this process.

Obtain Levels of Support. The department director is responsible for gaining the support of hospital administration and for conveying feedback between staff and administration. The respiratory therapy department must obtain levels of support from staff, physicians, administrators, and the entire organization to minimize CTDs. If the director is unsure of the mindset of the staff, an anonymous survey can reveal the current status and any underlying CTDs. The presence of CTDs should be seen as an opportunity for improvement.

IMPLEMENTATION: WHY A TRANSITION IS NEEDED

Failing to prepare is preparing to fail.
                    —John Wooden, UCLA basketball coach

CRITICAL CONTENT

PRE-TRANSITION ASSESSMENT

- Evaluate productivity, efficiency, and quality prior to implementation
- Develop strategies to minimize CTDs
- Create an environment that is accepting of critical thinking and time and resource management

Primary Issues During Transition

Primary issues for the implementation team that require considerable thought and effort include:

- Education: the first and last steps in implementation
- Central planning to keep implementation on track
- Motivation of staff to expand their roles, learn new skills, and contribute effort needed
- Development of strategies to overcome barriers early in the process
- Refinement of the program based on early results, new technology, changing physician consensus, and cost considerations to facilitate long-range ongoing support
- Surveillance: a major issue in the implementation process
- Identification of trends and their potential impact on implementation
- Identification of opportunities for improvement.

Monitoring the performance of individual respiratory therapists and of the department as a whole is an essential component of the implementation process. Defined mechanisms can ensure that respiratory therapists are using their skills appropriately and are able to make appropriate adjustments in care plans.

Time and resource management, and other critical thinking skills, can serve an educational function for physician and nursing staff as well as respiratory therapists. Collaboration of medical center personnel is essential, particularly where multidisciplinary assessments occur.

If the respiratory care manager wants to implement an effective time and resource management system, where should he or she begin? A good starting point could be the medical director, who can offer a physician's perspective. Next, the respiratory care supervisors should be notified. Because they usually have more recent bedside experience than the manager, the supervisors can offer valuable feedback. Discussing the change with the medical director and supervisors can make known their position on critical thinking, and indicate the level of resistance the manager may face. Once the manager (or whoever is proposing the new system) sells the idea to the medical director and supervisors, a power base is established, and the idea can be conveyed to the staff respiratory therapists.

Once staff respiratory therapists buy into the concept of implementing time and resource management strategies, they should communicate the benefits to physicians and other health care workers.

Creating the Right Environment: Balancing Productivity with Quality of Care

To balance cost, quality, and customer service, hospitals often look for areas of added value (ie, those areas which add efficiency and increase quality of care or customer service over and above the actual cost in dollars). For example, a competent employee whose patients and their family members repeatedly have praise for his or her humanistic style not only gets the job done, but also projects a positive image for the institution. Getting the job done properly is an expected part of the therapist's work; the enhancement of the institution's image is an added benefit. This becomes a net gain for the institution since the employee receives the same pay whether or not the therapist does something extraordinary for the patient or their family.

Departments can also add value by eliminating unnecessary therapy, fixing longstanding problems, or finding more efficient means of delivering care. Respiratory therapists have great potential for

adding value because their skills, knowledge, and abilities are needed by medical centers.[3]

The Importance of Image and Self-Image. The respiratory care manager should be visible to staff, administrators, and key physicians. Developing business and political acumen involves effectively balancing strength with flexibility.

One very important challenge for the respiratory care manager is the creation of a learning organization (ie, a department that can adjust to a specified situation as well as unforeseen situations). Quite often the secret to creating a learning organization starts with enhancing self-image. Enhancing self-image can lead to loyalty, added value, and eventually to increased customer satisfaction. As employees gain confidence from their enhanced self-image, they are more prone to perform in ways that add value to the department and are less resistant to change.

CRITICAL CONTENT

DEVELOPING SELF-IMAGE

- Creating a learning organization starts with enhancing self-image
- Lack of self-image can limit creativity and motivation
- An employee with a good self-image brings added value to the department

---

When managers and staff have a positive self-image, they can project this image to others, increasing the credibility of the individual and the department. As the department's credibility is enhanced, the ability to implement time and resource management strategies and critical thinking skills is significantly improved.[3]

Helping New Respiratory Therapists. New respiratory therapists (ie, those with less than 2 years of experience) depend on experienced respiratory therapists for training, mentoring, and other forms of guidance. Allowing them to observe and providing on-site coaching are stellar examples of how to help the new member establish a foundation for time and resource management through critical thinking.

For example, a veteran respiratory therapist takes a newly hired respiratory therapist with her to perform a formal patient assessment. According to the department's approved prioritization protocol, the patient does not require any respiratory care. The veteran respiratory therapist then shows the newly hired respiratory therapist how to inform the physician that, since indications for the therapy are lacking, the procedure will not be performed.

Collective Critical Thinking.   Although the critical thinking of one individual can effect great change within a department, pooling resources develops a certain level of synergy (ie, the outcome is greater than the sum of the individual efforts). Collectively changing the mindset of the department involves applying critical thinking skills and selling concepts and ideas inside and outside the RT department. Brainstorming shouldn't be restricted only to the work setting. True professionals who are critical thinkers identify with their work.

Concepts Worthy of an In-Service (or Two)

Doing More with Less.   Time and resource management concentrates on making staff work smarter, not harder. Key to this concept is balancing productivity with quality of care. The image of the individual and the department are both enhanced when time and resource management is optimized.

Suppose you know that the physician order for a severe asthmatic patient of a 2.5 mg albuterol HHN treatment every hour should be converted to continuous nebulizer therapy. This more efficient therapy minimizes use of human and financial resources.

The Quality–Productivity Hybrid.   Though a manager cannot completely sacrifice productivity for the sake of quality, productivity is essential to the financial survival of the institution. Although quality care is the ultimate goal, the system of balancing productivity and quality must be objec-

tive (ie, measurable). Hence, a delicate balance is required. The balance weighs aspects of critical thinking such as idea generation and brainstorming against performing procedures in a quick, often suboptimal manner (usually with limited human resources).

When a department implements critical thinking (eg, a new model for performing ventilator checks), two key factors come into play: quality and productivity. While often viewed as opposing forces, or at the very least mutually exclusive concepts (ie, if you increase one by 20%, the other has to decrease in a roughly similar amount), this may not be the case.

The Quality Perspective.   Perhaps you are now willing to try integrating critical thinking into your daily routine and into your department, but you feel the time-honored traditions and robotic clinical behavior are habits too entrenched to change.

 Critical Thinking Exercise 4

REFLECTING

Group discussion:

a. How *do* you enhance quality via critical thinking?

b. How do you implement critical thinking into the daily routine? These are vital questions for both new graduates and seasoned professionals.

The Productivity Perspective.   Quality patient care is wonderful, but it is difficult to measure. Hospital executives must use objective measurements to determine how well a department is performing. As changes in time and resource management are implemented, the productivity perspective will change. Staff and management must both understand the interdependence between quality and productivity. One key marker to observe is productivity per unit cost.

For example, a respiratory therapy department's workload suddenly becomes very busy during the holiday season. Since vacations have already begun and registries are already depleted, overtime for full-time and per diem staff is initiated in an attempt to cover the workload. When the monthly reports arrive, the director of the RT department is summoned by the hospital administrator. She wants to know why the productivity/dollar ratio has decreased during the last month. The RT director explains that the productivity has not decreased. In fact, the staff worked extremely hard during a time when it was difficult to obtain help. The director explains that the productivity/dollar ratio has decreased because the dollar value has increased. The dollar value has increased because so much overtime had to be used. Since overtime is paid at $1\frac{1}{2}$ times the normal amount, it costs more to provide labor in such situations.

The Vicious Cycle.   The productivity/dollar ratio is a key element to the *vicious cycle*, a concept best defined by example. Say a department practices the traditional ventilator check model, and assuming that each therapist oversees 6 patients, respiratory therapists would feel obligated to complete 36 procedures per shift (6 patients × 6 checks each = 36 procedures).

This is based on the respiratory therapist mindset summed up by: "I need to do the most for as many patients possible." The result is often suboptimal performance with a definite focus on productivity. This mindset has been endorsed by the department as a whole, usually in an unconscious way. Some examples are shown below.

"Did You Get That New Start Done?"   A supervisor may simply be ensuring that a new start is performed, but the staff therapist could easily get the impression that he (and the department) is solely focused on productivity. New starts are usually an unanticipated addition to the overall workload for which the supervisor is responsible. To the staff therapist, the supervisor is asking about the new start because he does not want to field any complaints, but the opposite may be true. Therefore, the department needs to effectively communicate messages to the staff about the expectations and strategies to balance quality with productivity.

"The Fifth Floor Is Calling for a Stat Treatment."   To staff, this comment seems to be not merely a request to add one more procedure to their assigned shift workload, but also to do so immediately. This is a stress inducer.

"Don't Leave Any Undone Work for the Next Shift Because I'll Hear about It."   This comment definitely puts productivity above quality. Clinical situations often occur during a shift that justify the need to omit or delay lower priority therapy to one patient in favor of administering higher priority therapy to another.

Trying to do the most for as many patients as possible often results in a completion rate of at least 36 procedures/shift (all ventilator checks get done in spite of new starts, codes, etc.). This may sound good, but in reality a disservice may have been done to patients by cutting corners, and to the department by falsely inflating the productivity level. Cutting corners can lead to a monthly or quarterly report that shows a completion rate 15% higher than predicted, "proving" that they can do 15% more work without increasing staffing levels. Now the staff is expected to continue completing 15% more work with no increase in staffing levels, and this exacerbates the mindset of "forget the quality, crank out the work." Respiratory therapists are now really forced to cut corners to provide the expected productivity. Hence, the vicious cycle is likely to worsen even more with time if it is not addressed.

Interactions with the Administrators

The respiratory care manager should present a proposal to his or her superior based on the premise that he or she can improve the quality of patient care without increasing human resources. It should be difficult for the administrator to argue against such a premise. For example, Bob, the respiratory care manager, meets with his hospital administrator, Alice. Bob tells Alice that he has a proposal that is certain to enhance the image of the department and its staff. Of course, Alice will also benefit since she oversees the department. In more objective terms, Bob says that the proposal will improve the statistics in the quarterly and annual continuous quality improvement reports *and* is likely to generate positive subjective feedback from key physicians and possibly family members as well. Bob informs Alice that the proposal will probably cause a decrease in productivity. However, he justifies this decrease by explaining how the department is caught in a vicious cycle and cutting corners is becoming the rule rather than the exception. Alice says that the hospital cannot afford to hire more staff to make up the difference between workload and production. Bob replies that additional staff may not be necessary because he is going to closely manage time and resources. He will also implement a critical thinking program to encourage smarter rather than faster therapy.

Start by Implementing Critical Thinking in a Key Area. The critical thinking approach to time and resource management does not have to be implemented in all procedures simultaneously. Begin with a common procedure such as a ventilator check. Other procedures can be added over time.

Critical Thinking Exercise 5

REFLECTING

a. What type of procedure should Bob select to begin development of time and resource management and critical thinking skills?

b. Considering the continuous quality improvements that he told Alice would be outcomes of the proposal, should Bob select a high volume procedure (ie, one performed many times a day) to increase the chances of others noticing the change?

c. Should Bob implement the critical thinking and time and resource management changes department-wide? Why?

CRITICAL CONTENT

HEALTH CARE QUALITY OR QUANTITY?

- Critical thinking and time and resource management strategies may result in a slightly lower productivity level.
- Efforts to increase the quality of patient care may affect the quantity of care.

- Decreases in quantity are often worth the gains in quality.
- Even a slight decrease in productivity may cause concern for individuals who are fixated only on numbers.

Dealing with Resistance to Change

Converting traditional, longstanding mind-sets to new philosophies or management systems can be difficult. Most major cultural changes require mutual trust between management and staff. The staff must trust that management will give them the time and resources to implement critical thinking skills at the bedside. Respiratory care managers must trust the staff to use their time wisely and efficiently. Since staff and supervisors alike have been conditioned to focus on productivity, it is an area that needs to be addressed. Perhaps the new time and resource management mind-set is best explained graphically.

Let us revisit Fig. 10-1. Traditional productivity level had determined that 36 procedures was the optimum number per shift based on 2 hours between ventilator checks (6 patients × 6 vent checks per patient per shift = 36). The implementation of a new time and resource management system shows a slightly lower productivity level of 31. This slight decrease is a result of an increase in the quality of patient care, though it may cause concern for those who fixate on numbers.

Keep in mind that delivering quality does not always result in a decrease in productivity. In fact, many quick procedures can be performed appropriately with critical thinking and still yield a higher-than-expected productivity level.

POST-TRANSITION: TOOLS FOR MEASURING IMPROVEMENT

Follow-Up Measurements of Productivity

Since clinical time is managed differently after the implementation of a new time and resource management system, productivity values will vary significantly. This new system does not give staff respiratory therapists total control over the use of their time, but it does allow them to manage their time differently and in a more constructive manner. Gains made in efficiency are not an excuse for additional breaks or an increase in socialization time. Therefore, it is the manager's responsibility to ensure that staff do not abuse any new freedom and flexibility acquired under the new system. The manager should determine that staff is productive throughout their shifts as they apply their newly acquired time and resource management skills.

Consider the following example which examines hours of actual clinical work per number of procedures, also called workload units (WLUs). A staff respiratory therapist working a 12-hour shift gets three 15-minute breaks in addition to a half-hour unpaid lunch period. The staff respiratory therapist spends half-hour at the beginning of the shift and half-hour at the end of the shift receiving and giving reports, respectively. As a result, 10.25 hours remain for performing the other activities, performing procedures, gathering equipment, traveling, waiting for elevators, etc.

CRITICAL CONTENT

IMPLEMENTATION OF A TIME/RESOURCE SYSTEM

- Time management maximizes effective utilization of human resources.
- Respiratory therapists can manage their time differently and become more effective.
- Time and resources are used in a more constructive manner.
- Respiratory therapists and departments assess outcomes to justify the ways that resources are used, including personnel, finances, information, and materials.

After the implementation of a new form of time and resource management, the manager has the right and the responsibility to keep his or her staff busy using at least one of the methods described earlier.

Critical Thinking Exercise 6

REFLECTING

a. If the staff members are actually applying time and resource management skills and they have enough extra time to take longer lunches and breaks, what should the manager do?

b. What should the manager (or staff) do if some therapists have idle time and other therapists are behind in their work?

Since the method for measuring productivity changes with the advent of a new time and resource management system, the method for generating a work assignment must change also. For example, the acuity level can be used to adjust the workload. Most respiratory care departments need a system for ranking the acuity level of patients based on their overall condition or strictly from a pulmonary standpoint. Using the previous example of ventilator checks, an acuity system for prioritizing ventilator management would assist in the transition from traditional to critical thinking.

A more objective measure of ventilator patient acuity has been described recently.[27] Initially, the acuity system does not need to be complex, but it must be clear. For example, the highest priority might go to a ventilator patient who has great difficulty obtaining adequate ventilation and oxygenation, with few if any options for ventilator setting changes. Patients on mechanical ventilation who require frequent monitoring or setting changes, but are not unstable, could be placed in the second priority level. The third level would include ventilator patients who are very stable and require few if any setting changes and minimal monitoring.

The new time and resource management system may involve an acuity factor for shift assignments. For example, if four ventilators were assigned to a respiratory therapist in the traditional system, the new system might result in the therapist having two-ventilator high-priority patients or six third-level ventilator patients (these being considered equivalent assignments).

Follow-Up Measurements of Quality

Implementing a new time and resource management system can have effects on the quality of care. These effects can be analyzed at different levels and from a variety of perspectives. A comprehensive analysis of quality would include the following elements.

- *Traditional objective quality monitors:* This type of monitor provides concrete, objective results.
- *Competency testing:* The testing should include a standardized approach to patient assessment and optimization of therapy.
- *Subjective quality assessment:* Informal—verbal comments. Formal—written comments.
- *Other measures of quality:* Enhanced skills of staff in communicating, providing compassionate care, and showing commitment.

Post-Transition Assessment

The right work environment is essential to the successful outcome of a new time and resource management system. A post-transition assessment of the work environment can in itself be an overall determinant of the level of success of the implementation process. For critical thinking and time and resource management strategies to take hold, the work environment must be conducive to learning and accepting new ideas. If these conditions exist, chances are good that the implementation of time and resource management strategies will be successful. On the other hand, it is unlikely that critical thinking or time and resource management strategies would take hold in a work environment that was not conducive to learning or accepting new ideas.

Below are some specific aspects of the work environment that can be assessed.

- Communication systems

- Systems for addressing complaints and accepting new ideas
- The department's problem-solving mechanism
- Critical thinking deficits (CTDs)

Rewards

Staff respiratory therapists should be compensated appropriately for the skills they possess and those they acquire. This is not only fair, it makes financial sense. Appropriate compensation assists in recruiting additional staff and helps to retain therapists with advanced skills and seniority. When experienced personnel leave the department, there is a significant cost associated with training new staff.

TIME AND RESOURCE MANAGEMENT CASES

Time and resource management strategies are best illustrated by using examples. Use time and resource management strategies to address the issues in the following case scenarios.

Time and Resource Management Case 1. An 88 kg patient is on the following ventilator settings:

Volume ventilation; SIMV mode; respiratory rate: 12 bpm; Vt: 700 mL
Pressure support, 10 cm H_2O; PS Vt, 400 mL
PEEP, 2 cm H2O

The most recent ABG on these settings yielded these results: pH, 7.45; P_{CO_2}, 25; P_{O_2}, 85

 Critical Thinking Exercise 7

MAKING INFERENCES BY CLUSTERING DATA

a. Is this patient ready to wean? Why or why not? Use EBM to determine your answer and cite your sources.

b. What other data would you need to make your recommendation?

A review of the chart reveals the following: In the physician notes—"Patient has sepsis." Chest x-ray—"Total white-out from aspiration."

Critical Thinking Exercise 8

MAKING INFERENCES BY CLUSTERING DATA

a. Does this additional information change your respiratory care plan at all? Why?

b. How might a respiratory therapist obtain this information (besides looking in the chart)?

A review of the respiratory therapist's ventilator flow sheet reveals: total respiratory rate, 25 to 30 bpm. F_{IO_2}, 70%.

The aforementioned critical thinking exercise involves reflecting, thinking outside of the boundaries imposed by mere review of the ventilator settings and ABGs to determine the patient's pulmonary status. Critical thinkers do not make automatic assumptions—they investigate. If additional data support the initial assessment that the patient is able to wean, then do so. But assumptions should not be made automatically at first glance. The correct decision should be made using patient data and weaning protocols based on the best evidence.

The next patient assessment and ABG reveal: ABG: pH, 7.45; P_{CO_2}, 25; P_{O_2}, 85. Total respiratory rate: 30 bpm.

Critical Thinking Exercise 9

ANTICIPATION

a. How hard is the patient working to obtain these relatively normal ABGs?

b. What is the patient's acid-base balance?

c. What are the clinical concerns associated with a respiratory rate of 30 bpm?

d. If the patient gets fatigued and the rate drops from a total of 30 bpm to the back-up rate of 12 bpm, what do you predict will happen to the acid-base balance?

Group Critical Thinking Exercise 3

DECISION-MAKING

a. The patient's total respiratory rate is 30 bpm, which is a sign of severe respiratory distress. The patient is likely to become extremely fatigued and go into respiratory failure. If the patient had a minute ventilation of 15.6 L/min prior to respiratory failure, what would the minute ventilation be if the patient does not initiate any spontaneous breaths ?

b. Form two groups. Group 1 will discuss the merits of "resting" the patient on assist/control and group 2 will discuss the merits of "resting" the patient on SIMV. Each group should incorporate time and resource management strategies into their discussions. For example, one or more of the following should be included in the discussion:

- Protocols (ie, weaning protocol and EBM)
- Productivity
- Competency testing (ie, strong ventilator management skills)
- Similar ventilator orders as a sign of a CTD
- Limited variation in ventilator modes as a sign of a CTD
- Q2 ventilator checks as an attitude that fosters a CTD

Time and Resource Management Case 2. A patient with asthma is admitted to the ED. The physician orders 2.5 mg of albuterol via HHN Q4h. Before the treatment, you auscultate the patient and hear significant wheezing during inspiration and expiration. After the treatment, you hear wheezing during expiration only.

Critical Thinking Exercise 10

MAKING INFERENCES BY CLUSTERING DATA

a. How effective was the treatment?

b. What methods and criteria are you using to measure effectiveness?

c. Do you have any recommendations for the physician?

When you approach the patient for his second treatment, you notice that his condition has worsened. The patient is in a state of exacerbation.

Group Critical Thinking Exercise 4

COMMUNICATION AND NEGOTIATION

a. Form two or more groups. Each group should consider the most efficient (ie, the least labor intensive or the least expensive), yet most effective method of appropriately treating the patient. Each group will describe the evidence and how they will communicate with the physician. The groups should write the exact words they will use. By role playing, one individual from each group will contact the physician and make a recommendation. The class will consider all recommendations and discuss the optimal way of communicating with the physician.

b. A variation of this exercise would be to have the medical director interact with each person making the recommendation from each group (with the class observing).

Time and Resource Management Case 3. Compare Example 2 to the following case.

Another patient arrives in the ED during an asthma attack. The physician orders 2.5 mg of albuterol via HHN Q4h. Before the treatment is administered, the respiratory therapist auscultates the patient and hears significant wheezing. The respiratory therapist follows department philosophy and asks the physician if you can implement therapy using the protocol for MDI to deliver four puffs of albuterol, with an option to titrate the dose and/or frequency.

Group Critical Thinking Exercise 5

ANTICIPATION FOR NEGOTIATIONS

Group discussion:

a. If your respiratory therapy department has recently implemented a new protocol, how do you think most physicians will respond when you suggest using it?

b. If the physicians are reluctant to use the protocol, why do you think they are resistant?

c. If your department's newly implemented protocol allows the respiratory therapist to titrate the dose according to the patient's symptoms, why might a physician be resistant to accepting the protocol?

d. To what time and resource management strategies could you refer when trying to convince the physician to order the protocol?

e. Describe the advantages in terms of time and resources when an MDI is used instead of an HHN. Cite evidence and state reasons to support your conclusions.

After delivering four puffs of albuterol (ie, 2.5 mg), the respiratory therapist hears minimal expiratory wheezing (as in Example 2 above). However, because of the option to titrate the dose, the therapist administers four additional puffs. Breath sounds after eight puffs are clear. The patient in this example does not enter into a state of exacerbation because the titration prevented such an occurrence. The clinical advantage of increasing the dose before a problem occurs is obvious. From the perspective of time and resource management, titration prevented an increased frequency of treatments (eg, every 2 hours as in the previous example), minimizing costs of labor and supplies.

Time and Resource Management Case 4. A respiratory care supervisor spent hours each month reviewing paper charts to determine if cuff pressure was being measured at least once per shift, per department policy. The department purchased a respiratory care information management system. Now the same supervisor obtains the same information on 100 patients in a matter of minutes. Computerized charting systems and respiratory care information systems can significantly improve quality assurance monitoring. A query can be developed that searches the extensive database for all relevant information. The improvement in data accessibility may lead to a more extensive review of the care and charting provided by respiratory therapists.

Group Critical Thinking Exercise 6

PROBLEM SOLVING
AND DECISION MAKING

Form two or more groups.

a. Half of the groups will discuss what items are most important to monitor using an information management system. The other groups will discuss what aspects of time and resource management (and other forms of critical thinking) cannot be monitored well by an information management system.

b. Each group will describe methods for monitoring such clinical skills as assessment, prioritization, time management, and resource management. Each group will share its results with the entire class.

KEY POINTS

• Time and resource management provides the potential for the respiratory care profession to significantly change the way we go about our work giving "added value." By applying critical thinking skills, respiratory therapists can simultaneously increase efficiency, provide quality care, improve staff morale, *and* enhance a professional image.

• Time and resource management can facilitate critical thinking in respiratory care practice.

• Critical thinking leads to improved utilization of resources.

• The key to an effective utilization control system is standardization of patient assessment, prioritization, and communication.

• Once critical thinking and a time and resource management system are in place, it is important to prevent stagnation.

• Time and resource management strategies need to be routinely reviewed and rejuvenated.

• The process of growth and improvement is dynamic and never ending.

REFERENCES

1. Fan L. *Liao Fan's Four Lessons.* English translation by Li-Pen Chao, Los Angeles, 1998.

2. Moorhead G, Griffin R. *Organizational Behavior.* Boston: Houghton Mifflin Company; 1989.

3. Malinowski T, Wright J, Ford R, Mahlmeister M. Blueprint for the Future: Guidelines for Operating & Managing A Respiratory Care Department. Unpublished article presented at the CSRC State Convention, Monterey, California. June, 1996.

4. Kester L, Stoller JK. Ordering respiratory care services for hospitalized patients: practices of overuse and underuse. *Cleveland Clinic J Med.* 1992;59:581–585.

5. Browning JA, Kiaser DL, Durbin CG Jr. The effect of guidelines on the appropriate use of arterial blood gas analysis in the intensive care unit. *Respir Care.* 1989;34:269–276.

6. American Association for Respiratory Care. The AARC Clinical Practice Guidelines. *Respir Care.* 1991;36:1398–1401, 1992;37:882–906.

7. Zibrak JD, Rossetti P, Wood E. Effects in reduction of respiratory therapy on patient outcome. *N Engl J Med.* 1986;315:292–295.

8. Stoller JK. The rationale for therapist-driven protocols. *Respir Care Clin N Am.* 1996;2:1–14.

9. Konschak MP, Binder A, Binder RE. Oxygen therapy utilization in a community hospital: Use of a protocol to improve oxygen administration and preserve resources. *Respir Care.* 1999;44:506–511.

10. Goldberg R, Chan L, Haley P, et al. Critical pathway for the emergency management of acute asthma: effect on resource utilization. *Ann Emerg Med.* 1998;31:562–567.

11. Ford RM, Phillips-Clar JE, Burns DM. Implementing therapist-driven protocols. *Respir Care Clin N Am.* 1996;2:51–76.

12. Lierl MB, Pettinichi S, Sebastian KD, Kotagel U. Trial of a therapist-directed protocol for weaning bronchodilator therapy in children with status asthmaticus. *Respir Care.* 1999;44:497–505.

13. Wood G, MacLeod B, Moffatt S. Weaning from mechanical ventilation: physician-directed versus a respiratory-therapist-directed protocol. *Respir Care.* 1995;40:219–224.

14. Kollef MH, Shapiro SD, Silver P, et al. A randomized-controlled trial of protocol-directed versus physician-directed weaning from mechanical ventilation. *Crit Care Med.* 1997;25:567–574.

15. Kollef MH. Therapist-directed protocols: their time has come. *Respir Care.* 1999;44:495.

16. Shrake KL, Scaggs JE, England KR, et al. Benefits associated with a respiratory care assessment-treatment program: results of a pilot study. *Respir Care.* 1994;39:715–724.

17. Walton JR, Shapiro BA, Harrison CH. Review of a bronchial hygiene evaluation program. *Respir Care* 1983;29:174–179.

18. Nielson-Tietsort J, Poole B, Creagh CE, Repsher LE. Respiratory care protocol: an approach to in-hospital respiratory therapy. *Respir Care.* 1981; 26:420–436.

19. Stoller JK, Haney D, Burkhart J, et al. Physician-ordered respiratory care vs. physician-ordered use of a respiratory therapy consult service: early experience at the Cleveland Clinic Foundation. *Respir Care.* 1993;38:1143–1154.

20. Weber K, Milligan S. Conference Summary—Therapist-driven protocols: The state of the art. *Respir Care.* 1994;39:746–756.

21. Giordano S, Anderson H, Boroch M, et al. *Uniform Reporting Manual.* 3rd ed. rev. Dallas: American Association for Respiratory Care; 1993.

22. McPeck M, Tandon R, Hughes K, Smaldone GC. Aerosol delivery during continuous nebulization. *Chest.* 1997;111(5):1200–1205.

23. Shrestha M, Bidadi K, Gourlay S, Hayes J. Continuous versus intermittent albuterol, at high and low doses, in the treatment of severe acute asthma in adults. *Chest.* 1996;110:42.

24. Maslow AH. A theory of human motivation. *Psychol Rev.* 1943;50:370–396.

25. Maslow AH. *Motivation and Personality.* New York: Harper & Row; 1954.

26. AARC clinical practice guidelines: patient-ventilator checks. *Respir Care.* 1992;37:882–886.

27. Paret G, Ziv T, Barzilai A, Ben-Abraham R, et al. Ventilation index and outcome in children with acute respiratory distress syndrome. *Pediatr Pulmonol.* 1998;26:125.

PART

II

PATIENT PROBLEMS IN RESPIRATORY CARE

11

ASTHMA

Shelley C. Mishoe and Melvin A. Welch, Jr.

The beautiful thing about learning is
nobody can take it away from you.

B.B. KING

LEARNING OBJECTIVES

1. Describe facts, descriptions, and definitions related to asthma.
2. Discuss the etiology, pathophysiology, and clinical features of a patient with asthma.
3. Discuss the acute and long-term management of patients with asthma, including health promotion and quality-of-life issues.
4. Apply specific formulas and theories to assist in clinical decision making in the management of a patient with asthma.
5. Apply the critical thinking skills of prioritizing, anticipating, negotiating, communicating, decision making, and reflection by completing exercises and case examples of asthma.
6. Apply strategies to promote critical thinking in the respiratory care management of patients with asthma through completion of chapter exercises and group discussion.
7. Use clinical case examples in the chapter to perform an initial patient assessment, using a standardized system [SOAPs and inspection,

palpation, percussion, and auscultation (IPPA)] and the clinical data presented.

8. Interpret clinical data from the case examples including history, physical examination, and laboratory and radiographic data to make recommendations for respiratory care management.
9. Using the chapter case, develop an asthma care plan, including recommendations for therapy and disease management, with consideration of the cost, ethical, and quality-of-life issues.
10. Communicate facts, evidence, and arguments to support evaluations and recommendations proposed in the care plan for the patient with asthma.
11. Practice the skill of negotiating in an attempt to persuade acceptance of your proposed care plan for each patient case with asthma.
12. Evaluate treatment and outcomes of interventions to propose changes in the care plan.
13. Describe the role of the respiratory therapist in the diagnosis, treatment, and management of asthma.

KEY WORDS

Airway Hyperresponsiveness	Asthma	Exacerbation	Morbidity
Airway Remodeling	Atopic	Extrinsic	Mortality
Allergy	Bronchospasm	Impending Respiratory Failure	Obstructive Disease
	Chronic Airway Disease	Intrinsic	Pulsus Paradoxus
			Status Asthmaticus

INTRODUCTION

Asthma is a common respiratory disease in the United States and throughout the world. Ten to fifteen million people in the United States have asthma.[1,2] The incidence, morbidity, and mortality of asthma have greatly increased during the past two decades as highlighted in the critical content box. Children and the elderly are at greatest risk. More than 5000 people die every year from asthma.[3] Hospitalizations and mortality from asthma continue to increase, despite greater understanding of asthma pathology, new asthma drugs, and better methods of long-term management. Consequently, the National Asthma Education Program was established, later renamed the National Asthma Education and Prevention Program (NAEPP), to systematically address the complexities of dealing with asthma and its consequences for individuals and society.[2]

CRITICAL CONTENT

INCREASE IN ASTHMA PREVALENCE, DEATH, AND HOSPITALIZATION RATES IN THE LAST TWO DECADES

Prevalence rate: 75% increase

Death rate: 56% increase

Hospitalization rates:

  Total population: 3% increase

  Children, 0 to 4 years of age: 45% increase

  Children, 5 to 14 years of age: 13% increase

  African Americans: 37% increase

Asthma is the most common chronic respiratory illness in children, with an estimated 4.8 million children affected. Approximately 10% to 12% of children seek medical attention due to the severity of their symptoms.[4,5] Consequently, asthma accounts for the majority of children's missed school days or parents' lost wages due to respiratory illness. More than 10 million school days were missed due to asthma, accounting for an estimated $900 million in lost wages for caregivers.[6] The health care costs of asthma are significant.

Asthma can seriously affect quality of life because it is the major cause of limitation of activity from any chronic illness in children. Although asthma begins most frequently in childhood and adolescence, it can develop at any time in life.

CRITICAL CONTENT

ASTHMA IS SERIOUS!

• It is the most common chronic illness in children.

• It is a common chronic illness of adults.

• It affects 10 to 15 million persons in the US alone.

• Incidence, morbidity, and mortality from asthma have increased and continue to increase.

• Every year 5000 people die from asthma.

• Asthma accounts for the majority of missed school days and parents' lost wages.

• Health care costs of asthma are significant.

Effective management of asthma is based on four essential components: 1) monitoring with objective measures of lung function, 2) comprehensive pharmacologic therapy, 3) environmental control measures to reduce allergens, and 4) patient education.[1,3] Too often, we focus on pharmacologic interventions and fail to adequately address the specific questions, misconceptions, and concerns of our patients. It is critical that adequate asthma education is provided to address the issues of increasing morbidity and mortality, rising direct costs for medical care, substantial indirect costs associated with missed school and work, and adverse effects on quality of life for children and caregivers. The educational component of asthma management cannot be overemphasized. Patient and caregiver education can improve management and possibly decrease health care costs.[7–10] Respiratory therapists can provide ideal patient education and disease management across the continuum of health care.

CRITICAL CONTENT

Asthma education must address:
- Increased morbidity and mortality
- Rising costs for medical care
- Missed days from school and work
- Decreased quality of life

ETIOLOGY

One of the ongoing difficulties has been the difficulty in agreeing on a clear cut definition of asthma. Considerable overlap in signs and symptoms occurs between asthma and other obstructive pulmonary diseases. To clarify this problem, this working definition of asthma was proposed by the National Heart, Lung, and Blood Institute (NHLBI):

> Asthma is a chronic inflammatory disorder of the airways in which many cells and cellular elements play a role, in particular, mast cells, eosinophils, T lymphocytes, macrophages, neutrophils, and epithelial cells. In susceptible individuals, this inflammation causes recurrent episodes of wheezing, breathlessness, chest tightness, and coughing, particularly at night or in the early morning. These episodes are usually associated with widespread, but variable airflow obstruction. The airflow obstruction is often reversible either spontaneously or with treatment. The inflammation also causes an associated increase in the existing bronchial hyperresponsiveness to a variety of stimuli.[10]

From this working definition, one can see that asthma is a very complex disease, without an easily described single etiology.

Although the differences are not always clear cut, we think of asthma as having two primary subcategories: **Extrinsic** (atopic) asthma, whereby the inflammatory response of the airways is explained as an allergic reaction to exposure to specific, identifiable antigens; and **Intrinsic**, a form of asthma

precipitated by other factors, but not associated with an allergic response. Intrinsic asthma is frequently referred to as *adult-onset asthma*. In adult-onset asthma, allergens may also continue to play a role. However, these adults often have coexisting problems such as sinusitis, nasal polyps, and sensitivity to aspirin or related nonsteroidal antiinflammatory drugs. The mechanism for intrinsic asthma is not fully established, although the inflammatory process is similar to atopic asthma. Extrinsic asthma is the type most often seen in childhood. The asthmatic airways can easily be irritated by a variety of stimuli, and once irritated they respond with an inflammatory reaction described below. One of the more common causes of irritation that causes or triggers the development of the asthma attack is the presence of a respiratory tract infection.

CRITICAL CONTENT

COMMON TRIGGERS OF ALLERGIC ASTHMA

Indoor Allergens
- Dust mites
- Animal dander
- Cockroach allergen
- Indoor pollens and mold
- Irritants (ie, smoke from cigarettes, fireplaces, wood-burning stoves)
- Fumes from household materials (perfumes, sprays)

Environmental Allergens
- Pollens from trees, grass, and weeds
- Outdoor molds
- Pollution, including automobile exhaust fumes

PATHOPHYSIOLOGY AND RELATED THEORY

The pathophysiologic changes that occur with asthma are related to the highly variable degree of airway obstruction that occurs because of the inflammatory response of the airways. With different airways having different degrees of obstruction, the air will unevenly distribute during inspiration. This results in some regions of lung receiving less air than normal, while other less obstructed areas may get more air than normal. This causes ventilation-perfusion (V/Q) mismatching. V/Q mismatch results in the characteristic hypoxemia seen when the patient is breathing room air.

The airway obstruction caused by asthma is now thought to be due to four different mechanisms, all a result of the inflammatory process central to the disease.[2]

1. Acute spasm of the involuntary (smooth) muscle of the airway (ie, bronchoconstriction).
2. Swelling of the airway resulting in reduction of the internal lumen diameter (ie, airway edema).
3. Excessive production of mucus by the goblet cells lining the airway (ie, mucus plug formation).
4. Changes in airway structure (eg, increased numbers of goblet cells and deposition of interstitial collagens beneath the epithelium). These chronic changes are referred to as *airway wall remodeling*.

CRITICAL CONTENT

Airway changes with asthma:
• Bronchoconstriction
• Airway edema
• Mucus plug formation
• Airway remodeling

The natural tendency of airways is to narrow during exhalation. This is true for all lung structures, because the lung is getting smaller as it empties, so airways and alveoli all decrease in size during expiration. This natural narrowing combined with the various obstructive effects of airway inflammation cause the expiratory airflow resistance to increase, resulting in trapping of air in the lungs. Hence, the characteristic hyperinflation that occurs during an exacerbation. Now this overinflated state causes the person to have trouble exhaling, but with the lungs nearly full, the person will

also have trouble inhaling. The lungs in this hyperinflated state are overstretched and therefore have decreased compliance. The combination of increased airway resistance and decreased lung compliance leads to excessive work of breathing (WOB) and all the characteristic signs and symptoms of respiratory distress described below.

CLINICAL FEATURES

The typical patient suffering an asthma attack presents with the expected signs and symptoms of a person with the altered mechanics of breathing (airway resistance and lung compliance changes) described earlier. The patient frequently complains of the following symptoms (subjective data): shortness of breath, chest tightness, difficulty breathing, and coughing. The onset of these symptoms may be very rapid or they may progress over a period of days.

Physical examination will often reveal many of the following findings (objective data): The patient will appear anxious and/or agitated. If the attack is severe and/or prolonged, he or she may even demonstrate mental confusion. The patient may have difficulty speaking in complete sentences and often assumes a body position that allows maximal ventilatory effort. It is common to see the patient sitting and leaning forward slightly. He or she will be unable to lie down. Exhalation will tend to be prolonged due to the expiratory airflow obstruction.

The upper respiratory tract, chest, and skin are the focus of the physical examination for asthma. The finding of increased nasal secretions, mucosal swelling, and nasal polyps would increase the probability of asthma, as would any dermatitis, eczema or any other manifestation of an allergic skin condition.

Vital signs reflect the associated cardiopulmonary distress: tachypnea, tachycardia, hypertension, and sometimes a fever (if infection is a factor). Accessory muscle use is common. Diaphoresis (excessive sweating) from the excessive WOB and associated anxiety is also common. On inspection of the chest, you may find an increased anteroposterior diameter, reflecting the hyperinflated state of the lungs. Signs of significant drops in intrapleural pressure from the patient's inspiratory efforts can include tracheal descent, retractions of muscle and tissue around the intercostal spaces, and sometimes a noticeable drop in systolic blood pressure during inspiration, referred to as *pulsus paradoxus*. These signs all reflect the patient's increased WOB that accompanies the altered pulmonary mechanics of a severe attack.

Percussion of the chest would reveal hyperresonance from the hyperinflated state, unless there is a coexisting localized infiltrate from a precipitating bacterial infection, in which case a consolidation may be noted from the dull or flat percussion note. Wheezing may be audible without a stethoscope. Alternatively, wheezing may be present during auscultation on both inspiration and expiration. During the mildest attacks, wheezing is heard on expiration only.

CRITICAL CONTENT

TYPICAL SIGNS AND SYMPTOMS WITH ASTHMA

Vital signs: tachycardia, tachypnea, fever
   (with infection), hypertension
Level of consciousness: Anxious and agitated,
   mental confusion, or lethargy
Head and neck: increased nasal secretions, mucosal
   swelling, nasal polyps
Lungs: wheezes or silent chest, prolonged
   expiration, hyperresonance, air trapping, use of
   accessory muscles
Extremities: diaphoresis, dermatitis, eczema, allergic
   skin conditions

Typical Laboratory Findings

Chest radiographs may be performed to assist in differential diagnosis and to see what coexisting complications may be present. However, chest radiography has little role in the assessment of mild to moderate asthma. The degree of hyperinflation can be verified by radiograph, although this fact alone would not justify the performance of a chest

x-ray. If the presenting signs and symptoms are severe and/or complications are suspected, a chest film would then be indicated. Atelectasis, pneumonia, and pneumomediastinum or pneumothoraxes are complications of asthma.

Bedside spirometry is routinely performed to assess and compare to baseline data (if available) as well as to assess response to therapy. Peak expiratory flow rate (PEFR) and forced expiratory volume in 1 second (FEV_1) are considered objective assessments of airflow obstruction. Both of these objective measures of lung function are utilized for long-term management and acute care. Although they are both objective measures, the practitioner needs to remember they are both dependent on patient effort. Therefore it is essential that proper supervision and patient instruction be used to produce consistent data.

A severe exacerbation exists when:

1. The PEFR or FEV_1 is less than 30% to 50% of predicted or of the patient's personal best (preferable, if known), or
2. The adult PEFR value is less than 120 L/min or the FEV_1 is less than 1 L.[11]

Some patients are just too distressed to perform the procedure. In this situation, you just note this as one more indication of the severity of the patient's distress and proceed without the data. For patients with moderate to severe persistent asthma, education in self-testing is recommended to permit long-term daily monitoring.[2]

CRITICAL CONTENT

PERSONAL BEST PEFR

- Highest peak flow achieved during a 2- to 3-week period when asthma is under good control.
- Test at least twice a day for 2 to 3 weeks, in morning and mid-afternoon.
- Test before and after taking inhaled beta$_2$ agonist, if needed for quick relief.

Respiratory therapists and other health care professionals should continuously encourage and evaluate daily records of lung function. In order to step up therapy, patients should be instructed to use zones to assess whether their lung function as measured by peak flow is good (green zone), borderline (yellow zone), or poor (red zone).

C R I T I C A L   C O N T E N T

PEFR red, yellow, and green zone:
• Green zone: 80% of personal best
• Yellow zone: 50% to 80% of personal best
• Red zone: less than 50% of personal best

Arterial blood gases (ABGs) are usually unnecessary in the patient with mild to moderate asthma, but are of great value if the patient is experiencing severe distress.[11] Typical ABGs during a mild attack reflect the V/Q mismatch described earlier. Thus the patient will be hypoxemic on room air and will be mildly hyperventilating. The severity of the attack can be assessed by the degree of hypoxemia and the inability of the patient to continue to hyperventilate. Once the distress has progressed to causing moderate hypoxemia on room air (ie, Pao_2 less than 60 mm Hg), or the $Paco_2$ has reached normal values for a nondistressed person (ie, 40 mm Hg), the ABGs are indicating that the airway obstruction is severe and/or the patient is beginning to fatigue.

The extent to which a patient will exhibit any or all of the above findings depends to a large part on the severity of the exacerbation. An asthma exacerbation that is not responsive to normal interventions, and is therefore placing the patient at risk for developing respiratory failure, is referred to as a **status asthmaticus** attack. These patients need to be identified as early as possible to prevent life-threatening complications.

C R I T I C A L   C O N T E N T

STATUS ASTHMATICUS

Status asthmaticus is an asthma attack that does not respond to normal intervention, placing the patient at risk for respiratory failure. **Every asthma attack has the potential to be fatal, just as every asthma attack has the potential to be reversed!**

The clinician will need to consider the physical examination data, with the insight revealed from the history of present illness (HPI), past medical history, and spirometry to differentiate asthma from other causes of acute respiratory distress. Reversibility of airway obstruction by at least 15% after administration of a bronchodilator suggests the diagnosis of asthma. According to the most recent recommendations, the diagnosis of asthma requires clinicians to determine that 1) episodic symptoms of airflow obstruction are present, 2) airflow obstruction is at least partially reversible, and 3) alternative diagnoses are excluded.[2]

TREATMENT AND MANAGEMENT

The management of asthma centers on prevention of exacerbations and the recognition and early treatment of exacerbations when they do occur.[2] The best strategy for the management of an attack of asthma is early recognition and subsequent early treatment.

C R I T I C A L   C O N T E N T

Essential components of asthma management:
• Objective measurement of lung function
• Comprehensive pharmacologic therapy
• Environmental control
• Patient education

Since asthma is a chronic disease, this means the patient will likely be at home or work when they notice the worsening symptoms of an exacerbation; therefore, patient education is a mainstay of asthma management. Clinicians involved in the care of persons with asthma should focus on this fact during all of their interactions with these patients. Patients must be educated on how to avoid triggers, recognizing the early signs and symptoms of an exacerbation, and taking action in response to increased symptoms. Patients should have a written action plan developed with their physicians and medical management team. This action plan will help guide patients to properly self-manage exacerbations at home, and to seek appropriate medical care when needed.[2,11]

Long-term management should include actions to limit exposure to environmental allergens, in addition to pharmacologic therapy and daily monitoring of lung function. Several actions can limit the number and types of indoor allergens. For example, washing bedding in hot water with bleach will reduce dust mite allergen. Keeping the kitchen clean and free of exposed foods can help control cockroaches, as can regular visits from a pest control service. Using central air conditioning and exhaust fans can limit home humidity, which will decrease the amount of indoor mite and mold allergens. Keeping kitchens and bathrooms as dry as possible and regularly cleaning them to prevent mold build-up can help. In humid climates, use of dehumidifiers can also help. Removing carpeting, upholstered furniture, stuffed toys, draperies, and other fabrics can reduce dust mite allergen levels. Obviously, animal dander, especially from cats, can be eliminated if there are no pets in the home. If the family has pets, moving them outdoors can help decrease animal dander inside.

Exposure to outdoor allergens is more difficult to control. Generally, persons with allergic asthma should limit their time spent out-of-doors, especially during the peak season for pollens. Keeping windows closed will limit exposure to outside allergens while inside. Persons with sensitivities to molds, pollens, and grasses may limit outside activities such as gardening, mowing, and raking leaves.

As shown in Fig. 11-1, if appropriate prevention strategies and home therapy do not lead to resolution of symptoms, the person should seek additional care under medical supervision. The goals of treatment for an exacerbation at this stage are threefold: 1) correction of hypoxemia by administration of supplemental oxygen, 2) rapid reversal of airflow obstruction by repetitive or continuous administration of an inhaled beta$_2$ agonist, and 3) early administration of systemic corticosteroids to patients with moderate to severe exacerbations or to patients who fail to respond promptly and completely to an inhaled beta$_2$ agonist.[2]

CRITICAL CONTENT

GOALS OF ACUTE ASTHMA CARE

1. Correction of hypoxemia
2. Rapid reversal of airway obstruction using inhaled beta$_2$ agonists
3. Early treatment of airway inflammation using corticosteroids

Appropriate oxygen therapy can usually prevent severe hypoxemia. The goal of oxygen therapy is to maintain adequate arterial saturation (ie, Sao$_2$ >90%). You can usually adequately monitor oxygen saturation noninvasively with pulse oximetry. The V/Q mismatch caused by asthma is quite responsive to low to moderate elevations of the oxygen concentration. Rarely will oxygenation be a significant problem once oxygen therapy is initiated. If a patient with asthma does not respond to simple oxygen therapy, this is a strong clue that there a co-existing condition at work (ie, the patient is invariably experiencing complications that can cause direct intrapulmonary shunting). This would include such complications as atelectasis, pneumonia, or pneumothorax. This would be one of the indications to obtain the additional data of an ABG.

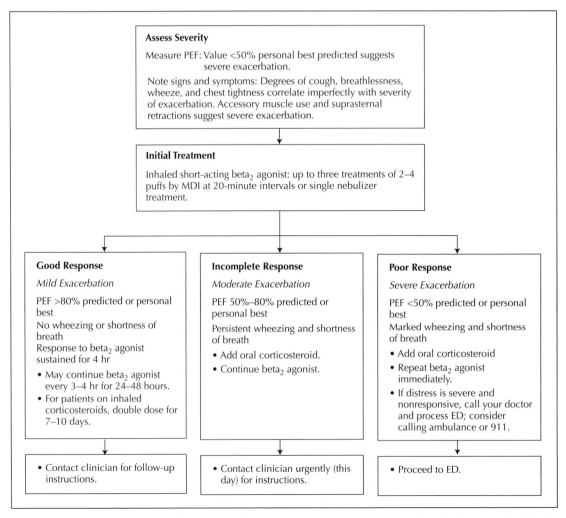

FIGURE 11-1   Management of asthma exacerbations: Home treatment. Patients at high risk of asthma-related death should receive immediate clinical attention after initial treatment. Additional therapy may be required. (*Source: National Heart, Lung, and Blood Institute.*[2])

Inhaled bronchodilator therapy can often achieve reversal of airflow obstruction. Inhaled beta$_2$ agonists are the drugs of choice to treat smooth muscle mediated bronchoconstriction in acute asthma.[2,11] They have rapid onset with relatively few side effects. Often repetitive doses (eg, three standard doses over the first 60 to 90 minutes) are effective. Continuous nebulization may be

more effective in children and severely obstructed adults.[12,13] Perform PEFR or FEV$_1$ pulmonary function tests to monitor response to therapy. The objective data from these tests more reliably indicate the severity of an exacerbation and response to therapy than do changes in the severity of symptoms.[2] Anticholinergic bronchodilators (ipratropium bromide) may be considered in addition to the nebulized beta$_2$ agonist bronchodilator regimen, particularly in patients who are not responding adequately to beta$_2$ agonists and steroids.[2,11]

Systemic corticosteroids are recommended if there is not an immediate and complete response to inhaled bronchodilator therapy. Corticosteroids can be given orally (prednisone), or if in the ED, intravenously (methylprednisolone) with equivalent effect.[14] The antiinflammatory effects as well as the potentiation of the effects of beta$_2$ agonists are essential beneficial effects of steroids that call for their use very early in a moderate to severe exacerbation. Frequent reassessment of the patient's status is critical to proper continuing management. Failure to respond adequately to appropriate therapy in the ED, or presenting with an initial severe clinical condition should lead to immediate hospitalization.

Determine objective improvement with serial measurement of pulmonary function. Return to >70% of the patient's baseline (personal best) or predicted pulmonary function is the ultimate goal that usually allows discharge.[2] Assessment of the patient's WOB, as assessed by the previously described physical examination parameters will usually indicate the direction the patient is heading. Many patients respond well to ED therapy and can be discharged within a short time. Before discharge, it is critical that you provide the patient appropriate education and directions for further follow-up care.

A small portion of patients will not respond well to initial therapy. Signs and symptoms of fatigue and/or declining mental clarity are a poor prognostic finding and may indicate the need for mechanical ventilation. The decision to intubate is based on expert clinical judgment, weighing such factors as previous history of exacerbations, current therapy and patient response to date, and in particular, the patient's clinical appearance. As described earlier, a $Paco_2$ that is approaching or greater than normal in a patient exhibiting continuing respiratory distress or obvious fatigue is a life-threatening condition. The health care team, including respiratory care professionals, must treat the patient aggressively.

Mechanical ventilation should be used with caution when a patient has status asthmaticus. Their prolonged exhalation times and altered pulmonary mechanics (described earlier) lead to potential complications of mechanical ventilation. Inadequate exhalation times can easily result in increased or inadvertent air trapping, which is often quantified as the measured auto-PEEP (self-controlled positive end-expiratory pressure). To reduce risks, some experts recommend ventilation with strategies that minimize exposure of the lung to high minute volumes and pressures.[15,16] This strategy, of focusing on minimizing lung hyperinflation even at the cost of hypoventilation, is referred to as *permissive hypercapnia*. These patients are monitored very closely, and particular attention is paid to maintaining an acceptable pH (ie, >7.20 to 7.25). This technique calls for use of lower minute volumes, through either low respiratory rates (achieved with sedation and sometimes muscle paralysis) and/or tidal volumes lower than traditional mechanical ventilator tidal volumes (eg, to 7 mL/kg). A common goal is to attempt to keep the static (plateau) pressure less than 30 cm H_2O, a level associated with less risk of barotrauma.

Some clinicians advocate alternate forms of mechanical ventilation to avoid the risks of barotrauma. The application of noninvasive positive pressure ventilation (NPPV) presents potential advantages over the more invasive requirements of traditional mechanical ventilation. The potential decreased need for intubation, sedation, and paralysis, and improved patient comfort all make this alternative attractive. However, the potential risks of aspiration, facial necrosis, and delay in securing a more stable airway weigh against this option. It is anticipated that additional research in the future will clarify the role of NPPV in asthma patients. Until the role of NPPV is clarified through clinical research, it remains an option to be utilized in selected individuals. One of the primary requirements for consideration of NPPV for acute asthma is that the respiratory care staff must have experience in the application and monitoring of this technique. Figure 11-2 provides an overview for ED and hospital-based asthma care.

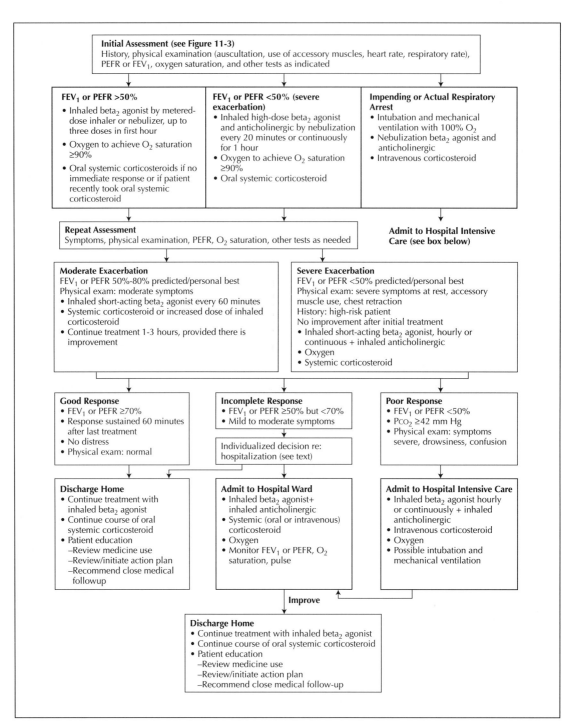

F I G U R E   1 1 - 2   Management of asthma exacerbations: Emergency department and hospital-based care. (*Source: National Heart, Lung, and Blood Institute.*[2])

SITE- AND AGE-SPECIFIC CONSIDERATIONS

There are special considerations in the diagnosis and management of asthma in different age groups. There are also site-specific strategies designed to be utilized in different health care delivery sites, including the home, clinic, physician's office, ED, and ICU. The following sections highlight the special considerations for various age groups and in various settings.

Infants and Young Children

Diagnosis. Asthma is most often underdiagnosed or misdiagnosed in infants and children less than 5 years of age.[2] Establishing a diagnosis of asthma in this age group is difficult. The process for diagnosis is similar to that used for older patients, but spirometry is not possible. The majority of children with asthma develop symptoms by their fifth birthday. However, these children often do not receive adequate treatment because physicians and other clinicians may misdiagnose their asthma. Common labels contributing to the underdiagnosis of asthma include chronic bronchitis, wheezy bronchitis, gastroesophageal reflux, and reactive airways. It is true that cough and wheeze in children can have other causes, such as congenital heart disease, foreign body aspiration, and cystic fibrosis. Clinicians should use caution to avoid giving prolonged asthma therapy when it is inappropriate.

Viral respiratory infections in children are the most common cause of asthma symptoms. The child who wheezes with viral infections will have either remission of symptoms by the preschool years or will have persistence of asthma throughout childhood. The factors most often associated with continuing asthma throughout childhood include family history of allergy or asthma and perinatal exposure to secondhand smoke.

Diagnosis of asthma in infants and young children is complex because you cannot obtain an objective measure of lung function. You may recall that objective measures of lung function are a cornerstone in the diagnosis and management of

asthma. With this age group, you must rely on a thorough evaluation, including history, symptoms, physical examination, and quality-of-life assessments. A therapeutic trial with asthma medications will help determine the diagnosis of asthma.[2]

CRITICAL CONTENT

Asthma in children under age 5:
- Asthma is often under- or misdiagnosed.
- Viral infection is the most common cause of asthma symptoms, and they lessen by age 5.
- Family history of asthma and secondhand smoke are strongly associated with childhood asthma.
- Thorough physical examination is important because you cannot obtain an objective measure of lung function.
- History, physical examination, therapeutic trial of medication, and quality-of-life measures are essential in diagnosing asthma in patients in this age group.

Treatment. Pharmacologic therapy is indicated in infants and small children if beneficial effects can be achieved, but there are few studies on medication use in this age group. Bronchodilators can be used for intermittent symptomatic relief. However, inhaled steroids are recommended whenever infants or children require symptomatic treatment more than two times per week. In general, physicians and other asthma specialists should not prescribe asthma medications if there is not a clear and obvious benefit.[2]

During asthma exacerbations, infants require special attention due to their greater risk of respiratory failure. Clinicians should use oral steroids early in the episode and monitor oxygen saturation by pulse oximetry. Oxygen saturation should be >95% at sea level. Assess infants for signs of serious distress, including use of accessory muscles, paradoxical breathing, cyanosis, a respiratory rate >60, or oxygen saturation <91%. A lack of response to beta$_2$ agonist therapy noted on physical examination or oxygen saturation is an indication for hospitalization. In hospitalized patients, intravenous methylxanthines are not beneficial in children with severe asthma, and their use remains controversial for adults. Chest physical therapy and mucolytics are not recommended. Antibiotics are not recommended for asthma treatment, but may be needed for coexisting conditions such as fever and purulent sputum, or with evidence of bacterial pneumonia. Assess fluid status and make appropriate corrections for infants and young children to reduce their risk of dehydration.

Geriatric Patients

As part of its continuing effort to promote improved asthma management in all population groups, the National Heart, Lung, and Blood Institute invited a working group of experts to further assess the issue of asthma management in the elderly population. A group of asthma specialists met to determine if elderly patients with asthma, their families, and the health professionals responsible for their care needed additional information and guidance.[17] Treatment of asthma in older patients should follow the recommendations for adults, but with a number of special considerations related to use of multiple medications, changes due to normal aging, and comorbid conditions that commonly occur in the elderly. Additional considerations concern the special educational efforts needed to encourage patient compliance and adherence in elderly patients with asthma.

Diagnosis.   Asthma can present in the elderly either as a primary occurrence or as a continuation of a disease entity that began in earlier years. The presentation of asthma in the elderly is similar to that of the young adult. At all ages, asthma is characterized by airflow obstruction, airway inflammation, and increased airway responsiveness to a variety of stimuli. Airflow obstruction with asthma can be partly or completely reversible, either spontaneously or with treatment. In elderly patients,

incomplete reversibility is becoming increasingly common. In the elderly, symptoms that mimic asthma, such as acute episodes of wheezing, coughing, shortness of breath, or chest tightness, may be due to other common conditions, such as myocardial ischemia or pulmonary embolism. Serum IgE and eosinophilia may be better indicators of asthma in the elderly, because older patients can have less skin-test sensitivity to allergens.

Differential diagnosis between asthma and chronic obstructive pulmonary disease (COPD) is important, especially in current and ex-smokers. Asthma has a different natural history than COPD, and a better prognosis with treatment. With asthma medication, the elderly, like other populations, are often able to achieve symptom relief and improved quality of life. A trial of systemic corticosteroid therapy is often useful to assess reversibility and determine an accurate diagnosis.

Treatment.   The four components of asthma care, including monitoring with objective measures of lung function, comprehensive pharmacologic therapy, environmental control, and patient education also pertain to the elderly, only with special considerations.

The goal of asthma treatment is to achieve an optimal level of activity and quality of life. More specific goals include optimizing pulmonary function, controlling cough and nocturnal symptoms, preventing exacerbations, promoting prompt recognition and treatment of exacerbations, reduction in the need for ED visits or hospitalizations, avoiding aggravation of other medical conditions, and minimizing adverse effects from medications.[17] These goals may be more difficult to achieve in elderly patients. For example, normal lung function may be either unattainable or attainable only with high, potentially dangerous doses of medications. Conversely, elderly patients may have unnecessarily restricted their lifestyles to accommodate their asthma. Further restriction of activity can pose additional health risks and problems for the elderly.

It is essential that the older patient learn how to detect symptoms of worsening asthma and that a written plan be developed in advance for dealing with exacerbations. The plan should specify thresholds for medical supervision, particularly because heart disease and other coexisting conditions or their therapy can confound symptoms and treatment of asthma exacerbations. Providing education about management to family and any caregivers also promotes compliance with therapy. Elderly patients may require additional education to understand the proper use of their medications. For example, metered dose inhaler (MDI) techniques can be increasingly difficult to master with advancing age, due to decreased hand strength and arthritis, and may require different inhalation devices and spacers.

For all elderly patients with asthma, lung function monitoring (with FEV_1 or peak expiratory flow rate [PEFR]) should be performed in the physician's office every 3 to 6 months. Daily PEF monitoring is important, especially for patients who do not perceive symptoms early. Elderly patients in particular may mistakenly attribute their worsening signs and symptoms to the effects of aging rather than deteriorating asthma. However, for some patients, home PEFR monitoring may be limited by age-related factors that compromise the effort required for accurate measurements. Symptom monitoring and using diaries may help elderly patients better assess their progress and become more sensitive to worsening asthma. Key indicators of worsening asthma include nocturnal or early morning awakenings with wheeze or cough, increased cough, increased use of or diminished response to beta$_2$ agonists, and decreased tolerance to exercise, including activities of daily living.

The same factors that trigger acute asthma exacerbations also affect the elderly with asthma, although sensitivity to inhaled allergens is less prevalent. Among the most common asthma triggers for elderly patients are respiratory infections and medications for other diseases.[17] The elderly with asthma should have regular immunizations, against pneumococcal infections and yearly influenza vaccination (flu shots). Smoking or exposure to tobacco smoke and other environmental allergens should be avoided.

The risk of adverse effects from asthma treatment increases with age and often limits the choice, dosage, and frequency of medications for the elderly. A stepwise approach to pharmacologic therapy is appropriate for asthma management in patients of all ages, including the elderly. Treatment of exacerbations also follows a stepwise approach to therapy, with frequent administration of inhaled beta$_2$ agonists, early administration of systemic corticosteroids, and oxygen supplementation. The elderly require some special considerations due to an increased likelihood of coexisting diseases treated with medications and possible drug interactions. They can also have adverse reactions or greater susceptibility to side effects. For example, systemic corticosteroids pose increased risks because they have a lower metabolic clearance rate in elderly patients.

Respiratory therapists can provide the education needed to raise the expectations of asthma treatment for the elderly to the highest possible levels. In defining individual treatment goals for elderly patients with asthma, respiratory therapists should pay significant attention to quality-of-life issues, including the restoration, maintenance, and extension of an independent, active, and personally satisfying lifestyle. Patient education must focus on working jointly with patients to set realistic, achievable goals. Together, the respiratory therapist and patient should develop a specific treatment plan to reach those goals and to establish the basis for a partnership in care.

CONSIDERATION OF COSTS AND ETHICAL ISSUES

It is estimated that the total economic costs for asthma in 1990 were $6.2 billion, including health care expenditures, mortality, lost school days, and days missed from work.[6] Consequently, the NAEPP has broadened its focus beyond clinical and biomedical asthma management to the economics of asthma management.[18] It has been shown that the costs for asthma prescriptions increase whenever there is better patient education and management. Does this mean that disease management costs more? The best answer is "not really." How can this be? It has been shown that the costs for ED visits and hospitalizations go down in those patients who have increased costs for asthma medications, so the net result is savings in health care costs. You and your colleagues must work together to consider these comprehensive costs for management of asthma. This also holds true for any chronic disease management. It is important to look at the complete picture over an extended period to accurately assess the total costs of health care.

What are the key cost considerations in the management of asthma? Who pays for the health care? Are less expensive treatments available? What are the most cost-effective strategies in the long-term management of asthma? How can respiratory therapists help control the costs of asthma management? These are the types of questions we need to ask. Specifically answer these questions when you discuss the case study in this chapter.

Despite the need for information by clinical and health system decision makers, too little evidence is available on the cost effectiveness of alternative asthma management strategies. Indeed, even the NAEPP therapeutic recommendations lack economic justification, although increasing numbers of studies are reporting data on the cost effectiveness of asthma care.[18] Faculty, students, and respiratory therapists should read current journals for original studies reporting on the cost effectiveness of the numerous asthma strategies for acute and long-term management.

PATIENT EDUCATION, HEALTH PROMOTION, AND QUALITY-OF-LIFE ISSUES

Health education must be incorporated into asthma care to effectively manage this chronic disease. Table 11-1 shows the recommended components for implementing an effective asthma education program to encourage wellness and improve quality of life for persons with asthma. Figure 11-3 shows a self-management form to monitor key indicators of asthma control.[2] Figure 11-4 shows an example of an action plan for persons with asthma to follow in response to any changes in these key indicators.[2] It is unfortunate that the health care system and health care providers often do not adequately address the educational needs of patients with asthma.

Patient compliance with care plans is a real concern in the management of chronic diseases, including asthma. Even when adequate patient education is provided, many patients do not follow through with recommendations. Lack of patient compliance interferes with quality of life and can result in near-fatal or fatal asthma exacerbations. Patients at greatest risk for noncompliance include teenagers, especially males, persons from minority groups, those of low socioeconomic status (SES), and inner city dwellers.

Asthma decreases quality of life due to restriction of normal activity, school absences, and lost wages of the caregivers. Until recently, assessment of disability from chronic diseases such as asthma has been based primarily on physiologic measures of impairment, such as pulmonary function testing. While physiologic indices of asthma remain important, there is increased attention paid to determining the impact of patient symptoms and the ability of patients to function in their day-to-day lives. There is growing interest on the part of investigators and clinicians in determining how clinical interventions affect quality of life. Health-related quality of life (HRQL) is increasingly being used as an outcome measure in clinical trials and disease management to determine effectiveness of asthma care. HRQL outcomes are used as a means of determining how clinical interventions affect the physical function, social function, and mental health of patients with asthma.[19]

The acute and chronic aspects of asthma are distressing to children and adults. A chronic illness like asthma can produce considerable stress that can affect physical and emotional health, school achievement, and social activities. The potential for an asthma attack and the care required in day-to-day living are stress producers.[20,21] This stress can affect the emotional life of the patient and the family. In addition, emotional stress has long been recognized as a factor exacerbating or precipitating asthma attacks,[22] and this can create a vicious cycle. Difficulty in breathing can arouse the fear of

TABLE 11-1 COMPONENTS OF EFFECTIVE ASTHMA EDUCATION

Basic facts about asthma

The contrast between asthmatic airways and normal airways

What happens to the airways during and after an asthma attack?

Roles of medications

How medications work

Long-term control: Medications that prevent symptoms, often by reducing inflammation

Quick relief: Short-acting bronchodilators relax muscles around airways

Stress the importance of regular use of long-term-control medications and warn not to expect quick relief from them

Skills

Inhaler use (have the patient demonstrate proper use)

Spacer/holding chamber use (have the patient demonstrate proper use)

Symptom monitoring, PEFR monitoring, and recognizing early signs of deterioration

Documentation of daily record of pulmonary function and symptoms

Appropriate response to key indicators by stepping up or stepping down treatment

Environmental control measures

Identifying and avoiding environmental precipitants or exposures

Describe actions taken to avoid exposure to indoor and outdoor allergens

When and how to take rescue actions

Describe correct response to changes in asthma severity (daily self-management plan and action plan)

death in anyone. In the child, fear of asthma may promote a sense of inferiority and helplessness, and this fear can impede the development of independence.[23] Perception of illness can be quite different from the actual condition, so it is important to understand the patient's perceptions and to individualize care accordingly.

The ways people cope with stressors may be more directly related to health and illness than the frequency and severity of the stressors themselves. The presence of psychological problems correlates with poorer outcomes in asthma, including sudden death, more than the severity of asthma symptoms.[24] Emotional responses such as panic and stress can affect physiologic measures, including pulmonary function, rehospitalization rates, and intensity of discharge treatments.[21] Respiratory

therapists must educate patients to help them cope with their chronic disease. HRQL instruments are important to evaluate the long-term management of asthma.

Table 11-2 describes quality-of-life instruments that can be utilized in the long-term management of asthma.[21,25–34] These instruments ask questions related to the patient's symptoms and physical health including activity limitations, but they also assess psychological and emotional well-being. Note that it is also important to assess the quality of life of the caregivers when dealing with children who have asthma. It is equally important to directly assess the child's quality of life and not rely solely on the caregiver's assessment, in order to maximize patient education, compliance, and well being.[35]

ASTHMA SELF-MANAGEMENT PLAN FOR _____
                                                                  (Name)

YOUR TREATMENT GOALS

_____ Be free from severe symptoms day and night, including sleeping through the night

_____ Have the best possible lung function

_____ Be able to participate fully in any activities of your choice

_____ Not miss work or school because of asthma symptoms

_____ Not need emergency visits or hospitalizations for asthma

_____ Use asthma medications to control asthma with as few side effects as possible

Add personal goals here: _____

_____

_____

YOUR DAILY MEDICATIONS

Daily Medication   How Much to Take   When to Take It

_____

_____

_____

_____

RECORD DAILY SELF-MONITORING ACTIONS in the asthma diary your doctor gives you.

Peak flow: At least every morning when you wake up, before taking your medication, measure your peak flow and record it in your diary. Bring these records to your next appointment with your doctor.

Symptoms: Note if you had asthma symptoms (shortness of breath, wheezing, chest tightness, or cough) and rate how severe they were during the day or night: mild, moderate, severe.

Use of your quick-relief inhaler (bronchodilator): Keep a record of the number of puffs you needed to use each day or night to control your symptoms.

Actual use of daily medications

Activity restriction

F I G U R E   1 1 - 3   Asthma daily self-management plan. (_Source: National Heart, Lung, and Blood Institute._[2])

Name _____ Date _____

ASTHMA ACTION PLAN

It is important in managing asthma to keep track of your symptoms, medications, and peak expiratory flow rate (PEFR). You can use the colors of a traffic light to help learn your asthma medications:

A. Green means Go: Use preventive (antiinflammatory) medicine.

B. Yellow means Caution: Use quick-relief (short-acting bronchodilator) medicine in addition to the preventive medicine.

C. Red means STOP! Get help from a doctor.

---

a. **Your GREEN ZONE is _____ 80% to 100% of your personal best. GO!**

Breathing is good with no cough, wheeze, or chest tightness during work, school, exercise, or play.

ACTION:

Continue with medications listed in your daily treatment plan.

---

b. **Your YELLOW ZONE is _____ 50% to less than 80% of your personal best.**
CAUTION!

Asthma symptoms are present (cough, wheeze, chest tightness).

Your peak flow number drops below _____ or you notice:

• Increased need for inhaled quick-relief medicine

• Increased asthma symptoms upon awakening

• Awakening at night with asthma symptoms

• _____ .

ACTIONS:

Take _____ puffs of your quick-relief (bronchodilator) medicine _____ .

Repeat _____ times.

Take _____ puffs of _____ (antiinflammatory) _____ times/day.

Begin/increase treatment with oral steroids:

Take _____ mg of _____ every a.m. _____ p.m. _____ .

Call your doctor (phone) _____ or emergency room _____ .

---

c. **Your RED ZONE is 50% or less of your best. DANGER!!**

Your peak flow number drops below, or you continue to get worse after increasing treatment according to the directions above.

ACTIONS:

Take _____ puffs of your quick-relief (bronchodilator) medicine _____ .

Repeat _____ times

Begin/increase treatment with oral steroids. Take _____ mg now.

Call your doctor now (phone _____). If you cannot contact your doctor, go directly to the emergency room (phone _____).

Other important phone numbers for transportation _____ .

AT ANY TIME, CALL YOUR DOCTOR IF:

Asthma symptoms worsen while you are taking oral steroids, or inhaled bronchodilator treatments are not lasting 4 hours, or

Your peak flow number remains or falls below _____ in spite of following the plan.

Physician
Signature _____

Patient's/Family Member's
Signature _____

FIGURE 11-4 Asthma action plan. (*SOURCE: National Heart, Lung, and Blood Institute.*[2])

TABLE 11-2   ASTHMA OUTCOME ASSESSMENT INSTRUMENTS

Pediatric asthma

- *About My Asthma:*[21,22] The About My Asthma Questionnaire is a disease-specific instrument designed to assess the number and types of stressors affecting the quality of life in children with asthma. The questionnaire asks children to rate how often they have certain thoughts and feelings that contribute to stress and decreased quality of life.

- *Childhood Asthma Questionnaire:*[26] The CAQ is a disease-specific instrument to assess children's perceptions of both active and passive aspects of living with asthma, together with their perceptions of its severity and any associated distress.

- *Functional Severity Index:*[27] The Functional Severity Index is a measure of functional impairment (ie, symptoms and restrictions) caused by asthma in school-aged children.

- *KINDL:*[28] The German KINDL is a generic, reliable, valid, and practical instrument to assess the HRQOL of children with chronic illness. This instrument should be supplemented by disease-specific asthma assessments.

- *Pediatric Asthma Caregiver's Quality of Life Questionnaire:*[29] The Pediatric Asthma Caregiver's Quality of Life Questionnaire (PACQLQ) is a 13-item disease-specific instrument designed to measure the impact of children's asthma on their primary caregiver's quality of life, and specifically how it affects normal daily activities and contributes to anxieties and fears.

- *Pediatric Asthma Quality of Life Questionnaire:*[30] The PAQLQ measures the impact of asthma on children's daily lives. It is intended to be administered to children aged 7 to 17, preferably by an interviewer, but a self-administered version is also available.

Adult asthma

- *Asthma Quality of Life Questionnaire—Juniper:*[31] The Asthma Quality of Life Questionnaire—Juniper is a disease-specific HRQOL instrument developed by Juniper and colleagues that assesses both the physical and emotional aspects of asthma.

- *Asthma Quality of Life Questionnaire—Marks:*[32] The Asthma Quality of Life Questionnaire—Marks is a self-administered questionnaire for adults. The respondents are asked to describe how troubling particular items have been over the previous 4 weeks. It covers both physical and emotional aspects.

- *Living With Asthma Questionnaire:*[33] The Living With Asthma Questionnaire is a disease-specific health-care–related quality-of-life questionnaire designed to evaluate the patient's subjective experiences with asthma, including both functional limitations and distress. It addresses the domains of social/leisure, sport, sleep, holidays, work and other activities, colds, mobility, effects on others, medication use, sex, dysphoric states, and attitudes.

- *Perceived Control of Asthma Questionnaire:*[34] The Perceived Control of Asthma Questionnaire is a disease-specific instrument designed to measure the individual's perceived ability to deal with asthma and its exacerbations.

- *St. George's Respiratory Questionnaire:*[35] The St. George's Respiratory Questionnaire is designed for use by patients with fixed and reversible airway obstruction to measure impact on overall health, daily life, and perceived well-being. It addresses the frequency and severity of symptoms, activities that cause or are limited by breathlessness, and impacts regarding social functioning, and psychological disturbances that are the result of airways disease.

INTRODUCTION TO THE CASE STUDY

Now you proceed into the most exciting part of this chapter by working your way through a hypothetical case. Your instructor will direct you to identify learning issues, answer specific case questions, and prepare for individual and/or group exercises. Your instructor will determine the approach to problem-based learning (PBL) and the choice of assignments. Both will depend on the available time, types of patients you are likely to encounter in your clinical rotations, and resources available. Please check with your instructor to verify how to proceed with the case. Please do not read the case ahead of time or without specific instructions. PBL is a process, but a textbook is a product; therefore, the way you use this text will depend on the approach adopted by your faculty. Please follow your faculty's instructions carefully so you can maximize the benefit from the learning experience. We hope your learning will transcend the content in this section.

The following questions and exercises are designed to help you expand your knowledge of asthma, and to prepare you for situations you will likely encounter in your respiratory care practice. The overview of asthma gave you the background necessary to work on the exercises and to answer some of the questions. However, to really provide a thorough and up-to-date response to many of the questions and exercises, you will need to consult additional resource materials. Of course, you are prepared for this, since this is one goal of PBL. You will learn by working through patient problems that require you to go out and find the resources to solve them.

The chapter incorporates the following to allow you to apply your understanding of asthma. The case asks specific questions to assess your understanding of the diagnosis, treatment, and long-term management of asthma. The case should challenge you to evaluate age-specific considerations, patient education needs, health care costs, and ethical concerns of asthma management. Whenever possible, the case will prompt more than one recommendation for patient care to allow comparisons of the advantages, disadvantages, and limitation of various approaches to asthma management. Furthermore, cases in this textbook are designed for small and large group discussion to facilitate critical thinking skills and traits.

CASE STUDY 1

KNIGHT COFFMAN

Initial Case Scenario

A 23-year-old male visits the emergency department (ED) with the chief complaint being shortness of breath. When you enter the ED, you see the patient sitting forward at the edge of the examining table. His respirations appear rapid and shallow. He appears to be having great difficulty breathing.

 Critical Thinking Exercise 1

PRIORITIZING PATIENT CARE

Explain how you would prioritize your patient assessment and treatment during the first few minutes of Mr. Coffman's arrival to the ED.

Case History

Your initial assessment verifies that Mr. Coffman has a history of asthma. He complains of dyspnea, nighttime coughing, and tightness in his chest over the past 1 or 2 days. Three days earlier, he developed a sore throat, swollen glands, rhinitis, and a low-grade fever. His wife experienced a similar respiratory illness earlier that week. He also developed congestion and a productive cough in the mornings with yellow-tinged sputum. The patient says, "I spent most of the night trying to sleep in a chair because I couldn't breathe easily when lying down." His usual treatment for asthma management includes albuterol via MDI (two puffs PRN). Mr. Coffman reports that he usually ends up using his inhaler "about daily,

---

occasionally two or three times on a bad day." He said over the past 48 hours he used his albuterol inhaler seven to nine times during the day and three to four times overnight. He came to the ED because his inhaler would not work and he was short of breath. Mr. Coffman is sitting on the edge of the examining table and leaning forward slightly. His speech is fragmented when he tries to answer your questions.

Critical Thinking Exercise 2

MAKING INFERENCES BY CLUSTERING DATA

a. Describe what is meant by an inference.

b. What inference can you make about Mr. Coffman's work of breathing (WOB)?

c. Practice clustering data that leads you to this inference.

Critical Thinking Exercise 3

ANTICIPATING PHYSICAL EXAM FINDINGS

a. What symptoms are you looking for in this patient?

b. What signs of respiratory distress are likely to be present?

c. What abnormalities would you anticipate in PEFR, oxygenation, and ventilation?

Evaluate the following clinical data and further assess your patient.

CLINICAL DATA ON ADMISSION

Signs and symptoms

HR	126
RR	28

Diaphoretic
Inspiratory and expiratory wheezes
Unable to lie supine

ABG (21%)

pH	7.34
$Paco_2$	38
HCO_3^-	20
Sao_2	92%
Hgb	15

PFT

PEFR	<60% of predicted
FEV_1	<60% of predicted

Mr. Coffman has been in the ED for 4 hours now, and has received the usual respiratory care. Here is the current clinical information available based on his most recent assessment.

CLINICAL DATA 4 HOURS LATER

Signs and symptoms

HR	126
RR	30

Very diminished breath sounds
Pulsus paradoxus 20 mm Hg

ABG 6 LPM NC

pH	7.32
$Paco_2$	40
Pao_2	60
Sao_2	90%
HCO_3^-	5.2

PFT

PEFR 43% of predicted, fails to improve by 10%
FEV_1 39% of predicted

CASE STUDY 1   *(continued)*

Mr. Coffman has been admitted to the ICU and has been receiving oxygen, bronchodilators via continuous nebulization, and corticosteroids. The following are the most recent data available.

CLINICAL DATA 8 HOURS AFTER ARRIVAL TO ED

Signs and symptoms

HR   130
RR   33
Silent chest
Pulsus paradoxus 22 mm Hg
Pt. is drowsy

ABG 6 LPM NC

pH   7.23
$Paco_2$ 44
Pao_2 60
Sao_2 90%
HCO_3^- 20

PFT

PEFR   160 L/min
            25% of predicted
            (636 L/min)
FEV_1 39% of predicted

Based on the new data provided, perform the following exercise.

Critical Thinking Exercise 4

ANTICIPATING PROBLEMS AND SOLUTIONS

The ability to foresee or anticipate problems is a very important critical thinking skill.

a. Based on the clinical data most recently collected and your analysis of this data, what problems do you anticipate in this case and what would you propose as a solution?

b. What problems would you anticipate based on Mr. Coffman's response so far?

c. What actions would you anticipate at this time or in the immediate future?

Based on the entire case, perform the following exercise.

Critical Thinking Exercise 5

REFLECTION ON YOUR DECISIONS AND ACTIONS TO IMPROVE CLINICAL DECISION MAKING

a. Describe why and how you would reflect on this case in order to figure out retrospectively what worked or did not work.

b. How would you use this information to manage cases in the future?

c. Why is reflection important to your practice?

Group Critical Thinking Exercises

The following exercises are intended to allow the learner to apply numerous strategies to enhance critical thinking in clinical practice. We suggest that the learner work on these exercises in small groups. The learners and PBL facilitator should work together to determine which of the following exercises would be most beneficial. If possible, we suggest that all of these exercises be completed during some portion of the curriculum. It is likely that certain exercises would be incorporated within a particular course within the curriculum. However, these exercises can be interwoven throughout the curriculum and be revisited in future courses, labs, and clinical experiences.

Group Critical Thinking Exercise 1

THE PRO/CON TEAM DEBATE

a. Use this case to present the argument that Mr. Coffman needs to be intubated and mechanically ventilated 4 hours after admission to the ED. Provide data, evidence, and reasons to support your group's recommendation. Explicitly state the special circumstances, needs, and considerations at this point in the case management. Be sure to explain why this deci-

CASE STUDY 1 *(continued)*

sion is the best one at the time and what could happen if there are any further delays. Have one team (three to five students) prepare this recommendation to intubate and ventilate, while a different team prepares the opposite recommendation.

b. This anti-intubation team uses the same case and data to develop the argument that Mr. Coffman should not be intubated or ventilated at this point in this ED admission. Again, they should provide data, evidence, and reasons to support their recommendation to delay intubation at this point. The instructor acts as the discussion facilitator, keeping the discussion going, but not supporting either position.

c. The debate can be presented to a third group if the class is large enough. This group can serve as judges to express their opinions on the persuasiveness of the arguments presented by the two debating sides of the issue.

d. After the exercise, as a combined group, the entire class can discuss which team appeared to make the more persuasive case. How and why was their case made more effectively?

**Variation of
Group Critical Thinking Exercise 1**

In this variation the teams above switch sides, with each arguing the opposing side of the debate. Was one group or the other able to make a more persuasive argument? Remember, the more able you are to see both sides of a position, the more effective a critical thinker you are likely to become.

**Other Variations to
Group Critical Thinking Exercise 1**

Other variations to group exercise 1 include debating issues with a narrower focus. The following questions will allow debate on one particular aspect of the respiratory care of status asthmaticus.

a. Follow the same directions as in group exercise 1, but have the opposing groups debate this issue: application of NPPV versus conventional intubation/ventilation for Mr. Coffman, 4 hours after admission to the ED.

Group Critical Thinking Exercise 2

**DECISION MAKING:
RECOMMENDING AN ACTION PLAN**

Based on the clinical data presented after 8 hours in the ED, what would probably be the best action to recommend at this point in the patient's management? Support your decisions with your reasons for making your recommendation(s).

Group Critical Thinking Exercise 3

**PROBLEM SOLVING
AND REFLECTION**

a. This exercise is designed to have the learner apply what they learned about ABGs to another example. The exercise further challenges your creative abilities because it asks you to actually come up with an example of an arterial blood gas analysis. Through the process of creating another example, you can test your understanding of ABGs while further developing your reflection and problem solving skills.

CASE STUDY 1 *(continued)*

b. Reflect on the complete description of the blood gas interpretation for the case of Mr. Coffman to explain why it is insufficient to rely on the numbers alone when interpreting an ABG. Then use your problem-solving skills to figure out the following example of a blood gas analysis that can have more than one interpretation based on the specific case.

First, what is the interpretation of the following ABG based strictly on the data (patient is on 30% oxygen): pH = 7.52, $Paco_2$ = 42 mm Hg, Pao_2 = 85 mm Hg, BE = +10, HCO_3^- = 34.5 mEq/L.

Now propose a different interpretation by identifying how additional clinical and historical data may completely change your initial interpretation.

Group Critical Thinking Exercise 4

DECISION MAKING—DEVELOPING A CARE PLAN

a. Use the information from case 1 to develop a long-term care plan with Mr. Coffman to manage his asthma. Describe your care plan for discharge from the hospital and for long-term care including follow-up visits.

b. Describe what outcome measures you will utilize to assess the effectiveness of Mr. Coffman's disease management. This exercise gives the learner the opportunity to make decisions involving the long-term management of Mr. Coffman's asthma. The exercise further asks you to consider how you will successfully measure the health care outcomes.

Group Critical Thinking Exercise 5

COMMUNICATION AND NEGOTIATION

Describe how you would communicate and negotiate with other members of the health care team in the overall management of the patient in case 1. In particular, discuss what you would do if your recommendations were not accepted.

Group Critical Thinking Exercise 6

DECISION MAKING INVOLVING COSTS AND ETHICS

Discuss the cost considerations in the immediate treatment and long-term management of Mr. Coffman's asthma. Also, describe strategies to decrease Mr. Coffman's out-of-pocket expenses for his asthma management as well as the total costs for the health care provider.

This exercise is designed for you to consider the costs of health care from two perspectives: 1) what are the actual out-of-pocket expenses for the patient? and 2) what are the actual health care costs for the providers? To determine Mr. Coffman's expenses for long-term management of his chronic disease, you will need to consider what insurance coverage he has and what he would actually be billed for various services. To understand health care costs from the perspective of the provider you will need to understand the difference between the actual costs (direct and indirect costs) of care as compared to the actual charges appearing on the bill.

CASE STUDY 1 *(continued)*

Group Critical Thinking 7

DECISION MAKING AND RELATED ETHICAL ISSUES

Now, consider what you would do (decision making) if you find that Mr. Coffman smokes cigarettes every day? How will this information affect your long-term management plan? What are the ethical considerations?

Group Critical Thinking Exercise 8

BECOMING A PROFESSIONAL— HAVING A BROAD PERSPECTIVE OF YOUR PRACTICE AND YOUR PROFESSION

Discuss the role of the respiratory therapist in asthma education and disease management. This exercise is designed to give you the opportunity to think about the broader perspectives of the department, the organization, and the profession.

KEY POINTS

- Asthma is the most common chronic illness in children and a common chronic disease for adults, affecting 10 to 15 million people in the US.

- Asthma is the most misdiagnosed and under-diagnosed illness in children under 5 years of age, probably due to an inability to obtain objective measures of lung function.

- Approximately 5000 people die every year from asthma.

- The incidence, morbidity, and mortality have increased, despite better understanding of effective asthma management and improved asthma medications and treatments.

- Asthma accounts for the majority of missed school days and parents' lost wages, which accounts for a significant amount of the total health care costs.

- Asthma has a major impact on the quality of life of children, adults, and caregivers.

- The airway obstruction caused by asthma is now thought to be due to four different mechanisms, all a result of the inflammatory process central to the disease: 1) acute spasm of the involuntary (smooth) muscle of the airway (ie, bronchocon-

striction), 2) swelling of the airway resulting in reduction of the internal lumen diameter (ie, airway edema), 3) excessive production of mucus from the goblet cells lining the airway (ie, mucus plug formation), and 4) changes in airway structure (eg, increased numbers of goblet cells and deposition of interstitial collagens beneath the epithelium).

- Every asthma attack has the potential to be fatal, just as every asthma attack has the potential to be reversed!

- There are the four aspects of asthma management to prevent exacerbations: 1) objective measures of lung function, 2) comprehensive pharmacologic therapy, 3) environmental control measures to reduce allergens, and 4) patient education.

- These are the goals of acute asthma care: 1) correction of hypoxemia, 2) rapid reversal of airway obstruction using an inhaled beta$_2$ agonist, and 3) early treatment of airway inflammation using corticosteroids.

- Status asthmaticus is a serious exacerbation that does not respond to initial therapy, placing the patient at risk of respiratory failure.

- Status asthmaticus requires aggressive treatment for reversal of airway obstruction and to provide adequate ventilation (ie, continuous nebulization, heliox, NPPV, mechanical ventilation).

SUGGESTED RESOURCES

http://www.nhlbi.nih.gov/guidelines/asthma/asthgdln.htm

http://www.nhlbi.nih.gov/health/prof/lung/index.htm

http://allergy.mcg.edu/physicians/manual/manual.html

REFERENCES

1. Centers for Disease Control and Prevention. Asthma —United States, 1989-1992. *MMWR*. 1995;43: 952–955.

2. National Heart, Lung, and Blood Institute. Expert panel report II: Guidelines for the diagnosis and management of asthma. National Asthma Education and Prevention Program, 1997.

3. Adams PF, Marano MA. Current estimates from the National Health Interview Survey, 1994. *Vital Health Stat*. 1995;10:94, or Lee DA, Winslow NR, Speight ANP, Hey EN. Prevalence and spectrum of asthma in childhood. *Br Med J*. 1983;286: 1256–1258.

4. Weiss KB, Gergen PJ, Hodgson TA. An economic evaluation of asthma in the United States. *N Engl J Med* 1992;326:862–866.

5. Fowler MG, Davenport MG, Garg R. School functioning of US children with asthma. *Pediatrics*. 1992;90:939–944.

6. Walton JR. Understanding the cost of health care with specific attention to respiratory care. *Respir Care*. 1997;42:54–70.

7. McFadden ER Jr, Elsandi N, Dison L, et al. Protocol therapy for acute asthma: therapeutic benefits and cost-savings. *Am J Med*. 1995;99: 651–661.

8. Lawrence G. Asthma self-management programs can reduce the need for hospital-based asthma care. *Respir Care*. 1995;40:39–43.

9. Wilson SR, Scamagas P, German DF, et al. A controlled trial of two forms of self-management education for adults with asthma. *Am J Med*. 1993;94: 564–576.

10. National Heart, Lung, and Blood Institute. *Global Initiative for Asthma*. National Institutes of Health. (NIH Publication No. 95-3659): 1995.

11. Corbridge TC, Hall JB. State of the art: The assessment and management of adults with status asthmaticus. *Am J Respir Crit Care Med*. 1995;151: 1296–1316.

12. Lin RY, Sauter D, Newman T, et al. Continuous versus intermittent albuterol nebulization in the treatment of acute asthma. *Ann Emerg Med*. 1993;22: 1847–1853.

13. Kelly HW, Murphy S. Beta-adrenergic agonists for acute, severe asthma. *Ann Pharmacother*. 1992;26: 81–91.

14. Rowe BH, Keller JL, Oxman AD. Effectiveness of steroid therapy in acute exacerbations of asthma: a meta-analysis. *Am J Emerg Med*. 1992;10:301–310.

15. Feihl F, Perret C. Permissive hypercapnia-how permissive should we be? *Am J Respir Crit Care Med*. 1994;150:1722–1737.

16. Kacmarek RM, Hickling KG. Permissive hypercapnia. *Respir Care*. 1993;38:373–384.

17. National Heart, Lung, and Blood Institute. NAEPP Working Group Report: Considerations for Diagnosing and Managing Asthma in the Elderly. (NIH Publication No. 96-3662): 1996.

18. National Heart, Lung, and Blood Institute. National Asthma Education and Prevention Program Task Force on the Cost Effectiveness, Quality of Care, and Financing of Asthma Care. (NIH Publication No. 55-807): 1996.

19. Wilson IB, Cleary PD. Linking clinical variables with health-related quality of life. *JAMA*. 1995; 273:59–65.

20. Mishoe SC, Baker RR, Poole S, et al. The development and evaluation of a new instrument to assess stress levels and quality of life for children with asthma. *Am J Respir Crit Care Med*. 1996;153:A549.

21. Mishoe SC, Baker RR, Poole S, et al. The development of an instrument to assess stress levels and quality of life in children with asthma. *J Asthma*. 1998;35:553–563.

22. Miller BD, Wood BL. Psychophysiologic reactivity in asthmatic children: A new perspective on emotionally triggered asthma. *Pediatr Asthma Allergy Immunol*. 1995;9:133–142.

23. Richards JM, Hemstreet MP. Measures of life quality, role performance, and functional status in asthma research. *Am J Respir Crit Care Med*. 1994; 149:S31–S39.

24. Sly RM. Increases in deaths from asthma. *Ann Allergy*. 1984;53:20–25.

25. French DJ, Christie MJ, Sowden AJ. The repro-
    ducibility of the childhood asthma questionnaires:
    measures of quality of life for children with asthma
    aged 4–16 years. *Qual Life Res*. 1994:3;215–224.

26. Rosier MJ, Bishop J, Nolan T, et al. Measurement
    of functional severity of asthma in children. *Am J
    Respir Crit Care Med*. 1994;149:1434–1441.

27. Ravens-Sieberer U, Bullinger M. Assessing health-
    related quality of life in chronically ill children with
    the German KINDL: first psychometric and content
    analytical results. *Qual Life Res*. 1998;7:399–407.

28. Juniper ER, Guyatt GH, Feeny DH, et al.
    Measuring quality of life in the parents of children
    with asthma. *Qual Life Res*. 1996;5:27–34.

29. Juniper EF, Guyatt GH, Feeny DH, et al. Measuring
    quality of life in children with asthma. *Qual Life
    Res*. 1996;5:35–46.

30. Juniper EF, Guyatt GH, Epstein RS, et al.
    Evaluation of impairment of health-related quality
    of life in asthma: development of a questionnaire
    for use in clinical trials. *Thorax*. 1992;47:76–83.

31. Marks GB, Dunn SM, Woolcock AJ, et al. An eval-
    uation of an asthma quality of life questionnaire as
    a measure of change in adults with asthma. *J Clin
    Epidemiol*. 1993;46:1103–1111.

32. Reid LD, Nau DP, Grainger-Rousseau TJ. Evalu-
    ation of patient's health-related quality of life using
    a modified and shortened version of the Living with
    Asthma Questionnaire (MS;LWAQ) and the med-
    ical outcomes, short form 36 (SF-36). *Qual Life
    Res*. 1999;8: 491–499.

33. Katz PP, Yelin EH, Smith S, et al. Perceived control
    of asthma: development and validation of a ques-
    tionnaire. *Am J Respir Crit Care Med* 1997;155:
    577–582.

34. Jones PW, Quirk FH, Baveystock CM, et al. The St.
    George's Respiratory Questionnaire. *Respir Med*.
    1991;85:25–31.

35. Baker RR, Mishoe SC, Harrell LM, et al. Assess-
    ment of caregiver's knowledge of asthma and qual-
    ity of life. *Am J Respir Dis Crit Care Med*. 1996;
    153:A754 (suppl).

12

EMMA SEEMA AND FRIENDS: CASES INVOLVING COPD

Salvatore A. Sanders and Leslie C. Patzwahl

The mind once stretched by a new idea
can never return to its original dimensions.
OLIVER WENDELL HOLMES
1809–1894

LEARNING OBJECTIVES

1. Describe facts, descriptions, and definitions related to chronic obstructive pulmonary disease (COPD).
2. Discuss the etiology, pathophysiology, and clinical features of a patient with COPD.
3. Discuss the acute and long-term management of patients with COPD including health promotion and quality-of-life issues.
4. Apply specific formulas and theories to assist in clinical decision making in the management of a patient with COPD.
5. Apply the critical thinking skills of prioritizing, anticipating, negotiating, communicating, decision making, and reflection by completing exercises and case examples involving patients with COPD.
6. Apply strategies to promote critical thinking in the respiratory care management of patients with COPD through completion of the case exercises and participation in group discussion.
7. Use clinical case examples in the chapter to perform an initial patient assessment, using a standardized system (SOAP) and the clinical data presented.
8. Interpret clinical data from the case examples including: history, physical examination, lab data, and radiographic data to make recommendations for respiratory care management.
9. Develop a care plan for the patients in each case example, including recommendations for respiratory care management.
10. Communicate facts, evidence, and arguments to support evaluations and recommendations proposed in the care plan for the patient with COPD.
11. Practice the skill of negotiating in an attempt to persuade others to accept your care plan for each case.
12. Evaluate treatment and outcomes of interventions to propose changes in the care plan for each patient with COPD.
13. Describe the role of the respiratory therapist in the diagnosis, treatment, and management of COPD.

KEY WORDS

Air Trapping
Airway Obstruction
Alpha$_1$-Antitrypsin
Chronic Obstructive
  Pulmonary Disease
  (COPD)
Chronic Bronchitis

Durable Powers of Attor-
  ney for Health Care
Emphysema
Hyperinflation
Irreversible Airway
  Obstruction
Living Will
Pursed-Lip Breathing

CHAPTER DESCRIPTION

This chapter provides an overview of chronic obstructive pulmonary disease (COPD), including discussion of its etiology, pathophysiology, and related theory, as well as the clinical features, laboratory findings, and an overview of treatment associated with COPD. Three patient case studies are presented. Case 1 presents a patient with exacerbation of COPD and guides the reader through issues related to the patient's inpatient management, as well as considerations for home care and rehabilitation. The second case reveals the pulmonary function test results of two patients and asks the reader to classify the severity of the patients' COPD and interpret the results of pulmonary function tests, discussing the type and severity of dysfunction suggested. A third case study offers an additional opportunity to interpret pulmonary function test results and includes diffusion studies and flow volume loops. The case studies are designed to present the reader with realistic information and an opportunity for practical application of knowledge gained through review of the chapter and through independent investigation on the part of the student.

INTRODUCTION

Chronic obstructive pulmonary disease (COPD), as the name implies, is characterized by obstruction of the airways. COPD is not a single disease, but a term describing a collection of respiratory disorders that often coexist. COPD is defined by the American Thoracic Society (ATS) as: "A disease state characterized by the presence of airflow obstruction due to chronic bronchitis or emphysema; the airflow obstruction is generally progressive, may be accompanied by airway hyperactivity, and may be partially reversible."[1] Previous definitions of COPD also included asthma. Although asthma is not specifically mentioned in the ATS definition, this does not mean that asthma does not coexist with emphysema and chronic bronchitis, or that persons with asthma may not develop the largely irreversible obstruction associated with COPD (see Fig. 12-1).[1] In fact, approximately 10% of patients diagnosed with COPD are said to also have asthma.[2] Another recently published definition states that COPD is a collection of diseases that includes asthma, emphysema, and chronic bronchitis, which can exist separately or coexist to varying degrees, and that this group of diseases is characterized by limiting expiratory flow rates.[3] For purposes of this textbook, asthma will be discussed in a separate chapter (see Chapter 11).

According to criteria provided by the American Thoracic Society, a person with chronic bronchitis presents with "a chronic, productive cough for 3 months in each of two successive years," and other causes for this cough are ruled out. Emphysema is defined by the presence of abnormal anatomic changes. "Emphysema is defined as abnormal permanent enlargement of the airspaces distal to the terminal bronchioles, accompanied by destruction of their walls and without obvious fibrosis."[1]

Chronic obstructive pulmonary disease ranks fourth, just behind cerebrovascular diseases, as a cause of death in the United States and accounted for 160,431 US deaths in 1996.[4] The mortality rate for COPD has been increasing throughout the 1990s.[4]

ETIOLOGY

Factors leading to the development of COPD can be divided into environmental and hereditary factors. Cigarette smoking is the greatest risk factor associated with COPD. Other environmental risk factors include second hand smoke from cigarettes,

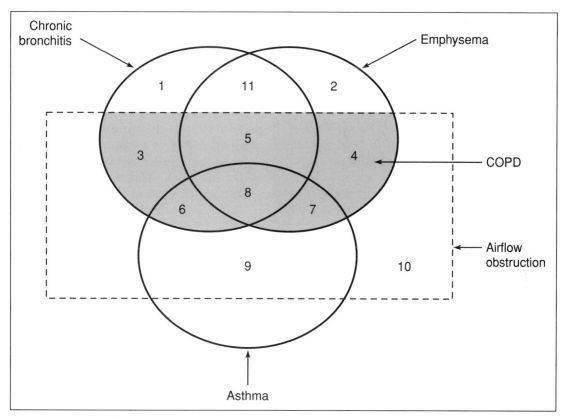

FIGURE 12-1 Schema of chronic obstructive pulmonary disease. This nonproportional Venn diagram shows subsets of patients with chronic bronchitis, emphysema, and asthma. The subsets comprising COPD are shaded. Subset areas are not proportional to actual relative subset sizes. Asthma is by definition associated with reversible airflow obstruction, although in variant asthma special maneuvers may be necessary to make the obstruction evident. Patients with asthma whose airflow obstruction is completely reversible (subset 9) are not considered to have COPD. Because in many cases it is virtually impossible to differentiate patients with asthma whose airflow obstruction does not remit completely from persons with chronic bronchitis and emphysema who have partially reversible airflow obstruction with airway hyperreactivity, patients with unremitting asthma are classified as having COPD (subsets 6, 7, and 8). Chronic bronchitis and emphysema with airflow obstruction usually occur together (subset 5), and some patients may have asthma associated with these two disorders (subset 8). Individuals with asthma exposed to chronic irration, as from cigarette smoke, may develop chronic productive cough, a feature of chronic bronchitis (subset 6). Such patients are often referred to in the United States as having *asthmatic bronchitis* or the *asthmatic form of COPD*. Persons with chronic bronchitis and/or emphysema without airflow obstruction (subsets 1, 2, and 11) are not classified as having COPD. Patients with airway obstruction due to diseases with known etiology or specific pathology, such as cystic fibrosis or obliterative bronchiolitis (subset 10), are not included in this definition. (From American Thoracic Society: Standards for the diagnosis and care of patients with chronic obstructive pulmonary disease. *Am J Respir Care Crit Care Med.* 1995;152:S78.)

occupational dusts, gases, and air pollution. Hereditary risk factors include sex (COPD is more common in males than females), race (Caucasians show a higher mortality rate than non-Caucasians), and the presence of homozygous alpha$_1$-antitrypsin deficiency (AAT).[1,5] Recent evidence suggests that other pulmonary enzymes and inhibitors may also play a role in the development of emphysema.[6] Even apart from AAT, COPD appears more frequently in certain families.[1,5]

PATHOPHYSIOLOGY AND RELATED THEORY

Emphysema and chronic bronchitis are the two main components characterizing COPD. For the purpose of this discussion they will be addressed separately, though they commonly coexist. This section will briefly outline the pathophysiology of chronic obstructive pulmonary disease as well as significant theory that will be useful in understanding how the changes resulting from this disease may affect the patient and the patient's clinical presentation.

Emphysema

The destruction of alveolar tissue, loss of elastic recoil, and weakening of the airways that occurs with emphysema allows the airways to narrow and collapse prematurely. This decreased elastic recoil of the lung results in decreased driving pressure for expiratory flow. The associated loss of alveolar attachments to the small airways as alveolar walls are destroyed in emphysema contributes to the irreversible component of airflow obstruction seen with this disease.[1,6] This decrease in driving pressure combined with early airway closure results in an increased amount of air being trapped in the lungs.[7] This narrowing and early closure of the airways is more pronounced during exhalation. This is a result of the natural increase in pleural pressure that occurs during exhalation, causing the pressure surrounding the airways to increase. Thus obstruction to airflow is greater during expiration than inspiration for all the disease processes that cause airflow obstruction.

It should be noted that airway obstruction is not distributed consistently throughout the lungs, resulting in an uneven distribution of ventilation and perfusion.[8] Gas exchange may also be affected by the presence of bullae (enlarged air spaces) that are ventilated less than normal areas of the lung. This too results in uneven distribution of ventilation and perfusion. This mismatching of ventilation with perfusion results in hypoxemia from areas of the lung where the V/Q ratio is low and increased wasted ventilation (dead space) from areas where the V/Q ratio is high.[7,8]

In patients with emphysema the diffusing capacity is often reduced, whereas patients with chronic bronchitis (without emphysema) commonly have normal diffusing capacity.[7] Fick's law relates that surface area is directly proportional to the rate of diffusion of a gas. In emphysema, the destruction of alveolar walls affects diffusion, because there is less surface area available for gas exchange to take place. In chronic bronchitis there is no loss of alveolar-capillary membrane, and hence no loss in diffusion capacity.

Chronic Bronchitis

Pathologic and structural changes seen with chronic bronchitis include inflammation of the airways, increased mucus production, an increase in the size of bronchial glands, and bronchospasm.[8] Varying degrees of obstruction of the airway may occur due to mucous plugging. This causes alveoli distal to some plugs to contribute to air trapping, while complete obstruction of some airways may lead to small areas of microatelectasis.

As a result of these disease processes, there are many areas of lung that receive reduced ventilation, and a relatively few areas that may receive no ventilation at all. These areas often have relatively normal perfusion, thus creating areas of lung that have a decreased ventilation to perfusion (V/Q) ratio or in the areas of microatelectasis, alveolar shunting. Low V/Q ratios cause hypoxemia, and are probably the primary cause of hypoxemia in chronic bronchitis. Chronic bronchitis may contribute more often to the occurrence of hypoxemia than emphysema, probably due to the increased number of low V/Q areas, as well as the presence of a few areas of microatelectasis as described above. With emphysema there is a loss of alveolar capillaries (decreased perfusion) associated with destruction of the alveolar tissue, whereas in chronic bronchitis the perfusion remains relatively normal while ventilation is decreased to areas supplied by diseased airways.[7]

COPD

Structural changes and other factors cause obstruction to airflow in COPD. The structural changes include inflammation of the airways,[1,6,8,9] fibrosis,[1,8] and an increase in the size of bronchial mucous glands and the number of mucus-producing cells that results in increased mucus production.[1] Airway hyperactivity is found in about 30% of patients.[1,8]

The obstructive dysfunction observed in COPD is caused by disease affecting the small airways that is partially due to inflammation of the airways, and partially due to the loss of support to the small airways that occurs when the alveolar septa are destroyed by emphysema. This obstruction to air movement is largely irreversible. Bronchoconstriction due to inflammation provides a reversible component of obstruction in COPD that has been observed to show a significant response to bronchodilator treatment in approximately one-tenth[2] to one-third of patients with COPD.[1]

Poiseuille's law suggests that as airways narrow, the driving pressure needs to increase if flow through the airways is to remain the same. One can appreciate the increased work of breathing and frustration a patient with COPD experiences as the work of breathing increases due to airway narrowing. The ability to increase driving pressure to keep air flowing through these narrowed airways may be further impaired by decreased elastic recoil resulting from loss of lung tissue. In addition to these problems, air trapping associated with COPD also decreases the efficiency of the diaphragm in moving air during inspiration. As air trapping flattens the diaphragm it makes each contraction mechanically less effective.[7]

CRITICAL CONTENT

- **Chronic Obstructive Pulmonary Disease (COPD):** The American Thoracic Society (ATS) defines COPD as "a disease state characterized by the presence of airflow obstruction due to chronic bronchitis or emphysema; the airflow obstruction is generally progressive, may be accompanied by airway hyperactivity, and may be partially reversible."

- **Chronic Bronchitis:** The ATS defines chronic bronchitis as "the presence of chronic productive cough for 3 months in each of two successive years in a patient in whom other causes of chronic cough have been excluded."

- **Emphysema:** The ATS defines emphysema as "abnormal permanent enlargement of the airspaces distal to the terminal bronchioles, accompanied by destruction of their walls and without obvious fibrosis."

CLINICAL FINDINGS

Many of the clinical findings exhibited by patients with COPD are similar to those found in patients with asthma. These findings include signs of increased work of breathing, bronchoconstriction, increased production and retention of secretions, hyperinflation, and in some cases signs of hypoxemia such as cyanosis. Some of these signs may not be observed in patients with mild COPD, but will be more readily apparent as the disease progresses or during an exacerbation.

History

Historical data should be considered when determining the patient's problems and when deciding if tests such as pulmonary function studies or arterial blood gas (ABG) analysis are warranted. Most patients are diagnosed with COPD at 50 or more years of age when the signs and symptoms become more pronounced. COPD is a progressive disease and patients will likely progress to the point of experiencing dyspnea on exertion around the age of 60 or older. Other historical factors may include occupational exposure to dusts, fumes, gases, and smoke; description of a chronic productive cough, dyspnea, and morning headache (suggestive of hypercapnia, and/or severe hypoxemia); and a history of smoking. Patients with COPD often have a history of 20 or more pack-years of smoking before symptoms are noted.[1] Research indicates that more than 30 pack-years of smoking is one of three variables shown to be useful in diagnosing obstructive airways disease—the other two being diminished breath sounds and a decreased peak flow (<350 L/min).[10]

Physical Assessment

Findings on physical assessment are described in the subsequent sections. These findings have been grouped by the physical assessment technique by which they are commonly identified. Possible problems related to each sign are enclosed in parentheses.

Inspection.   Observations may include: pursed-lip breathing, presence of retractions, tripod posture, use of accessory muscles, nasal flaring, diaphoresis (indicative of increased work of breathing), abdominal paradox (indicates fatigue of the respiratory muscles), dependent edema (possible heart failure), cyanosis (suggestive of hypoxemia), digital clubbing (suggestive of carcinoma), hemoptysis (possible carcinoma, likely mucosal erosion), jugular venous distension (JVD) (heart failure), and purulent sputum (infection/exacerbation).[1]

Palpation.   Findings may include: bilateral reduction in tactile and vocal fremitus (air trapping/hyperinflation), decreased chest expansion (air trapping/hyperinflation), dependent edema (possible heart failure), reduced extrathoracic tracheal length (hyperinflation of chest cage), and active neck muscles (accessory muscle use).

Percussion.   Findings may include: hyperresonant percussion note over the chest and low diaphragmatic position (indicative of air trapping/hyperinflation).

Auscultation.   Findings may include: decreased intensity of breath and heart sounds (air trapping/hyperinflation), wheezing and crackles (bronchoconstriction and/or accumulation of secretions), prolonged expiratory phase (airway obstruction), and decreased vocal resonance (air trapping/hyperinflation).[11]

TYPICAL LABORATORY FINDINGS

Radiographic Assessment

The chest radiograph of a patient with COPD may depict hyperinflation. Signs of hyperinflation include flattened diaphragm, increased retrosternal airspace on lateral films, appearance of a long, narrow heart shadow, and increased lung volumes evidenced by enlarged intercostal spaces. The chest radiograph of a patient with locally severe emphysema may include the appearance of bullae. In regard to identifying emphysema using chest radiographs, the ATS relates that studies show that emphysema is consistently diagnosed when the disease is severe, but is missed when disease is mild, and the success rate of diagnosis based on x-ray is about 50% for those cases between mild and severe.[1]

Pulmonary Function Measurements

Pulmonary function tests (PFTs) are not necessarily indicated during an acute exacerbation of COPD, but are necessary for diagnosis and tracking of the progression of the disease. Periodic testing of pulmonary function is needed to follow the patient's disease over time. PFTs are also indicated for evaluating the response to bronchodilator therapy. The ATS recommends measurement of forced expiratory volume in 1 sec (FEV_1) for staging the severity of COPD.[1]

Pattern of Dysfunction.   Patients with COPD display an obstructive pattern of dysfunction. A decreased FEV_1/forced vital capacity (FVC) ratio (<70%) and a reduced FEV_1 characterize this pattern. Lung volume studies typically reveal increased total lung capacity (TLC), functional residual capacity (FRC), and residual volume (RV). The vital capacity (VC) may also be decreased.[1] In addition to the obstructive pattern of dysfunction, subjects with emphysema will likely show a decreased value for D_{co}. Diffusion capacity of carbon monoxide (D_{co}) is also useful for differentiating possible causes of COPD. D_{co} values will likely be reduced in patients having emphysema as the primary disease, whereas if chronic bronchitis is the main problem the D_{co} will often be normal.[12]

CRITICAL CONTENT

PFT RESULTS SUGGESTING OBSTRUCTIVE DYSFUNCTION

- FEV_1/FVC ratio decreased
- FEV_1 decreased
- TLC, FRC, and RV increased or normal
- VC may be decreased or normal
- D_{co}: normal in chronic bronchitis; reduced value likely with emphysema

Response to Bronchodilators. Response to bronchodilator testing can assist in the diagnosis of COPD and in determining appropriate therapy. A significant response to bronchodilator testing is defined as a 12% or greater improvement in FEV_1 or FVC compared to predrug values, and a 200 mL increase in either FVC or FEV_1.[13] ATS standards do not include criteria for peak expiratory flow rate (PEFR) measurements in determining bronchodilator response, yet because of its ease of measurement, PEFR may be the only pulmonary function test performed in the ED. When only PEFR measurements are available, they still provide a way to quantify changes in airflow rates that may indicate a significant response to bronchodilator therapy. Clear guidelines have been set forth for the use of PEFR in the evaluation of asthma by the National Asthma Education and Prevention Program (NAEPP). Use of the NAEPP criteria (poor response: <50% of personal or predicted best; incomplete response: ≥50% but <70% of personal or predicted best; and good response: >70% of personal or predicted best) may be useful when only PEFR measurements are available.[14]

Another use of bronchodilator response testing is to differentiate chronic obstructive bronchitis from asthmatic bronchitis. Subjects with chronic obstructive bronchitis have obstructive dysfunction, but do not respond positively to bronchodilator therapy, while subjects with asthmatic bronchitis show significant reversibility in response to appropriate medication.[5] Keep in mind only about 10%[2] to 33%[1] of patients with COPD will display a positive response to bronchodilator therapy.[2] Continued use of bronchodilator therapy should be independent of the results of bronchodilator tests, according to the ATS, European Respiratory Society, and British Thoracic Society.[15] Thus patients often receive bronchodilator therapy even if they do not demonstrate significant improvement via PFT evaluation.

Staging Criteria. The American Thoracic Society proposes use of staging criteria to classify the severity of COPD. This criterion utilizes postbronchodilator FEV_1/FVC% to classify the severity of COPD. An FEV_1/FVC% ≥50% would be classified as stage I, while a value <50% and ≥34% would be stage II, and a value <34% would be classified as stage III.[1] Note that as the patient progresses from stage I to III, the patient's health-related quality of life is affected more and more by the disease. The associated per capita health care costs increase as patients reach stage III.[1,8] For example, airflow obstruction resulting in a stage I classification will usually result in only mild dyspnea and hypercarbia or hypoxemia are rarely seen; whereas a patient with stage III disease is likely to complain of severe dyspnea, hypercarbia may be observed, and hypoxemia is likely. A point to emphasize in regard to these stages is that if the patient's signs and symptoms are not compatible with the stage they are in, then additional testing may be required and evaluation by a respiratory specialist is recommended.[1] The additional testing and evaluation are needed to identify other health problems (eg, congestive heart failure [CHF], bronchogenic carcinoma) that may coexist with the patient's COPD.

CRITICAL CONTENT

ATS STAGING CRITERIA FOR SEVERITY OF COPD
- Stage I—FEV_1/FVC <50%
- Stage II—FEV_1/FVC 35% to 49%
- Stage III—FEV_1/FVC <35%

Note: If the patient's signs and symptoms are not compatible with the stage they are in, then additional testing may be required and evaluation by a respiratory specialist is recommended.

Blood

Arterial blood gas analysis (ABG) may be useful in the management of patients with COPD to determine ventilation, oxygenation, and the acid-base status of the blood. In the early stages of COPD, blood gases are likely to reveal mild to moderate hypoxemia with normal or even slightly reduced carbon dioxide tension. Hypercapnia presents along with more severe hypoxemia as the disease runs its course and the patient's disease enters ATS stage III. Guidelines recommend that patients with stage II or III COPD have ABG measurements performed while breathing room air.[1]

In addition to ABGs, blood may be analyzed for various factors that provide useful diagnostic and patient management information. Blood can be analyzed for hematocrit (Hct) to provide evaluation of the oxygen-carrying capacity as well as the effectiveness of long-term oxygen therapy. Patients with chronic hypoxemia often have an elevated Hct because the bone marrow is stimulated to increase red blood cell production in response to the hypoxemia. Appropriate oxygen therapy can reverse the increased Hct that occurs as a result of the chronic hypoxemia.

Monitoring of serum electrolytes can be especially useful when the patient is using diuretics as therapy for coexisting conditions such as congestive heart failure. For example, some diuretics cause the body to excrete greater amounts of potassium (K^+), thereby lowering serum levels. Monitoring electrolyte levels provides useful information for replacement therapy. Maintaining proper electrolyte levels is necessary to ensure optimal muscle function, including that of the heart and respiratory muscles.[16]

Thyroid function tests should be done on patients whose symptoms are worse than their disease state indicates it should be, because hypothyroidism and hyperthyroidism can give rise to fatigue and dyspnea.[17] A serum test for alpha$_1$-antitrypsin (AAT) deficiency is generally indicated if the patient has COPD and is a nonsmoker, has COPD before age 50, or has a family history of alpha$_1$-antitrypsin deficiency or early COPD.[1]

Sputum

Analysis of the sputum of patients with COPD may provide information that can be useful in determining acute care and long-term management. Sputum should be evaluated for color, consistency, quantity, and the presence of odor. Sputum of certain colors and the presence of odor can indicate an infection. However, routine bacteriologic sputum studies are not necessary in stable patients.[8] Sputum should also be inspected for the presence of blood. Hemoptysis may simply be due to mucosal damage from forceful or frequent coughing or mucosal erosion. However, the presence of hemoptysis may also be observed in patients with bronchogenic carcinoma, which is found more frequently in patients with COPD and a history of smoking.[1]

CRITICAL CONTENT

CLINICAL AND LAB FINDINGS IN COPD

- History of smoking
- Increased work of breathing
- Bronchoconstriction (airway obstruction)
- Increased production and retention of secretions
- Hyperinflation
- Hypoxemia
- Hypercapnia (in severe cases; eg, stage III disease)

The cellular makeup of sputum may shed additional light on the COPD patient's disease process. A larger number of neutrophils than is seen in normal or asthmatic subjects suggests that COPD is present. COPD patients presenting with a large number of eosinophils are also likely to demonstrate airway hyperactivity. Patients with increased sputum eosinophils may benefit from initial therapy with steroids, while patients whose sputum reveals increased neutrophils may initially benefit more from antibiotic therapy during an exacerbation of COPD.[16]

TREATMENT AND MANAGEMENT

The therapeutic goals of treatment are to restore the patient to baseline health as quickly as possible. By optimizing the patient's airflow and functional status, avoiding the need for intubation and mechanical ventilation (and their associated risks), and avoiding other complications of therapy, morbidity and mortality may be minimized.[1] The precipitating event for an episode of exacerbation must be identified. Common events include infection, deep venous thrombosis (DVT) or pulmonary emboli, chronic heart failure (CHF), and inhalation of environmental irritants.

Drug therapy should be adjusted according to the following variables: (1) the degree of reversible bronchospasm; (2) prior therapy of the stable patient; (3) recent drug use and evidence of potential toxicity; (4) the ability of the patient to appropriately self-administer inhaled medications; (5) the presence of contraindications to any specific medications; and (6) specific causes or complications related to the exacerbation (eg, withholding sedation, anticoagulation, or antibiotics).[18]

The American Thoracic Society has established clinical guidelines regarding pharmacologic therapy for COPD. These guidelines are organized according to the severity of disease and the patient's tolerance for specific drugs. The goals include inducing bronchodilation, decreasing the inflammatory reaction, and promoting expectoration.[1,18]

There are new medical and surgical treatments being developed nationwide. Surgical options include lung volume reduction, bullectomy, and lung transplantation. Patients are selected based on an extensive evaluation. Currently, there are multiple centers participating in a randomized study of lung volume reduction surgery (LVRS). This study, known as the National Emphysema Treatment Trial (NETT), seeks to collect data regarding the effectiveness of LVRS as a treatment for emphysema.[19]

Bronchodilators

Beta$_2$ adrenergic agonist aerosols are usually given as first-line treatment of airflow obstruction in acute exacerbations and stable COPD. Albuterol, pirbuterol acetate, metaproterenol sulfate, terbutaline sulfate, isoetharine, bitolterol mesylate, or salmeterol are available in metered-dose inhaler and several are available for the nebulizer (eg, metaproterenol, albuterol, and isoetharine). Inhalation is generally preferred to oral or parenteral routes of administration. Subcutaneous administration is preferred when inhalation is not possible, but caution should be exercised in patients with coronary artery disease. Due to the potential for a shortened functional half-life of these medications during acute exacerbations, dosing and frequency of supervised administration may be increased to hourly as needed. Close monitoring for systemic sympathomimetic effects such as tremors, nervousness, and tachycardia is appropriate.[1,18]

Anticholinergic Bronchodilators

Although the information available on the efficacy of anticholinergic agents is limited, it does suggest bronchodilator efficacy equal to that of the adrenergic agonists. Ipratropium bromide is available in metered-dose inhalers and as a nebulizer solution. These drugs generally have a longer time to maximal bronchodilation and a longer duration of action. The appropriate dosage is every 6 to 8 hours, and they are not recommended to be given more frequently. Clinical trials have shown that Combivent, a combination of ipratropium bromide and albuterol sulfate, is more effective in treating patients with COPD than either of these drugs used alone.[20]

Methylxanthines

Theophylline's potential for toxicity has led to a decline in its popularity, though it is of value for less compliant or less capable patients who cannot use aerosol therapy. Its ability to improve respiratory muscle function, stimulate the respiratory center, and enhance activities of daily living can be important to patients who are significantly limited by their disease. Patients with COPD and cardiac disease or cor pulmonale may experience an improvement in cardiac output, reduction of pulmonary vascular resistance, and an improvement in perfusion of ischemic heart disease. There is evidence that theophylline has some antiinflammatory effects, and that adding it to the combination of albuterol and ipratropium bromide can result in the greatest benefit in stable COPD.[1]

Antiinflammatory Therapy

Corticosteroids have been prescribed frequently in management of acute COPD exacerbations, but patients should be weaned quickly, since the older population is susceptible to complications.[1] The ATS recommends considering the use of oral steroids for patients with mild to moderate continuing symptoms, and intravenous steroid administration for severe exacerbations of COPD.[1] A review of clinical research pertaining to patients with stable COPD found that nearly all short-term studies found no significant effect on FEV_1. However, one study (of patients receiving treatment for 2 to 2.5 years) revealed a significant improvement in pre-bronchodilator FEV_1, and multicenter research found improvement in lung function, ability to walk, and a decrease in moderate and severe exacerbations with inhaled steroid use. Additionally, there is a small amount of evidence that oral prednisone is more effective than inhaled beclomethasone dipropionate in patients with less-than-severe COPD.[21]

Oxygen Therapy

Correction of hypoxemia and the prevention of tissue hypoxia are essential in the treatment of COPD. Oxygen administration with an optimal acute and long-term treatment regimen can improve survival in patients with COPD. When determining the best oxygen delivery method, the practitioner must also consider other oxygen transport issues, including adequate hemoglobin, cardiac output, and tissue perfusion. There are several options for low-flow oxygen delivery devices and the settings should be adjusted for rest, exertion, and sleep in order to meet the patient's needs. The standards for long-term oxygen therapy based on ATS recommendations are:

Absolute—$Pao_2 \leq 55$ mm Hg or $Sao_2 \leq 88\%$
In presence of cor pulmonale:

- Pao_2 55 to 59 mm Hg or $Sao_2 \leq 89\%$
- EKG evidence of "P" pulmonale, hematocrit >55%, congestive heart failure (CHF)

Only in specific situations:

- $Pao_2 \geq 60$ mm Hg or $Sao_2 \geq 90$
- With lung disease and other clinical needs such as sleep apnea with nocturnal desaturation not corrected by CPAP

If the patient meets criteria at rest, O_2 should also be prescribed during sleep and exercise, appropriately titrated. If the patient is normoxemic at rest, but desaturates during exercise or sleep ($Pao_2 \leq 55$ mm Hg), O_2 should be prescribed for these indications. Nasal continuous positive airway pressure (CPAP) or bilevel positive airway pressure (BiPAP) can be considered as additional treatment for situations in which patients fail to respond to oxygen therapy alone.[1]

Mechanical Ventilation

Invasive and noninvasive ventilation should be considered with patients experiencing an acute exacerbation of COPD when pharmacologic and other nonventilatory treatments do not correct clinically significant respiratory failure. Assisted ventilation may be indicated when there is evidence of respiratory muscle fatigue, worsening acidosis, and/or deteriorating mental status.[1] The goals of assisted ventilation in managing acute respiratory failure in COPD are to rest ventilatory muscles and restore gas exchange to a stable baseline. Weaning and discontinuance of mechanical ventilation should be initiated as soon as possible.

The respiratory clinician should be aware of the major hazards associated with mechanical ventilation: pneumonia, pulmonary barotrauma, and laryngotracheal complications associated with artificial airways. Ventilating patients with COPD can be particularly difficult. Patients with chronic hypercapnia may be overventilated, resulting in acute respiratory alkalemia. Systemic hypotension may result from complex pulmonary and cardiovascular interactions. Auto-PEEP may be created with dynamic airflow obstruction or with inadequate expiratory time.

Common ventilatory modes used with COPD patients include: assist-control ventilation (ACV), synchronized intermittent mandatory ventilation (SIMV), pressure support ventilation (PSV), and pressure control ventilation (PCV). Clinical reports offer support for each of these modes of ventilation, though no direct evidence exists indicating that patient outcomes are improved using a particular mode. The selection of ventilatory mode still appears to be one made mostly by familiarity and personal choice.

Once intubated and mechanically ventilated, patients with COPD who have been optimized in the management of their bronchospasm, fluid status, sedation, or inadvertent overoxygenation, may be successfully extubated without a prolonged period of weaning. Other patients may require gradual weaning after prolonged mechanical ventilation.

There are a variety of objective physiologic indices designed to evaluate patients for extubation. Measured values for maximal inspiratory pressure (MIP) (also called negative inspiratory force [NIF]), VC, and respiratory frequency/tidal volume ratio (f/V$_T$; also called the rapid shallow breathing index) may be helpful in identifying which patients can be weaned and extubated from mechanical ventilation. A f/V$_T$ of >105 is associated with difficulty in maintaining effective spontaneous ventilation.

Currently, the *American Journal of Respiratory and Critical Care Medicine* does not recommend elective use of invasive ventilatory support in ambulatory patients with COPD and hypercapnia. They suggest additional investigations into other methods of ventilation, such as a nasal mask or other noninvasive forms of ventilatory assistance.

Noninvasive Positive Pressure Ventilation. Noninvasive positive pressure ventilation (NPPV) refers to the delivery of assisted ventilatory support without the use of an endotracheal tube. It may be delivered using a facial or nasal mask along with a volume-controlled ventilator, a pressure-controlled ventilator, a BiPAP ventilator, pressure-support ventilation (PSV), or a CPAP device. Many clinicians appear to prefer use of a pressure-based mode such as PSV or its counterpart BiPAP for NPPV.

Issues that should discourage noninvasive ventilation for acute exacerbations of COPD include copious secretions, unstable hemodynamics, inability to protect the airway, altered mental status, and poor patient cooperation.[1] A high degree of staff skill is required to monitor patients receiving noninvasive ventilation. Intubation and positive pressure ventilation still remains the therapy of choice for acute respiratory failure.

In general, NPPV should be initiated early, before severe symptoms develop if at all possible. The initial change in arterial partial pressure of carbon dioxide (Paco$_2$) and mask tolerance may be predictors of successful NPPV. Several recent trials indicate that when ventilated with NPPV, patients with acute respiratory failure due to COPD may have fewer complications, and their hospital length of stay may be reduced.[22–24]

SITE- AND AGE-SPECIFIC CONSIDERATIONS

The majority of COPD patients are adults aged 50 and over. Age-specific considerations in these patients include taking into account decreased function and changes that occur in the body due to the aging process. It may be necessary to speak louder to them, or to ensure that a functional hearing aid is in place for patients suffering hearing loss (don't forget to check the batteries). Decreases in visual acuity may make instructional materials with large print necessary. Age-related changes, disease progression, and other circumstances may leave COPD patients with diminished ability to effectively provide self-care (see Chapter 9 for more on patient education).

When self-care is not possible or appears to be inadequate, patients with COPD who have adequate health care coverage can choose from a variety of care options, including hospitals, skilled nursing facilities (SNFs), and other extended care facilities. Generally, the goal is to have the patient receive care in the least intensive (and least costly) environment that will provide care appropriate for the patient's current needs. Care in an acute care hospital should be utilized only when other options do not meet a patient's medical needs.

Comprehensive Outpatient Management of COPD

All patients diagnosed with COPD should be provided with information that will allow them to actively participate in their therapy, with emphasis on preventive care (ie, immunizations), and maintaining an active, healthy lifestyle. Patients who continue to smoke must be encouraged to participate in a comprehensive smoking cessation program.

A successful smoking cessation program includes a strong social support system as well as physician and pharmacologic intervention. Protocols for smoking cessation include initiation of the program, early follow-up, continuing reinforcement, and additional support should the patient fail to quit smoking.

The patient's airway obstruction should be treated pharmacologically according to the severity of their disease. Patient education must include identifying the signs, symptoms, and severity of their disease, as well as the recommended pharmacologic treatment. As the ATS put it, "Collaborative self-management allows the patient to modify therapy according to symptoms and disease severity."[1] The guidelines for pharmacologic therapy have been outlined in this chapter. Hypoxemia should be assessed and treated with prescribed oxygen as described earlier.

Periodic reassessment of therapy is essential. If a patient requires more than two hospital or ED visits per year, or if their symptoms become severe, they may be referred to a multidisciplinary rehabilitation program. Education programs should be tailored to the individual patient. Instruction may include group discussions, didactic presentations, visual aids, and printed material. Educational elements should be incorporated into every patient contact, even when they are in the acute care hospital. Education should not be limited to formal rehabilitation programs.

COSTS AND ETHICAL ISSUES

It seems appropriate to consider cost and ethical issues together, for as with other medical matters, patients afflicted with COPD and their families are faced with many decisions, all of which have associated costs and benefits. Costs in terms of money and time, as well as quality of life, should be considered in the decision-making process. Health care workers including respiratory therapists are also faced with ethical decisions related to the management of COPD. Like those of patients and their families, decisions made by health care professionals have costs associated with them.

It is beyond the scope of this chapter to attempt to offer the reader a comprehensive overview of this complex, multidisciplinary issue (see Chapter 8 for a more detailed examination of this topic). What follows are excerpts from the American Association for Respiratory Care (AARC) Code of Ethics and Professional Behavior and some points about end-of-life issues for the reader to consider at work and while completing the case exercises.

Ethics and End-of-Life Decisions

The AARC code of ethics specifies several important factors that define ethical behavior for a respiratory therapist (RT). Several that appear most applicable in relation to the care of a patient with COPD appear below.

- RTs must respect and protect the legal and personal rights of patients they treat, including the right to informed consent and refusal of treatment.
- RTs must divulge no confidential information regarding any patient or family member unless such disclosure is required for responsible performance of duty or is required by law.
- RTs must provide care without discrimination on any basis, with respect for the rights and dignity of all individuals.
- RTs must promote disease prevention and wellness.[25]

End-of-life decisions are inevitable. The majority of COPD patients seeking medical care in the hospital setting for acute exacerbation will survive, while some will present with end-stage disease with little hope for a successful outcome. There is a lack of accurate models to predict outcomes for COPD patients. In light of this uncertainty it may be advantageous to use a decision-making process involving the patient, the physician, and the patient's family for end-of-life judgments. The use of advanced directives (durable powers of attorney for health care and living wills) can be beneficial during this decision-making and planning process.[26] See Chapter 8 for additional discussion of this topic.

Costs

COPD is common, and this illness is quite costly. National Heart, Lung, and Blood Institute figures for 1993 reveal national costs for COPD of $23.9 billion, and approximately 81% of this money was spent for direct health care costs.[5] The American Thoracic Society's three-tiered staging system reflects that as a patient is more adversely affected by COPD, moving from stage I to stage II for example, the per capita expense for health care increases.[1]

Cigarette smoking has been shown to be responsible for approximately 80% to 90% of the risk of developing COPD, and it also produces a greater decrease in FEV_1 for patients already afflicted with COPD.[1] It makes sense to prevent smoking whenever and wherever possible, and also to eliminate smoking in patients already diagnosed with COPD who continue to smoke, in order to slow the rate of progression of the disease. It appears that smoking cessation can improve the health of patients and save money in health care costs.[1]

The following exercises are case-based and designed to help students expand their knowledge of COPD and prepare them for situations they will likely encounter in respiratory care practice.

INTRODUCTION TO CASE STUDIES

Now you proceed with the most exciting part of this chapter, that of working through a real case. Your instructors will assign you to work on specific critical thinking exercises and group critical thinking exercises, depending on the available time, types of patients you are likely to encounter during your clinical rotations, and resources available. Please check with your instructors to verify which case(s) and exercises you should complete, working individually or in groups. Your instructors may also direct you to develop "learning issues" as part of your PBL process or assign specific, predetermined learning issues developed for this chapter. Please check with your program faculty before proceeding with the following case(s).

CASE STUDY 1

EMMA SEEMA

Initial Case Scenario

Ms. Seema presents to the ED with a chief complaint of increasing shortness of breath (SOB). She is 60 years old. You enter her room and discover the patient is sitting up, leaning forward so that her hands are flat on her bed and her arms are fully extended. You notice nasal flaring, retractions, and accessory muscle use. She is unable to speak in complete sentences, uttering only a word or two between breaths initially. Toward the end of the interview, she becomes barely able to speak. You also note that her lips are pursed during exhalation.

 Critical Thinking Exercise 1

PRIORITIZING PATIENT CARE

a. Explain what actions you would take to assess and manage Ms. Seema during the first few minutes of interaction with her.

b. What would your priorities be? Why?

Case History

Ms. Seema tells you she was diagnosed with COPD approximately 6 years ago. She complains of chronic SOB and difficulty breathing (which has gotten worse over the last 2 weeks) along with chest tightness. She also states that she feels tired. Her medical record reveals she has been admitted in the past for exacerbation of COPD. She denies any fever or chills, production of sputum, occurrence of cough, or hemoptysis.

Critical Thinking Exercise 2

MAKING INFERENCES BY CLUSTERING DATA

a. What inference can you make about Ms. Seema's work of breathing? Practice clustering data that supports this inference.

b. Is her condition improving, deteriorating, or remaining stable? How do you know?

Critical Thinking Exercise 3

ANTICIPATING PHYSICAL EXAMINATION FINDINGS

a. What symptoms are you anticipating this patient will relate, given the working diagnosis of exacerbation of COPD?

b. Given the diagnosis of exacerbation of COPD, what signs do you expect this patient will reveal?

Critical Thinking Exercise 4

ANTICIPATING PROBLEMS

What ventilation and oxygenation problems might develop over the next 24 hours? (Explain how and why you anticipate these problems may develop.)

Initial data and clinical presentation on admission to ED:

Vital signs

HR	120/min	SpO_2	% N/A
RR	32/min	Temp.	36.0°C
BP	129/63		

ABG 4 L/M NC

pH	7.32	HCO_3^-	35.0
PCO_2	68	BE	+9
PO_2	156	SaO_2	99.8%

General

Patient is alert, oriented × 3 and anxious. Sitting upright, slightly forward, with palms on knees. No cyanosis, no JVD.
Skin dry; ht, 5'6"; wt, 96 kg.

Chest auscultation

Decreased bilaterally, diffuse expiratory wheezing bilaterally. No crackles noted.

Labs

Hb	14.2 gm/dL
Hct	41.5%

PFT

VC	1.26 L

RADIOLOGY

AP Chest	See Fig. 12-2 for Ms. Seema's admission chest film.

Based on the ED admission data above, perform the following CT exercises:

Critical Thinking Exercise 5

DECISION MAKING—DEVELOPING A PLAN OF CARE

a. What therapy would you initially recommend?

b. What is your interpretation of the chest radiograph?

CASE STUDY 1 (continued)

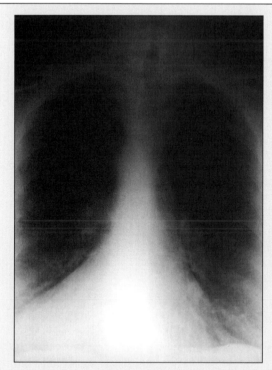

FIGURE 12-2 Chest radiograph of Ms. Seema. (Chest x-ray film courtesy of The Respiratory Therapy Section of the Pulmonary and Critical Care Medicine Department of the Cleveland Clinic Foundation.)

Vital signs

HR	114/min	SpO_2	89%
RR	32/min	Temp.	N/A
BP	N/A		

ABG 4 L/M NC

pH	7.36	HCO_3^-	35.0
PCO_2	60	BE	+9
PO_2	60	SaO_2	90.8%

Chest

Auscultation   Wheezes and diminished bilaterally, although improved.

Labs

Hb 14.2 gm/dL, Hct 41.5%, platelets 279 K/μL, neutrophils 86.6%, lymphocytes 10.3%

PFT

VC   1.26 L

Critical Thinking Exercise 7

ANTICIPATING PROBLEMS AND SOLUTIONS

a. What problems would you anticipate based on the actions and events so far?

b. What solutions do you anticipate may be applied?

Group Critical Thinking Exercise 1

PRO/CON DEBATE

Review Ms. Seema's clinical data and oxygenation status including the oxygen therapy she is currently receiving. Divide the class into two groups. One group will argue that Ms. Seema's oxygenation status requires a change and cite what change they recommend, as well as evidence and references to support their recommendation. The second group will argue that her oxygenation needs are being met with the current oxygen therapy and that no changes in this therapy are necessary. This group will also cite evidence and/or appropriate references to support

Critical Thinking Exercise 6

ASSESSING AND MODIFYING THE PLAN OF CARE

a. What response(s) to each recommended therapy would you expect?

b. How will you evaluate these expected responses?

c. How will you modify the treatment plan?

Additional data in the ED, 2 hours after admission: Ms. Seema has been treated in the ED for 2 hours and has received therapy as recommended. Her current clinical information follows:

CASE STUDY 1   *(continued)*

maintaining the oxygen therapy as is. The debate can be done before the full class. After the presentations, the class can weigh the strengths and weaknesses of the two sides of the debate. Was there a clear winner?

The physician has written the following orders as Ms. Seema is admitted to a general nursing floor after 5 hours in the ED:

VS: Q shift
Activity: As tolerated
Allergies: NKA
Nursing: I/O Q shift
Medication: Atrovent/Albuterol may be delivered by small volume nebulizer (SVN) or MDI. The frequency and dosage may be increased to hourly depending on the severity of the patient's symptoms. Solumedrol 40 mg IV Q8, Paxil 20 mg PO QD, Vasotec 5 mg PO BID, O_2 N.C. to keep SpO_2 >90%.

Her clinical presentation and available lab data 24 hours after admission are seen below.

Vital signs

HR	89/min	SpO_2	90%
RR	26/min	Temp.	N/A
BP	N/A		

ABG 4 L/M NC

pH	7.34	HCO_3^-	33.0
PCO_2	62	BE	+8
PO_2	69	SaO_2	94.8%

Inspection

Cough is noted to be moist-sounding, but nonproductive

Auscultation

BS diminished bilaterally, course crackles are noted at the bases of both lungs

Labs

WBC   20.9 K/μL

PFT

VC   1.26 L

Utilizing the above information, answer the following CT exercises and group CT exercises as assigned by your instructor:

Group Critical Thinking Exercise 2

GENERALIZING KNOWLEDGE TO OTHER CASES

Patients with COPD might respond differently to the same treatment. Have two or more groups discuss how a patient might respond in a different manner to treatment similar to that received by Ms. Seema and why they might respond the way you propose. Have each group then present the various scenarios they came up with to the full class. Were the scenarios plausible? Was one more realistic than another? Why is it useful to do this type of exercise?

Critical Thinking Exercise 8

DECISION MAKING—DEVELOPING A LONG-TERM CARE PLAN

You need to develop a long-term care plan in preparation for a patient's discharge.

a. What issues need to be addressed or questions answered in accomplishing this task?

b. What research is currently being conducted to potentially improve the COPD patient's quality of life?

Critical Thinking Exercise 9

REFLECTION ON YOUR DECISIONS AND ACTIONS TO IMPROVE CLINICAL DECISION MAKING

Describe how you would reflect on the information gathering and management techniques you proposed in this case to determine what was useful and had successful outcomes and what did not. This is fun; after all, hindsight is always 20/20. Keep in mind the important thing is to make what you've learned available to you so you can use it when you manage future cases.

a. What are three things have you learned so far by studying this case?

b. How would you utilize what you have learned to manage a similar case tomorrow?

Group Critical Thinking Exercise 3

THE PRO/CON DEBATE

Use the data for Ms. Seema on initial presentation to the ED, except assume that the first ABG on 6 LPM nasal cannula are pH: 7.22, P_{CO_2}: 88.0 mm Hg, P_{O_2}: 156 mm Hg, HCO_3^-: 35.5 mEq/L, BE: +4, SaO_2: 99%. One group of students should take the pro position and one group take the con position and prepare their arguments for a debate.

Pro: Utilize the framework and story line of the case of Ms. Seema to justify immediate intubation and mechanical ventilation upon her arrival at the ED. Be sure to give the rationale for your decision and state your reasons why intubation is the only viable option at that time.

Con: Same as above, but argue that Ms. Seema does **not** require intubation or mechanical ventilation. Convince the emergency room physician that one or more viable alternatives exist and give the rationale for delaying mechanical ventilation until other treatment(s) have been attempted.

Each group should use evidence-based medicine literature searches to prepare their arguments. Present the debate in front of the entire class. Discuss the strengths and weaknesses of the various arguments presented. Did one group clearly win the debate? Was this based on the quality of the references or on the quality of the verbal presentation? Discuss the importance of communication and negotiation skills when making clinical recommendations.

Group Critical Thinking Exercise 4

RECOMMENDING A STRATEGY— COSTS, BENEFITS, AND ETHICS

You are a registered respiratory therapist at the Managed Care Medical Mutual Center (MCMMC). Once again you find yourself caring for one of Dr. Usealot's patients, Ms. Eae Z. Breathin, age 50, who has just come from the recovery room and has orders to receive aerosol treatments with 0.5 cc of Proventil and 2.5 cc NS every 4 hours. A review of the patient's medical record reveals that Ms. Breathin had reconstructive surgery on her right foot to correct a problem with pain in that foot. You enter her room and find her alert, sitting up in bed watching television. You explain that Dr. Usealot ordered an aerosol treatment with albuterol for her. During your interview she says she is here because her foot problem causes her a great deal of pain whenever she walks more than a few hundred yards. She continued by revealing that she never really had any health problems other than this foot pain and certainly no problems with her breathing. She did smoke once or twice about 35 years previously, but never cared much for it.

Her initial assessment reveals the following:

Vital signs

HR	90/min	SpO_2	99%
RR	17/min	Temp.	36.8°C
BP	120/83 mm Hg		

Inspection

On 4 L/m NC, no cyanosis, no JVD, cough is moist sounding, but nonproductive

Auscultation

Breath sounds: Clear and equal to anterior and posterior auscultation

Labs

Hb	15.2 gm/dL	Hct	46.0%

CASE STUDY 1   *(continued)*

Ms. Breathin says, "I don't think I need any medicine to help me breathe." What do you think? How would you respond to Ms. Breathin?

You contact your supervisor to relate that you feel the aerosol therapy ordered for Ms. Breathin is not indicated and explain that you wish to discuss discontinuing this therapy with the surgeon, Dr. Usealot. Your supervisor suggests that because you are hired here as a per diem therapist, you may want to carefully consider getting aerosol treatments discontinued for any of the patients. After all, fewer aerosol treatments means less work, and less work means less need for per diem therapists.

What actions would you take in this situation? Specifically, to whom would you speak and what would you say?

Ms. Seema's hospital course was uncomplicated. After appropriate bronchial hygiene, patient education, and pharmacologic management she was discharged to home 8 days later.

The following two patients have had pulmonary function studies recently performed. The following exercise allows you to compare and contrast the results of these tests as well as apply your knowledge of classification of pulmonary disorders.

CASE STUDY 2

MS. COCO BASILA AND MR. CHARLES OSCAR P'DEE

Consider the pulmonary function tests for the following patients, Ms. Basila and Mr. P'Dee. For each patient, interpret the pulmonary function test results and respond to the critical thinking exercises.

Ms. Basila

Ms. Coco Basila arrives at the outpatient clinic where you work. She is here for pulmonary function testing. She explains, "I feel fine most of the time and I'm not having any trouble breathing today." She reports that she currently takes no medications other than an occasional painkiller for headache. She says, "My doctor ordered this breathing test for me, but I have no idea why." During your interview she states, "I have never worked outside the home," and adds "Running a home is certainly work enough."

Pulmonary Function Report

Name: Ms. Coco Basila
Height: 60 inches (152 cm)
Dyspnea: No
Smoker: Yes: 30 years, 4 pks/day
Age: 54 years
Weight: 97 lb (44 kg)
Cough: No
Quit Smoking: Yes/2 years ago
Race: Caucasian

ABG

pH	7.50
P_{CO_2}	42.4 mm Hg
P_{O_2}	72.0 mm Hg
HCO_3^-	33.0 mEq/L
BE	+9.3
Sa_{O_2}	95.2%
FI_{O_2}	.21%
HbCO	1.1

CASE STUDY 2 *(continued)*

Spirometry	Pred.	Pre-Tx Best	%Pred	Best	Post-Tx %Pred	%Change
FVC (L)	2.75	2.10	76	2.60	94	24
$FEV_{0.5}$ (L)	1.85	0.77	42	0.99	53	29
FEV_1 (L)	2.06	1.07	52	1.34	65	25
FEV_1/FVC %	75	51		52		
$FEF_{25\%-75\%}$ (L/sec)	2.53	0.38	15	0.45	18	18
Lung Volumes						
VC (L)	2.75			2.86	104	
TLC (L)	4.14			6.25	151	
RV (L)	1.46			3.39	232	
RV/TLC %	36			54		
FRC (L)	2.61			4.46	171	
Diffusion						
D_{CO}sb mL/min/mm HG	15.5			14.2	92	

Mr. P'Dee

Mr. Charles Oscar P'Dee, a retired conference organizer and plumber, is visiting the outpatient clinic at the hospital where you work. You interview him to obtain a brief history prior to beginning his pulmonary function testing. He tells you that his nephew owns a home care company, and because of this, he gets a really good price on his oxygen (which he uses when he's home) and his Proventil inhaler. He tells you, "I always carry my inhaler with me." Upon auscultation of his lungs you hear crackles in both lung bases. He states, "I cough all the time, but nothing comes up." Mr. P'Dee has experienced no other significant health problems other than this breathing problem. He says, "I don't do much now that I'm retired. I never liked physical activity much and I'm afraid to do too much now with this breathing thing and all. I like watching daytime television and I catch a movie whenever I can."

Name: Mr. C.O. P'Dee
Height: 68 inches (173 cm)
Dyspnea: Yes, for 1 year
Smoker: Yes: 60 years × 4 pks/day
Age: 72 years
Weight: 210 lb (95 kg)
Cough: Yes, for 2 years
Quit Smoking: No
Race: Caucasian
Productive: No

ABG

pH	7.40
P_{CO_2}	39.0 mm Hg
P_{O_2}	69.0 mm Hg
HCO_3^-	24.9 mEq/L
BE	−0.5
Sa_{O_2}	96.0%
F_{IO_2}	.21%
HbCO	5.6

continued

CASE STUDY 2 *(continued)*

Spirometry	Pre-Tx Pred.	Best	%Pred	Post-Tx Best	%Pred	%Change
FVC (L)	4.02	2.81	70	3.00	75	7
$FEV_{0.5}$ (L)	1.91	1.47	74	1.52	79	8
FEV_1 (L)	2.69	1.78	66	1.93	72	8
FEV_1/FVC %	68	63		64		
$FEF_{25\%-75\%}$ (L/sec)	2.47	0.81	33	0.90	36	11
Lung Volumes						
VC (L)	4.02			3.42	85	
TLC (L)	6.0			6.13	102	
RV (L)	2.44			2.71	111	
RV/TLC %	41			44		
FRC (L)	3.16			3.46	110	
Diffusion						
D_{CO}sb mL/min/mm HG	22.1			15.5	70	

Critical Thinking Exercise 1

DECISION MAKING—EVALUATING PULMONARY FUNCTION

a. Does either patient have restrictive dysfunction, obstructive dysfunction, or a combination of both? Rate the severity of the dysfunction: is it mild, moderate, or severe?

b. Is there a significant response to bronchodilator therapy revealed by either patient's pulmonary function test results? Explain the rationale for your answer.

c. Discuss which of these patients is most likely to have COPD as compared to COPD with asthma? Give reasons to support your conclusions.

d. Assume that both patients have COPD, and rate the stage of COPD for each patient.

e. How would you determine the stage of COPD for each patient?

Group Critical Thinking Exercise 1

DECISION MAKING—DEVELOPING A LONG-TERM CARE PLAN AND SMOKING CESSATION

Develop a long-term care plan for Mr. P'Dee. What is of immediate concern? What suggestions could you offer to Mr. P'Dee for his consideration to decrease medical costs for him and his health care provider?

Mr. P'Dee is referred to the outpatient pulmonary rehab clinic where you are currently employed. He has agreed to quit smoking. What are some smoking cessation strategies and techniques that you can employ to help Mr. P'Dee kick the habit?

CASE STUDY 3

MS. WEE ZEN

Initial Case Scenario

Chief Complaint: Shortness of Breath

You are a registered respiratory therapist working in an outpatient center that offers pulmonary function testing and pulmonary rehabilitation services to patients on an outpatient basis. Ms. Zen has not found it necessary to seek medical care since she was admitted to a local hospital 4 years ago for a severe case of pneumonia. Her past medical history includes hypertension. See Fig. 12-3 for the PFT graphics for Ms. Zen.

She states, "Three days ago I became increasingly short of breath and developed a cough. I kept coughing up clear mucous, which occasionally looked yellow or white. I've also noticed that my ankles are all swollen at times." She says she has no trouble getting around, but her grandson who brought her in says, "She's been having more trouble walking. She's taken to leaning on a walker in order to get around. The past couple of days she won't walk anywhere without using that walker."

Name: Ms. Wee Zen
Sex: Female
Dyspnea: Yes
Smoker: Yes: 48 years, 1 pk/day
Age: 67 years
Height: 66 inches (152 cm)
Cough: No
Quit Smoking: Yes, 4 years ago
Race: Caucasian
Weight: 102 lb (46 kg)

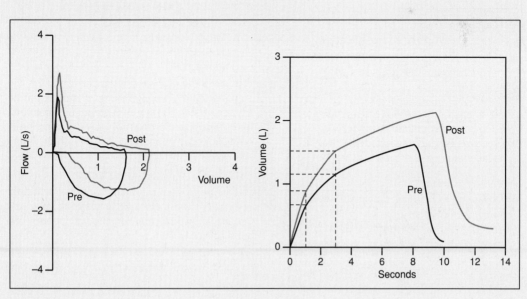

FIGURE 12-3   Pulmonary function test graphics for Ms. Zen.

CASE STUDY 3 *(continued)*

Spirometry	Pre-Tx Pred.	Best	%Pred	Post-Tx Best	%Pred	%Change
FVC (L)	2.95	1.63	55	2.14	72	31
$FEV_{0.5}$ (L)	1.84	0.44	24	0.57	31	30
FEV_1 (L)	2.33	0.67	29	0.88	38	33
FEV_1/FVC %	79	51		52		
PEFR (L/sec)	5.80	1.97	34	2.80	48	42
$FEF_{25\%-75\%}$ (L/sec)	3.08	0.27	9	0.35	11	27
MVV (L/min)	59	19	29			
Lung Volumes						
VC (L)	2.95	1.64	56	2.03	69	24
TLC (L)	5.02			4.52	90	
RV (L)	2.07			2.49	120	
RV/TLC %	41			55		
FRC (L)	2.93			3.15	108	
Diffusion						
D_{CO}sb mL/min/mm HG	18.63			10.26	55	
DL/VA	5.06			3.50	69	

Her vital signs, focused physical exam, and data given here. PFTs reveal the:

Vital signs

HR	118/min	SpO_2	87%
RR	24/min	SpO_2	87%
BP	138/88 mm Hg		

Inspection

Chest appears symmetrical and an increase in A-P diameter is noted.
No cyanosis or clubbing noted. Pt. has mild pedal edema.

Auscultation

Breath sounds: Diminished bilaterally with minimal wheezing.

Group Critical Thinking Exercise 1

PRO/CON DEBATE— DECISION MAKING

Have two groups debate the next course of action for the care of Ms. Zen.

Pro (hospitalization): One group prepares the argument that Ms. Zen should be admitted to an acute care hospital for evaluation and treatment. Be sure to give the rationale for your group's recommendation, stating why hospitalization is the best option at this time.

Con (hospitalization not required): This group should prepare the argument that the patient does not require an acute level of care at this time. Prepare to give reasons why the patient could be appropriately cared for without the need for hospitalization.

KEY POINTS

- COPD is typically viewed as a collection of diseases that includes asthma, emphysema, and chronic bronchitis, which can exist separately or coexist to varying degrees.

- COPD ranks fourth as a cause of death in the United States.

- COPD is more common in males than females.

- Cigarette smoking is the greatest risk factor associated with COPD.

- About 10–33% of patients with COPD will display a positive bronchodilator response.

- COPD is a progressive disease and patients will likely progress to the point of DOE around the age of 60 or older.

- Patients with COPD display an obstructive pattern of dysfunction including decreased FEV_1/FVC.

- Severity is classified according to "Staging Criteria" proposed by the ATS; Stage 1: FEV_1/FVC >50%, State 2: FEV_1/FVC 35–49%, Stage 3: FEV_1/FVC <35% (most severe).

- ABGs reveal mild to moderate hypoxemia with normal or slightly reduced $Paco_2$ with Stage 1 COPD, hypercapnia is not likely until Stage 3 is reached.

- Common precipitating events for a COPD exacerbation include infection, DVT, CHF, and inhalation of environmental irritants.

- Goals of pharmacologic therapy in COPD include bronchodilation, reducing the inflammatory reaction, and promoting expectoration.

- Correction of hypoxemia and the prevention of tissue hypoxia are essential in the treatment of COPD.

- Assisted ventilation (invasive and noninvasive) may be considered when there is evidence of muscle fatigue, worsening acidosis, and/or deteriorating mental status.

- NPPV should probably be avoided with acute exacerbations in the face of copious secretion, unstable hemodynamics, inability to protect the airway, altered mental status, and poor patient cooperation.

- All patients with COPD should actively participate in their therapy, with an emphasis on preventive care and maintaining an active, healthy lifestyle.

SUGGESTED REFERENCES

In addition to several web sites listed in the references, these sites provide information and resources that may be useful in learning more about COPD and how to assist others in living with this disease.

American Association for Respiratory Care Clinical Practice Guidelines: http://www.aarc.org/professional_resources/cpgs/cpg_index.html

AARC Quit Smoking Information: http://www.aarc.org/patient_education/tips/quitsmok.html

Alpha to Alpha support group: http://www.alpha2alpha.org/

American Lung Association—Chronic Bronchitis: http://www.lungusa.org/diseases/lungchronic.html

American Lung Association—Emphysema: http://www.lungusa.org/diseases/lungemphysem.html

American Thoracic Society: http://www.thoracic.org/

American Thoracic Society Position Papers: http://www.thoracic.org/statementframe.html

National Emphysema Foundation: http://www.emphysemafoundation.org/

National Emphysema Treatment Trial (NETT): http://www.nhlbi.nih.gov/health/prof/lung/nett/lvrsweb.htm

National Center for Health Statistics: http://www.cdc.gov/nchs/datawh.htm

REFERENCES

1. American Thoracic Society: Standards for the diagnosis and care of patients with chronic obstructive pulmonary disease. *Am J Respir Care Crit Care Med.* 1995;152:S78.

2. Barnes PJ. Mechanisms in COPD: Differences from asthma. *Chest.* 2000;117:S10–S14.

3. Rennard SI. COPD: Overview of definitions, epidemiology, and factors influencing its development. *Chest.* 1998;113:S235–S241.

4. Births and Deaths: United States, 1996. Monthly Vital Statistics Report. Vol. 46. No. 1 (S2). Available at http://www.cdc.gov/nchswww/products/pubs/pubd/mvsr/supp/46-45/mv46_1s2.htm

5. Petty TL. Definitions, causes, course, and prognosis of chronic obstructive pulmonary disease. In: Heffner JE, Petty TL, eds. *Respir Care Clin North Am.*1998;4:345–357.

6. Senior RM, Anthonisen NR: Chronic obstructive pulmonary disease (COPD). *Am J Respir Care Crit Care Med.* 1998;157:S139–S147.

7. Weinberger SE. *Principles of Pulmonary Medicine.* Philadelphia: Saunders; 1992:97.

8. Celli B. Pathophysiology of chronic obstructive pulmonary disease. In: Heffner JE, Petty TL, eds. *Respir Care Clin North Am.* 1998;4:359–370.

9. Des Jardins T, Burton GG. *Clinical Manifestations of Respiratory Disease.* St. Louis: Mosby-Year Book; 1995.

10. Badgett RG, Tanaka DJ, Hunt DK, et al. The clinical evaluation for diagnosing obstructive airways disease in high-risk patients. *Chest.* 1994;106:1427–1431.

11. Wilkins RL. Physical examination of the patient with cardiopulmonary disease. In: Wilkins RL, Krider SJ, Sheldon RL, eds. *Clinical Assessment in Respiratory Care.* 3rd ed. St. Louis: Mosby-Year Book; 1995:47–77.

12. Madama VC. *Pulmonary Function Testing and Cardiopulmonary Stress Testing.* Albany, New York: Delmar; 1998.

13. American Thoracic Society. Lung function testing: selection of reference values and interpretive strategies. *Am Rev Respir Dis.* 1991;144:1202–1218.

14. National Asthma Education Program. *Practical Guide for the Diagnosis and Management of Asthma.* US Department of Health and Human Services (NIH Publication No. 97-4053). 1997.

15. Ferguson GT: Recommendations for the management of COPD. *Chest.* 2000;117:S23–S28.

16. Chu LW, Wilkins RL. Clinical laboratory studies. In: Wilkins RL, Krider SJ, Sheldon RL, eds. *Clinical Assessment in Respiratory Care.* 3rd ed. St. Louis: Mosby Year Book; 1995:79–101.

17. Phillips YY, Hnatiuk OW. Diagnosing and monitoring the clinical course of chronic obstructive pulmonary disease. In: Heffner JE, Petty TL, eds. *Respir Care Clin North Am.* 1998;4:371–389.

18. Stoller JK, Lange PA. Inpatient management of chronic obstructive pulmonary disease. In: Heffner JE, Petty TL, eds. *Respir Care Clin North Am.* 1998;4:425–438.

19. National Emphysema Treatment Trial (NETT). National Emphysema Treatment Trial (NETT): Evaluation of lung volume reduction surgery for emphysema. Available at http://www.nhlbi.nih.gov/health/prof/lung/nett/lvrsweb.htm

20. Wilson JD, Serby CW, Menjoge SS, et al. The efficacy and safety of combination bronchodilator therapy, *Eur Respir Rev.* 1996;6:286–289.

21. Kerstjens HA. Clinical evidence: Stable chronic obstructive pulmonary disease. *BMJ.* 1999;319:495–500.

22. Hess DR. Noninvasive positive pressure ventilation for acute respiratory failure. *Int Anesthesiol Clin.* 1999;37:85–102.

23. Rabatin JT, Gay PC. Noninvasive Ventilation. *Mayo Clin Proc.* 1999;74(8):817–820.

24. Confalonieri M, Gazzaniga P, Gandola L, et al. Haemodynamic response during initiation of non-invasive positive pressure ventilation in COPD patients with acute ventilatory failure. *Respir Med.* 1998;92:331–337.

25. American Association for Respiratory Care: AARC Statement of Ethical and Professional Conduct. Available at http://www.aarc.org/professional_resources/position_statements/ethics.html

26. Heffner JE. End-of-life ethical issues. In: Heffner JE, Petty TL, eds. *Respir Care Clin North Am.* 1998;4:541–559.

Sheena Mari Ferguson and Joseph A. Morelos

Heroes may not be braver than anyone else.
They're just braver for five minutes longer.

RONALD REAGAN
40th US President

LEARNING OBJECTIVES

1. Describe the major defect caused by mutations in the cystic fibrosis gene and how this disorder is associated with carrier and noncarrier.

2. Using a case example, identify the subjective report, physical assessment findings, pulmonary function tests, and laboratory data that identify the individual with a cystic fibrosis exacerbation in need of the so-called "tune-up."

3. In selecting respiratory care and airway clearance techniques, identify the key factors in making those choices.

4. Discuss potential barriers to adhering to a plan of care for a patient with cystic fibrosis.

5. Identify mechanisms that may facilitate patient adherence to the plan of care.

6. As a team member, develop a method to track a patient's health and evaluate outcomes of selected interventions.

7. Discuss techniques to explore quality-of-life and end-of-life issues with an individual with cystic fibrosis.

8. Describe the role of the respiratory care practitioner as an integral member of the multidisciplinary team. Include assessment, treatment, evaluation, and patient/family education in your discussion.

9. Apply the critical thinking skills of prioritizing, anticipating, negotiating, communicating, decision making, and reflection by completing exercises and a case example with a patient who has cystic fibrosis.

10. Apply strategies to promote critical thinking in the respiratory care management of patients with cystic fibrosis through completion of chapter exercises and group discussion.

KEY WORDS

Adherence	Gene	Leukocytosis	Permanent Tube Feeding
Airway Clearance	Genotype	Liposomes	Apparatus (PEG)
Techniques (ACT)	Hemoptysis	Meconium Ileus	Phenotype
Chromosome	Hepatobilary	Mutation	Sinopulmonary
Epistaxis	Immunosuppressant	Nasal Polyp	Ursodeoxycholic Acid
Exocrine Gland	Inherited	Osteopenia /Osteoporosis	

INTRODUCTION

Cystic fibrosis (CF) is a common genetically inherited disease, predominantly affecting Caucasians. The National Patient Registry conducted by the Cystic Fibrosis Foundation follows over 20,000 individuals in this country alone,[1] although 30,000 individuals are believed to be affected. In the United States it occurs with an incidence of 1 in 3000 among Caucasians.[2,3] It affects other ethnic groups less commonly, at an incidence of 1 in 15,000 among African Americans,[4,5] 1 in 30,000 among Asian Americans,[6] 1 in 8500 among Hispanics,[7,8] and 1 in 11,000 among Native Americans.[9] Of significance, some Native American tribes have no reported cases of CF, while others have a significantly higher incidence and carrier rate than that reported in the literature for whites (eg, the Zuni Pueblo Indians with a 1 in 5 carrier rate).[10] The carrier rate refers to the number of persons who have the CF gene, and could potentially pass it on to their children. (See the critical content box in the etiology section for more details.)

The disease was described as a discrete clinical entity in 1938 by a pathologist, Dr. Dorothy Andersen, who first named the disorder "cystic fibrosis of the pancreas."[11] She further correlated her findings of intestinal obstruction, nutritional malabsorption, failure to thrive, and pancreatic changes with the respiratory infections and changes in the lung tissues. In 1953, di Sant'Agnese and colleagues[12] described the abnormal electrolyte composition of sweat in individuals with cystic fibrosis that leads to excessive loss of sodium.

The exocrine glands throughout the body are affected by the genetic mutation, leading to multiple organ dysfunction. Although multiple organs are affected, progressive respiratory failure is the cause of death in over 90% of individuals with cystic fibrosis. Intensive surveillance, combined with aggressive treatment plans implemented by multidisciplinary health care teams have increased median life expectancy from less than 1 year in 1940, to over 30 years by 1997. Key to this improvement in survival is the triad of nutrition (pancreatic enzymes), antibiotics (infection), and airway clearance techniques (bacterial load) suggested by Matthews and co-workers[13] in 1964.

CRITICAL CONTENT

INTRODUCTION TO CYSTIC FIBROSIS

• Most common genetically inherited disease in Caucasians
• All exocrine glands are affected
• Respiratory failure is the predominant cause of premature death
• A multidisciplinary team approach improves survival
• Median life expectancy has increased dramatically in recent years

ETIOLOGY

Cystic fibrosis is an inherited disease. The inheritance pattern is autosomal recessive; therefore, individuals with cystic fibrosis have inherited two affected genes, one from each parent (each parent being a carrier). Those who have only one affected gene are called *carriers* and a carrier is asymptomatic, leading a healthy life. The cystic fibrosis gene contains the DNA code for the large protein that controls the movement of salts (ions) through the exocrine glands that secrete fluid. This large protein is called the cystic fibrosis transmembrane conductance regulator or CFTR.

The result of this genetic mutation is that patients who have cystic fibrosis have a malregulation of the salt composition of their exocrine gland secretions. This genetic defect ultimately causes the viscosity of these fluids to be abnormally high. This viscous fluid causes obstruction and inflammation of the ducts of the affected organs, resulting in the various dysfunctions seen in CF.

Recent research has led to a more thorough understanding of the specific genetic defect found in CF. In 1989 the affected chromosome, number 7, was identified as the culprit in CF.[14,15] (An abnormality within a gene is called a *mutation*.) There are over 800 mutations that have now been identified that are associated with CF. Most of these mutations occur relatively infrequently and some of them are associated with particular ethnic groups. It is because of these various genetic mutations that there are variations of the disease itself within the CF population.

The most common genetic mutation is the delta F508, delta meaning deletion, F representing phenylalanine (the amino acid configuration), at position 508 on the CFTR protein of chromosome number 7.[9] This specific mutation is carried by 70% of individuals with cystic fibrosis in the US. The severity of the disease manifestation is called the *phenotype*. The correlation between genotype (type of genetic mutation) and phenotype (clinical severity) is not clear for all of the affected organs. For example, the clinical expression or phenotype of pancreatic insufficiency in an individual with CF having two of the delta F508 mutations is very strong, yet this same group of patients may have a wide range of pulmonary function.[9,16] Prediction of the severity of lung disease based on the genotype is not possible.

When an offspring inherits one normal gene and one abnormal gene, the individual is known as a carrier. This individual is not affected by the disease, but can pass the abnormal gene to an offspring. See the critical content box for an example of risk calculation based on each parent being a carrier as well as carrier rates for selected populations.

DIAGNOSIS

Most CF patients are diagnosed at birth with meconium ileus (18%),[9] or as infants with failure to thrive due to malabsorption (50%) secondary to pancreatic insufficiency (PI). However, some 8% to 10%

CRITICAL CONTENT

RISK OF INHERITANCE WHEN EACH PARENT IS A CARRIER

Three potential scenarios:

- Offspring inherits neither mutated gene and is neither affected nor a carrier = 25% risk
- Offspring inherits one mutated gene and is not affected, but is a carrier = 50% risk
- Offspring inherits both mutated genes, is affected and will pass on gene = 25% risk

Note that the probability is the same for each pregnancy.

Carrier rates in selected groups, US population: 1 in 20 Caucasians, 1 in 65 for African Americans, and 1 in 5 for Zuni Pueblo Indians.[10]

of adolescents and adults are diagnosed later in life. This group of patients tends to fall into the pancreatic sufficient (PS) group. Thus, although the classical picture of cystic fibrosis is well recognized, the respiratory therapist should recognize that the large number of genetic mutations is expressed in a wide array of clinical presentations, such that a clear cut diagnosis of cystic fibrosis can be difficult in some cases.

Diagnostic criteria for CF include clinical features as well as evidence of CFTR dysfunction. The diagnosis of cystic fibrosis as described by Knowles and colleagues[16] includes clinical features such as sinopulmonary disease with chronic cough, sputum production, chronic infection of characteristic bacteria (*Staphylococcus aureus* and *Pseudomonas aeruginosa*), airflow obstruction, sinus disease and nasal polyps, and chronic x-ray abnormalities. It also includes evidence of dysfunctional CFTR such as elevated sweat chloride greater than 60 mEq/L, two genetic mutations (genotype), and bioelectric abnormalities in the nasal epithelium (nasal potential difference or PD).[16,17]

DIAGNOSIS OF CYSTIC FIBROSIS

- Meconium ileus
- Sinopulmonary disease
- Characteristic pathogens in sputum
- Airflow obstruction
- Elevated sweat chloride level
- Positive genotyping

PATHOPHYSIOLOGY

The tissues in exocrine (ductal) glands regulate the movement of water and electrolytes (Na^+ and Cl^-) across their cellular membranes via a process called membrane transport. The exocrine glands (secretory epithelium) are distributed throughout the body; thus, numerous organ systems are affected by this disease (Table 13-1). Normally, membrane transport allows these tissues to maintain the appropriate concentrations of water, electrolytes, and macromolecules such that the exocrine secretions are sufficiently fluid to perform their functions of lubrication, protection, secretion, and digestion.

In cystic fibrosis the various mutations of the CFTR gene result in an abnormal chloride channel that causes a decrease in chloride conductance at the surface of the secretory epithelium. This malregulation of the salt concentration causes changes in the consistency of the various organs' secretions. This abnormality in the composition of secretions from the various exocrine organs of an individual with cystic fibrosis eventually leads to obstruction of their ducts and/or channels, leading to various types of organ dysfunction. The specific mechanism is not completely understood, nor is one explanation necessarily sufficient to explain all of the pathophysiologic results seen with this defect. In light of the variety of ways the ducts of the exocrine gland organs can become dysfunctional from obstruction, it becomes clear that an extensive treatment plan is necessary to maintain health and well-being.

A secondary pathophysiologic change occurs in the lungs as a result of the abnormal secretions. The inflammation caused by chronic bacterial infection (described later) and the resultant persistent infiltration of neutrophils with the subsequent release of their enzymes (elastases) leads to destruction of the airway walls. The loss of structural integrity of bronchial walls leads to a condition called *bronchiectasis*. The bronchiectatic wall is prone to collapse in high flow conditions and contributes to airflow obstruction and air trapping seen with this disease.

CLINICAL MANIFESTATIONS AND TREATMENT

Sinus Disease and Polyps

Over 90% of individuals with CF have evidence of paranasal sinus opacification on radiographs. Despite this significant finding, a much smaller percentage of these patients report daily symptoms (10% to 24%).[18] Headache, facial pain, nasal obstruction, foul breath, purulent drainage, postnasal drip, and fever are common. Treatment is directed toward treatment of the sinusitis with appropriate antibiotics (local or systemic) based on recent sputum cultures. Additional measures such as nasal irrigation and decongestants may also be beneficial. Nasal polyps are remarkably common, although the symptomatology varies widely. Presenting symp-

TABLE 13-1   EXOCRINE GLAND DISTRIBUTION

Eyes	Lacrimal glands
Mouth	Salivary glands
Nose/throat	Mucous glands
Bronchi	Goblet cells, mucous glands
Liver	Hepatobiliary ducts
Pancreas	Acinar/ductal cells
Intestines	Brunner's glands
Cervix	Mucous glands
Vas deferens	Ductal abnormalities
Skin	Sweat glands

toms (25% of individuals with CF) include nasal air-flow obstruction, polyps visibly protruding from the nares, purulent discharge, foul breath, and epistaxis. Treatment is directed toward reducing the chronic irritation of the nasal mucosa that occurs in sinusitis, as polyps develop secondary to this inflammatory process. Nasal corticosteroids may have some benefit in reducing this chronic irritation.

Pulmonary Disease

The airways of a CF patient are coated with extremely viscous secretions that are difficult for the mucociliary escalator to clear. This fact, combined with the fact that the lungs of individuals with CF are particularly receptive to several organisms (*Staphylococcus aureus*, *Haemophilus influenzae*, and *Pseudomonas aeruginosa*), result in the typical clinical picture of CF. Periodically, the bacterial load of these chronic infections overwhelms the individual and an exacerbation occurs. It is important to note that between these acute exacerbations, many afflicted individuals have relatively normal lives, a fact that many health care providers do not always appreciate.

An acute exacerbation may be manifested by the following: increased severity and/or frequency of cough, increased volume of sputum production, change in sputum color, the presence of "streaking" or frank hemoptysis, fatigue, dyspnea, weight loss, declining pulmonary function tests, decreased exercise tolerance, increase in baseline oxygen requirement, increased presence of adventitious breath sounds, leukocytosis, fever, and radiographic density. Of note, many health care providers unfamiliar with cystic fibrosis will look for the presence of standard markers of pulmonary infection: leukocytosis, fever, and radiographic changes, as the only evidence of an acute exacerbation.[19,20] These three findings may not be present. When present, fever is usually low-grade, leukocytosis is atypical, and chest x-rays are not generally useful.

If the exacerbation is considered mild, then oral (quinolones, such as ciprofloxacin) or inhaled antibiotics [aminoglycosides, such as Tobramycin (TOBI)] combined with increased attention to airway clearance techniques (ACTs), rest, and increased caloric intake may suffice. Moderate to severe exacerbations generally require intravenous antibiotics (double therapy, such as an aminoglycoside with a cephalosporin) with increased ACTs and a more concerted nutritional regimen.

Timely follow-up is essential when the individual with a mild exacerbation is treated at home. This ensures that the patient is returning to baseline and no further antibiotic therapy is indicated. Evidence of improving symptomatology, decreasing sputum volume, increasing pulmonary function tests, and stable or increasing weight should be demonstrated. Additionally, following an exacerbation a careful assessment of the precipitating factor(s) is warranted. For example, was a decrease in financial support hampering the individual's ability to respond? Was inability to obtain medications or failure to devote adequate time in the daily schedule for treatments responsible? All of these factors should be reviewed with a patient to learn from the experience in hopes of reducing the frequency and severity of future exacerbations.

CRITICAL CONTENT

TYPICAL CLINICAL MANIFESTATIONS OF CF EXACERBATION

- Increase in cough frequency
- Increase in sputum volume
- The presence of streaking or frank hemoptysis
- Fatigue
- Dyspnea
- Declining pulmonary function tests
- Decrease in exercise tolerance
- Weight loss
- Increase in baseline oxygen requirement
- Presence or increase in adventitious breath sounds

MARKERS OF INFECTION OFTEN *NOT* PRESENT IN CF EXACERBATION

- Leukocytosis
- Fever
- Chest radiograph density

A frequent problem in management of CF exacerbations is the development of antibiotic-resistant microorganisms, particularly pseudomonas. Treatment guidelines should include suitable sputum specimens with organism-specific antibiotics based on detected susceptibilities. Specific microbiology labs around the country specialize as referral centers for certain organisms that have become resistant, or are particularly lethal to the CF population. In addition to multiple bacterial infections, these patients may also have fungal infections (*Aspergillus fumigatus*), and atypical or nontuberculous mycobacteria (NTM). As a consequence, these are screened for routinely in CF patients.[21]

CRITICAL CONTENT

SIGNIFICANT PATHOGENS IN CF

- Bacterial: *Staphylococcus aureus, Haemophilus influenzae, Pseudomonas aeruginosa*
- Fungal: *Aspergillus fumigatus*
- Atypical and nontuberculous mycobacteria

Airway Clearance Techniques (ACTs)   There are two major issues to deal with when it comes to airway clearance techniques and the cystic fibrosis patient. The first deals with selection of appropriate ACTs for each CF patient, appropriate techniques being those that work best in removing secretions for that individual patient. A number of useful techniques have been developed and advocated over the years. Consistent with the problem-based learning (PBL) focus of this text, and the intent of these chapters to provide an overview of the diseases and their treatment options, the reader should look to additional resources for more extensive coverage of these techniques.

The second major issue is that the patient must be willing to use the techniques that have been identified for them, as prescribed. There are many factors that may affect the patient's adherence to

their prescribed ACT regimen. These include having appropriate equipment, proper patient education, adequate energy, sufficient airflow, and necessary time, as well as the patient's perception of the importance and effectiveness of the various techniques (does the patient think the technique works well enough for them to make it worth the bother to take time to do it?).

Chest physiotherapy (CPT) with postural drainage (PD) is but one method of many available to these patients. Positive expiratory pressure (PEP), autogenic drainage (AD), oscillating PEP (flutter valve), forced expiration technique (FET), high frequency chest oscillation (vests), and intrapulmonary percussive ventilation (IPV or IPPV, not to be confused with IPPB) are all methods with their proponents among patients and practitioners. A review of the literature has not shown any method to be clearly superior over the others.[25] Depending on the circumstances, more than one method may be used by an individual at different times, though the key is finding an ACT with which the individual is comfortable and compliant to use.

CRITICAL CONTENT

AIRWAY CLEARANCE TECHNIQUES OF POTENTIAL USE IN CF

- Chest physiotherapy (CPT)
- Positive expiratory pressure (PEP)
- Autogenic drainage (AD)
- Oscillating PEP (flutter device)
- Forced expiration technique (FET)
- High frequency chest oscillation (vests)
- Intrapulmonary percussive ventilation (IPV)

Aerosol Therapy.   A significant number of patients with CF have some degree of bronchial hyperactivity. As a result, many are treated with bronchodilators, and some with aerosol antiinflammatory agents. These needs should be individualized to the patient according to the clinical findings and the patient's demonstrated degree of responsiveness.

Although there is a lack of research evidence, mucolytics and hypertonic saline are often used in an attempt to thin and mobilize the extremely thick pulmonary secretions. DNase is another aerosol agent that has documented benefit in liquefying secretions.[22] This is an aerosol enzyme that cleaves the DNA found in very high levels in the sputum of individuals with cystic fibrosis and thus improves sputum viscosity and clearance.

There are a variety of potential treatments (see critical content box) and it is unreasonable to expect the patient to consistently perform each. The practitioner must keep in mind the amount of time and effort it takes to complete these treatments when developing and reviewing the respiratory care plan. For example, using a nebulizer compressor and medication delivery device to administer the medications the most efficaciously, yet in the shortest time, helps with patient compliance.

CRITICAL CONTENT

TREATMENT CONSIDERATIONS: HOW MANY NEBULIZER TREATMENTS COULD (WOULD) YOU DO IN A DAY?

Typical daily regimen:

    Albuterol with cromolyn sodium or saline:

      4 per day

    DNase: 1 per day

    TOBI: 2 per day

20 to 30 minutes each $\times$ 7 = $3^1/_2$ hours total

RECOMMENDED ORDER OF MEDICATION ADMINISTRATION

- Bronchodilator
- Antiinflammatory agent (nebulizer or MDI)
- Mucolytic
- ACT of choice
- Antibiotic

Note: Bronchodilator may be mixed with cromolyn sodium. DNase and antibiotic each needs its own nebulizer cup and they should not be mixed.

Pancreatic Disease

Approximately 85% of individuals with CF are pancreatic insufficient, thus 15% can be characterized as pancreatic sufficient.[23] The pancreatic disease results in impaired digestion of fats, which leads to malabsorption and loss of fat in the stool (steatorrhea) often resulting in poor weight gain and growth curves. Blockage of the small bile ducts to the small intestine occurs due to the failure of sodium bicarbonate and water secretion. Proteins and complex carbohydrates are also not properly digested. The fat soluble vitamins A, D, E, and K must be supplemented to prevent secondary complications (see critical content box for importance of these vitamins).

Abdominal bloating, cramping, and discomfort result from increased intestinal bulk because an inadequate amount of pancreatic lipase makes its way to the small intestine. Individuals with CF must take supplemental pancreatic enzymes throughout the day to correct this malabsorption. Enzymes come in varying strengths, such as MT-10 and MT-20. Each MT-10 capsule has 10,000 U of lipase and each MT-20 capsule has 20,000 U of lipase. Each capsule also contains protease to break down proteins and amylase to break down complex carbohydrates.

About now you might be asking yourself why the pancreatic function of a patient with CF should be of concern to the respiratory therapist. First and foremost, the correlation between body weight and lung function is unique. For example, does lung function follow weight loss, or does weight fall as pulmonary function deteriorates? Inadequate muscle mass and diaphragm strength have implications for respiratory performance, and the anorexia and loss of appetite associated with exacerbations can quickly lead to an unacceptable degree of weight loss. Additionally, abdominal bloating and discomfort can interfere with the ability to perform ACTs and/or breathing. Chronic pain syndromes resulting from bone disease impact exercise tolerance, activity level, and comfort in performing airway clearance, particularly with a rib fracture caused by coughing. Vitamin K deficiencies are of concern because severe frank hemoptysis is common.

Another problem associated with pancreatic disease is the development of cystic fibrosis-related diabetes mellitus (CFRDM).[24] As the exocrine function of the pancreas is impeded by inspissated secretions, the pancreas becomes fibrotic. This coupled with fatty infiltration of the organ results in destruction of some but not all of the islets, thereby affecting endocrine function. This results in the diminished secretion of pancreatic hormones.

CRITICAL CONTENT

IMPORTANCE OF FAT SOLUBLE VITAMINS

Vitamin A: deficiency can cause diseases of the eye and night blindness

Vitamin D: critical in bone and tooth health, prevents osteoporosis

Vitamin E: important for reflexes and gait

Vitamin K: necessary for the liver to make clotting factors

Hepatobiliary Disease

The primary site of CFTR expression in the liver is the intrahepatic duct epithelium.[25] The abnormal electrolyte transport results in altered bile composition. This altered bile is not as effective in the digestion of fats and is another mechanism precipitating malabsorption malnutrition. As bile stasis obstructs the smaller bile ducts, the hepatic tissue is damaged and the liver enzymes become elevated. This results in cirrhosis, portal hypertension, and in some cases, liver failure. Although the long-term benefits are not clear, patients with elevated liver function tests may have a satisfactory response to ursodeoxycholic acid, but some patients will require a liver transplant.

Intestinal Disease

Approximately 18% of newborns with CF are diagnosed by the presence of meconium ileus. This is the blockage of the intestine with meconium, and the treatment is emergent surgery. Older patients may also develop blockage of their intestines due to impaired clearance of the macromolecules. Once called meconium-ileus equivalent (MIE), this disorder is now called distal intestinal obstructive syndrome (DIOS). Treatment includes measures aimed at prevention such as optimal enzyme intake, avoiding constipation, and adequate hydration. For obstructive events, high-volume oral balanced electrolytes (such as Golytely) are effective.

Reproductive Issues

The two major abnormalities of the reproductive system in individuals with CF are a delay in the onset of puberty and reduced fertility. Advances in nutrition and overall attention to health have somewhat improved the growth and stature of patients. Still, for a variety of reasons, menarche is about 2 years later in patients with CF than in their unaffected peers.

Although difficult to quantify, fertility in women with CF is decreased. The same pathophysiologic mechanism that alters other organ secretions is also present in the cervical mucus. The cervical mucus has less water and is more viscous, and can cause a delay in sperm migration. Many adolescent females with CF believe that they are infertile and should be counseled as well about the need for protection from STDs.

Women with CF who become pregnant face all of the same physiologic changes as women without CF, and there are obviously other issues to consider. The couple should have genetic counseling and the significant other should have genotyping to evaluate carrier status. With over 800 mutations, not all of the mutations can be detected, but the appropriate panel based on their ethnic background will be evaluated. Recent studies suggest that pregnancy in women with CF is not a significant risk in and of itself. All adults considering having children should give consideration to a plan for the care of their offspring in the event of a catastrophic incident.

Women with CF who become pregnant also face the added burden of difficulties with weight gain, added fatigue, and the need to complete their daily regimen of ACTs, which can affect pulmonary function. Additionally, if they have a respiratory exacerbation, the decision of what antibiotics to prescribe must also consider the risks of side effects to the fetus. Women with CF can successfully breast-feed their infants. As with any new mother, fatigue is an issue and pre-delivery counseling should include provisions for child care assistance that enable the mother to receive adequate sleep, nutrition, and time for her daily ACT regimen. It is recommended that both the CF team and a high-risk OB team provide the prenatal care.

Males with CF make sperm, but over 95% of individuals are infertile. This is due to absence, obstruction, or atrophy of the vas deferens and/or seminal vesicles. Because the male makes sperm, a procedure called MESA (microsurgical epididymal sperm aspiration) allows the sperm to be injected into the ova of the female partner. Again, genetic counseling is important as the offspring will be a carrier, and the partner should have genetic screening.

Skin and Sweat Gland Abnormalities

Long before there was a sweat chloride test, children with salty-tasting skin were recognized as having a shorter lifespan. This is the basis for the diagnostic sweat chloride test, and can also be explained by the abnormal CFTR pathway and the impermeability to Cl⁻ and Na⁺.[26] Due to the faulty reabsorption of Na⁺ and Cl⁻, individuals with CF are at increased risk of dehydration and heatstroke, particularly in hot climates. Dehydration can have a negative impact on sputum and bowel clearance as well as other secretions.

Pain

The previous sections have highlighted the multiple systems affected by CF. As each of these systems becomes affected, or during acute exacer-

bations, there are many different mechanisms for individuals with CF to experience pain or pain syndromes. Additionally, with the threat of premature death and the chronic nature of this disease, there are issues of fear, anxiety, and loss, which contribute to lack of control or ability of the patient to verbalize their needs. As part of each encounter, careful questioning and assessment with regard to pain are important, including emotional or psychiatric distress. Untreated pain affects quality of life and may often explain lack of adherence or lack of interest in the treatment plan.

CRITICAL CONTENT

CF IS A MULTISYSTEM DISEASE

Note: Number in parentheses (%) = incidence in CF population

- Sinus: chronic sinusitis (90%) and polyposis (25%)
- Pulmonary: chronic infection, bronchiectasis/bronchitis, pneumonia, pneumothorax (1%, up to 20% of adults), mucus plugging/atelectasis, hemoptysis (massive, 300 cc in 24 hours, 1%), airflow obstruction, respiratory failure (cause of death in 94%)
- Pancreatic: insufficiency (85%), fat malabsorption, fat soluble vitamin deficit, osteopenia/osteoporosis, CF-related diabetes mellitus (15% to 20%), pancreatitis (10%)
- Hepatobiliary: fat maldigestion, cirrhosis (5%), liver disease (19%)
- Gastrointestinal: reflux/GERD (25%), meconium ileus (18%), distal intestinal obstruction syndrome (4%), constipation (12% to 15%)
- Reproduction: decreased fertility, male infertility (95%), maternal-fetal concerns
- Skin: decreased Na⁺ and Cl⁻ secretion/reabsorption, dehydration
- Arthopathy/arthritis (12%)
- Pain: Physical and psychosocial

Evolving Treatment Strategies

There is no cure for cystic fibrosis. Screening and genetic counseling are important, but new mutations continue to be identified. The treatment triad (nutrition, ACTs, and antibiotics) has increased life expectancy, but the treatment plan is rigorous and limited. New therapies are being developed through the Cystic Fibrosis Foundation's Therapeutic Development Network. Two categories of investigation include gene therapy as a way to reverse the defect, and pharmacologic advances that focus on ways to eliminate the altered electrolyte transport.

With the gene therapy, the goal is to introduce corrected genes into the cells. Various means of transporting the corrected genetic material into the affected cells are being investigated, including viruses and liposomes. Pharmacologic targets include agents to thin the mucus, combat the damage caused by the inflammatory process, and maximize ion transport through the defective chloride channels.

Lung transplantation is a complex and involved decision for individuals with end-stage lung disease. However, because the waiting period is somewhere between 18 and 24 months, individuals who may be candidates for this procedure should be referred earlier rather than later. There are several excellent consensus documents available for the respiratory therapist who desires more specific information.[27,28] Based on the 1996 International Lung Transplant Registry, the 5-year survival rate for transplant recipients with cystic fibrosis is 48%. It is important to remember that the transplant does not reverse the multisystem disease of CF, but it does provide the patient with undamaged lungs, albeit at a price. As with other organ transplants, these patients must take immunosuppressant medications, and posttransplant infections and organ rejection can be catastrophic events.[29,30]

THE CYSTIC FIBROSIS FOUNDATION

The Cystic Fibrosis Foundation is a tremendous resource for health care professionals attending to individuals with cystic fibrosis. Created in 1955 by parents of children with CF, this organization provides extensive support through education of professionals, resources for patients, the development of treatment guidelines, partnerships with industry for pharmacologic and gene therapy advances through the Therapeutic Development Network, fundraising (over 50 chapters) for support of research, and the accreditation of both adult and pediatric centers (over 100) for state-of-the-art patient care. Additionally, the organization sponsors the national/international annual meeting where the latest research and advances are shared with providers and researchers from around the world. The Foundation also supports the development of consensus documents on many aspects of CF care. These documents are developed by panels of experts and based on best available evidence.

MULTIDISCIPLINARY TEAM MANAGEMENT

Having reviewed the multisystem clinical manifestations and treatment of CF, it becomes apparent why a team approach has extended life expectancy and quality of life for CF patients. It should also be clear why the respiratory therapist is an integral member of the CF treatment team. Considering that until recently CF was considered a pediatric disease, as the life expectancy of CF patients has increased, there has developed a need for health care team members caring for adults to have knowledge of CF as well. The overall plan should include, at a minimum, the following on the adult and pediatric teams: Dieticians, nurses, physicians (pulmonary and gastroenterology), respiratory therapists, and social workers, each with CF expertise. In addition, ENT, endocrine, CDE, rheumatology, interventional radiology, physical therapy, surgery, genetic counseling, primary care, and high-risk obstetrics are extremely important. The Cystic Fibrosis Foundation has specific requirements for accreditation of care centers. Obviously, the patient and family are also important components of the team.

Team management includes trending patient parameters, considerations for transitioning between programs, infection control plans, and end-of-life care planning, as well as routine clinic visits and in-hospital management. Protocols and guidelines can also facilitate early intervention by identifying for the team what each member is responsible for, and what interventions each member will initiate. The University of New Mexico Health Sciences Center utilizes a Clinic Encounter Form (Fig. 13-1) to guide team members in a multisystem approach to patient care.

As the section on clinical manifestations described, there are multiple organ systems involved, requiring multiple interventions. In order to be able to track outcomes as well as therapeutic trials, a specific method for tracking is necessary. A shadow file, either a sectioned notebook or computer database, is used by many centers. This allows members to record their findings, interventions, and outcomes. It is useful in team meetings and can follow the patient throughout care.

Trending such parameters as height and weight, pulmonary function tests (PFTs), labs, SpO_2, microbiology, antibiotics, medications, diagnostics, ACTs, referrals, genetic counseling, immunizations, well-person care, and counseling are critical to avoid oversights and complications, but it also gives the team feedback on its progress. The University of New Mexico Health Sciences Center utilizes a Clinic Flow Sheet (Fig. 13-2) that can be used by the CF team to monitor patients in the adult cystic fibrosis program.

SITE OF CARE AND AGE-SPECIFIC CONSIDERATIONS

Health care providers often fail to recognize that individuals with CF have an involved daily regimen to maintain after discharge from the hospital. The bulk of their care occurs in the home. When one thinks about it, there are airway clearance devices, nebulizer compressors, bilevel positive airway pressure (BiPAP) machines, oxygen concentrators, feeding tubes and pumps, intravenous (IV) supplies, and numerous medications to deal with. For adolescents or young adults away at college, these

differences, which set them apart from their peers and particularly from the opposite sex, can make adherence to a regimen difficult when trying to fit in. For a young adult with a permanent IV access (port) or permanent tube feeding apparatus (PEG) and other special needs, intimacy can be difficult due to the altered body image and/or increased self-consciousness. These issues, as well as precautions for safe sex and pregnancy, must be addressed when providing counseling to patients.

Often an admission to the hospital follows failed oral antibiotic therapy, or insufficient resources to provide adequate airway clearance and nutritional intake, particularly as the individual moves into young adulthood and leaves the parents who have been the primary caregivers. A hospitalization may be viewed as a respite for the patient when illness and subsequent exhaustion prevent even basic self-care. In fact, college and expanded occupational requirements can be extremely difficult without assistance from others during acute exacerbations.

When considering the selection or changes in airway clearance techniques, an individual who has always had a parent provide manual percussion may now need an independent type of ACT, such as an oscillating vest. Remember that changes in insurance coverage over the last 5 years have meant that many services that can be delivered in the home are no longer covered, particularly services provided by respiratory therapists. However, the importance of a home care visit by the respiratory therapist cannot be overemphasized. Seeing the individual's surroundings, including cleanliness, type of equipment, safety issues, and other aspects of the physical environment (ie, stairs or contaminants from pets) can provide the practitioner with a wealth of information about potential problems or adherence issues.

The very young patient can also present treatment challenges to the health care team. Many clinics cannot provide PFTs for infants and very young children due to the difficulty in evaluating PFTs and subjective symptoms in patients who are unable to cooperate or verbalize. An infant PFT machine with conscious sedation capabilities can

UNIVERSITY OF NEW MEXICO CYSTIC FIBROSIS CENTER, ADULT PROGRAM
Building 5-ACC, 2211 Lomas NE, Albuquerque, NM 87131-5271
Telephone: (505) 272-4751   FAX: (505) 272-8700

CLINICAL ENCOUNTER RECORD   **VISIT DATE** _____

DATE OF LAST VISIT	AGE	PURPOSE OF VISIT: ☐ ROUTINE ☐ SICK ☐ SICK FOLLOW-UP ☐ HOSPITAL FOLLOW-UP ☐ NEW PATIENT OTHER:_____

LAST ADMISSION	LAST IV ANTIBIOTICS	LAST ORAL ANTIBIOTICS

HISTORY

PMH CF Related Liver Disease ☐ Cirrhosis ☐ Elevated Liver Function Tests ☐ CF Related Diabetes Mellitus ☐ Atypical Mycobacterial Disease

REVIEW OF SYSTEMS

COUGH FREQUENCY SINCE LAST VISIT:	☐ NONE	☐ OCCASIONAL	☐ DAILY
SPUTUM PRODUCTION SINCE LAST VISIT:	☐ NONE	☐ OCCASIONAL	☐ DAILY

SPUTUM CHARACTERISTICS:	HEMPTYSIS ☐ NO ☐ YES
AMOUNT	☐ SCANT (streaking) ☐ SUBMASSIVE (less than 1 cup in 24 hr) ☐ MASSIVE (more than 1 cup in 24 hr)

ABDOMINAL:	☐ CHANGE IN BOWEL HABITS	☐ BLOATING	☐ CRAMPING	STOOLS number per day, consistency
ACTIVITY:	☐ WORK ☐ SCHOOL ☐ HOME		☐ FULL TIME ☐ PART TIME ☐ NOT WORKING OR GOING TO SCHOOL	
PHYSICAL ACTIVITY:				

MEDICATIONS

ANTIBIOTICS (ORAL) ☐ NO	START: FINISH:	CIPROFLOXACIN	TMP/SMX	CEPHALOSPORIN	OTHER
ANTIBIOTICS (IV) ☐ NO				START: FINISH:	
ANTIBIOTICS (INHALED) ☐ NO		TOBRAMYCIN (TOBI) ☐ ON MONTH ☐ OFF MONTH		COLY-MYCIN	
BRONCHODILATORS ☐ NO		ALBUTEROL ☐ MDI ☐ NEB	SALMETEROL (Serevent)		
ANTI-INFLAMMATORY ☐ NO		CORTICOSTEROID (INHALED)	CROMOLYN	TILADE	IBUPROFEN
PULMOZYME ☐ NO	2.5 mg NEB ☐ QD ☐ BID		OXYGEN _____ LPM ☐ Q24 ☐ QHS ☐ WITH EXERTION		
PANCREATIC ENZYMES ☐ NO		BRAND	STRENGTH	NUMBER WITH MEALS	NUMBER WITH SNACKS
VITAMINS & MINERALS ☐ NO	ADEK	MULTIVITAMIN	VITAMIN K	VITAMIN E	CALCIUM
NUTRITIONAL SUPPLEMENTS ☐ NO	ORAL	ENTERAL		PARENTERAL	
H2 ANTAGONIST ☐ NO	FAMOTIDINE (Pepcid)	RANITIDINE (Zantac)	CIMETIDINE (Tagamet)		
OTHER:	URSODIOL (Actigall)	INSULIN	ORAL HYPOGYCEMIC		

AIRWAY CLEARANCE TECHNIQUES

	MANUAL PERCUSSION	MECHANICAL PERCUSSOR	FLUTTER	EXERCISE	THERAVEST	PHYSICAL ACTIVITY	BREATHING TECHNIQUES
FREQUENCY							

PRIMARY CARE PROVIDER _____   PATIENT NAME _____
                                                DOB   MR No.   *Continued*

FIGURE 13-1   The University of New Mexico Health Sciences Center clinic encounter form used to guide team members in a multisystem approach to patient care.

PHYSICAL EXAMINATION

TEMP	PULSE	RESPIRATION	BP	OXYGEN SATURATION	WEIGHT	KG LB	PREVIOUS WEIGHT

GENERAL	CHEST	CARDIAC	ABDOMEN	OTHER
	☐ Crackles			☐ Clubbing
	☐ Wheezing			

LABORATORY

SPIROMETRY

	CURRENT		PREVIOUS, DATE _____	
FVC	_____ L (%)	FVC	_____ L (%)
FEV$_1$	_____ L (%)	FEV$_1$	_____ L (%)
FEF$_{25-75}$	_____ L (%)	FEF$_{25-75}$	_____ L (%)

☐ STABLE   ☐ SICK

MICROBIOLOGY

	CULTURE TYPE	ROUTINE	AFB	FUNGAL
DATE ___/___/___ M D Y	☐ SPUTUM ☐ THROAT ☐ BAL ☐ OTHER	☐ NOT DONE ☐ NO GROWTH ☐ GROWTH, CODE_____ SENSITIVITIES	☐ NOT DONE ☐ NO GROWTH ☐ GROWTH, CODE_____	☐ NOT DONE ☐ NO GROWTH ☐ GROWTH, CODE_____
DATE ___/___/___ M D Y	☐ SPUTUM ☐ THROAT ☐ BAL ☐ OTHER	☐ NOT DONE ☐ NO GROWTH ☐ GROWTH, CODE_____ SENSITIVITIES	☐ NOT DONE ☐ NO GROWTH ☐ GROWTH, CODE_____	☐ NOT DONE ☐ NO GROWTH ☐ GROWTH, CODE_____

ORGANISM CODES:
1. No growth/Normal flora
2. P. aeruginosa (non-mucoid)
3. P. aeruginosa (mucoid)
4. P. aeruginosa (multiply resistant)
5. B. cepacia
6. Other Pseudomonas
7. X. multiphilia
8. Other gram negative bacilli
_____
9. S. aureus
10. H. influenza
11. Candida
12. Aspergillus
13. Atypical mycobacterium
14. Other organisiums
15. Methacillin resistant S. aureus (MRSA)
16. Mycobacterium avium intra-cellulare complex (MAC)

NUTRITIONAL ASSESSMENT_____

_____

_____

_____

ASSESSMENT AND PLAN _____

_____

_____

_____

_____

_____

_____

_____

_____

ATTENDING _____   PROVIDER_____

RETURN TO ADULT CYSTIC FIBROSIS CLINIC (CHEST CLINIC) ON: _____

FIGURE 13-1   Continued

UNIVERSITY of NEW MEXICO HEALTH SCIENCES CENTER							First Name	Last Name
CYSTIC FIBROSIS CLINIC FLOW SHEET								
AGE_____(DOB / /19)				UNMHSC MR# ___ ___ ` ___ ___ ___ ___ ___				

DATE						
Symptoms						
PARAMETER	PARAMETER	PARAMETER	PARAMETER	PARAMETER	PARAMETER	PARAMETER
WEIGHT						
IDEAL WT						
SpO2						
FEV1						
FVC						
FEV1/FVC						
GLUC /HbA1C /	/	/	/.	/	/	/
ALT /AST /	/	/	/	/	/	/
GGT/ALK PHOS /	/	/	/	/	/	/
BILI T/D /	/	/	/	/	/	/
CHOLESTEROL						
MEDICATION	MEDICATION	MEDICATION	MEDICATION	MEDICATION	MEDICATION	MEDICATION
TESTS	TESTS	TESTS	TESTS	TESTS	TESTS	TESTS
PROCEDURES	PROCEDURES	PROCEDURES	PROCEDURES	PROCEDURES	PROCEDURES	PROCEDURES
HOME IV TX						
HOSPITAL TX						
RT / RD / SW						
OTHER:						

CFCI INIC7/96   *Continued*

FIGURE 13-2   The University of New Mexico Health Sciences Center clinic flow sheet used by the CF team to monitor patients in the adult cystic fibrosis program.

Adult Cystic Fibrosis Clinic - Problem List

Date   Problems/Needs:

____   **1.** _____

            _____

____   **2.** _____

            _____

____   **3.** _____

            _____

____   **4.** _____

            _____

____   **5.** _____

            _____

____   **6.** _____

            _____

____   **7.** _____

            _____

FIGURE 13-2   Continued

provide the team with the ability to obtain PFTs in this population.[31]

For families with one, two, or even three affected children, their ability to provide treatments, deal with financial difficulties, and attempt to maintain some degree of normalcy can be very taxing. Some states have funding to provide respite capabilities, and hospitalization is sometimes the only way for these families to cope with a very sick child.

PATIENT AND HEALTH CARE PROVIDER EDUCATION

Respiratory therapists can have a tremendous impact on the education of health care providers and direct patient education. There are many complexities involved in the management of CF, hence the need to be prepared with the needed information at your fingertips. To accomplish this we recommend

a rapid-response file system. This is a cabinet containing articles for both providers and patients. One drawer holds journal references for house staff, home care agencies, and community caregivers, as well as insurance providers.

A second drawer holds patient education materials with a section for each member of the team. As patients are introduced to the clinic, each is given a notebook with sections for phone numbers or business cards, an overview of CF, and sections on each aspect of their care. There is a place to note and trend their own parameters, including weight and PFTs.

A third drawer includes videos that may be checked out by staff or patients. This allows the team to quickly respond to requests for information during clinic or rounds. The patient is encouraged to bring their notebook to clinic for review with any of the team members and also to write down questions that they may have to be reviewed during clinic.

Across hospitals, clinics, and care centers, there is a wide variation as to what health care teams require for infection control. Some facilities do not allow two CF patients in the same waiting area; patients are given a pager at a check-in point and paged when they are to come to clinic. Some clinics cohort patients with certain organisms (such as *Burkholderia cepacia*) on separate clinic days. Others provide thorough cleanings in examination rooms between patients. Although the Cystic Fibrosis Foundation will sponsor a consensus conference in early 2001, at present clear-cut guidelines are not available. Certainly, handwashing is of paramount importance, as is the cleaning of equipment (compressors, oscillating vests, G-5, PFT equipment, SpO_2 and blood pressure devices) between patients with the assumption that the health care team will not always know when a patient develops MRSA or *B cepacia*. Established protocols as recommended by the Centers for Disease Control and Prevention and hospital epidemiology are also critical.

In previous sections, the specific organisms that can threaten the health of individuals with CF were discussed. These pathogens are not a concern for the healthy and unaffected; however, transmission to others with CF is a real concern. Lung transplant may be ruled out as a treatment option for individuals colonized with certain organisms (*Burkholderia cepacia*, methicillin-resistant *Staphylococcus aureus*), as these infections can put the immunosuppressed transplant recipient at risk if antibiotic therapy is not an option. Simply the development of a highly resistant pseudomonas infection can worsen an individual's clinical course. Because of these risks, clinic, hospital, and social situations must be considered. CF organizations ask that patients with *B cepacia* or MRSA refrain from attending these events. Additionally, they may request submission of a microbiology report verified by the patient's physician. Many patients will request masks and waterless antibacterial soaps when attending these events.

Although infection control issues such as transmission of virulent bugs, particularly *Burkholderia cepacia*, has discouraged CF summer camps, "family days" that are limited to adult patients or parents of pediatric patients (who take infection control precautions) are still very helpful in disseminating information, both with regard to CF treatment options and to advocacy issues. There are also many professional and patient/family-oriented chat rooms on the Internet that may be accessed.

HEALTH PROMOTION AND QUALITY OF LIFE

When discussing the daily regimen of an individual with CF, discussions have centered on airway clearance techniques, medications, and nutrition, the so-called triad of therapy. However, as the life expectancy of these patients increases, attention to other body systems becomes essential as secondary complications of CF become apparent. Certainly smoking has a negative effect on the individual's already affected lungs, thus the need for avoidance of this habit will be obvious to the patient with CF. However, since liver dysfunction is not as obvious in all CF patients, a more vigorous amount of health education and promotion activities may be needed to keep the CF patient from adding to the insidious damage that often occurs from CF (cirrhosis and other liver disease). Chronic alcohol consumption may further stress an already stressed liver, and now that CF patients are living longer life spans this is yet another new health education issue that should be addressed.

Despite attempts at weight gain and vitamin D supplementation, CF patients remain at risk for osteoporosis and spontaneous fractures. Exercise as a means of developing cardiopulmonary fitness is increasingly recognized as being essential to good health and emotional well-being. For the individual with CF, not only are treatments, medications, and weight gain often a full-time job, but they must also integrate a proactive healthy lifestyle as well.

The individual's quality of life is obviously impacted by these many therapies, medications, and concessions of time. Additional stressors such as financial concerns, fear of a premature death, pain, lack of intimacy, and differences with their peers also affect one's satisfaction with life and ability to meet personal goals. To accurately measure the impact of these measures on patients with the unique condition of cystic fibrosis, a specific quality-of-life tool was recently developed.[32] As the validity and reliability of this instrument is evaluated, providers will be able to identify which interventions help CF patients to have the highest quality of life possible.

CONSIDERATION OF COSTS AND ETHICAL ISSUES

The implementation of life-prolonging treatments (oscillating vests and tube feeding devices), medications (TOBI and DNase), and services (home IV treatment and physical therapy) costs a great deal of money. Considering the relatively small number of individuals with CF (20,000 in the US and 70,000 worldwide) in relation to the millions of dollars necessary for drug development, one can see that orphan drugs (drugs for use in a small group of patients) can be costly. As an example, oscillating vests cost about $15,000 each, inhaled antibiotics about $600 per month, and an IV antibiotic course costs several thousand dollars. For individuals with insurance that has a limited lifetime capitation these numbers quickly add up. Lung transplants may cost several hundreds of thousands of dollars, and the benefit offered by the insurance company may not cover those costs. Coverage for infertility procedures may also be an issue for both males and females with CF. Some may argue that these costs should not be covered, particularly when there is the risk of the conceived child also having CF.

In addition to the costs of developing these therapeutic measures, one must also consider the ramifications of providing them. Lung transplants are extremely intricate treatment decisions, given that the patient is often trading one set of health concerns for another. The regimen is complex and the patient still has the other manifestations of cystic fibrosis to manage. Concerns in the health care community regarding the development of gene therapy to correct the CFTR defect remain unanswered.

For the individual who is not a candidate for lung transplant and is too ill to participate in new studies, ethical issues may be as simple (or complex) as the use of intubation and mechanical ventilation in an individual with severe lung disease.

Other ethical issues to be addressed include the use of end-of-life therapies. For example, health care providers may see a combination of therapy categories being used that may not fit the usual view of end-of-life care. Levels of care may be divided into several categories: disease prevention (calcium or vitamin supplementation), therapeutic intervention (ACTs or antimicrobials), and/or palliative management (oxygen or morphine). A combination of these types of care is often indicated, and they are not mutually exclusive. Communication among the health care team members, patient, and family are critical to ensure that the individual's needs are addressed. One cannot overemphasize the importance of discussions with regard to advance directives and designation of alternate decision makers. A key point here is that each person needs to consider these personal decisions, including the public and the members of the health care team. Unfortunately, many patients interpret these discussions as a sign that their disease is progressing rather than a discussion that everyone should participate in to ensure that the patient's wishes are carried out.

INTRODUCTION TO CASE STUDIES

The following two cases are included in this chapter to allow the learner to apply his or her understanding of critical concepts in the management of patients with cystic fibrosis. The questions are designed to allow the learner to practice gathering information and building assessment skills, as well as learn to formulate treatment plans and work as a team member. Please refer to the specific assignments made by your faculty. You may be asked to address particular exercises rather than all of them, due to time or priority constraints. Please see your faculty for specific directions regarding when and how to use the following cases.

CASE STUDY 1

MS. HEATHER PHLEM

An 18-year-old woman from Zuni, Pueblo is referred for the first time to your pulmonary clinic for evaluation of a chronic cough that she has had since age 2. The cough varies in frequency and productivity of sputum. Currently, the cough occurs throughout the day and she is producing about 2 tablespoons of thick, green phlegm per day. The woman was last hospitalized at age 8 for a lower respiratory tract infection. She is currently 6 months pregnant and has had poor weight gain. Her usual weight is 102 lb and her height is 62 inches. Her current medications are beclomethasone inhaler 4 puffs, twice per day; albuterol inhaler 2 puffs every 4 hours as needed, and a prenatal vitamin.

Critical Thinking Exercise 1

PRIORITIZING AND PATIENT ASSESSMENT

Given the initial history, explain how you would prioritize your patient assessment of Ms. Phlem upon her arrival to the clinic.

a. What diseases would you include in your differential diagnosis?

b. What additional history or physical assessment information would you like to know?

c. What additional diagnostic information would you obtain?

The following additional history and data are now obtained:

General   Her weight has been relatively stable over most of her life, 85% of ideal body weight. She has no abdominal bloating or cramping. She has three formed bowel movements a day with floating stools. She has never smoked. She has a brother with asthma. There has been no history of tuberculosis or known exposure to individuals with active tuberculosis. Her ear, nose, and throat exam is normal and there are no polyps. There is a slight increase in the P_2 cardiac sound. Abdominal exam is normal without liver or spleen enlargement and is consistent with a gravid uterus. There is no clubbing present.

Chest   Her breath sounds are clear.

Labs   Her chest radiograph reveals mild streaky infiltrates in the upper lobes. Serum analysis shows a normal white blood count, clotting studies, and chemistry. The microbiologic profile of her sputum shows the presence of *Staphylococcus aureus* and *Stenotrophomonas maltophilia*. The culture was negative for fungal and acid-fast bacillus species. Her genotyping reveals 3849+10kbC–T/3849+10kbC–T mutations.

Vital signs

HR	87/min
RR	18/min
BP	116/68
SpO_2	93%
Temp.	Afebrile

Pulmonary function tests show:

PFT data

FEV_1	2.07 L (68%)
FVC	2.96 L (93%)
FEV_1/FVC	.70
$FEF_{25\%-75\%}$	1.44 L/s (42%)

Based on the additional history and data above, please do the following exercise.

Critical Thinking Exercise 2

ASSESSMENT
OF DATA/MAKING INFERENCES

a. How do the additional history and physical assessment findings assist you with your preliminary diagnosis?

b. What would you infer from the additional laboratory data?

c. How would you interpret the pulmonary function tests?

In the team discussion, you have been asked to develop an airway clearance regimen for this woman.

Ms. Phlem was placed on a comprehensive airway clearance therapy protocol as recommended by the respiratory therapist. This included the addition of the use of a flutter device twice a day and a spacer on her two MDI medications (albuterol and beclomethasone). She was also coached in her coughing technique, and her nutritional regimen was evaluated. One pancreatic enzyme (Ultrase) was added to each meal and snack, as was an ADEK vitamin every day, and a high-calorie supplement three times a day. Her weight gain stabilized. Additionally, her cough diminished and there was a reduction of her daily sputum load. She went on to deliver a healthy male infant weighing 6 lb 13 oz at 39 weeks gestation. There were no complications for the mother or the infant.

Critical Thinking Exercise 3

ANTICIPATING/PRIORITIZING CARE

a. What factors will you consider as you develop her treatment plan?

b. What treatment considerations do you anticipate the other members of your team to initiate?

c. What patient teaching issues are of primary importance? of secondary importance?

d. What are the priorities in her care?

Critical Thinking Exercise 4

ANTICIPATING FUTURE HEALTH
CARE/HEALTH EDUCATION NEEDS

a. Do you believe Ms. Phlem has cystic fibrosis? Why or why not? What data would you need to review to make that determination?

b. What do you anticipate will be Ms. Phlem's future respiratory care needs?

c. Develop a long-term health care plan for Ms. Phlem including attention to health promotion.

CASE STUDY 2

MR. JEFFREY MUCOID

Initial History

A 34-year-old patient presents to the outpatient clinic with the following information initially available:

General   Mr. Mucoid is a 34-year-old male who was diagnosed with CF at the age of 6 months. He had a meconium ileus at birth and a positive family history for CF. He works full-time as an engineer. His sister, who also had CF, died when she was 12 years old. He is seen in clinic today for a routine scheduled visit, but he is complaining of a worsening cough for the last 3 weeks. He is producing more than $1/_2$ cup of dark green and brown phlegm per day. His daily CF regimen includes: Pulmozyme 2.5 mg nebulized every day, Ultrase MT-20 enzymes 6 by mouth with each meal and 3 to 4 by mouth with each snack, and albuterol 2.5 mg nebulized twice a day, ADEK one by mouth every day, and oxygen 1 to 2 L/min by nasal cannula, which he wears at night.

Labs   His sweat chloride test was 96 mEq/L. His genotype performed last year showed that he was homozygous for the delta F508 mutation.

Critical Thinking Exercise 1

ASSESSMENT AND DECISION MAKING

a. What additional information collected through the interview process is necessary in order to formulate an impression of his overall status?

b. What diagnostic tests would you obtain at this time?

You are evaluating Mr. Mucoid's respiratory care needs while he is in the clinic. As part of the routine assessment that you perform with each clinic patient, you assess his prescription for airway clearance therapy while other members of the team are obtaining additional data. In addition to your evaluation, he is being seen by the pulmonologist, clinical nurse specialist, dietician, and social worker. After their evaluation of Mr. Mucoid, each team member above noted that they feel that he has some issues that require intervention.

These are the data obtained during the team's assessment: Mr. Mucoid reveals that he has had no change in intermittent blood streaking in his sputum over the last 3 to 4 months. His weight has decreased. His chest examination shows slight retractions with breathing. For airway clearance, he admits to using the vest twice a week, and he walks 30 minutes the other 5 days. (This is not what you had previously recommended or what was prescribed by his physician.) He also has more shortness of breath and admits that this is why he has quit doing his ACTs as prescribed. On examination, the following is noted:

General   Clubbing is present in the digits. He has bilateral crackles in the upper lung fields, and the breath sounds are slightly diminished over the rest of his chest. There is no wheezing. His chest radiograph reveals a slight worsening of the cystic changes seen on his previous film 6 months earlier with some increased streaking infiltrates bilaterally (see Fig. 13-3).

Labs   The microbiologic profile of his sputum is negative for fungus or acid-fast bacilli. Gram's stain shows moderate gram-negative bacillus and a final report shows *Pseudomonas aeruginosa* (PA) and a mucoid *Pseudomonas aeruginosa* (PAM). See Table 13-2 for the antibiotic sensitivities.

CASE STUDY 2 *(continued)*

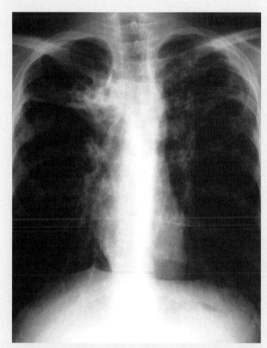

FIGURE 13-3 Chest radiograph reveals cystic changes that appear worse than on the film made 6 months earlier, with some increased streaking infiltrates bilaterally.

Pulmonary function tests show:

PFT data

FEV$_1$	.88 L (21%)
FVC	1.82 L (37%)
FEV$_1$/FVC	.48
FEF$_{25\%-75\%}$	24 L/s (5%)

Vital signs

HR	118/min
RR	28/min
BP	130/78
SpO$_2$	86% (room air)
Temp.	99.3°F orally

TABLE 13-2   ANTIBIOTIC SENSITIVITIES FOR CULTURE FROM MR. MUCOID

ANTIBIOTIC	PS	PAM
Amikacin	R	R
Cefepime	R	I
Ciprofloxacin	R	S
Gentamycin	R	R
Imipenem	S	R
Piperacillin	S	S
Tobramycin	S	S

R = resistant; I = intermediate; S = susceptible.

PS = *Pseudomonas aeruginosa*;
PAM = mucoid *Pseudomonas aeruginosa*.

Critical Thinking Exercise 2

ASSESSMENT AND DECISION MAKING

a. How would you categorize his current respiratory status?

b. Would you admit Mr. Mucoid to the hospital? Give the reason(s) why you would or would not recommend admission at this time, using an evidenced-based approach to practice.

Mr. Mucoid somewhat reluctantly agrees to be admitted to the hospital, but only for "a couple of days." He shares with you his feeling that he knows you really can't help him.

CASE STUDY 2 *(continued)*

 Critical Thinking Exercise 3

DECISION MAKING: DEVELOPING A TREATMENT PLAN

a. What should constitute the respiratory care plan for this patient?

b. What interventions can you initiate to improve adherence to the ACT regimen?

c. Given the data in Table 13-2, what would likely be recommended for Mr. Mucoid?

d. What else should be included in Mr. Mucoid's plan of care?

 Critical Thinking Exercise 4

ASSESSMENT

Now that Mr. Mucoid has been admitted to the hospital, what other diagnostic test(s) would you recommend?

SECOND DAY OF HOSPITALIZATION

The next morning when you follow-up with Mr. Mucoid as an inpatient, he reports that he is still feeling short of breath. You are continuing to assess his respiratory status and you inquire if the ACT prescription is helping him with his sputum load. He responds that it doesn't matter, because he is going to "die like my sister."

 Critical Thinking Exercise 5

ANTICIPATING PROBLEMS AND SOLUTIONS

a. What are the long-term options for treatment of Mr. Mucoid's lung disease?

b. What interventions are available to treat his dyspnea?

c. Should he be referred for a lung transplant?

 Group Critical Thinking Exercise 1

NEGOTIATION, COMMUNICATION, AND ETHICAL ISSUES

The following exercises can be performed by either the individual student, or preferably, by a group assigned to discuss and arrive at a group decision on the best answer for each of the following questions. In either situation, the faculty should remind students to use the THINKER approach and determine which responses to include during the class discussion of the issues generated by these exercises.

a. How would you respond to his statement that he is going to "die like his sister"?

b. Should you negotiate with Mr. Mucoid in an attempt to get him to change his mind and accept the therapy?

c. Is this patient competent to make his own decisions?

d. What would you tell him about advance directives?

e. What is the role of the respiratory therapist in discussing code status?

f. Should Mr. Mucoid have as his code status listed as Do Not Resuscitate?

This hospitalization lasted 10 days. Multiple interventions by the team were initiated, including addressing his hopelessness, fear of death, and anxiety over his dyspnea, as well as major nutritional interventions. A meticulous daily educational session about progressive ACTs and pharmacologic therapy by the respiratory therapist combined with nocturnal BiPAP was also initiated. This, in combination with IV antibiotics, significantly improved his pulmonary function. Additionally, the team explored with Mr. Mucoid what his treatment options were and what the team could offer him. He was diagnosed with CFRDM, and this was also treated. Three months later, he had been evaluated for lung transplant and been listed. He has gained weight and his pulmonary function has continued to show a **1** slight improvement. He reports an improved outlook on life and an increase in his activities.

KEY POINTS

- It is estimated that 30,000 individuals, mostly Caucasian, are affected with this genetically inherited disease.

- All exocrine glands are affected

- Respiratory failure is the cause of death in over 90% of individuals with CF.

- Median life expectancy has increased dramatically in recent years.

- Key to improved survival is the triad of nutrition, antibiotics, and ACTs.

- A malregulation of the salt composition of exocrine glands makes their secretions viscous, resulting in obstruction and inflammation of the ducts of the affected organs resulting in various forms of organ dysfunction.

- There are over 800 mutations of the CF gene, causing differing degrees of dysfunction of the various organs, as a result, not all patients with CF have the same clinical picture.

- Most CF patients are diagnosed early in life, in infancy or early childhood, however, 8% to 10% are diagnosed as adolescents or adults.

- Diagnosis is made by a combination of clinical features as well as evidence of CFTR (meconium ileus, cough/sputum production, characteristic pulmonary pathogens, sinus disease, nasal polyps, airflow obstruction, elevated sweat chloride, chronic chest radiograph changes, and bioelectric abnormalities in the nasal epithelium).

- Acute exacerbation of the pulmonary disease does not always result in the traditional markers of leukocytosis, fever, and chest radiograph densities.

- Typical causes of resistant pulmonary infection include the bacteria; *Staphylococcus aureus, Haemophilus influenzae, Pseudomonas aeruginosa,* nontuberculous atypical mycobacteria or fungal infections with *Aspergillus fumigatus.*

- ACTs must be individualized to activities and procedures to which the patient will adhere and usually include such things as CPT and PD, PEP, AD, PEP, flutter valves, high-frequency vests, and possibly IPV.

- A patient may spend 3 to 4 hours a day to administer their daily regimen of therapy and procedures.

- Eighty-five percent of patients are pancreatic insufficient, leading to fat absorbtion problems and necessitating fat soluble vitamin and pancreatic enzyme supplementation.

- CF is a multisystem disease affecting to varying degrees the sinus, pulmonary, pancreatic, hepatobiliary, GI, reproductive, and skin organ systems.

- Evolving treatments strategies and categories of investigation include gene therapy, pharmacologic improvements, and lung transplants.

- With multisystem disease, the CF patient is ideally treated by a multidisciplinary team at a specialty center.

- The bulk of care for the CF patient occurs at home.

- Respiratory therapists provide much patient education on self-care to patients affected with CF.

- As the CF population ages, other general health promotion activities are becoming of increasing importance.

ACKNOWLEDGMENTS

The authors would like to thank the Adult Cystic Fibrosis Center team members for their contributions to the case studies: David S. James, MD, Director; Kyla Boswell, RRT, Respiratory Therapist; and Jan Esparza, MS, RD, Dietician. We would also like to thank "Heather" and "Jeffrey" for sharing their lives with us and with the next generation of health care providers.

REFERENCES

1. Cystic Fibrosis Foundation. Cystic Fibrosis Patient Registry. Bethesda, Md: CFF; 1999.

2. Hammond K, Abman S, Sokol R, et al. Efficacy of statewide neonatal screening for cystic fibrosis by assay of trypsinogen concentrations. *N Engl J Med.* 1991;325:769–774.

3. Gregg R, Wilfond B, Farrel P, et al. Application of DNA analysis in a population screening program for neonatal diagnosis of cystic fibrosis. *Am J Hum Genetics.* 1993;52:616–626.

4. Hamosh A, Fitzsimmons S, Macek M, et al. Comparison of the clinical manifestations of cystic fibrosis in black and white patients. *J Pediatr.* 1998;132:255–259.

5. Macek M, Mackova A, Hamosh A, et al. Identification of common cystic fibrosis mutations in African Americans with cystic fibrosis increases the detection rate to 75%. *Am J Hum Genetics.* 1997; 60:1122–1127.

6. Kazazian H. Population variation of common cystic fibrosis mutations: the CF Genetic Analysis Consortium. *Hum Mutat.* 1994;4:167–177.

7. Grebe T, Seltzer W, DeMarchi J, et al. Genetic analysis of Hispanic individuals with cystic fibrosis. *Am J Hum Genet.* 1994;54:443–446.

8. Arzimanoglou I, Tuchman A, Li Z, et al. Cystic fibrosis carrier screening in Hispanics. *Am J Hum Genet.* 1995;56:544–547.

9. Murphy T, Rosenstein B. Advances in the science and treatment of cystic fibrosis lung disease. Durham, NC: Duke University Medical Center; 1999:1. Monograph, first published 1995:1.

10. Kessler D, Moehlenkamp C, Kaplan G. Determination of cystic fibrosis carrier frequency for Zuni Native Americans of New Mexico. *Clin Genet.* 1996;49:95–97.

11. Andersen D. Cystic fibrosis of the pancreas and its relation to celiac disease. *Am J Dis Childhood.* 1938; 56:344–399.

12. di Sant'Agnese P, Darling R, Perera G, et al. Abnormal electrolyte composition of sweat in cystic fibrosis of the pancreas. *Pediatrics.* 1953;12:549–566.

13. Matthews L, Doershuk C, Wise M, et al. A therapeutic regimen for patients with cystic fibrosis. *J Pediatr.* 1964;65:558–575.

14. Rommens J, Iannuzzi M, Kerem B-S, et al. Identification of the cystic fibrosis gene: chromosome walking and jumping. *Science.* 1989;245: 1059–1065.

15. Riordan G, Rommens J, Karem B-S, et al. Identification of the cystic fibrosis gene: cloning and characterization of complementary DNA. *Science.* 1989;245:1066–1073.

16. Knowles M, Friedman K, Silverman L. Genetics, diagnosis, and clinical phenotype. In: Yankaskas J, Knowles M, eds. *Cystic Fibrosis in Adults.* Philadelphia: Lippincott-Raven; 1999:27–42.

17. Cystic Fibrosis Foundation. The diagnosis of cystic fibrosis: consensus statement. Bethesda, Md: CFF; 1996:1–15.

18. Stern R, Jones K. Nasal and sinus disease. In: Yankaskas J, Knowles M, eds. *Cystic Fibrosis in Adults.* Philadelphia: Lippincott-Raven; 1999:221–231.

19. Stutts M, Boucher R. Cystic fibrosis gene and functions of CFTR: Implications of dysfunctional ion transport for pulmonary pathogenesis. In: Yankaskas J, Knowles M, eds. *Cystic Fibrosis in Adults.* Philadelphia: Lippincott-Raven; 1999:3–26.

20. Schidlow D, Taussig L, Knowles M. Cystic fibrosis foundation consensus report on pulmonary complications of cystic fibrosis. *Pediatr Pulmonol.* 1993; 15:187–198.

21. Cystic Fibrosis Foundation. Consensus conference: Microbiology and infectious disease in cystic fibrosis. Bethesda, Md: CFF; 1994:1–26.

22. Ramsey B, Dorkin H. Consensus committee: practical applications of Pulmozyme. *Pediatr Pulmonol.* 1994;17:404–408.

23. Ramsey B, Farrel P, Pencharz P. Consensus committee: Nutritional assessment and management in cystic fibrosis. *Am J Clin Nutr.* 1992;55:108–116.

24. Cystic Fibrosis Foundation. Consensus document: Diagnosis, screening, and management of cystic fibrosis-related diabetes mellitus. Bethesda, Md: CFF; 1999:1–25.

25. Cystic Fibrosis Foundation. Consensus document: Recommendations for management of liver and biliary tract disease in cystic fibrosis. Bethesda, Md: CFF; 1999:1–22.

26. Quinton P. The sweat gland. In: Yankaskas J, Knowles M, eds. *Cystic Fibrosis in Adults*. Philadelphia: Lippincott-Raven; 1999:419–438.

27. Yankaskas J, Mallory G, and the Consensus Committee. Lung transplantation in cystic fibrosis. *Chest.* 1998;113:217–226.

28. Joint Statement from American Society for Transplant Physicians (ASTP)/American Thoracic Society (ATS)/European Respiratory Society (ERS)/ International Society for Heart & Lung Transplantation (ISHLT). International guidelines for the selection of lung transplant candidates. *Am J Respir Crit Care Med.* 1998; 158:335–339.

29. Mallory G. Lung transplantation in cystic fibrosis patients. *J Respir Care Pract.* 1999;5:41–45.

30. Mallory G. Lung transplants in patients with cystic fibrosis. *New Insights Cystic Fibrosis.* 1996;4:1–11.

31. Gibbons M. Infant pulmonary function testing. *Adv Managers Respir Care.* 2000;1: 46–47.

32. Gee L, Abbott J, Conway S, et al. A disease specific health related quality of life measure for adults with CF. *Pediatr Pulmonol.* 1999;S19: 326.

ACUTE PEDIATRIC UPPER AIRWAY EMERGENCIES

Bruce A. Feistner and Mary L. Reinesch

Tell me, and I'll forget. Show me, and I may not remember. Involve me, and I'll understand.
—NATIVE AMERICAN PROVERB

LEARNING OBJECTIVES

1. Describe facts, descriptions, and definitions related to acute pediatric upper airway emergencies.
2. Discuss the etiology, pathophysiology, and clinical features of pediatric patients with acute upper airway emergencies.
3. Describe the acute care and long-term management of pediatric patients with acute upper airway emergencies.
4. Apply specific formulas and theory to assist in clinical decision making involving patients with acute pediatric upper airway emergencies.
5. Apply the critical thinking skills of prioritizing, anticipating, negotiating, communicating, and decision making to a case example of acute pediatric upper airway emergencies.
6. Through performance of critical thinking exercises and group discussion of case questions, apply strategies that promote critical thinking to the respiratory care management of a patient with an acute pediatric upper airway emergency.
7. Use the clinical data and a case example to perform an initial patient assessment using a standardized system.

8. Interpret clinical data from case examples, including history, physical examination, laboratory data, and radiographs to make recommendations for respiratory care management.
9. Develop a care plan for a patient with an acute pediatric upper airway emergency, including recommendations for therapy and disease management with consideration of the costs, as well as ethical and quality-of-life issues.
10. Communicate facts, evidence, and arguments to support evaluations and recommendations proposed for the care of a pediatric patient with an acute upper airway emergency.
11. Practice the skill of negotiating in an attempt to persuade acceptance of a proposed plan of care for a pediatric patient with an acute upper airway emergency.
12. Evaluate treatment and outcomes of interventions, giving attention to health promotion and quality-of-life issues.
13. Describe the role of the respiratory therapist in the assessment, treatment, management, and education of the patient with an acute pediatric upper airway emergency.

CHAPTER DESCRIPTION

This chapter allows students to learn about management of pediatric airway emergencies by completing a series of exercises and cases with discussion questions. The chapter includes two typical pediatric cases: acute laryngotracheobronchitis (subglottic croup) and acute epiglottitis (supraglottitis). Although the beginning of this chapter includes basic etiology, pathophysiology, and management, it is presented in an abbreviated format to give a general introduction. Students are expected to refer to more detailed resources in order to perform the exercises and answer all the questions as part of the problem-based learning (PBL) process.

This chapter provides key learning resources to assist students with answering the case questions. The real learning is meant to take place by having students research and work through the exercises, questions, and cases. Students can work through this chapter individually or in groups. It is hoped that the students can draw parallels between the pathology background, the individual cases, and their own clinical rotations. Once the students can apply the newly acquired knowledge to patient care, the cases will take on a new, exciting aspect. Our intent is that this chapter and PBL will stimulate students to explore new techniques to apply their knowledge for managing pediatric airway emergencies.

INTRODUCTION

In the pediatric population, it is common for the larynx to become obstructed due to its location and structure. Obstruction frequently involves inflammation of the laryngeal structures secondary to an infection. Causative processes include croup (laryngotracheobronchitis or subglottic croup), epiglottitis (supraglottic croup), and other noninfectious processes such as aspiration of a foreign body, allergic or traumatic laryngeal edema, cancer, congenital conditions, vocal cord dysfunction, and burns affecting the upper airway.[1]

The following sections provide a brief overview of various etiologies of acute upper airway obstruction in the pediatric population.

ETIOLOGY

Foreign Body Obstruction

Children, especially toddlers, can have foreign body obstruction from a number of objects. Parents and care providers must be watchful for this danger, and should "child-proof" their homes by putting small objects out of reach of toddlers. In the event of aspiration and obstruction, it is critical that the parent or care provider knows CPR, because they may be the only one nearby able to dislodge the object and save the child's life.

If the foreign body is smaller than the airway, a "bypass valve" effect is created, in which air is allowed to enter on inspiration, but becomes trapped on exhalation. If the object is larger than the airway, a complete blockage is created—air cannot get in or out during inspiration or expiration. A foreign body is more commonly found in the right main stem bronchus, since it has a more vertical alignment and foreign bodies can travel that way more easily.[2]

Young children may easily aspirate certain foods (nuts, seeds, or popcorn) and small objects (buttons or beads). Such objects may cause either partial or total airway obstruction. Small toys, marbles, pins, rocks, or anything else small enough for infants or toddlers to put in their mouths can be swallowed. If a swallowed object traverses the esophagus and into the stomach without obstruction, it will probably pass through the entire digestive tract in several hours.

The symptoms the child exhibits depend on the size of the foreign body. There may be sudden choking and acute respiratory distress, or there may be delayed symptoms with cough, wheezing, and possibly hemoptysis. If the object is small, the patient could suffer recurring pneumonias.

Inspiratory and expiratory posteroanterior chest films or airway fluoroscopy are most helpful in diagnosing foreign body obstruction. On the expiratory film, there is air trapping on the affected side and mediastinal shift away from this side. On the inspiratory film, there is mediastinal shift toward the affected side as the other lung expands normally. On the decubitus film, the affected side will not collapse when it is placed in a dependent position. Pneumomediastinum and pneumothorax will rarely be seen.[2]

Anaphylactic Reactions

Even though it is rarely seen, infants and toddlers can have anaphylactic reactions to drugs such as penicillin, cephalosporin, and sulfa drugs, as well as food sensitivities, insect stings, and many other chemical or environmental allergens. If hypotension is observed, it is usually due to other causes such as shock from sepsis or dehydration. Wheezing is usually due to reactive airway disease, infection, or a foreign body. Drooling, hoarseness, and stridor indicate upper airway narrowing, which is usually due to infection in children.[3] If any of these symptoms are observed, the child should be immediately transported to the emergency department (ED).

Other symptoms may be observed in a child with an anaphylactic reaction, including anxiety, itching of the skin, headache, nausea and vomiting, sneezing and coughing, abdominal cramps, hives and swelling of the lips or joints, diarrhea, shortness of breath and wheezing, low blood pressure, seizures, and loss of consciousness. The child's eyes may itch, water, and swell. It is possible to observe symptoms including itching of the mouth and throat, hoarseness, change of voice, nasal congestion, chest pain and/or tightness, and flushing and redness of the skin.[4]

Most reactions occur with 30 minutes following allergen exposure, although the onset of symptoms can vary from several seconds to hours. The earlier the onset of symptoms after exposure to the antigen, the more severe the subsequent reaction. Anaphylaxis can affect all body systems, including the skin, respiratory tract, cardiovascular system, eyes, and bladder. Since this is a true medical emergency, rapid transport to a medical facility is indicated.

A common result of an anaphylactic reaction is swelling of the airway mucosa with the possibility of total obstruction. The best way to treat the pediatric victim of a life-threatening reaction such as this is to call 911 immediately, or take the victim to the nearest ED if one is nearby. Parents usually do not have the advanced knowledge necessary to treat anaphylactic reactions, so their best response is to get the child to medical care as soon as possible. Unless the parents have epinephrine in an auto-injector Epi-pen Jr. or similar device, and know how to use it, the best thing they can do is arrange immediate transport to a hospital.

CRITICAL CONTENT

SYMPTOMS OF ANAPHYLACTIC SHOCK

- Anxiety
- Headache
- Nausea and vomiting
- Shortness of breath
- Wheezing
- Hoarseness
- Change of voice
- Nasal congestion
- Sneezing
- Coughing
- Itching of the skin, eyes, mouth, and throat
- Hives
- Abdominal cramps
- Diarrhea
- Swelling of the lips or joints
- Flushing or redness of the skin
- Low blood pressure
- Chest pain and/or tightness
- Seizures
- Loss of consciousness

Trauma

Pediatric trauma is a major threat to the child's life. If unrestrained in a vehicle, during a crash a child is thrown about violently in the car, or the child can be ejected. As a result of the crash, trauma to the upper torso, neck, head, or spine can occur. Trauma can cause mucosal edema and easily compromise the airway. If the EMS unit has advanced life support capabilities, they can use a jet ventilator to ventilate the child until arrival in the ED. If the airway is already badly swollen, the emergency staff may be unable to intubate. If the child needs CPR and the airway is traumatized, even if the parents know what to do, they may be unable to ventilate. Advanced life support is the only hope for the child. See Chapter 19 for a more detailed discussion of this subject.

Cancer

Neoplastic lesions in the pediatric population sometimes result in airway obstruction. If the child has a tumor growing in the airway mucosa or adjacent to it, the mass may project into the airway and compromise ventilation. Depending on the doubling time of the mass, the child's airway problems could advance at a significant rate. The child (and parents) would notice progressive shortness of breath, possibly cyanosis, and lack of energy in the child. If these signs are noticed, the child should be taken in for evaluation.

Congenital Abnormalities

Congenital defects in the airway are usually manifested at birth. Any number of events could occur, including agenesis of a lung, congenital airway stenosis, choanal atresia, or improper development of lobes or segments. Surgical correction is usually curative for these conditions.

Vocal Cord Dysfunction

In the early 1980s, doctors discovered a new condition that mimics asthma. They named this condition vocal cord dysfunction (VCD). VCD causes asthma-like symptoms due to abnormal closing of the vocal cords. It can cause a person to have diffi-

culty breathing and may even cause wheezing. Based on these symptoms, many people with VCD may have been diagnosed with asthma and treated with asthma medications. Since VCD is *not* asthma, the symptoms will not improve with this treatment. To further complicate matters, some people have both asthma and VCD.[5]

Vocal cord dysfunction can be life threatening. Under normal conditions, the adductor muscles of the vocal cords move the cords toward each other to produce speech. If the function of these muscles is impeded, bilateral vocal cord paralysis could result. Glottic closure could also be produced as a result of increased activity of the adductor muscles.[4] If this occurs during inspiration, it could lead to partial airway obstruction.

The patient admitted to the hospital with VCD is often diagnosed with a status asthmaticus-like condition (asthma that does not improve with treatment). The patient exhibits wheezing from inspiratory adduction of the vocal cords (as they move toward each other) that causes stridor. Triggers for this condition include upper respiratory infection, exercise, and stress, but sometimes a cause is not evident.[6] VCD may also be present concurrently with other pulmonary disease.

Diagnosing vocal cord dysfunction is very difficult. A flow-volume loop is useful in demonstrating VCD, especially the inspiratory loop. A drawback to the flow-volume loop is that it is only valuable if the patient is symptomatic. A laryngoscopy is also valuable in diagnosing VCD. This test also needs to be done when the patient is symptomatic so the doctor can witness the abnormal cord movements.

The patient is largely responsible for treating VCD. A common treatment for the condition is speech therapy to increase awareness of abdominal breathing and create conscious relaxation of the throat muscles. The exercises are best practiced when the patient is asymptomatic, so when an attack occurs the techniques can easily be recalled and applied. Counseling also plays an important role in helping the patient deal with the stress and adjust to the diagnosis and the new treatment program.

CRITICAL CONTENT

ESSENTIALS OF VOCAL CORD DYSFUNCTION

- VCD causes asthma-like symptoms but does *not* respond to asthma therapy.
- Some people have both asthma and VCD.
- Vocal cord dysfunction can be life threatening.
- VCD is often diagnosed as a status asthmaticus-like condition.
- Triggers for VCD include upper respiratory infection, exercise, and stress.
- Diagnosis is difficult. Inspiratory flow-volume loop may be helpful if patient is symptomatic at the time of testing. Laryngoscopy is also valuable in diagnosing the symptomatic patient.
- Speech therapy (relaxation exercises) may be helpful.

Burns

Burns in the pediatric population can be life threatening, especially if they occur around the head and neck of the child. An upper airway burn may be suspected if a fire victim has singed nasal hair and soot or burn markings in the nose and/or mouth. The superheated gases that enter the mouth, nose, and upper airway cause mucosal edema of the upper airway, ciliary sloughing, and destruction of the epithelial cells. Immediate intubation is often necessary since the edema could lead to acute respiratory failure and respiratory arrest. Since the airway could become totally obstructed, intubation at a later time may be impossible to achieve. Once adequate airway control has been guaranteed, other problems such as the burns themselves may be addressed.

When dealing with a possible airway burn, your highest priority is to carry out immediate assessment and treatment on the scene, because time is the enemy. If the airway is not intubated,

more invasive procedures (emergency cricothyrotomy or tracheotomy) must be done, with their associated higher risks. See Chapter 20 for a more extensive discussion of this topic.

CRITICAL CONTENT

NONINFECTIOUS PROCESSES THAT CAN CAUSE UPPER AIRWAY OBSTRUCTION

- Aspiration of a foreign body
- Allergic or traumatic laryngeal edema
- Malignant growths (cancer)
- Congenital conditions
- Vocal cord dysfunction
- Airway burns

Croup

Croup has proven to be the most common cause of subglottic edema in children in the age group spanning 6 months to 6 years.[4] Croup (also called laryngotracheobronchitis or LTB) is usually spread by the airborne route or by contact with infected secretions. Croup affects the area below the glottis, whereas epiglottitis actually affects the epiglottis. Both conditions cause upper airway obstruction through swelling of the involved areas, the difference being where the edema is located.

Since the subglottic area is the narrowest part of the larynx in an infant, even an extremely small amount of edema can significantly reduce the lumen. Furthermore, the rigid cricoid cartilage prevents external swelling when fluid leaks into the tissues of the laryngeal area. Without this ability to expand externally, as the swelling process advances, the effect is to rapidly reduce the inner lumen of the already narrow airway. This process also impairs the ability of the vocal cords to move apart on inspiration, which further diminishes the cross-sectional area of the airway.[7]

Acute Epiglottitis

Acute epiglottitis is a life-threatening emergency. The inflammation of the supraglottic region does not involve other areas such as the pharynx, trachea, or other subglottic structures. As the condition worsens, the edges of the epiglottis start to curl, and the tip protrudes posteriorly and inferiorly. Then, when the child inhales, the negative pressure pulls the epiglottis over the laryngeal inlet, and may even totally block it.[7]

Since there are so many different potential causes of upper airway emergencies in the pediatric population, it would not be practical to discuss each in depth in this chapter. Now that we have briefly highlighted some of the potential noninfectious causes of airway emergency, we will now focus on the more classic forms of acute upper airway obstruction in the pediatric population—croup (acute LTB or subglottic croup) and epiglottitis (acute supraglottitis).

CRITICAL CONTENT

INFECTIOUS PROCESSES THAT CAN CAUSE UPPER AIRWAY OBSTRUCTION

- Croup (laryngotracheobronchitis; LTB) or subglottic obstruction
- Epiglottitis-glottic obstruction

Upper Airway Assessment and Auscultation

All of the causes of acute upper airway emergencies can potentially produce clues as to what is occurring in the airway by creating specific abnormal breath sounds. Auscultation of breath sounds is an important part of the assessment in any patient presenting with respiratory distress. This can be confusing because different diseases or processes may produce similar breath sounds, including stridor, wheezing, grunting, or breath sounds that are decreased, absent, or unequal. Even though an upper airway obstruction may be recognized through auscultation of breath sounds, the specific differential diagnosis (croup, epiglottitis, foreign body, etc.) may be difficult to determine.

INFECTIOUS CAUSES OF UPPER AIRWAY OBSTRUCTION

There are many etiologies for upper airway obstruction in the pediatric population. Some (LTB or acute epiglottitis) have a bacterial or viral source, while others (such as trauma) do not. Knowing the various disease processes can help narrow your differential diagnosis. Consideration of the child's recent medical history can also facilitate your decision making.

Laryngotracheobronchitis is a viral infection caused most commonly by the parainfluenza viruses 1, 2, and 3, with type 1 being the most common. LTB may also be caused by influenza A and B, respiratory syncytial viruses (RSV), rhinovirus, and adenoviruses. **Acute epiglottitis**, however, has a bacterial origin, usually from *Haemophilus influenzae B* (Hib). *Streptococcus pneumoniae*, *Staphylococcus aureus*, though *Haemophilus parainfluenzae* may also rarely be the cause.

Parainfluenza viruses are large RNA viruses called paramyxoviruses. Four types have been identified. Type 1 causes most viral croup infections and usually occurs in the fall, while type 3 is generally seen in the spring and summer. The virus has an incubation period of 2 to 6 days. The child may become reinfected at any age, but overall symptoms are milder. The organism can be cultured from nasopharyngeal secretions, using immunofluorescent and ELISA methods. However, since it is a virus, current treatment is only supportive, not curative.[8]

The asymptomatic child may be colonized with *Haemophilus influenzae* type b, and transmission is by direct contact from person to person or inhalation of respiratory droplets. Although the incubation period is unknown, occurrences peak during the fall (October/November) and the spring (February through April).[9]

Before an effective vaccine became available, there were an estimated 20,000 invasive Hib infections per year in the US, which caused up to 1000 deaths, but the number of reported cases has markedly dropped since 1990. Hib invasive disease has not been totally eliminated, and the incidence is not uniform among all socioeconomic groups. The occurrence of Hib invasive disease is related to a number of factors, such as children not getting immunized, vaccine failure, a failure to build up immunity in very young children, and infection by non-type b *H influenzae*. Certain populations are at higher risk for infection, including urban dwellers, children in day care, American Indians and Eskimos, African Americans, and patients with diseases such as immunodeficiency syndromes, sickle cell anemia, and cancer.[9]

If a child has had epiglottitis previously, it is imperative that all respiratory infections be treated early and aggressively under medical supervision. All children should also be immunized against *Haemophilus influenzae*, which would help further decrease the number of new cases of epiglottitis seen every year. Recurrences of epiglottitis are unusual, but the child should still be immunized against it.

Epiglottitis is associated with several serious complications, including pneumonia, meningitis, pericarditis, and cellulitis.[10] If epiglottitis is promptly diagnosed and treated, the patient should recover fully. But if it goes untreated, complete airway obstruction and death could occur quickly, even within hours.

Pathophysiology and Related Theory

As previously described, croup (LTB or subglottic croup) has a viral origin. The virus causes inflammation and narrowing of the subglottic airway that leads to partial or total obstruction of the local airway and larynx. An anteroposterior (AP) film will show proximal subglottic airway narrowing, sometimes known as the "steeple sign," where there is loss of the subglottic tracheal shape. A lateral film of the airway is indicated to rule out other diseases with a differential of inspiratory stridor, especially epiglottitis. Differential diagnosis could include diseases such as congenital subglottic stenosis, a foreign body in the airway or esophagus, or epiglottitis. About one quarter of epiglottitis patients have subglottic airway narrowing, which could complicate the diagnosis.[11] When a virus infects the mucosa of the larynx and trachea, the reaction is to secrete mucous that narrows the airways. The secretions soon dry and thicken, making it even more difficult for the child to breathe. Hydrating the dried airway secretions with steam may be all that is needed to make the child more comfortable. A child's normal growth progressively widens the airways, which decreases the incidence of croup.[12]

Although relatively uncommon, spasmodic croup exists, which is characterized by a short episode of cough and stridor with no fever. Infectious LTB is the more classic form of croup, and typically presents with a fever after one half to 3 days and a persistent cough and coryza.

Epiglottitis is an infection of the epiglottis. Like croup, it causes a progressive obstruction of the airway secondary to the swollen mucosal membranes. Since the epiglottis is swollen, the child's voice will usually be muffled. Lateral neck x-rays exhibit a characteristic swelling of the epiglottis. This is also known as the "thumb" sign, since it resembles the size and shape of a human thumb. The AP film will usually be normal. Spasm may cause the airway to acutely close, and death may follow in minutes. Because of this, no attempts should be made to look in the mouth if epiglottitis is suspected in a child.

Epiglottitis is always a medical emergency and should not be taken lightly. A child with croup symptoms that are not improving, who cannot swallow saliva, drools, or sits upright and does not want to be laid down, or who shows any sign of dyspnea even when quiet needs immediate medical attention.[13] The differential diagnosis should be made as rapidly as possible so the respiratory therapist should be familiar with the typical presenting clinical features of each condition.

Clinical Features

Even though croup is usually a mild illness, it can quickly become so severe that hospitalization of the child is needed. Acute epiglottitis is extremely dangerous, and can rapidly become a life-threatening condition. Although the signs and symptoms associated with these two conditions are not very similar, they are usually recognizable by the parent, and these observations must be described to the health professional by telephone or in the ED.

An examination of the child with croup reveals chest retractions with breathing. Chest auscultation shows prolonged inspiration or expiration, wheezing, and diminished breath sounds. A reddened epiglottis may be visualized on direct laryngoscopy.

The child with croup has a barking cough and noisy breathing caused by swelling in the upper airway. The child's breathing becomes more difficult and requires more and more effort. The child may be physically tired, but cannot rest because of the increased work of breathing.

Croup symptoms usually worsen at night. The child will probably have a barking cough with pale or cyanotic, cool and clammy skin. There may also be a low-grade fever. The cough sounds like that of a seal or puppy. The child may be exhibiting dyspnea, and inspiratory or expiratory stridor may be heard. The child may also exhibit intercostal and subcostal retractions. The episode is frightening, since the child cannot move air into and out of the lungs without great effort. The onset of croup symptoms can commonly follow another illness such as a cold or sore throat.

The child with epiglottitis will appear quiet, will not cough, and will lean forward to breathe. The chin may be extended and the mouth will be open to try and maintain the airway lumen. The skin is commonly pale, but may also be flushed, with a high temperature. The child will be drooling and unwilling to swallow. A barking cough will not be heard with epiglottitis, but rather an expiratory "purr" is heard. Other types of noisy breathing may also be noted. The child may be so worn out from the work of breathing that he or she may be close to respiratory failure. Epiglottitis has a rapid onset,

usually progressing within only 1 to 2 hours to fully developed, life-threatening distress.

When diagnosing epiglottitis, be suspicious if the child exhibits dysphagia or voice changes, begins to drool, and develops respiratory distress. Even though croup and epiglottitis affect the same general region of the body, they display marked differences as summarized in Table 14-1.[14]

Typical Laboratory Findings

The radiograph is valuable when diagnosing upper airway obstruction in children. Although croup is usually diagnosed clinically, it can be identified on a lateral or frontal view of the airway, where subglottic narrowing is seen. The characteristic finding is called the pencil point sign or steeple sign, in which there is *gradual* widening of the subglottic airway instead of the rather *abrupt* widening seen normally.[15]

Acute epiglottitis can also be diagnosed with a *lateral* soft tissue neck film. The characteristic finding on this type of x-ray is an enlarged epiglottis and edematous aryepiglottic folds, which produce the upper airway obstruction and dyspnea.[15] The epiglottis may actually swell to three to four times its normal size.

In the child with epiglottitis, direct visualization of the epiglottis should not be attempted without an anesthesiologist and/or otolaryngologist present, because the airway may become further compromised secondary to the procedure. Examination of the larynx may show an enlarged, reddened epiglottis, and the child may be exhibiting audible stridor. Blood or throat cultures may demonstrate *Haemophilus influenzae* or other bacteria, and the white blood cell count may be elevated.

The child with signs and symptoms of epiglottitis should have direct visualization of the supralaryngeal area with a laryngoscope or bronchoscope. The diagnosis of epiglottitis is based on identifying swollen, cherry-red supraglottic structures, which usually include the epiglottis. The aryepiglottic folds and arytenoid cartilages are thickened. These structures form the lateral and posterior aspects of the larynx and actually cause the upper airway

TABLE 14-1   CHARACTERISTICS OF VIRAL CROUP AND ACUTE EPIGLOTTITIS

CHARACTERISTICS	VIRAL CROUP	ACUTE EPIGLOTTITIS
Age	3 months–5 years	2–7 years
Organism	Viral	*H. Influenza*, type b
Incidence	Common	Rare
Clinical presentation	Gradual onset	Sudden onset
	Mild URI symptoms	Drooling
	Barky cough	Sitting forward
	Low fever	High fever
Physical examination	Respiratory distress	Toxic appearance
	Inspiratory stridor	"Hot potato" voice
X-ray and projection	Steeple sign on	Thumb sign on
	A/P view	lateral view
Treatment	Humidification	Epiglottitis protocol[a]
	Racemic epinephrine	
	Steroids (controversial)	

[a]Although protocols vary between institutions, this would generally include a lateral neck x-ray (to differentiate between croup and epiglottitis), bronchoscopy (also to differentiate croup from epiglottitis), intubation, and transfer to ICU.

obstruction in acute epiglottitis. The thickened aryepiglottic folds and arytenoid cartilages are what produce the classic thumb sign on the x-ray.[16]

Treatment and Management

Vaccination to prevent *H influenzae* disease began in 1985 in the US for children 24 months or older, but in October 1990, *H influenzae* type b conjugate vaccines were approved for children 2 months of age and older. Any child less than 2 years of age experiencing *H influenzae* disease such as epiglottitis should be vaccinated, because they might not acquire natural immunity from the infection. If the child is older than 2 years, the disease itself most likely will cause natural immunity, and immunization is therefore not needed.[16]

Since a virus causes croup, antibiotics will not treat it. The virus that most commonly causes croup does not usually predispose to secondary bacterial infection, and antibiotics are rarely indicated. The virus that causes croup is considered to be relatively contagious. Children with recurring episodes of croup should be seen by a pediatrician

to diagnose the underlying cause. Remember that good handwashing technique helps prevent the spread of this and many other illnesses.

An attack of acute epiglottitis requires that the child be hospitalized immediately, since it is a medical emergency and could be life threatening. However, if a child has an attack of croup at home, a parent or caregiver can help the child get through the acute phase, calm down, and breathe easier.

It is of critical importance that the caregiver of a child with croup not panic when the child starts exhibiting the frightening signs of respiratory distress. By remaining calm, the caregiver will help the child stay calmer, which can potentially help him or her through the acute phase. Panic and fright only serve to worsen the situation. To help the child stay relaxed, it is a good idea for the caregiver to remain in the child's room. Knowing that the parent is close by reassures the child and allows them to relax, which in turn allows the parent to relax.

Another recommendation is to start a cool mist room humidifier for the child with croup. Cool mist humidifiers are safer because an accidental burn is always possible when using a heated humidifier. The cool mist humidifier is just as effective as a heated humidifier, but much safer. Since not all homes have humidifiers, simply taking the child into the bathroom, starting the shower, and having the child breathe the steam can relieve symptoms. The mist from the shower will closely approximate the mist from a room humidifier. Since you should always remain aware of the burn potential, it may be advisable to run the shower with a cooler water temperature. If the shower idea does not work, taking the child out into the cool night air can sometimes help. Again, this will simulate the cool room humidifier or cool, steamy shower. Not only does the cool air make it easier for the child to breathe, but it may also have a calming effect. Both factors help to reassure the child, a big advantage in the early treatment phase.

Coughing may make the dyspnea worse and increasingly frighten the child. Administration of a cough suppressant to prevent harsh coughing episodes is recommended. These episodes have the potential to quickly make the situation worse if they go untreated. Also encourage the child to drink plenty of fluids. If the airway mucosa remains hydrated, the secretions will not become dry, which can stimulate coughing. Secretions that are in a hydrated state have a much lower potential of causing airway obstruction than if they are dry, sticky, and hard to clear.

If the child is having trouble clearing secretions, it is possible that he or she will also have a fever. It is safe to administer a fever medication if necessary. Bringing the child's body temperature down will slow the breathing rate, calm the child, and possibly allow more effective air exchange.

Serious episodes of croup require hospitalization. If the child exhibits continuing or increasing breathing difficulty, or becomes fatigued or cyanotic, this indicates that the child needs medical attention or hospitalization. Oxygen and humidity may be given via an oxygen tent or by face mask. If the airway develops progressive obstruction, the child may need to be intubated. Intravenous fluids can help treat dehydration, and corticosteroids may also be used to improve the child's condition.

Another treatment option is nebulized racemic epinephrine. This drug stimulates the alpha-adrenergic receptors in the blood vessels of the airway walls and causes vasoconstriction, which decreases mucosal edema. The usual dosage administered to croup patients is 0.25 to 0.50 mL of a 2.25% solution of racemic epinephrine in 2 to 3 mL normal saline. The effect lasts from 30 minutes to 1 hour, and the treatment can be repeated as often as every hour. Even though racemic epinephrine does not shorten the course of croup, it gives the patient symptomatic improvement and rapid relief from dyspnea.

Occasionally, the child given one to two nebulizer treatments with racemic epinephrine shows enough improvement to be discharged. If the child's croup is more severe and racemic epinephrine does not improve symptoms, he or she may need to be admitted to the hospital, and additional medications added to the treatment regimen.

There are several signs that should alert one to the fact that the child with croup needs to be taken to the ED. If the parent or caregiver has been attempting the home treatments (hydration, steam, and calming) and it does not seem to be improving the child's breathing after 15 to 20 minutes, or if the problem actually gets worse instead of better, a trip to the hospital is warranted.

Evaluating the condition of the upper airway visually also gives valuable clues about what should be done. For example, if the child starts to drool and has increasing trouble swallowing, the situation is worsening. If this is coupled with central cyanosis and anxiety on the part of the child, one must again realize that these are bad signs, and immediate transport to an ED is indicated.

Additional symptoms of the child with croup include a high fever (>103°F), inability or unwillingness to bend the neck forward, leaning forward and desperately gasping for air, retracting, flaring the nostrils, stridor, inability to talk or cry, and an anxious, frightened appearance.[17] These very descriptive findings should provide clues about the worsening condition of the child. Any of these symptoms could indicate a much more serious situation than could be handled at home, and may mean that the child's airway is becoming dangerously narrowed and treatment in the hospital is necessary.

The role of steroids in the treatment of croup is still debated, even though it has been evaluated in more than a dozen clinical trials over the past 30 years. Steroid usage in the hospitalized child with croup should reduce the need for intubation and help the child's airway condition to improve more quickly. An increasing number of doctors are now using steroids early in the course of severe, hospitalized cases of viral croup with good success.

A recent randomized double blind, placebo-controlled trial was done to determine the added clinical benefit of nebulized budesonide (a steroid) in children with mild to moderate croup treated with 0.6 mg/kg oral dexamethasone.[18] The study was carried out in the ED of a tertiary-care pediatric hospital with 47,000 visits per year. Participants were children 3 months to 5 years of age with a syndrome consisting of hoarseness, inspiratory stridor, and barking cough, and a croup score of 3 or greater after at least 15 minutes of mist therapy. See the accompanying critical content box for the details of the croup scoring system utilized in this study.

CRITICAL CONTENT

SCORING SYSTEM USED TO DETERMINE THE SEVERITY OF CROUP[18]

Stridor: 0, none; 1, audible with stethoscope at rest; and 2, audible without stethoscope at rest

Retractions: 0, none; 1, mild; 2, moderate; and 3, severe

Air entry: 0, normal; 1, decreased; and 2, severely decreased

Cyanosis: 0, none; 4, with agitation; and 5, at rest

Level of consciousness: 0, normal; and 5, altered

All patients received 0.6 mg/kg oral dexamethasone and were randomly assigned to receive 4 mL (2 mg) of budesonide solution ($n = 25$) or 4 mL of 0.9% saline solution ($n = 25$) by updraft nebulizer. The primary outcome measure was the proportion of patients in each group who had clinically significant changes (2 points) in the croup score during the 4 hours after treatment. Eighty-four percent ($n = 21$) of the patients who received budesonide had clinically important responses, compared with 56% ($n = 14$) in the placebo group. The conclusion reached was that despite receiving simultaneous oral dexamethasone, pediatric outpatients with mild to moderate croup have additional, clinically significant improvement in respiratory symptoms after treatment with budesonide.[18] Budesonide acts rapidly and has a prolonged effect that may be effective against subglottic inflammatory edema, but must be used cautiously in the treatment of patients with immunodeficiency, tuberculosis, or recent exposure to varicella.[19]

Since acute epiglottitis is a medical emergency, the child should be taken to a hospital without delay. Keeping the child calm during the ride and opening the car windows can make breathing a little easier. It is important to not give the child food or water during this acute phase. The child can be in any comfortable position, usually leaning forward and held by a parent. The child will not want to lie down, since this increases anxiety due to the increased work of breathing. Do not attempt to examine the child's throat en route to the hospital, since a reflex laryngospasm could occur, causing total obstruction and possibly respiratory arrest.[17]

When the child with acute epiglottitis arrives in the ED, critical personnel that should be in attendance include an anesthesiologist who is skilled at executing pediatric intubation, an endoscopist to assist with difficult intubations with direct visualization, and an intensivist for postoperative management. To diagnose epiglottitis, direct visualization of the supralaryngeal area is immediately carried out with a laryngoscope or bronchoscope. The child is taken to the operating room and usually put under a general anesthetic. An IV line is started, and blood is sent to the lab for culture and CBC. The larynx and supraglottic tissues are then inspected. From the OR, the child goes to the ICU, where mechanical ventilation continues. Systemic antibiotics such as ampicillin, chloramphenicol, ceftri-axone, or cefotaxime should be started as soon as possible. Mechanical ventilation should be continued until the edema diminishes, which usually occurs over the first 1 to 2 days. The child must be kept in respiratory isolation for the first 24 hours of antibiotic treatment.[16]

Control measures for *H influenzae* type b are very important since asymptomatic carriers are quite numerous. Prophylactic treatment with rifampin once a day for 4 days kills *H influenzae* in most (approximately 95%) carriers. Rifampin prophylaxis should be given to all household members regardless of age if at least one child is positive for *H influenzae* and at least one child is less than 4 years of age. A nasopharyngeal culture should be done before treatment. Chemoprophylaxis should be instituted as soon as possible after diagnosis of *H influenzae* type b is made. Guidelines for the treatment of day care personnel and children have been set by the American Academy of Pediatrics.[16]

CRITICAL CONTENT

INDICATIONS THAT A CHILD NEEDS MEDICAL ATTENTION OR HOSPITALIZATION FOR CROUP

- Repeated episodes of croup should be assessed by a pediatrician
- Continuing or increasing breathing difficulty, or the child becomes fatigued or cyanotic
- No response to or deteriorating condition with home treatment
- If the child starts to drool and has increasing trouble swallowing
- High fever (>103°F) or inability or unwillingness to bend the neck forward
- Leaning forward and desperately gasping for air, retracting
- Flaring the nostrils, stridor, inability to talk or cry
- An anxious, frightened appearance with central cyanosis

Consideration of Costs and Ethical Issues

Monetary costs for treating croup or epiglottitis can range from those of a few hours in the ED to those of several days in the hospital. If the parent recognizes the symptoms of croup, and is successful with basic treatments such as cool night air or steam from a shower, the child may not need an ED admission. If home treatments do not relieve the child's symptoms, or if the croup attack becomes more severe, a hospital admission may be required. Depending on the child's response to therapies for croup given in the ED, he or she may go home in a few hours or be admitted for a few days.

Epiglottitis, however, may progress so rapidly that the only option parents have is rapid transport to a hospital for emergency treatment. Even though the number of cases of epiglottitis is decreasing, it is usually associated with higher costs than croup, since a hospital admission is often necessary. Vaccination against *H influenzae* can prevent occurrences of epiglottitis, and this may significantly reduce the number of hospital admissions, with resulting savings of thousands of dollars in hospital costs.

Epiglottitis has not been eradicated. Though the vaccine against *H influenzae* has been available for several years, many children have not been immunized due to limited access to medical care, or due to socioeconomic issues. This keeps the number of new cases of epiglottitis low but still constant, as seen in overall ED admissions. This brings us to an ethical dilemma: We have the resources to eradicate this potentially life-threatening disease, but can we as a society exert the collective desire to implement a plan to see that this is done?

Many of the diseases of childhood and many of the causes of acute airway obstruction in the pediatric population discussed in this chapter could be reduced or eliminated by better health care education and by focusing more health care resources on prevention. Improved funding for prenatal maternal education, education of families about preventive health care practices, and immunization of *all* children against common pediatric diseases are examples of actions that could go a long way to reduce morbidity and mortality in the pediatric population. Can our society make this a national health care priority?

INTRODUCTION TO CASE STUDIES

Now you proceed with the most exciting part of this chapter, that of working through two hypothetical cases. Your instructors will assign you to work on specific critical thinking exercises and group

critical thinking exercises, depending on the available time, the types of patients you are likely to encounter during your clinical rotations, and resources available. Please check with your instructors to verify which case(s) and exercises you should complete, working individually or in groups. Your instructors may also direct you to develop learning issues as part of your PBL process, or assign specific, predetermined learning issues developed for this chapter. Please check with your program faculty before proceeding with the following case(s).

CASE 1

BILLY BARKER

Initial Case Scenario

A 2-year-old white male is admitted to the ED at 8:00 AM on October 26, with a harsh cough and fever. When you enter the room, you see a child in moderate distress with RR of 28, pulse of 124, and BP 124/60. Intercostal and subcostal retractions and stridor are observed.

History

The patient started having difficulty with a cough and fever spanning 2 to 3 days. The symptoms progressively worsened, so he was seen in a medical clinic. The physician felt Billy had bronchitis, so he prescribed amoxicillin and clavulanic acid. His symptoms subsided during the day, but in the evening he worsened with increased difficulty breathing and trouble sleeping. His parents took him to the ED, where they said that he could not keep fluids down because of trouble with his breathing. He has had a runny nose, but has not complained of a sore throat or earache.

   The child is sitting up in bed, exhibiting moderate difficulty breathing with frequent coughing. His cough has a barking, nonproductive character, and Billy seems to be tiring. His breath sounds

reveal transmitted upper airway noise, but no rales, crackles, or wheezes.

 Critical Thinking Exercise 1

PRIORITIZING PATIENT CARE

a. Explain the steps you would need to follow to complete an initial patient assessment, ie, what is your first priority?

b. What would be your initial recommendation for a therapeutic intervention?

 Critical Thinking Exercise 2

MAKING INFERENCES BY CLUSTERING DATA

a. What inferences can be made about his barking cough, fever, and difficulty swallowing?

b. How does one cluster data leading to this inference? In this exercise, look critically at each fact relating to Billy's signs and symptoms, and then determine how they fit together to reach your differential diagnosis.

CASE 1 *(continued)*

Critical Thinking Exercise 3

INFORMATION GATHERING AND DECISION MAKING

a. During your patient assessment, what data should be obtained to complete the patient profile?

b. Based on this initial assessment and your evaluation of it, what additional lab tests or data are needed to assist in the care of this patient?

Critical Thinking Exercise 4

ANTICIPATING FINDINGS

Given the working diagnosis of croup, what physical assessment and lab data do you anticipate?

CLINICAL DATA ON ADMISSION

Vital signs

HR	124/min
RR	28/min
BP	124/60
SpO$_2$	RA 96%
Temp.	103.4°F

PHYSICAL EXAMINATION

General	Appearance: Some respiratory distress, diaphoretic, slight runny nose, no cyanosis, weight 13.8 kg
HEENT	Eyes: PERRLA, EOMs (extraocular eye muscles) intact, and fundi benign;
	Ears: TMs (tympanic membranes) clear;
	Nose: Has some clear rhinorrhea; Pharynx: Clear
Chest	Lungs: Coarse sounds with decreased air exchange; marked stridor with intercostal and subcostal retractions
CV	Heartbeat: Regular
Abdomen	Soft and nontender
GU	Within normal limits
Extremities	Within normal limits

AUTOMATED LEUKOCYTE DIFFERENTIAL

Date	10-26	Normal
Time	1315	Ranges
Neutrophils (%)	54.9	15.0–85.0
Lymphocytes (%)	33.4	12.0–50.0
Monocytes (%)	7.4	3.0–15.0
Eosinophils (%)	0.4	0.0–5.0
Basophils (%)	0.3	0.0–3.0

LAB DATA ON DAY OF ADMISSION

Hematology			
Date	10-26	10-26	Normal
Time	0900	1315	Ranges
WBC (1000 per mm^3)	8.7	7.7	4.3–10.8
RBC (1000 per mm^3)	5.17	5.17	4.8–5.4
Hgb (g/dL)	14.2	14.0	12.0–16.0
Hct (%)	43.2	42.6	42.0–47.0
Platelets (1000 per mm^3)	227	226	150–350
MCV (fL)	83.5	82.3	80.0–94.0
MCH (pg)	27.4	27.0	27.0–32.0
MCHC (g/dL)	32.8	32.8	32.0–36.0
RDW (%)	14.1	14.0	11.5–14.5

CASE 1 *(continued)*

MANUAL LEUKOCYTE DIFFERENTIAL

	10-26 0900	10-26 1315	Normal Ranges
Segments (%)	29	38	34–75
Band (%)	27	18	0–8
Lymphocytes (%)	31	38	12–50
Monocytes (%)	13	6	3–15
Platelet (est)	Adequate	Adequate	
Morphonucleocytes	NL	NL	
Atypical lymphocytes	Few		

IMMUNOLOGY— INFECTIOUS DISEASE SEROLOGY

Date	Time	RSV by EIA	DFA Resp Viral
10-26	0830	Negative	Positive*

*Parainfluenza virus type 1 detected by DFA. RSV, respiratory syncytial virus; EIA, electro-immunoassay; DFA, direct fluorescent antibody.

Critical Thinking Exercise 5

PROBLEM SOLVING USING CLINICAL DATA

a. How does the appearance of the radiographs in Figs. 14-1 and 14-2 relate to the patient's signs and symptoms?

b. How does the appearance of the radiograph in Fig. 14-3 modify your differential list?

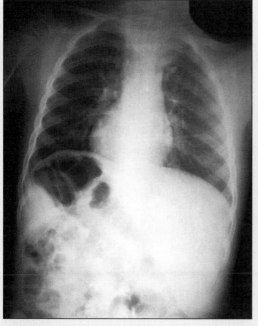

FIGURE 14-1 Posteroanterior chest x-ray of Billy B.

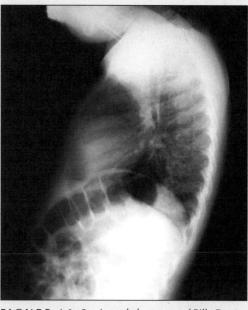

FIGURE 14-2 Lateral chest x-ray of Billy B.

CASE 1   *(continued)*

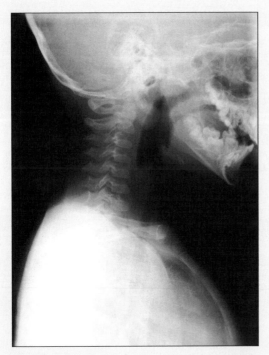

FIGURE 14-3   Spine-cervical soft tissue x-ray of Billy B.

  Critical Thinking Exercise 6

TROUBLESHOOTING/APPLYING PHYSIOLOGY TO CLINICAL PRACTICE AND COMMUNICATION

Billy's oxygen saturation is being questioned by the nurse. He feels that with the amount of respiratory distress the child is exhibiting, the reading is too high and that the pulse oximeter must not be working properly. Answer the following.

a. Do you suspect a malfunction of the oximeter?

b. Does acute upper airway obstruction predictably lead to serious difficulty with oxygenation? Explain the physiology to support your answer.

c. Describe what you would communicate to Billy's nurse and how you would do so.

  Group Critical Thinking Exercise 1

DECISION MAKING: ASSESSMENT OF DATA AND DEVELOPING A PLAN OF CARE

Have your group discuss Billy Barker's current status, reviewing all known data. Given the patient's current condition, have your group address the following.

a. What would you recommend for a care plan?

b. What results would you expect from each therapy?

c. How would you know that the patient was benefiting from these therapies?

d. What side effects or adverse reactions might result from the therapies?

e. How would treatment be modified in case of an adverse reaction?

  Group Critical Thinking Exercise 2

ANTICIPATING PROBLEMS AND SOLUTIONS

a. Discuss the unique challenges for intubation and airway management during any episode of pediatric acute upper airway obstruction. What are the risks and complications?

b. Discuss how you would evaluate and manage a child who requires intubation for an acute episode of upper airway obstruction.

The following clinical data were obtained 4 hours after treatment was started.

CLINICAL DATA FOLLOWING INITIAL TREATMENT

Vital signs

HR	102/min
RR	24/min
BP	120/65
Spo_2	N/A
Temp.	101.1°F

CASE 1 *(continued)*

Chest inspection	Some retractions noted, but fewer than previously observed. The child's color is pale, with no cyanosis. His coughing is barky, but less frequent, and his breathing does not appear as labored.
Auscultation	Breath sounds remain coarse, but stridor is decreased after therapy.

Over the next 96 hours, Billy continues to receive appropriate care, including respiratory care. He improves relatively quickly and is discharged on day 5, with a follow-up visit with his pediatrician scheduled for the following week.

 Group Critical Thinking Exercise 3

REFLECTION ON YOUR DECISIONS AND ACTIONS TO IMPROVE CLINICAL DECISION MAKING

a. Discuss why and how you would reflect on this case in order to decide retrospectively what was or was not effective.

b. How would you use this information to manage cases in the future?

c. Why is reflection important to your development as a professional?

CASE 2

DEBBIE DRUELER

Initial Case Scenario

A 2-year-old female who had been previously healthy was admitted to the ED at 11:15 PM on November 20. Her chief complaint is an acute onset of respiratory distress. When you enter the room, you notice a young child in moderate respiratory distress, with mild retractions and tachypnea. Her vital signs are: temperature 103°F, pulse 130, respiratory rate 40, and BP 110/60.

History

She has not had any previous hospitalizations. Her mother states that the child became irritable the day prior to admission and started wheezing and having difficulty breathing in the morning. She was taken to her family physician, started on amoxicillin, and sent home. She continued to have problems with breathing with increased wheezing and distress. Within a few hours she was returned to her physician, where a lateral soft tissue radiograph of the neck and AP and lateral films of the chest were ordered. The radiograph of the neck showed a clas-

sic thumb sign. This finding, and the patient's rapidly deteriorating condition with onset of both inspiratory and expiratory stridor, suggested the possibility of epiglottitis.

She was transferred to a larger regional hospital by air ambulance. Upon arrival in the ED, the patient presented in obvious distress. She was sitting upright in bed in the sniffing position. It was noted that her tongue was protruding from her mouth and drooling was present. She did not want to move her neck, and was resistant to any attempt at moving her.

 Critical Thinking Exercise 1

PRIORITIZING PATIENT CARE

a. Explain the steps you would need to follow to complete an initial patient assessment, ie, what is your immediate concern?

b. What would be your initial recommendation for a therapeutic intervention?

CASE 2 *(continued)*

Critical Thinking Exercise 2

MAKING INFERENCES
BY CLUSTERING DATA

a. What inferences can be made about Debbie's protruding tongue, drooling, respiratory distress, and reluctance to move her neck?

b. How does one cluster data leading to this inference? In this exercise, look critically at each fact relating to the child's signs and symptoms, and then see how they fit together to reach your differential diagnosis.

Critical Thinking Exercise 3

INFORMATION GATHERING
AND DECISION MAKING

a. During your patient assessment, what data should be obtained to complete the patient profile?

b. Based on this initial assessment and your evaluation of it, what additional lab tests or data are needed to assist in the care of this patient?

Critical Thinking Exercise 4

ANTICIPATING FINDINGS

Given the working diagnosis of epiglottitis, what abnormal physical assessment and lab data do you anticipate?

CLINICAL DATA ON ADMISSION

Vital signs

HR	130/min
RR	40/min
BP	110/60
SpO$_2$	RA 86%
Temp.	103°F

PHYSICAL EXAMINATION

General	Moderate respiratory distress, mouth breathing, drooling; pt. appears frightened, weight approx. 25 lb
HEENT	Head: Normocephalic and atraumatic; Eyes: PERRLA, EOMs intact; Ears: Within normal limits; Nose: Within normal limits; Throat: Mildly erythematous. Patient had her mouth open while breathing.
Chest	Lungs essentially clear to auscultation and percussion with obvious inspiratory and expiratory stridor. There are some coarse inspiratory crackles in the left base.
CV	Normal rate and rhythm without S3, S4, rubs, or murmurs.
Abdomen	Abdomen: Soft and nontender without organomegaly.
GU	Within normal limits.
Extremities	Within normal limits.
Neurologic	Cranial nerves II to XII grossly intact. The DTRs (deep tendon reflexes) were 2+ and bilaterally symmetric. Motor, sensory, and cerebellar exams were grossly within normal limits.

Critical Thinking Exercise 5

PROBLEM SOLVING
USING CLINICAL DATA

a. How does the appearance of the radiographs in Figs. 14-4 and 14-5 relate to the patient's signs and symptoms?

b. How does the appearance of the radiograph in Fig. 14-6 modify your differential list?

CASE 2 *(continued)*

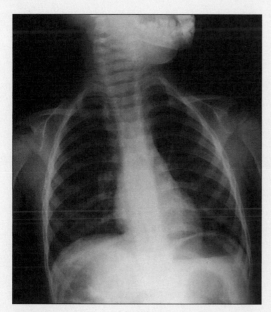

FIGURE 14-4 Posteroanterior chest x-ray of Debbie D.

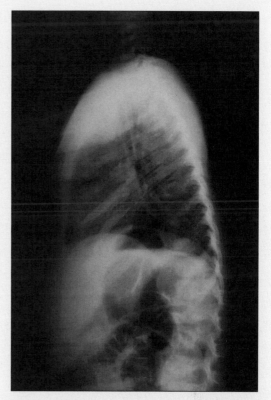

FIGURE 14-5 Lateral chest x-ray of Debbie D.

 Group Critical Thinking Exercise 1

ANTICIPATING PROBLEMS AND SOLUTIONS

a. Discuss the unique challenges for intubation and airway management during any episode of pediatric acute upper airway obstruction from epiglottitis. What are the risks and complications?

b. Discuss specifically where and by whom intubation for an acute episode of epiglottitis should be performed.

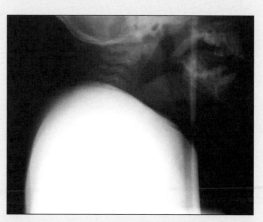

FIGURE 14-6 Spine-cervical soft tissue x-ray of Debbie D.

CASE 2 *(continued)*

Debbie was intubated and placed on a mechanical ventilator and put in isolation for the first 24 hours. The following clinical data were obtained.

Vital signs

HR	144/min
RR	16/min
BP	98/52
SpO$_2$	N/A
Temp.	99.6°F

PHYSICAL EXAMINATION

General	Skin color is pink, with no cyanosis observed. She does not require suctioning more often than every 4 to 5 hours, at which time clear secretions are aspirated. No retractions are noted at this time.
Chest	Breath sounds reveal some scattered crackles, but stridor is absent.

CLINICAL DATA FOLLOWING PATIENT STABILIZATION

Hematology

Date Time	11-21 0205	11-21 0630	11-29 0730	12-1 0715	Normal Ranges
WBC (1000 per mm³)	13.2	16.2	5.8	6.2	5.0–13.0
RBC (1000 per mm³)	3.97	3.99	4.4	4.32	4.7–6.1
HGB (g/dL)	10.5	10.5	11.8	11.4	11.0–15.0
Hct (%)	34.2	33.5	36.4	35.5	28.0–45.0
Platelets (1000 per mm³)	177	188	297	247	140–500
MCV (fL)	86	84	83	82	75.0–95.0
MCH (pg)	25.4	25.3	25.8	25.4	24.0–32.0
MCHC (g/dL)	33.7	31.3	32.4	32.0	30.0–36.0

MANUAL LEUKOCYTE DIFFERENTIAL

Date Time	11-21 0205	11-21 0630	11-29 0730	12-1 0715	Normal Ranges
Segments (%)	78	84	17	14	34–75
Bands (%)	4	0	5	1	0–8
Lymphocytes (%)	17	8	75	84	12–50
Monocytes (%)	1	8	2	1	3–15
Platelets (est)	Adequate		Adequate		
Morphonucleocytes	NL		NL		

CASE 2 *(continued)*

ARTERIAL BLOOD GASES

Date:	11-21 0600	11-21 0950	11-22 0530	11-22 0600
pH	7.37	7.36	7.41	7.38
$Paco_2$	38	41	34	42
HCO_3^-	22	23	21	24.5
BE	−3	−2	−2	−0.5
Pao_2	64	91	99	97
Sao_2	92	95	98	98
Fio_2	0.3	0.4	0.35	0.3

Debbie received appropriate antibiotic therapy and the upper airway swelling rapidly resolved over the next 2 days. Mechanical ventilation was maintained for the following 48 hours, after which Debbie was rapidly weaned from the ventilator and successfully extubated. Her remaining hospital stay was uneventful and she was discharged after 12 days of hospitalization.

Group Critical Thinking Exercise 2

THE PRO/CON DEBATE

Using Debbie's case that was just presented, one group of students will be assigned to support the argument that the child needs to be immediately trached when she arrives in the ED. This group will need to use facts such as lab data, clinical signs, and symptoms to build a strong case. Be sure to clearly indicate why this child needs an emergency tracheostomy at this time. The group should explain why its decision is the correct one, and what could potentially happen to Debbie if the tracheostomy is delayed.

Now, the second group of students is going to take the exact *opposite* position. This group will make the case that Debbie does *not* need to be trached upon admission to the ED, but rather should be intubated in the OR. This group should explain and support why its decision is the correct one, and what could happen to Debbie if she is not immediately intubated in the OR. Each group should include all data necessary to support its position.

Group Critical Thinking Exercise 3

REFLECTION ON YOUR DECISIONS AND ACTIONS TO IMPROVE CLINICAL DECISION MAKING

Discuss why and how you would reflect on this case in order to figure out retrospectively what did or did not work. How would you use this information to manage cases in the future? Why is reflection important to your practice?

KEY POINTS

- Pediatric airway obstruction has a wide and varied etiology.

- Noninfectious causes of airway obstruction include foreign body obstruction, anaphylactic reactions, trauma, cancer, congenital abnormalities, VCD, and burns.

- Croup (also called laryngotracheobronchitis or LTB) affects the subglottic area, while acute epiglottis affects the supraglottic region.

- Croup has a viral origin, while acute epiglottis has a bacterial origin.

- Development of the *Haemophilus influenzae B* vaccine (in October 1990) has greatly decreased the incidence of acute epiglottis.

- Since a virus almost always causes croup, antibiotics are not an effective treatment option.

- Acute epiglottitis is always a medical emergency, but croup can also deteriorate into a life-threatening condition.

- X-ray diagnosis of croup is made by presence of the "steeple" sign, while the "thumb" sign identifies acute epiglottitis.

- A "barking cough," gradual onset, and low grade fever is seen with croup, while epiglottis is associated with rapid onset, drooling, an expiratory "purr," and high grade fever.

- Parents or caregivers can greatly assist the child in upper airway distress by remaining calm.

- Nebulized steroids (budesonide) may be effective in the treatment of croup.

- Treatment of croup or acute epiglottitis may range from conservative to aggressive.

REFERENCES

1. Farzan D, Farzan S. *A Concise Handbook of Respiratory Diseases*, 4th ed. Norwalk, Conn: Appleton & Lange; 1997:131–133.

2. D'Alessandro MP. Foreign body, trachea. 1998. Available online at http://indy.radiology.uiowa.edu/Providers/TeachingFiles/PAP/ChestDiseases/FBTrachea.html: accessed July 11, 2000.

3. Andrews B. Pediatric anaphylaxis. 1998. Available online at http://www.vgernet.net/bkand/state/panaph.html: accessed July 11, 2000.

4. American Academy of Allergy, Asthma and Immunology. Anaphylaxis. 1998. Available online at http://www.allergy.or.kr/mirror/aaai/tip18.html: accessed October 27, 1998.

5. National Jewish Medical and Research Center. Vocal cord dysfunction. No date. Available online at http://www.njc.org/mthtml/vcd_mf.html: accessed October 29, 1998.

6. Shreve M. Vocal cord dysfunction. 1997. Available online at http://www.peds.umn.edu/divisions/pccm/teaching/vcd.html: accessed July 11, 2000.

7. Des Jardins T, Burton G. *Clinical Manifestations & Assessment of Respiratory Disease*. 3rd ed. St. Louis: CV Mosby; 1995:221–222.

8. Santer DM, D'Alessandro MP. Discussion of parainfluenza virus. 1998. Available online at http://www.vh.org/Providers/Textbooks/ElectricAirway/Discussion/DiscParaflu.html: accessed July 11, 2000.

9. Santer DM, D'Alessandro MP. Discussion of *H influenzae* type b. 1998. Available online at http://www.vh.org/Providers/Textbooks/ElectricAirway/Discussion/DiscHFlu.html: accessed October 25, 1998.

10. RxMed. Epiglottitis. (No date). Available online at http://www.rxmed.com/illnesses/epiglottitis.html: accessed July 11, 2000.

11. D'Alessandro MP. Croup (acute laryngotracheobronchitis). 1998. Available online at http://indy.radiology.uiowa.edu/Providers/TeachingFiles/PAP/ChestDiseases/Croup.html: accessed July 11, 2000.

12. American Institute of Preventive Medicine. Croup. 1995. Available online at http://www.healthy.net/library/Books/Healthyself/croup.htm: accessed July 11, 2000.

13. Unknown. Epiglottitis. 1996-2000. Available online at http://sleeptight.comEncyMaster/E/epiglottitis.html: accessed July 11, 2000.

14. Santer DM, D'Alessandro MP. Table of characteristics of viral croup and acute epiglottitis. 1992-2000. Available online at http://www.vh.org/Providers/Textbooks/ElectricAirway/TableText/TableCharCroupEpi.html: accessed July 11, 2000.

15. Barnhart SL, Czervinske MP. *Perinatal and Pediatric Respiratory Care*. Philadelphia: Saunders; 1995:49, 90–91.

16. Santer DM, D'Alessandro MP. Acute Epiglottitis. 1998. Available online at http://www.vh.org/Providers/Textbooks/ElectricAirway/Text/Epiglottitis.html: accessed July 11, 2000.

17. Women.com Networks. Croup: Chasing off a scary cough. 1998. Available online at http://www.rprevention.com/children/remedies/croup.html: accessed October 25, 1998.

18. Klassen TP, et al. The efficacy of nebulized budesonide in dexamethasone-treated outpatients with croup. Pediatrics. 1996;97:463–466.

19. Medical Sciences Bulletin. Nebulized budesonide for croup. 1994. Available online at http://pharminfo.com/pubs/msb/budeson.html: accessed July 11, 2000.

OBSTRUCTIVE SLEEP APNEA

Brian H. Foresman and Pamela Minkley

*He who knows others is clever; he who
knows himself is enlightened.*

LAO-TZU
604–531 BC

LEARNING OBJECTIVES

1. Describe the basic terminology related to sleep-related breathing disorders and commonly associated sleep disorders.
2. Discuss the etiology, pathophysiology, and clinical features of a patient with sleep-related breathing disorders.
3. Discuss the evaluation process and critical diagnostic issues that arise during evaluation of the patient suspected of having a sleep-related breathing disorder, and acute and long-term management of patients with sleep-related breathing disorders, including health promotion and quality-of-life issues.
4. Apply specific theories related to polysomnography and sleep medicine to assist in clinical decision making in the management of a patient with sleep-related breathing disorders.
5. Apply the critical thinking skills of prioritizing, anticipating, negotiating, communicating, decision making, and reflection by completing exercises and a case study of sleep-related breathing disorders.
6. Apply strategies to promote critical thinking in the diagnosis and respiratory care management of patients with sleep-related breathing disorders through completion of chapter exercises and group discussion.
7. Use the clinical case study in the chapter to perform an initial patient assessment, using a standardized system (SOAP notes and IPPA) and the clinical data presented.
8. Interpret clinical data from the case study, including history, physical examination, lab data, and polysomnographic data to make recommendations for respiratory care management.
9. Develop a care plan for the patient as the case progresses, including recommendations for issues important in the evaluation of the patient, taking into consideration the available methodology, cost, efficacy, and quality-of-life issues.
10. Communicate facts, evidence, and arguments to support the diagnostic decisions, evaluations, and recommendations proposed in the care plan for the patient with a sleep-related breathing disorder.
11. Evaluate treatment and outcomes of interventions to propose changes in the care plan.
12. Describe the role of the respiratory therapist in the diagnosis, treatment, and management of sleep-related breathing disorders.

KEY WORDS

Apnea
Apnea-Hypopnea Index (AHI)
Apnea Index (AI)
Arousals
Bilevel Positive Airway Pressure (BiPAP)
Continuous Positive Airway Pressure (CPAP)
Circadian
Electromyogram (EMG)
Electro-oculogram (EOG)
Excessive Daytime Sleepiness (EDS)
Hypopnea
Multiple Sleep Latency Test (MSLT)
Noninvasive Continuous Positive Airway Pressure (NCPAP)
Obstructive Sleep Apnea (OSA)

Periodic Limb Movements (PLM)
Periodic Limb Movement Disorder (PLMD)
Polysomnography (PSG)
Respiratory Disturbance Index (RDI)
Rapid Eye Movements (REM)
Respiratory-Event Related Arousals (RERA)
REM Sleep
Respiratory Disturbances
Sleep Disorders
Sleep-Related Breathing Disorder (SRBD)
Sleep Stages
Sleep Onset REM (SOREM)
Sleep-Related Breathing Disorders (SRBD)
Slow Rolling Eye Movements (SREM)
Slow Wave Sleep (SWS)

DEFINITIONS OF SELECTED KEY WORDS

10-20 System A system for EEG electrode placement that allows for a consistent placement of the electrodes.

AHI The number of apneas plus hypopneas per hour of sleep.

Alpha Activity EEG frequencies from 8 to 13 Hz. Usually seen with relaxed wakefulness with the eyes closed and during arousals.[1]

Apnea An event where measurable airflow through the nostrils and the mouth ceases at some point during the event with an event duration of 10 sec or more. The exact amount of reduction necessary to define "no measurable airflow" is controversial and is dependent upon the measurement technique employed. Criterion measures vary from 80% to 100% reduction from baseline and may include oxygen desaturation and/or arousal criteria.

Arousal An abrupt shift in EEG frequency, which may include theta, alpha, and/or frequencies greater than 16 Hz but not spindles and lasts a minimum of 3 sec. Arousals observed in the polysomnogram are scored by published scoring rules.[2]

Awakening An abrupt change from any sleep stage to wakefulness lasting 15 sec or more.[2]

Beta Activity EEG frequencies above 13 Hz. For sleep this usually means frequencies from 13 to 35 Hz.[1]

Cataplexy An involuntary sudden decrease in motor tone, not associated with a change in consciousness, that occurs while awake and results in muscle weakness, paralysis, or loss of motor function.

Delta Activity EEG frequencies less than 4 Hz.[1]

Hertz (Hz) Cycles per second.

Hypopnea Episodes of reduced airflow lasting 10 to 120 sec. The exact amount of reduction necessary is controversial and is dependent upon the measurement technique employed and the conditions of assessment. Criterion measures vary from 20% to 50% and may include oxygen desaturation and/or arousal criteria.

K Complex An isolated wave form that stands out from the background EEG with a well-delineated initial negative sharp wave followed by a high amplitude positive slow wave and with a duration of >0.5 sec. The slow wave does not need to meet 75 ϕV criteria required for SWS. Usually, recorded best over the vertex regions.

Limb Movements Arm or more typically leg muscle bursts. These bursts are evident on the polysomnogram in both wake and sleep and are scored and reported using a defined set of published rules.[3]

Morbidity The condition of being diseased. Statistically, the rate at which an illness occurs (number of sick divided by total people in the group).

Mortality The death rate of a particular disease, usually expressed deaths per 1000 or per 100,000 who have the disease.

Multiple Sleep Latency Test A test that consists of 4 to 5 daytime naps occurring every 2 hours.[4,5]

NREM Sleep Non-REM sleep includes sleep stages 1, 2, 3, and 4.

Periodic Limb Movements Myoclonic limb movements that typically occur during sleep, last from 0.5 to 5 sec, are separated by 5 to 90 sec, and occur in groups of four or more. A grouping of four or more is sometimes referred to as a "train" or "sequence" of PLMs.[3]

PLM Index The total number of PLMs divided by the hours of sleep.

RDI The number of respiratory disturbances per hour of sleep. This is often used interchangeably with the AHI. However, in the future it is likely that the RDI will include apneas, hypopneas, and RERAs thereby making such use inappropriate.

REM Rapid eye movements—these may occur during wakefulness or as part of REM sleep. Blinks are not physiologically the same as rapid eye movements.

REM Sleep The stage of sleep characterized by rapid eye movements, low voltage mixed EEG signal, and muscle atonia. This is characteristically the stage of sleep where dreaming occurs.

RERA Respiratory-event related arousals that terminate a period (at least 10 sec in duration) of increasing respiratory effort and that occur during sleep. Effort may be indicated by a variety of conventional measures with the most consistent and accurate being esophageal pressure monitoring.

Sleep Hygiene A system of principles and rules to promote optimum sleep and alertness.

Sleep Spindle Isolated bursts of EEG activity 0.5 to 1.5 sec in duration with a frequency of 12 to 14 Hz often with a waxing and waning of the amplitude (spindle). Recorded best over the vertex regions in contrast to 8–12 Hz alpha activity, which is typically longer in duration, a more

consistent aplitude and recorded best over the occipital region.[1]

SOREM Sleep onset REM. REM sleep that occurs in 20 min or less after sleep onset.

Theta Activity EEG frequencies from 8 to 13 Hz.[1]

Total Sleep Time The total amount of time spent in sleep from lights out to lights on as recorded on the polysomnogram.

Disorders[6]

Periodic Limb Movement Disorder A disorder characterized by frequent PLMs occurring at a rate of five per hour of sleep or more and associated with symptoms of insomnia or excessive sleepiness.

REM Behavior Disorder A sleep disorder whose hallmark is the lack of muscle atonia during REM sleep often associated with dream-related body movements or vocalizations.

Narcolepsy A disorder of unknown etiology that is characterized by excessive sleepiness that typically is associated with cataplexy and other REM sleep phenomena, such as sleep paralysis and hynagogic hallucinations.

Obstructive Sleep Apnea Syndrome A disorder characterized by repetitive episodes of upper airway obstruction that occur during sleep, usually associated with a reduction in blood oxygen saturation.

Sleep-Related Breathing Disorders A term generally used to encompass all described breathing disorders that pathologically occur during the sleep period.

INTRODUCTION

In the United States, estimates are that 10% to 15% of the general population experience frequent daytime sleepiness, and some populations may have an incidence approaching 35%.[7] In a large proportion of these individuals, the major causes for the sleepiness involve disorders that limit the amount of sleep achieved, behavior patterns that disrupt sleep, or disorders that interfere with achieving adequate amounts of consolidated sleep. Of the disorders that affect sleep and cause excessive daytime sleepiness, sleep-related breathing disorders (SRBD) are one of the most common, with obstructive sleep apnea (OSA) being the major disorder in this class. Within the general population these disorders are not trivial, affecting between 2% and 4% of women and 5% to 9% of men, depending on the measuring criteria employed.[8,9]

Sleep-related breathing disorders, (SRBDs) have been associated with excessive sleepiness, the development of several cardiovascular disorders, and an increase in accidents.[10] Recently, studies conducted through the National Institutes of Health (NIH) have begun to identify the relationship between OSA and the development of cardiovascular disease.[11] The findings have now identified OSA as an independent risk factor for the development of cardiovascular disease. Close associations with the development of hypertension and stroke further strengthened these findings and suggest that effective treatment may prevent the development of these disorders. Consequently, the identification and treatment of SRBDs may help prevent major accidents and prevent the morbidity and mortality associated with many cardiovascular disorders.

SLEEP PHYSIOLOGY

In order to understand the sleep-related breathing disorders it is necessary to understand basic sleep physiology and the effects of sleep on breathing. We begin by dividing sleep into two major states: non-REM sleep and REM or rapid eye movement sleep. Non-REM sleep is comprised of sleep stages 1, 2, 3 and 4.[1] Stage 1 sleep is typically the initial stage of sleep that is then followed by stage 2 sleep. These first two stages of sleep are commonly characterized as light sleep. Stages 3 and 4 are the stages of sleep referred to as slow wave sleep (SWS) due to the prominence of high-amplitude slow waves. As an individual progresses from stage 1 to stage 4, sleep becomes progressively deeper with a decrease in alpha and beta brain wave activity shown on EEG. The majority of dreaming occurs during REM sleep, and a number of characteristic physiologic changes also take place. The characteristics of each of these sleep stages is briefly reviewed in Table 15-1.

The pattern of sleep stages that occurs during a night's sleep constitutes the sleep architecture. Typically, an individual progresses from stage 1 to stage 2 to slow wave sleep and then to REM sleep in a recurring pattern. Each cycle, from the lighter stages of sleep through the end of REM, typically takes 60 to 90 minutes. As the night progresses each cycle contains less slow wave sleep and more REM sleep, until the final sleep cycle, which may have 30 to 50 minutes of REM sleep. The length of each sleep stage and the amount of sleep required by an individual changes with age, with significant decreases in slow wave and REM sleep occurring by age 20, followed by more gradual decreases thereafter. However, the characteristic stages of sleep are fairly consistent from approximately 1 year of age through adulthood. The other major change that occurs with aging is a decrease in the amount of sleep required. Newborn children require 14 to 16 hours of sleep a day, and the sleep periods are quite intermittent. The sleep requirement rapidly falls to 10 to 12 hours by early childhood, a period usually associated with youngsters taking an afternoon nap. Further reductions in sleep requirements occur, so teenagers and young adults will only need about 8 to 10 hours of sleep. For adults, the typical sleep requirement ranges from 6 to 9 hours. There are individuals who require more or less sleep than this average, but they represent less than 5% of the population. In general, someone who sleeps less than 6 hours each night should be viewed as being sleep deprived until otherwise proven to be a short sleeper.

The timing of sleep is important in the overall assessment of sleep disorders. Sleep is a physiologic requirement that is part of our *circadian rhythm*, a term given to the physiologic cycle of changes that occur during the course of each day. For most individuals this rhythm is about 26 hours in duration, and is synchronized with the daylight each morning when we arise. Three primary processes contribute to the synchronization of our physiologic rhythms. The first is exposure to light. The light stimulates neural signals to be generated from the retina as part of our visual process. Some of the neural fibers pass to the suprachiasmic nucleus, a structure in the brain that helps regulate our internal clock and biological rhythms. The second mechanism is the pattern of our daily activities. The stimulation arising from these activities and our interactions with other peo-

TABLE 15-1   SLEEP STAGE CHARACTERISTICS

BACKGROUND EEG		EMG	EOG	SPECIAL CHARACTERISTICS
Stage wake[a]	Mixed frequency with more than 50% of the epoch alpha with eyes closed	Relatively high tonic	Eye movements and blinks	May observe beta in EEG
Stage 1[a]	Low voltage, mixed frequency, less than 50% alpha, predominance of 2–7 Hz activity	Tonic EMG less than wake	SREMs in early portion	Occasional vertex sharp waves in EEG. Absence of spindles and K complexes
Stage 2[a]	Low voltage, mixed frequency may have some slow wave activity	Similar to stage 1 tonic EMG	Absence of REMs or SREMs	Sleep spindles[b] and/or intermittent K complexes[b] stand out from background
Stage 3[a]	Slow wave activity (<2 Hz) of 75 ΦV amplitude in 20%–50% of the epoch	Similar to stage 1 tonic EMG	Absence of REMs or SREMs	Clearly identifiable sleep spindles and K complexes are uncommon
Stage 4[a]	Same as stage 3 but greater than 50% of the epoch consists of delta waves	Same as stage 3	Same as stage 3	Same as stage 3; *clearly identifiable* K complexes are rare
Stage REM[a]	Low voltage, mixed frequency,[b] 5–7 Hz sawtooth waves frequently seen but not required	Low voltage, tonic EMG, lower than preceding stage[b]	Episodic REMs (phasic REM)[b]	Absence of sleep spindles and K complexes; may see intermittent alpha activity

[a]In all instances the eyes must be closed. For more details and exceptions see R&K criteria.[1]

[b]Characteristics that must be present.

A scoring epoch is typically 30 seconds. If paper systems are used, the paper speed is 10 mm/second.

EMG, electromyogram; REM, rapid eye movement; SREM, slow rolling eye movements.

ple reinforces the sleep-wake cycle. The final mechanism involves our patterns of eating. Food is a very potent stimulus with regard to our sleep-wake mechanisms. These three mechanisms are often referred to as *Zeitgebers* or "time givers." Through a series of complex interactions, these mechanisms affect sleep onset, the patterns of sleep, and the timing of REM sleep. Because sleepiness and sleep stages are linked to the circadian rhythms, polysomnography must be performed according to the individual's sleeping routine, otherwise misleading or inaccurate data may result. Such errors in determining proper sleep times can profoundly affect the accuracy and reliability of tests designed to assess daytime sleepiness (eg, multiple sleep latency testing).[4,5,12,13] Occasionally, the sleep period may be extended to provide additional time for sleep repletion if excessive sleepiness is thought to be related to insufficient sleep. Enforcing a sleep period for polysomnography to meet staffing demands rather than adapting polysomnography to the patient's routine is likely to render inaccurate results and should be avoided.

Each of the major mechanisms affecting our circadian rhythms, and indirectly our sleep, are affected by our patterns of activity. Patterns of behavior closely linked with sleep may facilitate good sleep or may disrupt sleep. The principles and rules for optimizing sleep are called *sleep hygiene*. If good sleep hygiene is practiced, sleeping and waking periods are generally well maintained and efficient. Please review the principles of good sleep hygiene as outlined in the following critical content box.

CRITICAL CONTENT

GOOD SLEEP HYGIENE

- Allow an adequate amount of time for sleeping each day.
- Keep a regular bedtime routine and time of arousal.
- Be active and get regular exercise.
- Maintain a quiet, comfortable sleeping environment.
- Keep the room a comfortable temperature.
- Reduce caffeine intake.
- Do not drink alcoholic beverages before going to bed.
- Do not go to bed hungry, but do not eat large meals just before bedtime.
- Do not try to catch up on lost sleep by sleeping late. It is better to go to bed early when you are sleepy.
- Reduce or eliminate the use of tobacco products, especially near bedtime.
- If you awaken at night, limit your light exposure and activity. Try not to count the minutes while waiting to go back to sleep.

Factors that limit or fragment sleep cause sleep deprivation. The major effect of sleep deprivation is to cause excessive sleepiness; however, studies by Rechtschaffen and colleagues[14] have shown that sleep is required for maintenance of good health.

Individuals who experience sleep deprivation consistently show moodiness, decrements in memory, difficulty in concentration, and progressive increases in daytime sleepiness. The reported effects are often dependent upon the type of sleep deprivation (total versus selective) and the amount of sleep deprivation (number of hours lost, and acute versus chronic).[15–19] A short sleep latency and increased sleep efficiency are characteristic of generalized sleep deprivation. Some disorders such as OSA may result in selective REM deprivation due to the physiologic changes that occur during REM sleep.[20–22] With continued REM sleep deprivation there is an increase in the physiologic need for REM, or so-called *REM pressure*. During the recovery phase the increased REM pressure can result in an increase in REM sleep; this is commonly referred to as *REM rebound*.

As an individual makes the transition from waking to sleep, the respiratory control relationships change (Table 15-2). With the onset of sleep the central mechanisms controlling blood levels of CO_2 and O_2 allow functionally higher and lower levels, respectively. In theory, the reason behind these changes is a shift to metabolic control of respiration and a change in the set points in the partial pressure of both gases. The set point changes allow the CO_2 to rise by 2 to 3 torr and the oxygen saturation to fall by 2% to 3%. If the transition to sleep is rapid, the change in set points can cause sleep-onset central apneas to occur (Fig. 15-1). These are generally considered a normal occurrence during sleep if there is no associated obstructive component, and an individual event may last up to 90 seconds. The pattern of respiration is generally more regular during slow wave sleep and may be quite erratic during REM sleep. REM sleep has one unique characteristic that significantly alters the mechanics of ventilation: muscle atonia. This occurrence during REM sleep decreases the contribution of the intercostal and accessory muscles of ventilation, leaving only the hemidiaphragms to maintain ventilation. Under some conditions like obesity, chronic obstructive pulmonary disease (COPD), and OSA, the loss of the intercostal and accessory muscles may make the maintenance of ventilation or oxygenation difficult.

TABLE 15-2　PHYSIOLOGIC CHANGES IN RESPIRATORY CONTROL WITH SLEEP

	TRANSITIONAL SLEEP[a]	STAGE 2 SLEEP	SLOW WAVE SLEEP	REM SLEEP
Major influence on breathing	Metabolic[b]	Metabolic	Metabolic	Nonmetabolic
Pattern of breathing	Periodic	Regular	Regular	Irregular
Central apneas/hypopneas	Often	Rare	Absent	Frequent
Response to metabolic stimuli	Variable	Mild decrease	Mild decrease	Moderate decrease
Chest wall movement	Phasic	Phasic	Phasic	Paradoxical

[a]Transitional sleep refers to the period of sleep between wakefulness and continuous stage 1 sleep.

[b]The metabolic regulation becomes predominant during the transition from wakefulness to sleep.

ETIOLOGY AND PATHOPHYSIOLOGY OF OSA

Obstructive sleep apnea is a disorder characterized by recurrent narrowing or closure of the upper airway, leading to repeated respiratory events that are often associated with reductions in airflow, desaturations, and fragmentation of sleep. The pathophysiologic mechanisms active in OSA are attributable to physiologic changes that occur during sleep and/or structural abnormalities of the upper airway. The sleep-related mechanisms include altered control of respiration, abnormal functioning of the pharyngeal dilator muscles, depressed arousal responses, and shifts in neuromuscular control. Problems caused by these mechanisms may be compounded by structural changes in the oropharynx that narrows the pharynx.

The pharyngeal muscles are composed of two functional groups of muscles: a pharyngeal dilator group and a pharyngeal constrictor group. At the initiation of each breath, the pharyngeal dilator mechanism is activated, thereby maintaining the patency of the pharynx throughout inspiration. With sleep onset there is a relative relaxation of the pharyngeal muscles that under normal circumstances causes a mild increase in airway resistance. In the majority of cases of OSA, the pharyngeal dilator mechanism is dysfunctional, resulting in partial or complete airway closure during sleep, as well as significant increases in airway resistance. The three sites where this narrowing commonly occurs (ie, the posterior nasopharynx, the posterior oropharynx, and the velopharynx or hypopharynx) are shown in Fig. 15-2. While narrowing may occur in only one location, more than 50% of patients with OSA have two or more areas involved in their disease.

Structural abnormalities such as micrognathia, macroglossia, and large tonsils may contribute to the development of sleep apnea through a reduction in the dimensions of the upper airway. Increased body fat, a condition common among OSA patients, also may contribute to airway narrowing and may further predispose to upper airway obstruction. In this regard, obesity should be considered a contributor to OSA, but not a common etiologic mechanism.

Arousal from sleep is a major function that protects against life-threatening respiratory compromise that occurs during sleep, independent of the etiology. Arousals due to respiratory compromise are usually associated with an increase in respiratory rate and sympathetic outflow, although the sympathetic outflow is attenuated by the increase in respiration. For asthma and early OSA, an increase in airway resistance without a reduction in flow can cause arousals and symptoms of sleepiness or fatigue.[23] In this instance, as airway resistance increases, the body responds by increas-

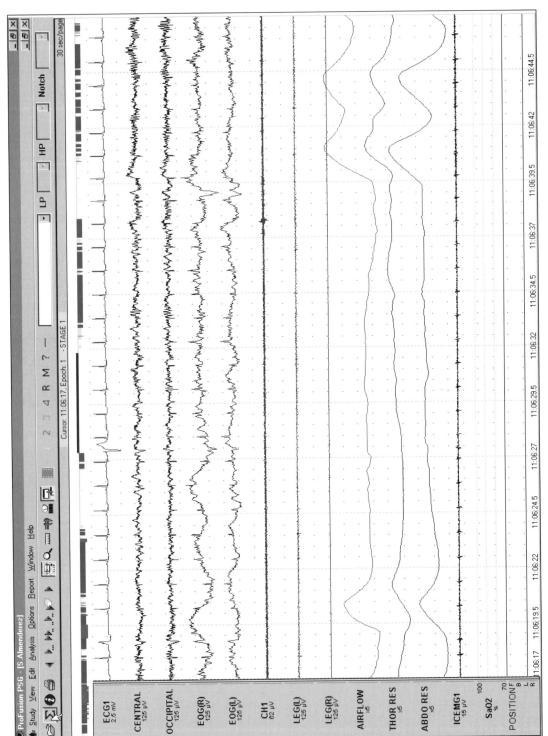

FIGURE 15-1   Sleep-onset central apneas.

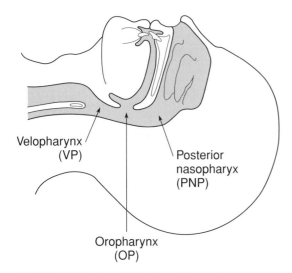

FIGURE 15-2 *Major sites of airway closure in OSA. Typical sites of pharyngeal obstruction contributing to OSA include the posterior nasopharynx (PNP), oropharynx (OP), and velopharynx (VP) (also known as the hypopharynx). Nasal polyps, septal deviations, macroglossia, and several other anatomic features that can lead to airway narrowing may contribute to increased upper airway resistance and obstruction.*

ing respiratory effort to maintain flow; however, the increased effort arouses the individual, and this is classified as a respiratory-event related arousal (RERA). As airway obstruction becomes more severe or hypoventilation ensues, flow is reduced and arterial desaturation and/or elevations of CO_2

may occur, thereby adding an additional stimulus for further arousals. Thus it appears that OSA progresses from the milder RERAs to apneas (Fig. 15-3). Factors that decrease the tendency to arouse will frequently worsen respiratory events related to OSA by prolonging events and delaying the resumption of normal respiration. Factors that may decrease the tendency to arouse include sedative agents, alcoholic beverages, hypnotic agents, and conditions that cause excessive sleepiness or sleep deprivation. All of these should be avoided in patients with OSA or other chronic respiratory diseases.

There are several adverse cardiovascular consequences of obstructive respiratory events. During these events excessive vagal tone results in bradycardia that is typically followed by tachycardia after resolution of the respiratory event. Sympathetic increases occurring with these events and the reactive tachycardia often cause a transient rise in blood pressure. Over time the increases in sympathetic tone become more persistent and may develop into hypertension.[24] In contrast, pulmonary hypertension is a relatively rare complication more commonly associated with chronic hypoxemia or hypoventilation.

Apneas may be divided into obstructive apnea, mixed apnea, or central apnea (Table 15-3). Obstructive and central forms of hypopneas may also be seen. Mixed apneas are characterized by an initial central component followed by an obstructive component with eventual resumption of breathing.

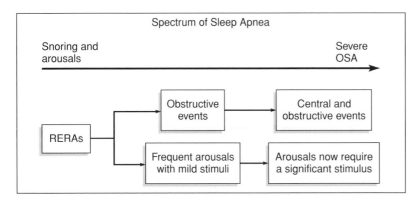

FIGURE 15-3
Spectrum of OSA.

TABLE 15-3   CHARACTERISTICS OF RESPIRATORY EVENTS

	DURATION	AIRFLOW	EFFORT	DESATURATION[a]	AROUSAL
Obstructive apnea	At lest 10 seconds	Absent at some point in the event	Proportionately greater than flow; crescendo effort common	Not required	Not required
Central apnea	At least 10 seconds	Proportional to respiratory effort; absent at some point in the event	Absent or proportionally decreased with airflow	Common but not required	Not required
Hypopnea	10–20 seconds, longer should be hypoventilation	Decreased by 50% relative to most recent airflow baseline	Proportionately greater than flow; crescendo effort common	Usually required if there is no arousal	Usually required if there is no desaturation
Respiratory-event related arousal[b]	At least 10 seconds; often several minutes	No significant change from baseline	Slight increase, may crescendo to end of event	Not required	Required; usually cyclic
"Hypoventilaton" period	Not an "event" but a long PERIOD of time	No significant, discernable change from baseline	No change or subtle decrease; respiratory rate may decrease	Gradual decrease from baseline; may last several minutes; may be severe	Hypoventilatory period usually ends with an arousal and resaturation
Cheyne-Stokes respiration	Series may last 15–30 minutes or more	Varies proportionate with the respiratory effort; may include apnea at lowest point	Crescendo-decrescendo pattern	Usually mild cyclic desaturations but not required	Not required

[a]Spo$_2$ desaturations must be defined and are dependent on the oximeters used. Typically a 3% drop in Spo$_2$ using an average response time of 3 seconds or 4 pulses is used.

[b]Associated with upper airways resistance syndrome (UARS).

Both apneas and hypopneas must have a duration of at least 10 seconds (Table 15-3) in order to be scorable.

A *hypopnea* is a period of reduced airflow typically lasting from 10 to 20 seconds. Reductions in airflow longer than this are typically characterized as *hypoventilation*. The exact amount of decrease in airflow necessary to identify the reduction varies,[25]

however, a minimum reduction of 30% to 50% is necessary in most circumstances in order to be detectable by the equipment used to measure airflow. In some centers, the reduction in airflow must be coupled with a desaturation or arousal in order to score as an event. The choice of criteria for scoring respiratory events varies widely and no one definition has been accepted as a standard. It is important to note that while these definitions are based on air-flow measurements, there are major technical limitations associated with the thermistors or transducers used to record airflow. Such airflow measurements represent an indirect measurement of airflow and the limitations imposed by the technology must be understood by the technologist and physician alike. Commonly used methods to record respiratory effort have similar limitations.[26]

The number of apneas that occur per hour of sleep is referred to as the apnea index (AI). The number of apneas plus hypopneas that occur per hour of sleep is referred to as the apnea-hypopnea index (AHI). In some instances the respiratory disturbance index (RDI) may be substituted for the AHI; however, the criteria for respiratory events has changed over the past 10 years,[26] and proposed changes in the definition will likely change the validity of such substitutions in the future. Typically an AHI or an RDI >5 is abnormal. In the past, some authors suggested that the RDI does not become clinically significant until it reaches >20; however, several studies have shown that the RDI does not correlate well with other measures of severity and should not be used as the only index of disease severity. More recent data from the Sleep Heart Health Study and other investigations[11,27,28] have shown that an AHI of 5 is closely associated with the development disease, and this number may increase as the individual ages. Thus symptomatic patients with an abnormal AHI (>5) should be treated.

CLINICAL FEATURES

Signs and Symptoms

The most common features of OSA are excessive daytime sleepiness (EDS), loud snoring, witnessed apneas, morning headaches, frequent nocturnal arousals, and weight gain. Usually the patient presents with a history of increasing daytime sleepiness that has been present for 2 to 5 years. This is usually associated with increasing weight and decreasing ability to perform daily activities. The patient

or their bed partner often reports that the patient's sleep is quite restless and associated with the frequent arousals related to snorting or snoring. These patients usually awaken unrefreshed and often take naps during the day or fall asleep spontaneously. The sleepiness associated with OSA can lead to accidents, interfere with activities of daily living, impair work performance, and lead to a general decline in satisfaction that is often perceived as depression. Additional symptoms or complaints may relate to a decline in vision, poor memory, irritability, dry mouth, chronic fatigue, weight gain, and male sexual dysfunction.

CRITICAL CONTENT

HISTORICAL CHARACTERISTICS OF OSA

- Excessive daytime sleepiness
- Loud snoring
- Weight gain
- Morning headaches
- Frequent nighttime arousals
- Awakening unrefreshed
- Difficulty concentrating
- Witnessed apneas
- Family history of sleep apnea
- History of cardiovascular disease

Individuals with OSA are frequently obese with a narrow or crowded oropharynx and increased neck girth. Men are two times more likely to have OSA than premenopausal women. These individuals often have macroglossia, micrognathia, tonsillar hypertrophy, or an enlarged uvula. Occasionally nasal obstruction, nasal polyposis, structural defects of the nose, or allergies may also contribute to airway obstruction. Ventilation may also be impaired due to moderate obesity when the patient is the supine position. Further physical examination often reveals that there is evidence of lower extremity edema, hypertension, or other cardiovascular disorders.[10] The family medical history often shows that other family members either have OSA or have a history of excessive sleepiness and snoring.

CRITICAL CONTENT

PHYSICAL CHARACTERISTICS OF OSA PATIENTS

- Frequently, but not always, obese
- Crowded oropharynx
- Increased neck girth
- Micrognathia
- Frequent hypertension
- Peripheral edema
- More commonly seen in men and postmenopausal women
- Increases with age

Laboratory Assessments and Typical Findings

When sleep-related breathing disorders (SRBDs) are suspected, definitive testing usually involves one or more forms of polysomnography. Polysomnography is performed not only to verify the diagnosis of a SRBD, most commonly OSA, but also to rule out other coexistent disorders that may complicate the treatment regimen.[29,30] These studies include physiologic measurements of eye movements, EEGs, oronasal airflow, pulse oximetry, ECG activity, chin and leg muscle activity, and snoring. Other physiologic measurements may also be included depending on the diagnoses under consideration. Such measurements could include esophageal pH monitoring for gastroesophageal reflux, esophageal pressure monitoring for upper airway resistance, or extended EEG montages for seizures. Recently, a wide array of multichannel recording devices has been developed for use in sites outside of the sleep laboratory. Because of the technical limitations of portable monitoring, these devices should be used sparingly and only by experienced technologists under the supervision of experienced, trained physicians. The use of these devices has been reviewed and clinical recommendations on their use have been published elsewhere.[31]

CRITICAL CONTENT

INDICATIONS FOR POLYSOMNOGRAPHY

Sleep-related breathing disorders
    Obstructive sleep apnea
    Central sleep apnea syndrome
    Obesity-hypoventilation syndrome
    Upper airway resistance syndrome
Neurologic and movement disorders
    Periodic limb movement disorder
    Seizure disorders
    Parasomnias (ie, sleepwalking, nocturnal movements)
    Narcolepsy or hypersomnolence
    REM-behavior disorder
Therapeutic indications
    CPAP titration
    Assess adequacy of sleep-related interventions
    Respiratory insufficiency [ie, amyotropic lateral sclerosis (ALS)] and the titration of noninvasive ventilatory support

CRITICAL CONTENT

POLYSOMNOGRAPHIC FINDINGS IN OSA

- Obstructive respiratory events
- Apneas and hypopneas >10 seconds long
- AHI >5 per hour
- Have one or more associated features:
  Sleep latency on MSLT <10 minutes (see below)
  - Frequent arousals
  - Arterial oxygen desaturations
  - Bradycardia or tachycardia
  - Other cardiac arrhythmias
  - Seizures

An AHI of 5 or more in association with arousals, brady- or tachycardias, arterial oxygen desaturations, or daytime sleepiness in addition to other symptoms of sleep apnea is diagnostic for OSA. Respiratory events are frequently worse during REM sleep or in the supine position. These conditions lead to a lengthening of the respiratory events and an accentuation of the arterial desaturations. Respiratory events are typically terminated by a snort and an arousal. During the event there may be a marked slowing of the heart rate followed by a brief tachycardia that occurs with the arousal. Desaturations that occur during respiratory events may be profound, with saturations reaching levels of less than 50%. Snoring is commonly noted even when there are no discernable respiratory events.

Assessment of sleepiness and diagnostic testing for narcolepsy constitute another major aspect of polysomnography. Sleepiness assessments may be categorized into assessments of physiologic sleepiness, manifest sleepiness, and perceived sleepiness. Physiologic sleepiness is the underlying tendency to sleep devoid of environmental stimuli. Manifest sleepiness is the tendency to fall asleep when trying not to or under conditions in which environmental stimuli are present. The impact of environmental stimuli and the individual's ability to enhance their alertness modify the underlying physiologic sleepiness, resulting in the manifest sleepiness. The most widely used test of sleepiness is the multiple sleep latency test (MSLT). The principal use for the MSLT has been to assess physiologic sleepiness and to diagnose narcolepsy.[5] The MSLT is performed using methods similar to the overnight polysomnogram; however, four to five naps are typically used instead of a full night's sleep.[4] The performance of the MSLT adheres to a relatively rigid protocol to assure the validity of the results. The naps are no longer than 20 minutes each and are principally assessed for the time until sleep onset and the occurrence of any sleep-onset REM periods. In preparation for an MSLT, some patients may be instructed to discontinue medications or alter their sleep period for several weeks. Also, an overnight polysomnogram is performed prior to the MSLT to rule out other disorders and to verify the amount of sleep immediately preceding the MSLT. Care must be taken to perform the testing at times synchronized with the patient's typical sleep periods to avoid erroneous diagnoses, unless there is a diagnostic or therapeutic reason to alter the sleep period. The performance standards and indications for MSLT testing have been reviewed elsewhere.[4,5]

CRITICAL CONTENT

COMMON DISORDERS OF EXCESSIVE DAYTIME SLEEPINESS

- Obstructive sleep apnea
- Narcolepsy
- Insufficient sleep syndrome
- Periodic limb movement disorder (PLMD)
- Restless legs syndrome
- Shift work sleep disorder
- Irregular sleep-wake pattern
- Time zone change syndrome ("jet lag")
- Central sleep apnea syndrome
- Hypnotic-dependent sleep disorder

TREATMENT AND MANAGEMENT

Once the diagnosis of OSA has been confirmed, an appropriate treatment regimen needs to be developed.[32-34] Therapy should first be directed at the primary disorder, and then consideration should be given to any secondary or confounding disorders. This step requires careful review of polysomnographic findings in light of the history and physical examination. Unusual or atypical components of the patients history, physical examination, or polysomnographic findings need to be noted and addressed as part of the treatment regimen. Simply treating obstructive sleep apnea without consideration of associated illnesses, behaviors, or circadian disturbances usually results in an inadequate treatment regimen and often leads to incomplete resolution of symptoms and nonadherence by the patient.

The most common treatment for OSA is positive airway pressure. This type of treatment applies air pressure to the upper airway either through the nose (nasal CPAP) or through the nose and mouth using a full face mask. The air pressure in the upper airway displaces the airway walls outward, providing a pneumatic splint to the areas of obstruction. This effect is diagrammed in Fig. 15-4. If effectively applied, this treatment will typically relieve the obstruction experienced by patients with OSA. There are two major methods for delivering positive airway pressure that are routinely used to treat OSA: continuous positive airway pressure (CPAP) and bilevel positive airway pressure (BiPAP). In both of these delivery patterns the pressure delivered to the patient during exhalation must be sufficient to maintain airway patency and not allow collapse of the oropharynx. These two forms differ in one significant respect: BiPAP increases pressure during inspiration when the tendency to collapse the airway is the greatest and CPAP does not.

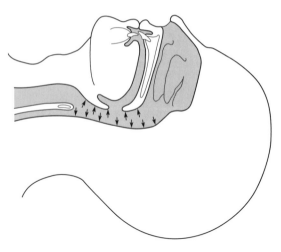

FIGURE 15-4 Effects of continuous positive airway pressure. Noninvasive positive airway pressure, either continuous or bilevel, acts as a pneumatic splint in the upper airway to maintain patency.

CRITICAL CONTENT

INDICATIONS FOR BiPAP

- Patient is intolerant to CPAP
- To reduce air leaks
- To improve tolerance
- To decrease mean airway pressure
- Patient's need for ventilatory assistance

In more recent years variations on CPAP have been attempted to improve tolerance, increase adherence, and adjust to day-to-day variations in the severity of OSA. Another goal has been to provide for improved monitoring of the use of CPAP. Initially, monitoring was performed using hour meters, which simply documented the number of hours the CPAP machine was turned on. More sophisticated devices have been developed using computerized algorithms to determine if the patient is actually using the machine. These algorithms are used in an attempt to eliminate times when the patient has the CPAP machine turned on but not in use, or times when the patient has inadvertently taken the CPAP mask off in the middle of the night. Recently, machines have been developed that can automatically vary the applied pressure, have the ability to report the time of use on a day-to-day basis, and can report alterations in pressure settings. These reports may be printed out and become part of the patient's chart. Such reporting can also be preserved in electronic format. The collection and distribution of such information is usually performed by a respiratory therapist or sleep technologist. Such information is quite useful during follow-up clinic visits when determining the patient's response to treatment.

In general, CPAP is a less expensive modality than BiPAP, although somewhat more sophisticated forms of CPAP may be more costly. BiPAP is more expensive because of an additional sensing mechanism and other mechanical modifications necessary to enable the bilevel delivery process.

The devices that sense partial airway obstruction and automatically increase CPAP pressure, so-called autotitrating CPAP, are more expensive than traditional CPAP because of the sensing mechanisms and computer algorithms necessary to achieve the automatic titration. Overall, each of these devices has an appropriate use and no one device is the universal solution for all situations.

CRITICAL CONTENT

CPAP OPTIONS

- Multiple pressure ramping options
- Built-in heated humidifiers
- Computerized compliance monitoring
- Follow-up assessments on-line
- Autotitration mechanisms

The choice of masks used for applying CPAP or BiPAP is important in the appropriate care of the patient with OSA. The masks are of three major formats: the nasal mask, the full face mask, and nasal prongs or pillows. Each of these formats has its advantages and disadvantages. The nasal mask is the most commonly used format and also has the advantage of being the most versatile. The nasal mask is able to tolerate most pressure settings and usually has the lowest air leaks of any format. However, it suffers from a somewhat higher incidence of pressure sores, typically over the bridge of the nose, and claustrophobia. These masks come in a wide variety of sizes and shapes; some may even be formed to fit the nose. The full face mask is often advantageous for individuals with a mustache or hard-to-fit nose. The major disadvantage of the full face mask is an increase in air leaks. Nasal prongs or pillows are often associated with less physical discomfort and are often preferred for patients with claustrophobia. The major limitation of nasal prongs is that the recommended pressure settings are generally less than 9 to 11 cm of pressure.

CRITICAL CONTENT

CPAP APPLICATION OPTIONS

- Nasal mask
- Gel-type interface
- Nasal prongs or pillows
- Modified nasal masks
- Full face masks

APPLICATION CONSIDERATIONS

- Adequacy of fit
- Patient comfort and tolerance
- Sensation of claustrophobia
- Air leaks
- CPAP pressures required

In order to adequately treat an individual with OSA, proper pressure settings must be determined. Most centers will attempt to determine an adequate pressure setting using a titration trial. Titration studies are frequently performed on a night following the diagnostic study for OSA. Some centers perform the diagnostic phase and the titration phase during the same study when they have appropriate patients. This type of study is referred to as a split-night study. Usually this requires that a patient have a minimum of 30 respiratory events within the first 2 to 3 hours of the study, although the specific protocol varies from center to center. Whatever protocol is employed, sufficient time must remain to perform the titration phase of the study. Some third-party (insurance) carriers require a total of 30 apneas before a titration study may be performed. Such criteria need to be considered in the development of policies and before performing a split-night study.

The goals of a titration study are to eliminate respiratory events, optimize oxygen saturations, and decrease arousals. Some centers will also try to eliminate snoring as part of the titration protocol. This may be appropriate since snoring may represent some residual upper airway resistance or partial closure. Other factors that need to be addressed as part of the titration protocol are summarized in Table 15-4.

Under some circumstances the positive airway pressure may cause an air leak around the mask or out of the mouth. These air leaks decrease the pressure to the area of obstruction and allow apneas to recur. However, in some instances adjusting the nasal mask to be free of leaks often requires considerable pressure on the nose or face. Consequently, we often attempt to find a balance between patient comfort and minimization of leaks. If air leaks are excessive, increased nasal dryness, sinus problems, and intolerance will typically result. There is no clearly defined acceptable air leak level; however, it is generally assumed that air leaks less than 10 L/min do not present a substantial problem.

Tracheostomy has been shown to be an effective therapeutic intervention for OSA. Studies performed following the introduction of nasal CPAP demonstrated an improvement in mortality[35] with both CPAP and tracheostomy. Today, a tracheostomy may be an appropriate intervention for individuals who cannot be well controlled with CPAP or BiPAP, or those who do not tolerate any positive airway pressure interventions. Surgical interventions such as uvulopalatopharyngoplasty (UPPP), hyoid advancement, and mandibular advancement are potential alternatives.[33] The reduction in respiratory events associated with these interventions, either alone or in combination, is significantly less than that associated with CPAP, but most series show that 40% to 50% of patients have cut the number of respiratory events in half. At present there is no reliable test to determine which patients will benefit from UPPP or other surgical interventions. There is also a tendency for individuals treated with surgery to relapse 3 to 5 years postsurgery. In contrast, maxillofacial surgery is effective and should be considered for those individuals with craniofacial abnormalities leading to airway obstruction. Laser-assisted uvulopalatoplasty (LAUP) has been applied in the treatment of OSA.[34] The literature shows it to be an ineffective modality for the treatment of OSA; however, it may be an effective modality for the treatment of snoring.

Oropharyngeal appliances are another modality that has shown some utility in the treatment of OSA.[32] Generally these appliances are best used with individuals who have mild OSA, or in situations in which patients do not have access to their CPAP for short periods. The choice of these alternative therapies requires knowledge of the patient's condition, the severity of their sleep apnea, the tolerance to previously attempted therapeutic interventions, and the patient's preference. No one modality works for all patients and the failure of a modality, such as CPAP, should not preclude its consideration again at some time in the future.

TABLE 15-4 **CONSIDERATIONS AND GOALS OF CONTINUOUS POSITIVE AIRWAY PRESSURE TITRATION**

Goals of CPAP titration	Eliminate or minimize apneas and hypopneas
	Improve oxygenation
	Elimination or reduction of snoring
	Reduction of arousals
	Optimize respiratory pattern
Considerations before or during the titration	Minimize air leaks
	Assess positional influence on the interventions
	Assess adequacy of settings during REM and when supine
	Address patient concerns and claustrophobia
	Perform patient education

CRITICAL CONTENT

EFFECTIVE THERAPEUTIC OPTIONS FOR OSA

- Continuous positive airway pressure
- Bilevel positive airway pressure
- Tracheostomy
- Orofacial surgery
- Oropharyngeal appliances

Ancillary measures are also needed when developing a treatment regimen. Weight loss, while rarely a cure for OSA, frequently reduces the severity of the disease and may reduce the CPAP pressure needed for effective control of respiratory disturbances. Some patients have clear worsening of their respiratory events when in the supine position. In these instances training the patient not to sleep supine, rather than increasing CPAP pressure, may be an effective adjunct, but rarely provides effective long-term treatment alone.

Supplemental oxygen may be necessary to control desaturations in some patients. However, supplemental oxygen must be used with caution in patients with CO_2 retention. These individuals may be prone to respiratory suppression due to a decline in hypoxic drive. However, less than 15% of patients who chronically retain CO_2 will be adversely affected by the administration of supplemental oxygen. Of those who do experience a significant rise in CO_2, most will improve with continued use, often through the improvement of the underlying disease and the attenuation of sleep deprivation.

AGE-SPECIFIC CONSIDERATIONS

The diagnosis and treatment of OSA in young children and geriatric patients may require adjustments in the technical aspects of polysomnography and the therapeutic interventions employed. In young children, the criteria for scoring respiratory events may require monitoring of end-tidal CO_2 and the RDI criterion is significantly lower than that of adults (eg, >1 per hour of sleep). Also, in children, surgical interventions may be more commonly employed and more effective than in the adult patient. However, children may also be treated effectively with CPAP. In contrast, geriatric patients are known to have more RDIs with fewer symptoms than their younger counterparts. This has caused debate as to proper age-adjusted criteria for the RDI or AHI.[36,37] Currently this clinical judgment is best made by an experienced sleep physician.

PATIENT EDUCATION, HEALTH PROMOTION, QUALITY OF LIFE, AND PUBLIC POLICY

The vast majority of the lay public and most health care professionals have little knowledge of, or training in, sleep medicine. For instance, most medical schools dedicate less than 4 hours to sleep medicine despite the prevalence of these disorders. For the lay public, most of their information on these disorders comes from the news media and the Internet rather than from peer-reviewed or scientific resources. In this regard patient education is badly needed. Once a diagnosis of OSA is made, patient education is necessary to avoid complications and optimize adherence to treatment recommendations. For the therapist interacting with the OSA patient, education needs to address OSA as a disease, treatment of OSA, and its potential complications (Table 15-5).

Patients with untreated OSA have a significantly increased risk of accidents.[38–41] This may include workplace accidents, incidents in the home, and accidents while driving. The laws regarding reporting of OSA vary from state to state and may be dependent upon the occupation of the afflicted patient. In some circumstances this may require reporting of the diagnosis to an appropriate administrative body such as the Federal Aviation Administration (FAA). Once under adequate treat-

T A B L E   1 5 - 5   PATIENT EDUCATION

	COMMENTS	EXAMPLES
OSA	Explain the details of the disease briefly and with regard to the patient's learning ability.	• Symptoms of OSA • Disorders associated with OSA • Complications of OSA
Treatment options	Discuss options cautiously and don't oversell the options. Avoid making specific recommendations with regard to one type of treatment or another. This may interfere with the physician's plan.	• CPAP • Oropharyngeal devices • Surgery (UPPP, LAUP, maxillofacial surgery, etc.) • Weight loss • Positional retraining
Humidity options	Humidification mechanisms need to be drained daily. Heated humidification may help those with frequent complications of CPAP.	• Cleaning issues • Alternate options for complicated cases • Cleaning agents • Need may be seasonal
Goals of CPAP titration	Explain the anticipated benefits of the intervention and a reasonable timeline in which to expect them. The most common reason for failure of therapy is nonadherence.	• Eliminate apneas and hypopneas • Improve oxygenation • Elimination of snoring • Reduction of arousals
Complications of CPAP	Complications can often be avoided or treated. Describe the common problems. Regular and frequent care and use are the basic measures for avoiding the complications.	• Nasal dryness or sinus problems • Skin irritation from mask • Air leaks • Exacerbation of asthma (rare)
Care and cleaning of CPAP	Instruct patients to rinse the equipment daily and to clean at least weekly. Discuss proper care.	• Type of cleaning agent to use • Frequency of cleaning • Frequency of equipment inspection/replacement
Follow-up	Detail outline of the care plan and the duration of home care in the plan.	• Home care involvement • Physician involvement • Ancillary issues
Health care giver roles	Explain the role of each health care giver in the delivery of the patient's care. Then explain who should or will handle problems or questions that arise. Most important message is to contact SOMEONE. If it is not the person most able to address the issue, they can direct patient to the appropriate person.	• Equipment problems • Travel needs • Billing issues • Complications • Changes in equipment • Return of symptoms

CPAP, continuous positive airway pressure; OSA, obstructive sleep apnea; LAUP, laser-assisted uvulopalatoplasty; UPPP, uvulopalatopharyngoplasty.

ment most professional drivers and pilots with OSA will require yearly assessments in order to maintain their active status. Each patient should be cautioned about these potential risks and follow-up should be tailored accordingly.

Of significant importance in improving quality of life and achieving an optimal outcome is the development of a comprehensive therapeutic regimen, adequate patient education, and compliance with the medical regimen. Regular follow-up is an important component in achieving adherence to any medical regimen and in addressing side effects. The most common side effects seen with nasal CPAP include nasal dryness, pressure sores, claustrophobia, nasal congestion, sinusitis, and skin allergies. Many aspects of discomfort can be corrected with the use of the newer heated humidification units. The therapeutic regimen should also address concerns of bed partners, parents, and other concerned individuals. Also, addressing issues that may complicate adherence, such as limitations to travel or occupational problems, may be very important to the patient.

Health Consequences and Public Policy

Important issues with regard to public policy and OSA include the development of cardiovascular disease and the prevention of accidents.[38,39] Recent data suggest that OSA is not only a cause of hypertension, it is also an independent risk factor for the development of cardiovascular disease. The relative risk for the development cardiovascular disease is approximately 1.2 to 1.5 and is likely to increase with advancing age.

To date, little is known about the effects of treating OSA on preventing the development or progression of cardiovascular disease. Despite this, it seems likely that effective interventions will have a significant impact. With regard to accidents, effective treatment for OSA has been clearly shown to reduce the risk of accidents. Despite the close association between driving accidents and sleep apnea, many individuals at risk for OSA are never evaluated. This may be in part due to the small amount of medical education time spent on studying sleep disorders. Recent efforts by the National Institutes of Health and several agencies including the American Academy of Sleep Medicine have begun to reverse this trend.

INTRODUCTION TO THE CASE STUDY

Now you proceed to the most exciting part of this chapter by working your way through a hypothetical case. Your instructor will direct you to identify learning issues, answer specific case questions, or prepare for individual and/or group exercises. Your assignment will depend on the available time, types of patients you are likely to encounter in your clinical rotations, and resources available. Please check with your instructor to find out how to proceed with this case. Please do not read the case ahead of time or without specific instructions. Problem-based learning (PBL) is a process, but a textbook is a product. Therefore your process for using this case will depend on the approach adopted by your school faculty. Please follow your instructor's instructions carefully so you will benefit the most from the learning experience. We hope your learning will transcend the content of this specific case!

The following questions and exercises are designed to help you expand your knowledge of sleep-related breathing disorders, and to prepare you for situations you are likely to encounter in your respiratory care practice. The overview of sleep-related breathing disorders at the beginning of this chapter gave you a start toward having the knowledge to work on the exercises, to identify learning issues, or to answer predetermined questions, as determined by the strategy employed by your instructor. However, to provide a thorough and up-to-date response to many of the questions and exercises, you will need to consult additional resource material. Of course, you are prepared for this—after all this is one goal of PBL! PBL helps you to learn by presenting you with problems that require you to go out and find the resources to solve them. There are many resources listed at the end of this chapter that can help you in this respect.

The following case is included here to allow you to apply your understanding of sleep-related breathing disorders. The case may be used to help you identify learning issues that will help develop your understanding of the diagnosis, treatment, and long-term management of SRBDs, or your instructor may assign you predetermined learning issues. The case challenges you to evaluate age-specific considerations, patient education needs, health care costs, and ethical concerns of management of SRBDs. Whenever possible, the case will prompt you for more than one recommendation for patient care, to allow comparisons of the advantages, disadvantages, and limitations of various approaches to patient care. Furthermore, some of the exercises in this case are designed for small and large group discussion to facilitate development of critical thinking skills and traits.

CASE 1

OLIVIA SALLY ANN SLEEPER

Initial Case Scenario

A 31-year-old Caucasian female with a 2-year history of excessive daytime sleepiness is referred for evaluation. This patient stands 5 feet 6 inches tall and weighs 120 pounds, and reports a history of mild snoring, restless sleep, and morning headaches. During the past 2 years she has been experiencing increasingly excessive daytime sleepiness, which has become significantly worse over the past 6 months. The major reason for seeking medical assistance is that the fatigue and sleepiness has begun to impact on her activities of daily living.

 Group Critical Thinking Exercise 1

PRIORITIZING AND ORGANIZING THE APPROACH TO THE PATIENT WITH SLEEP COMPLAINTS

Issues to address include whether this patient has insomnia or excessive daytime sleepiness (EDS) or has other issues that may direct the therapeutic approach. Note: Due to the complexity of the following issues, it is recommended that the following exercise be done collaboratively, with two or three students being assigned each of the following, and then the complete group coming together to discuss and decide on the best answers. Alternatively, the following may be assigned to each individual student. If individuals develop their own responses, it is recommended that a class discussion involving the entire class be held, in which student answers can be compared. See your instructor for specific instructions.

a. What are the major components of the sleep history that should be addressed with this patient?

b. Discuss the major categories of sleep complaints and how they affect the approach to the patient with a sleep complaint.

c. What major disorders should be considered in a patient with complaints of excessive sleepiness?

d. What components of the physical examination are important in the evaluation of patients with sleep complaints? Explain why each is important and how it might affect the evaluation process or interventions chosen.

C A S E   1   *(continued)*

Description of Sleep. She typically works until 11:30 PM and then goes home. She usually is in bed by 1 or 2 in the morning and arises between 9 and 10 in the morning. On weekends or days off the patient will go to bed at approximately the same time but may sleep until 1:00 in the afternoon. She frequently takes naps in the afternoon and recently has had difficulty remaining awake under conditions of low levels of activity. Her sleep is somewhat restless and she admits to awakening two to three times each night. When she does awaken she looks at the clock and goes to the bathroom. Upon returning to bed the patient is able to return to sleep quite quickly. The patient's husband confirms that she is a restless sleeper. He has witnessed the patient snoring and gasping for breath, and reports that her breathing will occasionally stop for 20 to 30 seconds. There's no history of sleepwalking, sleeptalking, or other parasomnias. The husband is concerned that some of her restlessness may be due to acting out her dreams. He specifically mentions having seen this discussed in a news program on REM behavior disorder and was concerned that his wife had this disorder.

The patient denies any symptoms consistent with periodic limb movement disorder or restless legs syndrome. The patient denies any history of difficulty falling asleep, anxiety concerning sleep, or any difficulty returning to sleep. When she does awaken at night, she always notes what time it is. When the patient awakens she does not eat or partake of any activities. There's no history of nocturnal smoking, eating in bed, reading in bed, watching TV late at night or in bed, or using the computer late at night.

Social History. The patient is married with one child who is 2 years of age. She drinks only socially and has never smoked. The patient denies any use of illicit drugs. She works as an air traffic controller at the nearby airport. She started working as an air traffic controller 5 years prior to her presentation. During the first 2 to 3 years on the job the patient reports that she had no significant difficulty in performing her duties; however, over the past 2 years she has been experiencing increasing difficulty with her job. Most recently she noted difficulties in maintaining concentration and responding quickly to situational changes. This has led to several administrative actions taken against her at work. Over the past 2 years she reports gaining 5 pounds.

Past Medical History. The patient has had the usual childhood diseases. There is no history of encephalitis, meningitis, fainting, or seizures. HEENT: patient has a history of rhinitis and some mild seasonal allergies. There is no history of dysphagia, dysphonia, or other ENT disorders. Respiratory: patient denies any history of asthma, bronchitis, or respiratory disease. Cardiac: patient has a history of hypertension for the past 2 years. No other cardiovascular disease was noted. GI: there is no history of nausea, vomiting, diarrhea, constipation, jaundice, melena, pain, or other GI disorders. GU: patient is para 1 gravida 1. There's no history of renal disease or recurrent urinary tract pathology. Neuromuscular: there is no history of motor, cerebral, cerebellar, or sensory dysfunction. There is no history of developmental abnormalities, seizures, or other neurologic problems that would account for the findings reported by the husband. Except for the chief complaint listed above, there are no other significant medical disorders reported by the patient or her husband. Allergies: patient has no known drug allergies. Medications: enalapril. Past surgical history: tonsillectomy and adenoidectomy.

CASE 1   *(continued)*

Critical Thinking Exercise 1

**ANTICIPATING PROBLEMS:
HISTORICAL ISSUES TO ADDRESS**

Once we have decided that the patient has EDS, we need to address the complicating issues and circadian problems.

a. What is the major category of sleep complaint in this patient? How does this affect the differential diagnosis?

b. What components of the history support a diagnosis of OSA?

c. What components of the history suggest diagnoses other than OSA?

d. Identify the major complicating issues associated with this patient and how they would affect our approach to the patient. Specifically address safety, behavioral, and follow-up issues.

Physical Examination. At the time of examination the patient was alert and oriented to time, place, and person. She was in no apparent distress but appeared sleepy. She answered questions easily and had no apparent difficulty with thought processes. Vital signs: blood pressure 130/90, respiratory rate 16, heart rate 78, weight 55 kg. Patient was normocephalic. Pupils were equally round and reactive to light and accommodation. The nose was intact and the nares were patent. The nasal mucosa was mildly hyperemic and there was a mild serous discharge. Sinuses were not tender. Ear canals were patent. The tympanic membranes showed evidence of mild otosclerosis. The oropharynx was mildly narrowed in both the anterior-posterior and lateral dimensions. No tonsillar hypertrophy was noted. No masses were noted. The gingiva and dentition were intact without gross abnormalities. There is no evidence of micrognathia or structural deformities of the jaw. The neck was intact and measured 13 inches around. The thorax was symmetrical and without gross abnormalities. The lungs were clear to auscultation. The heart rate and rhythm were regular. No murmurs, S_3, or S_4 were noted. The abdomen was flat, soft, nontender and without masses or other abnormalities. Bowel sounds were present in all four quadrants. The patient's extremities were intact and without edema, cyanosis, or clubbing. Distal pulses were 2¾ in all extremities. Neurologically there was no significant motor, cerebral, cerebellar, or sensory dysfunction noted. The patient's mentation was unremarkable. The patient's short- and long-term memory were intact.

Critical Thinking Exercise 2

**ANTICIPATING FINDINGS
FROM THE PHYSICAL EXAM**

The physical examination will aid in determining therapeutic options and in ruling out complicating illnesses.

a. What physical examination findings are important in the assessment of the patient with EDS and SRBD? How might these findings alter our approach to the patient before and during polysomnography?

b. What physical findings are typical of an OSA patient? How do these differ from those present in this patient?

c. What findings would suggest disorders that might be complicating the patient's condition? Have any complicating illnesses been adequately addressed?

CASE 1 *(continued)*

 Critical Thinking Exercise 3

ANTICIPATING CONFOUNDING OR COEXISTENT ISSUES

Commonly patients with sleep disorders will have problems stemming from habits, personal behaviors, and occupational issues. These need to be addressed during the evaluation and sometimes may best be addressed prior to further diagnostic work-up.

a. Describe how the patient's sleep pattern may be influencing her complaints.

b. Is the sleeping environment optimal? Describe the major components of good sleep hygiene. Is the patient adhering to them?

c. Discuss the potential for psychiatric or psychological issues and how these might influence the approach to the patient. Is there a potential for drug-related issues? If so, how would you approach them?

 Critical Thinking Exercise 4

CLINICAL ASSESSMENT AND DECISION MAKING

a. What study or studies should be ordered for this patient? Why?

b. What disorders should be treated in this patient before further diagnostic studies are performed? Why?

 Group Critical Thinking Exercise 2

ANTICIPATING PROBLEMS AND SOLUTIONS

Preparing for the sleep study in addition to preparing the patient are important in avoiding problems. As in Group Exercise 1, this exercise may be done collaboratively, or it may be assigned to the individual students.

a. What information, that may affect the preparation of a patient for a sleep study, should be specifically sought when evaluating a patient with a sleep disorder?

b. What disorders or behavioral issues might benefit from treatment before the sleep study? Describe your approach and your rationale.

c. What issues relevant to this patient should be considered that might affect the type of study performed or the manner in which it is performed? How might they alter our approach to this patient?

d. What pre-study preparations or instructions from the technologist should be performed prior to the study?

The physician decides to order the patient to have a sleep study (polysomnography) performed. In addition, it is decided that this be followed by the MSLT. A summary of the results of the polysomnography study is shown in Table 15-6.

CASE 1   *(continued)*

TABLE 15-6   POLYSOMNOGRAPHY SUMMARY REPORT: OLIVIA SALLY ANN SLEEPER

SLEEP STAGING SUMMARY			
Recording start time:	01:30:00	Recording end time:	10:30:30
Total recording time: (min)	540.5	Epoch size	30 seconds
Total sleep time:	519	Wake time after sleep onset (min):	19.5
Sleep efficiency:	96%	Number of awakenings/arousals:	22/173
Sleep onset latency (min):	1.5	Stage REM latency (min):	65
(Lights out to first epoch of 3 consecutive sleep epochs, stage 1, 2, 3, 4, or one epoch of REM)		(Sleep onset to first REM epoch)	

STAGING TABLE		
Sleep stage	Duration (min)	% Sleep time
Wake	21	
Stage REM	77.9	15
Stage 1	51.9	10
Stage 2	290.6	56
Stage 3–4 Slow wave sleep	98.6	19

RESPIRATORY EVENT SUMMARY					
	NREM	REM	Total	With Arousal	With Desat
Obstructive apnea	1	19	20	16	4
Mixed apnea	1	5	6	4	0
Central apnea	3	0	3	0	0
Hypopnea	9	12	21	20	0
RERA	40	0	40	40	0
Apnea index (AI)	0.7	18.5	3.4	2.2	.5
Hypopnea index (HI)	1.2	9.2	2.4	2.2	0
AHI (AI + HI)	1.9	27.7	6.8	4.4	0
RDI (AI + HI + RERAs)	7.3	27.7	10.4	8.4	0
SpO_2		Lowest	89%	Average	97%

LIMB MOVEMENTS			
	NREM	REM	TOTAL
Limb movements	16	0	16
Limb movements with arousal	2	0	2
Limb movements associated with respiratory events	1	11	12
Periodic limb movements (PLM)	0	0	0

Standard polysomnography was performed recording: central and occipital EEG, submental EMG, right and left outer canthus EOG, lead II ECG, right and left anterior tibialis EMG, SpO_2, respiratory airflow by thermocouple, and respiratory effort by piezoelectric belts and intercostal EMG. The study was performed in the sleep center attended by a registered sleep technologist with continuous video and audio monitoring.

Technologist's notes: Cyclic arousals noted. Many arousals were associated with crescendo snoring, some with paradoxing and crescendoing effort, but most without scorable, identifiable respiratory events or limb movements. These events were usually longer than 10 seconds in duration.

AHI, apnea-hypopnea index; desat, desaturation; EMG, electromyogram; EOG, electro-oculogram; NREM, non-REM sleep; RDI, respiratory disturbance index; REM, rapid eye movement sleep; RERA, respiratory-event related arousals.

TABLE 15-7 MEAN SLEEP LATENCY TEST (MSLT) RESULTS: OLIVIA SALLY ANN SLEEPER

	TIME	SLEEP LATENCY (MIN)	REM LATENCY
Nap 1	12:00	.5	12
Nap 2	14:01	3	No REM
Nap 3	16:17	7	No REM
Nap 4	17:59	1.5	No REM
Nap 5	20:02	4.5	No REM
Mean sleep latency		3.3	

Critical Thinking Exercise 5

PROBLEM SOLVING AND INTERPRETATION OF DATA

a. What were the pertinent negative findings of the PSG?

b. What were the pertinent positive findings of the PSG?

c. Do the majority of central apneas described in this report reflect the presence of an abnormality? If so what? How do you reach this conclusion?

d. Why might the patient's apneas and hypopneas be more frequent in REM sleep or in the supine position?

e. How do we explain the arousals and the husband's reports of nocturnal activity? Does she have REM behavior disorder?

f. What components of the history and physical exam information suggest disorders other than OSA? How might this alter the preparation of the patient for the study and the reporting during the study? Remember, in some circumstances accurate reporting of pertinent negatives or the presence of unusual occurrences may be extremely important to the clinician. Which are important here? How might these comments affect the interpretation and recommendations for additional treatment?

Following the sleep study, the patient is scheduled for and has an MSLT performed. The results of this study are shown in Table 15-7.

Critical Thinking Exercise 6

PROBLEM SOLVING AND INTERPRETATION OF DATA

a. What do the results of the MSLT suggest?

b. How might the SOREM that occurred during the MSLT be explained? Give several different interpretations that are plausible for this patient.

c. How do we interpret the sleep latency findings of the MSLT?

d. Has narcolepsy been ruled out? Is it a likely diagnosis?

CASE 1 *(continued)*

 Group Critical Thinking Exercise 3

PROS & CONS OF TREATMENT OPTIONS FOR OSA

Have a group that is assigned by the instructor research the various treatment options for OSA. The group should present the various options to the full class, when the pros and cons of each option should be thoroughly discussed. Is the appropriate option for Ms. Sleeper obvious? Have the class discuss and debate which of the various treatment options would be most appropriate for Ms. Sleeper. Give reasons why a particular option is being advocated for this patient. Was the class able to agree on what is most likely to be the most effective treatment?

 Group Critical Thinking Exercise 4

ETHICS AND PUBLIC SAFETY ISSUES

Discuss the implications of a public policy that would not allow persons with sleep disorders to drive or work in hazardous occupations until they have been adequately treated. Address the economic impact on the person, the potential for causing accidents in the workplace, and how "adequately treated" should be defined. This could be done by the whole class, or the class can be divided into two groups to debate the merits of such a policy. One group could support such a policy and the other could oppose it.

 Critical Thinking Exercise 7

DECISION MAKING AND DEVELOPING A CARE PLAN

a. Develop a plan to treat each of the major disorders in this patient. What interventions should be used to treat the patient? How do we assess adherence to our treatment regimen? How should effectiveness be monitored?

b. Should medications be used to treat the patient's sleepiness? Why or why not? How would you assess the response to any intervention directed at improving the patient's sleepiness?

c. What additional action needs to be taken to address the SOREM noted during the sleep study?

d. What options should be considered for addressing the patient's sleep hygiene and environmental issues?

e. What recommendations and follow-up should be undertaken pertinent to driving and working? Explain your rationale and any potential problems.

 Critical Thinking Exercise 8

PROBLEM SOLVING AND NEGOTIATION

Discuss the options for dealing with employer concerns regarding immediate actions to be taken and the future performance of this employee. Should the person be off work? For how long? How would the ability to return to work be assessed? What are the requirements for reporting and following such a patient, and how should this be addressed by the health care professionals involved in her treatment?

CASE 1 *(continued)*

Group Critical Thinking Exercise 5

PROBLEM SOLVING, COSTS, AND ETHICAL ISSUES

The following exercise is recommended to be performed as described in the instructions for Group Exercise 1, in small teams followed by a large group discussion.

a. Since OSA potentially affects 5% to 10% of the adult population, who is going to pay for the diagnosis and treatment of these individuals?

b. Is there a long-term benefit that outweighs the cost?

c. Because performing a polysomnogram is expensive and sleep disorders often overlap, should clinicians performing sleep studies be trained in all aspects of sleep disorders medicine? Is it cost effective and appropriate to perform a sleep study for OSA only? What kind of follow-up should be performed and to whom should it be reported?

d. In matters involving public safety, such as in the transportation industry, what are the considerations and concerns that should be addressed by the employer, the patient, and/or the health care providers? Do these vary by location? If so, how? Where might you find additional information?

Ms. Sleeper was scheduled for and completed a polysomnogram with CPAP titration. She began treatment with CPAP at 7 cm H_2O and reported a significant decrease in her sleepiness. Once she was established on, and compliant with, noninvasive CPAP therapy, she returned to the sleep center to assess improvement in her sleepiness and document her readiness to return to work. Her sleep architecture was very good with arousals and respiratory events well within the normal range. Her normal sleep architecture indicated that she indeed was compliant with her therapy and her MSLT indicated her pathologic sleepiness had improved with a 16.9 minute mean sleep latency. The sleep specialist documented the study results on the required FAA and Department of Transportation forms and released her to return to work as an air traffic controller.

One year later she continues to be compliant with her therapy, attends AWAKE group meetings, has implemented a fairly strict sleep hygiene routine, and appears to be maintaining her alertness quite well. She has no complaints of sleepiness and has received a promotion at work. She is currently exploring the options of noninvasive continuous positive airway pressure (NCPAP) with a maxillofacial surgeon due to her slightly short, narrow maxilla.

KEY POINTS

• Sleep-related breathing disorders are common in the general population. The typical patient is male, obese, and reports excessive sleepiness. However, many patients are not obese and the disease is also common in women.

• Patients with sleep apnea frequently present with excessive daytime sleepiness, snoring, and witnessed apneas that have been present from 6 months to several years. This may be associated with weight gain and decreased functional status.

• Attention should be given to the patient's sleep history, including the pattern of sleep and sleep hygiene issues when evaluating any patient with sleep complaints. These may be significant contributors to their underlying disease.

- Patients should be questioned about their occupation and activities of daily living as a part of the critical pathway for the evaluation. The recommendations and the implications may be affected significantly.

- Sleep-related breathing disorders contribute to the development of hypertension and other cardiovascular diseases. Therefore, patients with cardiovascular disease are at higher risk of having sleep apnea and may be prime candidates to benefit from treatment.

- Diagnostic polysomnography is usually done in the sleep laboratory; however, portable testing may be indicated in select populations.

- Although CPAP is an effective modality for the treatment of sleep disorders it may not be effective in all patients. Other recognized modalities either used alone or in concert with PAP include tracheostomy, orofacial surgery, and oral appliances.

- Sleep apnea is frequently associated with other behaviors and conditions. Therefore, all therapeutic regimens should be comprehensive and address comorbid illnesses.

RESOURCES FOR PRACTICE PARAMETERS AND STANDARDS OF PRACTICE RELATED TO POLYSOMNOGRAPHY

American Sleep Disorders Association. Practice parameters for the use of actigraphy in the clinical assessment of sleep disorders. *Sleep*. 1995;18:285–287.

American Sleep Disorders Association. Practice parameters for the treatment of snoring and obstructive sleep apnea with oral appliances. *Sleep*. 1995;18:511–513.

American Sleep Disorders Association. The ASDA Atlas Task Force: EEG arousals: scoring rules and examples. *Sleep*. 1992;15:174–184.

American Sleep Disorders Association. The ASDA Atlas Task Force: Recording and scoring leg movements. *Sleep*. 1993;16:749–759.

Chesson AL Jr, Littner M, Davila D, et al. Practice parameters for the use of light therapy in the treatment of sleep disorders. Standards of Practice Committee, American Academy of Sleep Medicine. *Sleep*. 1999; 22:641–660.

Chesson AL Jr, Wise M, Davila D, et al. Practice parameters for the treatment of restless legs syndrome and periodic limb movement disorder. An American Academy of Sleep Medicine Report. Standards of Practice Committee, American Academy of Sleep Medicine. *Sleep*. 1999;22:961–968.

Ferber R, Millman R, Coppola M, et al. Portable recording in the assessment of obstructive sleep apnea. ASDA standards of practice [see comments]. [Review.] [91 refs.] *Sleep*. 1994;17:378–392.

Mitler MM, Aldrich MS, Koob GF, et al. Narcolepsy and its treatment with stimulants. ASDA standards of practice. [Review.] [256 refs.] *Sleep*. 1994;17:352–371.

Polysomnography Task Force, American Sleep Disorders Association Standards of Practice Committee. Practice parameters for the indications for polysomnography and related procedures. *Sleep*. 1997;20:406–422.

Report of the American Sleep Disorders Association. Practice parameters for the treatment of obstructive sleep apnea in adults: the efficacy of surgical modifications of the upper airway. *Sleep*. 1996;19:152–155.

Standards of Practice Committee of the American Sleep Disorders Association. Practice parameters for the use of portable recording in the assessment of obstructive sleep apnea [see comments]. *Sleep*. 1994;17:372–377.

Standards of Practice Committee of the American Sleep Disorders Association. Practice parameters for the use of stimulants in the treatment of narcolepsy. *Sleep*. 1994; 17:348–351. [Published erratum appears in *Sleep*. 1994;17:748.]

Standards of Practice Committee of the American Sleep Disorders Association. Practice parameters for the use of laser-assisted uvulopalatoplasty. *Sleep*. 1994;17:744–748.

Standards of Practice Committee of the American Sleep Disorders Association. Practice parameters for the use of polysomnography in the evaluation of insomnia. *Sleep*. 1995;18:55–57.

Thorpy MJ. The clinical use of the multiple sleep latency test. The Standards of Practice Committee of the American Sleep Disorders Association. [Review.] [120 refs.] *Sleep*. 1992;15:268–276. [Published erratum appears in *Sleep*. 1992;15:381.]

RESOURCES FOR SLEEP PROFESSIONALS

Organizations

Association of Polysomnographic Technologists (APT)
8310 Nieman Road
Lenexa, KS 66214-1579
Phone: 913-541-1991
Website: www.aptweb.org

American Academy of Sleep Medicine (AASM)
6301 Bandel Rd, Suite 101
Rochester, MN 55901
Phone: 587-287-6606
Website: www.asda.org

National Sleep Foundation (NSF)
1522 K Street NW, Suite 500
Washington, DC 20005-1253
Phone: 202-347-3471
Email: nsf@sleepfoundation.org
Website: www.sleepfoundation.org

Credentialling

Board of Registered Polysomnographic Technologists (BRPT)
Professional Examination Services
111 8th Ave.
New York, NY 10011-5290
Phone: (212) 367-4360
Email: brpt@proexam.org

American Board of Sleep Medicine
6301 Bandel Road, Suite 101
Rochester, MN 55901
Phone: (507) 287-9819
E-mail: absm@absm.org

Websites

www.Sleepnet.com
Great information for all levels: personal, consumer, public, professional, and research. Links to just about anything related to alertness, sleep, and fatigue. Well maintained and updated.

www.bisleep.medsch.ucla.edu
Good information and links to professional and research information.

www.nhlbi.nih.gov/about/ncsdr/
Professional and research information including grant opportunities through the National Center for Sleep Disorders Research and other National Institutes of Health Centers.

ACKNOWLEDGMENT

This project was supported in part by the Clinical Investigator Development Award from the American Osteopathic Association.

REFERENCES

1. Rechtschaffen A, Kales A. *A Manual of Standardized Terminology, Techniques and Scoring System for Sleep Stages of Human Subjects.* 1st ed. Los Angeles: Brain Information Service/Brain Research Institute; University of California; 1968.

2. American Sleep Disorders Association. The ASDA Atlas Task Force: EEG Arousals: scoring rules and examples. *Sleep.* 1992;15:174–184.

3. American Sleep Disorders Association. The ASDA Atlas Task Force: Recording and scoring leg movements. *Sleep.* 1993;16:749–759.

4. Carskadon MA, Dement WC, Mitler MM, et al. Guidelines for the multiple sleep latency test (MSLT): a standard measure of sleepiness. *Sleep.* 1986; 9:519–524.

5. Thorpy MJ. The clinical use of the multiple sleep latency test. The Standards of Practice Committee of the American Sleep Disorders Association [Review.] [120 refs.] *Sleep.* 1992;15:268–276. [Published erratum appears in *Sleep.* 1992;15:381.]

6. American Sleep Disorders Association. *International Classification of Sleep Disorders, Revised: Diagnostic and Coding Manual.* Rochester, Minn: American Sleep Disorders Association; 1997.

7. Partinen M, Hublin C. Epidemiology of sleep disorders. In: Kryger MH, Roth T, Dement WC, eds. *Principles and Practice of Sleep Medicine.* 2nd ed. Philadelphia: WB Saunders; 2000.

8. Young T, Palta M, Dempsey J, et al. The occurrence of sleep-disordered breathing among middle-aged

adults [see comments]. *N Engl J Med.* 1993;328:1230–1235.

9. Young T. Analytic epidemiology studies of sleep disordered breathing—what explains the gender difference in sleep disordered breathing? *Sleep.* 1993;16:S1–S2.

10. Foresman B, Gwirtz P, McMahon J. Cardiovascular disease and obstructive sleep apnea: implications for physicians. *J Am Osteopath Assoc.* 2000;100:360–369.

11. Quan SF, Howard BV, Iber C, et al. The Sleep Heart Health Study: design, rationale, and methods. *Sleep.* 1997;20:1077–1085.

12. Carskadon MA, Dement WC. The multiple sleep latency test: what does it measure? *Sleep.* 1982;5 (Suppl 2):S67–S72.

13. Richardson GS, Carskadon MA, Orav EJ, et al. Circadian variation of sleep tendency in elderly and young adult subjects. *Sleep.* 1982;5(Suppl 2):S82–S94–S94.

14. Rechtschaffen A, Gilliland MA, Bergmann BM, et al. Physiological correlates of prolonged sleep deprivation in rats. *Science.* 1983;221:182–184.

15. Bliwise DL, Carskadon MA, Seidel WF, et al. MSLT-defined sleepiness and neuropsychological test performance do not correlate in the elderly. *Neurobiol Aging.* 1991;12:463–468.

16. Carskadon MA, Dement WC. Sleepiness and sleep state on a 90-min schedule. *Psychophysiology.* 1977;14:127–133.

17. Carskadon MA, Dement WC. Cumulative effects of sleep restriction on daytime sleepiness. *Psychophysiology.* 1981;18:107–113.

18. Friedman L, Bergmann BM, Rechtschaffen A. Effects of sleep deprivation on sleepiness, sleep intensity, and subsequent sleep in the rat. *Sleep.* 1979;1:369–391.

19. Philip P, Stoohs R, Guilleminault C. Sleep fragmentation in normals: a model for sleepiness associated with upper airway resistance syndrome. *Sleep.* 1994;17:242–247.

20. Clemes SR, Dement WC. Effect of REM sleep deprivation on psychological functioning. *J Nerv Ment Dis.* 1967;144:485–491.

21. Cohen H, Shane MD, Dement WC. Sleep and REM deprivation in the rat: effect of dexamethasone, a preliminary study. *Biol Psychiatry.* 1970;2:401–403.

22. Veasey SC, Hendricks JC, Kline LR, et al. Effects of acute sleep deprivation on control of the diaphragm during REM sleep in cats. *J Appl Physiol.* 1993;74:2253–2260.

23. Exar EN, Collop NA. The upper airway resistance syndrome. *Chest.* 1999;115:1127–1139.

24. Fletcher EC. Sympathetic activity and blood pressure in the sleep apnea syndrome. *Respiration.* 1997;64(Suppl 1):22–28.

25. Redline S, Sanders M. Hypopnea, a floating metric: implications for prevalence, morbidity estimates, and case finding. *Sleep.* 1997;20:1209–1217.

26. Loube DI, Gay PC, Strohl KP, et al. Indications for positive airway pressure treatment of adult obstructive sleep apnea patients: a consensus statement. *Chest.* 1999;115:863–866.

27. Young T, Peppard P, Palta M, et al. Population-based study of sleep-disordered breathing as a risk factor for hypertension. *Arch Intern Med.* 1997;157:1746–1752.

28. Young T, Finn L. Epidemiological insights into the public health burden of sleep disordered breathing: sex differences in survival among sleep clinic patients. *Thorax.* 1998;53(Suppl 3):S16–S19.

29. Standards of Practice Committee of the American Sleep Disorders Association. Practice parameters for the use of polysomnography in the evaluation of insomnia. *Sleep.* 1995;18:55–57.

30. Polysomnography Task Force, American Sleep Disorders Association Standards of Practice Committee. Practice parameters for the indications for polysomnography and related procedures. *Sleep.* 1997;20:406–422.

31. Standards of Practice Committee of the American Sleep Disorders Association. Practice parameters for the use of portable recording in the assessment of obstructive sleep apnea [see comments]. *Sleep.* 1994;17:372–377.

32. American Sleep Disorders Association. Practice parameters for the treatment of snoring and ob-

structive sleep apnea with oral appliances. *Sleep*. 1995;18:511–513.

33. American Sleep Disorders Association. Practice parameters for the treatment of obstructive sleep apnea in adults: the efficacy of surgical modifications of the upper airway. *Sleep*. 1996;19:152–155.

34. Standards of Practice Committee of the American Sleep Disorders Association. Practice parameters for the use of laser-assisted uvulopalatoplasty. *Sleep*. 1994;17:744–748.

35. He J, Kryger MH, Zorick FJ, et al. Mortality and apnea index in obstructive sleep apnea. Experience in 385 male patients. *Chest*. 1988;94:9–14.

36. Loube DI, Gay PC, Strohl KP, et al. Indications for positive airway pressure treatment of adult obstructive sleep apnea patients: a consensus statement [see comments]. *Chest*. 1999;115:863–866.

37. Young T. Sleep-disordered breathing in older adults: is it a condition distinct from that in middle-aged adults? [editorial; comment.] *Sleep*. 1996;19:529–530.

38. Mitler MM, Carskadon MA, Czeisler CA, et al. Catastrophes, sleep, and public policy: consensus report. [Review.] [41 refs.] *Sleep*. 1988;11:100–109.

39. Pakola SJ, Dinges DF, Pack AI. Review of regulations and guidelines for commercial and noncommercial drivers with sleep apnea and narcolepsy. *Sleep*. 1995;18:787–796.

40. Stoohs RA, Bingham LA, Itoi A, et al. Sleep and sleep-disordered breathing in commercial long-haul truck drivers. *Chest*. 1995;107:1275–1282.

41. Young T, Blustein J, Finn L, et al. Sleep-disordered breathing and motor vehicle accidents in a population-based sample of employed adults. *Sleep*. 1997;20:608–613.

CHAPTER

16

PNEUMONIA

Orna Molayeme and J. Michael Thompson

*Under the most rigorously controlled conditions
of temperature, pressure and humidity, the
microorganism will do as it darn well pleases.*
UNKNOWN
1965

LEARNING OBJECTIVES

1. Describe the pathophysiological changes and the expected arterial blood gas findings associated with pneumonia.
2. Identify complications associated with pneumonia.
3. Describe the clinical monitoring of a patient with pneumonia and develop a respiratory care plan based on specific patient data.
4. Discuss the etiology, pathophysiology, clinical features, and management of a patient with bacterial pneumonia.
5. Discuss the etiology, pathophysiology, clinical features, diagnosis, and management of a patient with aspiration pneumonia.
6. Describe the evaluation of a patient admitted to the emergency room with a diagnosis of bacterial pneumonia.
7. Apply the critical thinking skills of prioritizing, anticipating, negotiating, communicating, decision making, and reflection by completing case examples with pneumonia.
8. Describe the role of the respiratory therapist in the diagnosis, treatment, and management of the patient with pneumonia.

9. Interpret clinical data from the case examples including: history, physical examination, lab data, and radiographic data to make recommendations for respiratory care management.
10. Develop a care plan for the patient in each case, including recommendations for therapy and disease management, with consideration of cost, ethical, and quality-of-life issues.
11. Communicate facts, evidence, and arguments to support evaluations and recommendations proposed in the care plan for patients with pneumonia.
12. Practice the skill of negotiating in an attempt to gain acceptance of your proposed care plan for each patient with pneumonia.
13. Evaluate treatment and outcomes of interventions to proposed changes in the care plan.
14. Apply strategies to promote critical thinking in the respiratory care management of patients with pneumonia through completion of chapter exercises and group discussion.

INTRODUCTION AND DEFINITIONS

Despite modern antibiotic therapy, pneumonia ranks as the sixth leading cause of death in the United States and is associated with a 15% to 20% mortality rate among ICU patients.[1] In addition, the leading cause of death from hospital-acquired infections (also known as nosocomial infections) is hospital-acquired pneumonia (HAP).[2]

Pneumonia consists of an alveolar inflammation caused by infectious or noninfectious pathogens. Pneumonia is often classified based on the contaminant source, such as community-acquired, hospital-acquired, or aspiration pneumonia. Further classification may include the specific causative agent, such as bacterial, viral, fungal, or chemical. The lung segment involved, such as in lobar pneumonia, is included in the description when applicable.

COMMON CAUSES OF PNEUMONIA

Community-Acquired Pneumonia (CAP)

Community-acquired pneumonia generally refers to pneumonia contracted outside of the hospital environment. The microorganisms found in this environment differ from those seen in a medical inpatient environment, and as a result the causes of infection tend to be different. In addition, pneumonia of this origin is often treatable in an outpatient setting.

CAP strikes about 4 million people annually.[1] It is most common in the young, elderly, and patients with coexisting illnesses. The most common CAP pathogens are *Streptococcus pneumoniae, Haemophilus influenzae,* and *Mycoplasma pneumoniae.* Streptococcal pneumonia accounts for up to 75% of cases of CAP.[3] Community-acquired as well as nosocomial infections are commonly spread by fluid and contact transmission.

Hospital-Acquired Pneumonia (HAP)

The leading cause of nosocomial pneumonia is aspiration pneumonia[4] (see Table 16-1 for types of aspiration pneumonia). Bacterial aspiration pneumonia is often caused by colonization of the aerodigestive tract, and by aspiration of contaminated secretions into the lower airway. The presence of invasive devices, such as endotracheal or nasogastric tubes, predisposes the patient to gastric reflux and impairs coughing and swallowing, leading to aspiration.

Endotracheally intubated patients are 20 times more likely than nonintubated patients to aspirate.[5] Intubated patients receiving mechanical ventilation who develop a nosocomial pneumonia are considered a subset of HAP, and these infections are referred to as ventilator-associated pneumonia (VAP). When pneumonia occurs within 48 to 72 hours of endotracheal intubation, it is often caused by antibiotic-sensitive bacteria (ie, *Streptococcus pneumoniae, Staphylococcus aureus,* and *Haemophilus influenzae*). VAP with an onset of 72 hours or more after intubation is often caused by antibiotic-resistant pathogens (ie, oxacillin-resistant or methicillin-

TABLE 16-1 TYPES OF ASPIRATION PNEUMONIA

A. Chemical aspiration (can cause ARDS)
  1. Causes: hydrochloric acid with a pH <2.5, bile, mineral oil, gasoline
  2. Reaches pleura in about 18 seconds
  3. Type I alveolar cells die first, then type II alveolar cells
B. Inert fluid aspiration pH >3.0
  1. Causes: fresh water, saltwater, naso-gastric feedings
C. Particulate aspiration
  1. Causes: peanuts, teeth, food, etc.
  2. May result in obstructive atelectasis
  3. Chest x-ray may show mediastinal shift
  4. Bronchoscopy is usually needed to remove the material
D. Bacterial aspiration
  1. Causes: poor dental hygiene (eg, tooth or gum abscess); often results in mixed anaerobe bacterial pneumonia
  2. Usually seen in lower parts of upper lobes and upper parts of the lower lobe
  3. Common organisms aspirated:
    Gram-negative: *Klebsiella* and *Pseudomonas aeruginosa*
    Gram-positive: *Staphylococcus aureus* and *Streptococcus pneumoniae*

ARDS, acute respiratory distress syndrome.

resistant *Staphylococcus aureus*, *Pseudomonas aeruginosa*, *Acinetobacter* species, and *Enterobacter* species).[6,7]

Among all nosocomial infections, HAP is the second most common infection, although its mortality rate is the highest, ranging between 13% and 55%.[2,8] Hospital-acquired pneumonias are often caused by gram-negative organisms that tend to be more resistant to antibiotic therapy. The most common causes of bacterial and infectious nonbacterial pneumonia can be reviewed, along with key comments about each microorganism, by referring to the appropriate table (see Tables 16-2 and 16-3).

Neonatal Pneumonias

Categories of neonatal pneumonia depend on the route of acquisition and the age at presentation. Transplacental pneumonia is acquired in utero by the mother passing on the organism to the fetus. Aspiration pneumonia consists of aspirated amniotic fluid containing various agents capable of causing some form of pneumonia. Acquired pneumonia consists of transmission of organisms to the infant and is often due to poor handwashing. For more specific information on route, onset, and specific causes of neonatal pneumonias, see Table 16-4.

CRITICAL CONTENT

CHARACTERISTICS OF COMMUNITY-ACQUIRED PNEUMONIA

- It is often treatable in an outpatient setting.
- It strikes about 4 million people annually.
- Streptococcus pneumonia accounts for up to 75% of cases.

HOSPITAL-ACQUIRED (NOSOCOMIAL) PNEUMONIA

- The leading cause of HAP is aspiration.
- Intubated patients are 20 times more likely to aspirate and get HAP.
- Ventilator-associated pneumonia (VAP) a large subset of HAP.
- Among all nosocomial infections, HAP is the second most common infection, although its mortality rate is the highest.

PATHOPHYSIOLOGY

Pneumonia is a restrictive lung disease characterized by inflammation of lung parenchyma with exudative solidification or consolidation,[9] resulting in decreased lung compliance and abnormal gas exchange (V/Q mismatch or shunt). Areas of lung with partially obstructed airways will have decreased ventilation, resulting in V/Q mismatch, and other areas of lung with complete consolidation will create intrapulmonary shunts.

Permanent parenchymal lung damage may result from infection with some organisms (eg, staphylococcal and pseudomonal), depending on the degree of necrotizing action they have. As a group, gram-negative bacteria tend to have more necrotizing activity than most gram-positive bacteria. This is one of the traits of these bacteria that makes infection caused by them more serious.

In bacterial pneumonia there is often complete alveolar consolidation, in which areas of atelectasis or complete alveolar filling may alternate with hyperinflation. This, along with impaired mucocil-iary clearance, leads to decreased lung compliance, a rapid shallow breathing pattern, accessory muscle use, and shortness of breath. Viral pneumonia tends to affect the airways more than the alveolar spaces, thus leading to exhausting coughing episodes, but often without the same level of sputum production typically found with bacterial infections.

Aspiration pneumonia can lead to an acute mechanical airway constriction, creating partial airway obstructions caused by ball-and-valve (one-way) mechanisms within the airways. This process can create increased expiratory lung resistance and potential air trapping. Additionally, decreased lung compliance caused by regional atelectasis and V/Q mismatch, as well as disruption of surfactant function may occur. Autopsy findings of aspiration pneumonia patients may include: cellular debris in

TABLE 16-2   COMMON BACTERIAL CAUSES OF PNEUMONIA

Streptococcus pneumoniae	Most common cause of community-acquired pneumonia (CAP). Often present in heavy smokers, alcoholism, COPD, HIV, and nursing homes.
Staphylococcus aureus	Common strain resistant to the antibiotics methicillin (MRSA) or vancomycin (VRSA). Prevalent in structural disease of the lung (ie, bronchiectasis or cystic fibrosis) and injection drug use. Present in CAP and hospital-acquired pneumonia (HAP).
Mycobacterium tuberculosis	HIV, injection drug use.
Klebsiella pneumoniae	Most common cause of bacterial pneumonia in alcoholics.
Pseudomonas aeruginosa	Most common cause of bacterial pneumonia from contaminated respiratory therapy equipment. Often present in patients with structural diseases of the lung.
Haemophilus influenzae	Most common cause of bacterial pneumonia in COPD patients, heavy smokers, HIV, and nursing homes. Community-acquired.
Mixed anaerobes	Most common cause of bacterial pneumonia in patients who have aspirated.
Legionella	Relatively uncommon gram-negative pneumonia present in patients exposed to stagnant water in air conditioning ducts, swimming pools, and spa whirlpools.

COPD, chronic obstructive pulmonary disease; HIV, human immunodeficiency virus; MRSA, methicillin-resistant *Staphylococcus aureus;* VRSA, vancomycin-resistant *Staphylococcus aureus.*

TABLE 16-3 COMMON NONBACTERIAL INFECTIOUS CAUSES OF PNEUMONIA

Respiratory syncytial virus (RSV)	Immunocompromised pediatric as well as adult patients.
Mycoplasma	Most common cause of pneumonia in young healthy adults.
Pneumocystis carinii	Common in HIV patients or other immuno-suppressed patients.
Hantavirus	Frequently lethal in previously young, healthy adults exposed to mice bodily fluids.
Adenovirus	Common in conjunctivitis and nasopharyngitis.

HIV, human immunodeficiency virus.

airspaces between large airways and alveoli, along with evidence of an inflammatory response, consisting of macrophages, alveolar edema, and hyaline membrane formation. Additional findings may include necrosis of pulmonary microvasculature and lung parenchyma.

DIAGNOSIS

Laboratory and Radiographic

The specific causative pathogen of most pneumonias cannot be predicted based on clinical, radiologic, or laboratory examination. All current tests have low sensitivity and therefore are associated with a low diagnostic yield. Only 30% to 60% of pneumonia patients have the pathogenic organism identified.

The chest radiograph is essential not only to the diagnosis of pneumonia, but also to determine other radiographic abnormalities that may predict a complicated course, such as pleural effusion or pneumothorax. A list of various complications that can arise from pneumonias are summarized in the accompanying table (Table 16-5).

Pneumonia is often seen on radiographs as areas of increased density. Additionally, air bronchograms are often seen, which appear as airway shadows that stand out when the surrounding lung tissue is consolidated. See Fig. 16-1 for a chest radiograph demonstrating typical bilateral infiltrates and air bronchograms. Occasionally, lobar consolidation is seen in bacterial pneumonia. See Fig. 16-2 for the typical chest film appearance of a lobar pneumonia with air bronchograms.

Viral pneumonia frequently has unilateral or bilateral interstitial infiltrates. Gastric aspiration

TABLE 16-4 CATEGORIES OF NEONATAL PNEUMONIA

ROUTE	ONSET	CAUSE
Transplacental	Hours postbirth	Herpes simplex V, rubella, toxoplasmosis, *Listeria*, syphilis
Aspiration	Hours to days of life	Meconium, Streptococcus, *Klebsiella*
Acquired	First week of life	Respiratory syncytial virus, parainfluenza, influenza A and B, enteroviruses, rhinoviruses, aden oviruses, herpes simplex, *Chlamydia*

TABLE 16-5   POTENTIAL COMPLICATIONS OF PNEUMONIA

- Lung abscess
- Bronchiectasis
- Empyema
- Pericarditis and/or endocarditis
- Adult respiratory distress syndrome (ARDS)
- Formation of cysts and bullae
- Pneumothorax
- Pleural effusion (other than empyema)
- Respiratory failure
- Reye's syndrome (especially common in influenza B pneumonia) is associated with aspirin and affects the liver and brain
- Pulmonary fibrosis
- Blood sepsis and septic shock

pneumonia consists of bilateral patchy airspace consolidation, favoring perihilar or basal regions. Necrotizing pneumonias display areas of radiolucency caused by lung destruction. In the newborn, aspiration of meconium usually results in bilateral infiltrates, not consolidation. Syphilis causes a white-out pneumonia.

The appearance on chest films often does not correlate with the severity of clinical illness. The incidence of a false positive radiologic finding increases in the presence of underlying lung disease. False negatives are more likely in dehydration, neutropenia, early disease, and *Pneumocystis carinii* pneumonia.[10] It is often only after a dehydrated patient receives volume and fluid replacement that the lung infiltrate becomes obvious.

Patients with pneumonia typically are able to hyperventilate. They achieve this by increasing their minute volume in response to the effects of the pneumonia. In addition, they present with hypoxemia that may or may not be responsive to oxygen therapy. If there is significant alveolar consolidation present, it will produce alveolar shunting, which will make the hypoxemia unresponsive to oxygen therapy. If, however, the infiltrate causes mostly ventilation-perfusion mismatching,

the hypoxemia will be more responsive to oxygen administration. Thus, a respiratory alkalosis and hypoxemia are typically present in arterial blood gases. Acidosis is usually observed only in the presence of severe chronic obstructive pulmonary disease (COPD), neuromuscular weakness, or respiratory failure from an overwhelming pneumonia.

A complete blood chemistry and blood count is typically ordered. Leukocytosis is often initially prevalent in bacterial pneumonia. As the infection progresses, the number of immature white blood cells (bands) increases. In severe pneumonia, leukopenia is noted when the immune system has been compromised. In a nonbacterial pneumonia, the white blood count is usually normal.

Sputum culture specimens are collected prior to the administration of antibiotics for microbiological identification of the pathogen causing the pneumonia. A Gram's stain identifies the general category of the involved bacteria. Culture identifies the specific pathogen and sensitivity testing identifies the antibiotic that the bacteria is susceptible to. Sputum samples have low specificity and sensitivity.[11] In one study of CAP in the elderly popula-

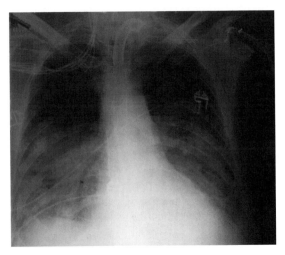

FIGURE 16-1   Typical bilateral infiltrates seen in a bacterial pneumonia. Notice that the shadows of a couple of the large airways stand out due to the contrast of the surrounding consolidated lung tissue. These are referred to as air bronchograms.

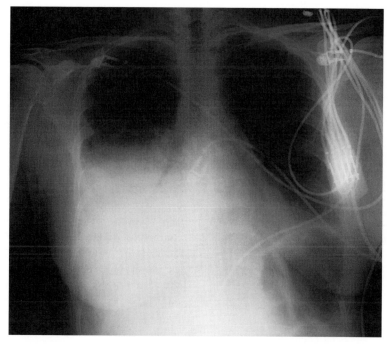

FIGURE 16-2 Typical appearance of a bacterial lobar pneumonia with air bronchograms.

tion, the causative agent was identified in only 42% of cases.[10] A sputum sample can be obtained via transtracheal or transthoracic bronchoscopy, or by lung biopsy if the patient is unable to expectorate. A sputum sample is considered uncontaminated with oral secretions when many polymorphonuclear cells (more than 25/LPF) and few epithelial cells are present.

Blood cultures are often used to establish the etiology of the infection, since many lung-infecting organisms will enter the bloodstream. Serologic tests are mostly indicated in the diagnosis of viral pneumonia, when influenza, parainfluenza, respiratory syncytial virus (RSV), or cytomegalovirus (CMV) pneumonitis are suspected.

Identification of viral organisms, such as CMV, RSV, adenovirus, herpes simplex virus, and varicella can be done with immunofluorescence and immunohistochemistry. Recent utilization of polymerase chain reaction and in situ hybridization allow cultures of respiratory secretions, cells, and blood.

History and Physical Examination

The general clinical manifestations of an acute bacterial pneumonia often include a sudden onset of symptoms, including chills, high fever, and a hacking cough producing purulent and abundant pink, brown, or yellow sputum. Other symptoms include headaches, skin rashes, nausea, or diarrhea. In the presence of underlying chronic pulmonary disease or when multiple lung fields are affected, chest pain, usually pleuritic, and dyspnea are present. Additional physical findings may include a unilateral chest expansion, tactile fremitus, and dullness to percussion due to a lobar consolidation. Auscultation may reveal decreased breath sounds, bronchial breath sounds, and rales or wheezes due to the inflammatory response from toxins or obstruction. Coarse crackles often represent a late sign of pneumonia. A pleuritic friction rub indicates an inflammation of the pleura. Moist crepitations, egophony, and pectoriloquy are often

TABLE 16-6 CLINICAL MANIFESTATIONS OF NEONATAL PNEUMONIA

Nonspecific	Changes in eating pattern, lethargy or irritability, poor color
Specific (tend to develop later)	Hypothermia, cough, grunting, tachypnea, dyspnea, cyanosis
Physical findings (possible to have a normal exam)	Nasal flaring, sternal and substernal retractions, decreased breath sounds, rales or wheezes

present. Cyanosis and accessory muscle use may be present. An increased heart rate and respiratory rate may be due to hypoxemia, fever, or a decrease in lung compliance.

In viral or mycoplasma pneumonia, a gradual onset of symptoms, a low-grade fever, and initially scant, mucoid sputum is present. Other symptoms such as significant changes in vital signs, chills, chest pain, lobar or segmental consolidation, or polymorphonuclear leukocytosis are uncommon.

In addition to the above, clinical manifestations of pneumonia in the infant, as well as in the elderly, may include changes in eating pattern, lethargy, irritability, or hypothermia (see Table 16-6 for clinical manifestations of neonatal pneumonia). However, in spite of the numerous signs and symptoms described above, it is possible to have a completely normal physical examination even in the presence of pneumonia.

CRITICAL CONTENT

DIAGNOSIS OF PNEUMONIA IS MADE BY:

1. Chest radiograph
2. Elevated polymorphonuclear cell count
3. Sputum culture and/or titers
4. History and physical examination

TREATMENT

Early recognition and treatment of this serious disease decreases patient morbidity and mortality. Most pneumonia patients can be treated as outpatients; however, in the presence of a severe infection or preexisting risk factors, such as age, underlying illness, hyperthermia, or leukopenia, the patient may require hospital admission.

Empiric broad-spectrum antibiotic therapy is often started before sputum and blood culture and sensitivity results are obtained.[12–14] In such cases, the antibiotic is chosen based on patient history and radiographic presentation. When culture results are obtained, the antibiotic most likely to be effective in eradicating the organism in question should be used. The drug of choice for gram-positive, elongated diplococci (usually pneumococci) and mixed anaerobes is penicillin. Ampicillin or a second generation cephalosporin is used for gram-negative coccobacilli.

Antiviral agents may be administered for the treatment of viral pneumonias. They work by either preventing viral replication or boosting the host's immune response. Generally they have been more successful in vitro than in vivo.

Contact isolation is initiated if antibiotic-resistant organisms are cultured. Respiratory isolation is also implemented if the mode of transmission is airborne, such as with influenza and tuberculosis.

Severe pneumonia requires general supportive measures, including fluid and nutritional therapy, as well as correction of acid-base disorders, hypothermia, and low glucose levels, if present. Oxygen therapy is initiated to maintain a pulse oximetry saturation (Spo_2) of greater than 92% and to decrease pulmonary hypertension. Aerosol therapy and airway clearance devices, such as PEP and flutter valves, are sometimes used, especially in patients with preexisting lung disease, to improve mucociliary clearance in patients who are unable to effectively spontaneously cough. Postural drainage and percussion can be implemented if it does not cause decreased oxygen saturation, and it meets the criteria established by the American Association for Respiratory Care

(AARC) clinical practice guidelines. Expectorants such as saturated solution of potassium iodide (SSKI) are usually not clinically effective. Mechanical ventilation may be instituted if respiratory failure ensues. Pain medications for chest pain, along with sedation or paralysis may be indicated. In the presence of worsening hypoxemia, high-frequency or jet ventilation, surfactant replacement therapy, and extracorporeal membrane oxygenation (ECMO) may be necessary. Inhaled nitric oxide is used if persistent pulmonary hypertension is identified. General measures for the treatment of pneumonia are summarized in the Table 16-7.

A careful reevaluation of the patient who shows poor progress must be made to rule out the possibility of tuberculosis, fungal infections, resistant organisms, cancer, pulmonary embolism, lymphoma, viruses, lipoid pneumonia, and vasculitis.[15] The proper diagnosis may be achieved via bronchoscopy with biopsy in addition to serologic studies. The mortality rate increases in the presence of malignancies or neurological illnesses such as

TABLE 16-8 FACTORS ASSOCIATED WITH FAILURE TO RESPOND TO THERAPY

- Inadequate host defenses
- Erroneous drug selection
- Erroneous dosage regimen or diagnosis
- Unusual pathogen
- Dual pathogen
- Complications (ie, empyema)

dementia, cerebrovascular disease, and multiple sclerosis.[15] Failure to respond to treatment can be ascribed to many different causes (Table 16-8).

If clinical improvement occurs, documentation of complete clearing of the infiltrate is not required unless the patient is at high risk of lung cancer, because the chest film may take as long as 3 months to resolve.[10,16,17] Complete recovery from pneumonia may take several months.[17] Discharge from the hospital occurs when the patient is responsive to treatment and is able to tolerate oral medications.

TABLE 16-7 GENERAL TREATMENT FOR INFECTIOUS PNEUMONIA

A. Appropriate antibiotic therapy:
   1. Gram-positive, diplococci, mixed anaerobes: penicillin
   2. Gram-negative, coccobacilli: ampicillin, cephalosporin

B. Bedrest

C. Oxygen if indicated

D. Pain medications as needed for chest pain

E. Aerosol therapy if indicated, ie: dry secretions and/or concurrent wheezes

F. Postural drainage and percussion per AARC clinical practice guidelines
   (if >25 mL of secretions per day and the patient is unable to effectively cough spontaneously)

G. Intravenous fluid therapy

H. Prevention

PREVENTION AND VACCINATION

To prevent the spread of hospital-acquired infections, careful handwashing, maintenance of sterile technique during suctioning, and flushing multiuse suction catheters with normal saline after each use are important measures. In addition, it has recently been postulated that decreasing the frequency of ventilator circuit disruptions will help prevent circuit contamination. Airway care measures used to prevent ventilator-associated aspiration pneumonia include routine mouth care to reduce accumulation of bacteria in the oropharynx and use of adequate endotracheal tube cuff pressures. Minimizing rainout (condensation) in ventilator circuits is important, not only because a warm, moist environment is an ideal breeding ground for bacteria, but also to prevent aspiration of condensation in the ventilator circuit.

Bacterial growth in the sinuses may predispose the patient to pneumonia through the aspiration of infected secretions from the nasal sinuses. Its risk can be minimized by replacing nasotracheal and nasogastric tubes with oral tubes and by avoiding prolonged nasal intubation (longer than 48 hours).[18] Other methods that may reduce the risks of nosocomial pneumonia include use of closed (multiuse) suction catheters; continuous subglottic suctioning; humidification with heat and moisture exchangers; and kinetic therapies that change the patient's position by the use of specialized medical beds or other devices.

The use of antacids and H_2 blockers to reduce the risk of stress ulcers increases bacterial growth in the stomach. Consequently, the use of contaminated enteral feedings, and/or regurgitation (through unnoticed aspiration) may cause pneumonia. Enteral feeding can increase the pressure inside the stomach and lead to regurgitation, especially since feeding tubes keep the gastroesophageal sphincter open. To minimize gastric pressure and the probability of regurgitation, intermittent rather than continuous tube feedings can be implemented. The head of the bed can also be elevated to a 30° to 45° angle to reduce aspiration risk.

Administration of gastric pH-altering drugs such as H_2 receptor antagonists and antacids to reduce the incidence of stress ulcers can increase bacterial gastric colonization and thereby increase the risk of VAP.[19] The drug sucralfate has been found to reduce stress ulcer bleeding without altering gastric pH, and is therefore associated with lower rates of VAP than are antacids or H_2 receptor antagonists.[20]

Strategies for the prevention of pneumonia by decreasing lower respiratory tract colonization by antibiotic-resistant organisms such as *P aeruginosa* and oxacillin-resistant *S aureus* include eliminating the unnecessary use of antibiotics[4,21,22] and alternating the antibiotic classes used for suspected infection.[23] Antibiotic prophylaxis for the prevention of VAP is not presently recommended,[24,25] except for ventilator patients with neutropenic fever due to their increased risk of both community-acquired and nosocomial infection.[26]

Oropharyngeal decontamination with chlorhexidine oral rinse has been associated with a decrease in bacterial accumulation in dental plaque and VAP.[27] Its use is recommended only for certain high-risk patients due to the risk of development and colonization of chlorhexidine-resistant pathogens.[28]

A single pneumococcal vaccination is strongly advised for any patient older than 65 years, especially if COPD, cardiac disease, diabetes mellitus, liver disease, or an immunocompromised state is present.[29-31]

Annual influenza vaccinations have been associated with a reduction of influenza infections by 58%.[17] Vaccination of health care providers in chronic care facilities may be as or more important than vaccination of the patients.[32] Vaccines tend to be less effective in immunosuppressed and asplenic patients.

SITE- AND AGE-SPECIFIC CONSIDERATIONS

Hospitals have historically been an efficient setting for the spread of resistant organisms, partly because they congregate patients at high risk of infection and expose them to an environment that makes extensive use of antibiotics and invasive procedures. To minimize the acquisition and spread of resistant organisms, invasive lines should be discontinued and the patient discharged as soon as the clinical situation permits it. As increased numbers of patients live in board and care or retirement homes, differences between community-acquired and hospital-acquired pneumonia become less well defined, making preventive maintenance an increasing challenge. The vaccination of high-risk patients should be considered during discharge planning to prevent nosocomial pneumonia. Although the hospital may not be a desirable place to keep the patient for the above reasons, evaluation of the home environment and support system must be made prior to discharge, in order to address any physical limitations, such as those due to the design of the home, and to facilitate home patient care.

Lower respiratory infections are estimated to affect 1 out of 18 people over age 65 each year.[15] The mortality rate from pneumonia in the elderly population is estimated to be 3 to 5 times greater that that of the younger population.[11] Half of all pneumonia cases[11] and 90% of deaths occur in the geriatric population.[10,33] Pneumonia is reported to be the most common infectious cause of death in older Americans.[33,34]

The clinical manifestations, diagnosis, treatment, and prognosis of pneumonia in older patients differ from those of younger patients[17] in that in elderly patients 43% have fever,[35] between 15% and 30% have lobar consolidation,[1] 25% have signs of congestive heart failure (CHF),[17] and 70% present with an altered mental status.[17] Delirium or acute confusion in the elderly has been reported to be due to pneumonia in up to 25% of cases.[17] The patient's cognitive impairment limits the ability for accurate history taking to identify pneumonia.

Radiographic findings in the elderly may have a low degree of specificity due to preexisting diseases. Sputum collection for Gram's stain and culture may not be possible, due to the patient's inability or unwillingness to cooperate; therefore blood cultures are often done to establish the infectious organism responsible for the pneumonia. Although very nonspecific, tachypnea may be a very early sign in pneumonia in the elderly.[17] The 30-day mortality rate of pneumonia in elderly patients is 11%.[15] Atypical presentation of pneumonia, characterized by altered mental status (AMS), lethargy, anorexia, and prior or current antibiotic use, increases the 30-day mortality rate.[15]

CRITICAL CONTENT

FACTORS THAT PLACE THE ELDERLY AT HIGHER RISK OF CONTRACTING PNEUMONIA

- Changes in pulmonary anatomy, such as a decrease in lung elasticity, diaphragmatic and intercostal muscle strength, cough reflex, and mucociliary clearance
- Preexisting illnesses are present in 80% to 90% of the elderly
- An increased likelihood of occult aspiration takes place in the elderly population
- Reduced effectiveness of immune system

Aspiration syndromes are an important cause of morbidity in the newborn. Diagnostic challenges in the infant include a limited physical assessment due to difficulty in percussing for dullness, and difficulty in differentiating cardiac from lung disease in the neonate. Laboratory tests as well as radiographic findings are less specific than at any other age. Their results are used to guide the therapy. Other details of neonatal pneumonia have been discussed earlier in the chapter.

COSTS AND ETHICAL ISSUES

Hospital-acquired pneumonia ranks as the second most common nosocomial infection after urinary tract infections (UTIs); however, it is the most deadly.[8] HAP is associated with prolonged hospitalization and higher medical charges than UTIs, with an estimated cost of $4 billion per year.[10] Due to the higher mortality associated with pneumonia in the elderly, the need for advance directives must be addressed. With a large portion of total health care expenditures occurring in the final few days of life, there is an increasing focus on the medical decisions that are made during these final days. It is critical that the patient makes clear what his or her health care wishes are regarding use of advanced life support measures.

With respect to the newborn, poor perinatal care and a poor maternal history can predispose the patient to an increased hospital length of stay. This brings up major social issues that do impact the health of the newborn. Maternal lifestyle decisions can also greatly influence the well-being of the fetus during pregnancy. The ethical issues behind provision of prenatal care and/or imposing some standards of health practice on pregnant women are complex, and the interested student is encouraged to pursue them.

PATIENT EDUCATION, HEALTH PROMOTION, AND QUALITY-OF-LIFE ISSUES

Education of the patient, family, and caregiver should include instructions on recognition of the signs and symptoms that require medical intervention, especially if the patient is elderly or an infant with underlying medical conditions. Adequate nutrition, exercise, and rest are necessary to strengthen the patient's immune response. Preventive measures such as vaccination are recommended.

Growing numbers of people are without family support systems and are therefore dependent on public institutions, which can lead to distancing the patient from the home environment. When the family is not directly involved in the provision of care outside the hospital environment, there are concerns that the quality of care may be affected. When the patient is discharged home, the readiness and ability of the caregiver to promote the patient's health by learning about the patient's condition and any necessary medical equipment are important.

All care provided to the patient in the home should promote the greatest degree of mobility possible. For example, a nasal cannula may be more restrictive than an oxygen conserving device in a stable, active home care patient. Attempts to maximize the patient's mobility will go a long way toward facilitating the patient's continued interaction with society, thus enhancing their quality of life.

INTRODUCTION TO CASE STUDIES

Now you proceed with the most exciting part of this chapter, that of working through two hypothetical cases. Your instructors will assign you to work on specific critical thinking exercises and group critical thinking exercises, depending on the available time, types of patients you are likely to encounter in your clinical rotations, and resources available. Please check with your instructor to verify which cases and exercises you should complete, individually or working in groups. Your instructor may also direct you to develop learning issues as part of your problem-based learning (PBL) process or assign specific, predetermined learning issues that have been developed for this chapter. Please check with your program faculty before proceeding with the following cases.

CASE STUDY 1

MS. CONNIE KONGESTED

Initial History

Ms. Kongested is a 74-year-old Caucasian female who lives in a senior citizen's residence. She was transferred to the ED this morning when the staff noticed she was very short of breath, slightly cyanotic, and coughing up yellow sputum. Upon admission to the ED, she was sweating, febrile, and complained of chest pain. She is a former cigarette smoker, but quit 5 years ago. Before she quit, she smoked 1 pack of cigarettes per day for 50 years. Ms. Kongested states "I felt fine until about 2 weeks ago, when I hurt my ankle and was unable to get out of bed." She then reports that about 1 week ago she began experiencing mild chest pain, night sweats, and shortness of breath.

 Critical Thinking Exercise 1

PRIORITIZING PATIENT CARE

How you would prioritize your assessment of this patient based on her age, history, and symptoms?

Physical Examination

Appearance: Acutely ill, elderly female in mild to moderate respiratory distress at rest, oriented to time, place, and person. Height, 65 inches; weight, 140 lb.

CASE 1 *(continued)*

Vital signs

HR	110/min
RR	22/min
BP	145/88
SpO$_2$	88% on RA
Temp.	39.2°C

HEENT	Lips are slightly cyanotic and some accessory muscle use noted.
Chest	Normal thoracic configuration.
Inspection & Auscultation	Bronchial breath sounds over right lower and middle lobes, clear but decreased sounds over remaining lung fields, large area of dullness to percussion in the right lower lobe posteriorly.
CV	Tachycardia with regular rhythm, no murmurs, rubs, or gallops heard.
Extremities	Warm and moist, cyanosis noted in fingertips, no clubbing or edema, pulses normal and symmetrical.

Critical Thinking Exercise 2

MAKING INFERENCES BY CLUSTERING DATA

What inferences can you make based on the data presented?

Critical Thinking Exercise 3

REFLECTING ON THE PROCESS OF MAKING INFERENCES

Go back and carefully consider how you arrived at the inference(s) you just made in the previous exercise. Answering the following will help you reflect on how you reached the conclusion(s) you did:

a. Which of the above pieces of data would you cluster together because you feel they point to the same inference?

b. Which of the above pieces of data were strongest in their implication of what inference you should draw?

c. Which pieces of data were only suggestive, but not conclusive, to the inference you reached?

d. What do you think was the main point of doing this particular exercise?

Critical Thinking Exercise 4

DATA GATHERING TO ASSIST IN PROBLEM SOLVING

What additional data would you recommend obtaining at this time? Give a brief reason for each test or piece of data you recommend obtaining.

The following tests were ordered and data obtained over the next hour.

CBC	Results pending
WBC	14,200/mm^3
Hgb	12.9 g/dL
Hct	39%
Electrolytes	Normal

CASE 1 *(continued)*

ABG room air

pH	7.47
P_{CO_2}	33 torr
P_{O_2}	56 torr
HCO_3^-	23 mEq/L
BE	+2 mEq/L
Sa_{O_2}	88%

Radiology

Portable AP Chest Film	Consolidation of the right lower lobe. Infiltrates in the right middle lobe. The cardiac border is absent on right side.

 Critical Thinking Exercise 5

DECISION MAKING: ASSESSMENT OF DATA AND DEVELOPING A PLAN OF CARE

a. What types of respiratory care would you recommend at this time, using an evidence-based approach?

b. What (in addition to the respiratory care) would be the focus of the plan of care?

Ms. Kongested is placed on nasal oxygen at 3 L/min and transferred to the medical ward. A sputum specimen is obtained and sent to the laboratory for Gram's stain, culture, and sensitivity. The Sp_{O_2} is 92% on 3 L/min of oxygen. Intravenous fluids and penicillin are started. Four hours later her initial sputum examination results show many gram-positive cocci present.

 Critical Thinking Exercise 6

ANTICIPATING A SPECIFIC DIAGNOSIS

a. Based on the clinical data obtained, what specific kind of pneumonia is this patient likely to have?

b. What specific care is being provided that is based on this hypothesis (what is the tentative diagnosis)?

Complete culture and sensitivity results are pending. Sp_{O_2} is now 89% on 3 L/min of oxygen. Updated physical examination data are as follows.

Chest

Auscultation	Expiratory wheezes in the right lower and middle lobes. Clear breath sounds over the remaining lung fields.

 Critical Thinking Exercise 7

ASSESSING AND MODIFYING THE PLAN OF CARE

Given the newest physical exam findings, what suggestions for therapy would you now have?

Eight hours after arrival to the ED the patient was given oxygen by heated aerosol mask 50%, which resulted in a Sp_{O_2} of 92%. The physician orders hand-held nebulizer treatments with albuterol followed by postural drainage and percussion every 4 hours.

Chest

Auscultation	Decreased wheezes
Cough	Dry, nonproductive

CASE 1 *(continued)*

EIGHT HOURS LATER

Chest
Auscultation   Clear.
Cough   Dry, nonproductive.

The postural drainage and percussion are discontinued.

24 HOURS LATER

Chest
Auscultation   Clear.
Cough   Productive.

The hand-held nebulizer treatments are discontinued.

Vital signs

HR	89/min
RR	17/min
BP	110/75
SpO_2	97%
Temp.	37.6°C

The oxygen is decreased to 2 L/min by nasal cannula.

Radiology

Portable AP Chest Film	Decreased consolidation in the right lower lobe and infiltrates in the right middle lobe.

Group Critical Thinking Exercise 1

REFLECTION AND DEBATE ON COMMON CLINICAL RECOMMENDATIONS

Given the current controversy surrounding the use of various treatments for this type of patient, have the class use current research, the THINKER strategy, and an evidence-based approach to discuss and debate both of the therapies that this patient received. The following should be considered during the class discussion/debate:

a. Reflect on the decision to initiate PD&P on this patient. Was the decision to initiate evidence based? Was there enough clinical data to clearly support the ordering of PD&P at the time it was ordered?

b. Should the bronchodilator have been started sooner? Should the treatments have been discontinued as quickly as they were? State your reasons and evidence.

The above exercise can be done by having the entire class enter into the discussion, or the instructor may choose to divide the class into pro and con groups and have them research their positions and then present their debate to the entire class.

Twenty-four hours later the SpO_2 is 94% on room air. Ms. Kongested is switched to oral penicillin. She is discharged and scheduled for a follow-up visit with her physician 1 week later.

Critical Thinking Exercise 8

DECISION MAKING: HEALTH PROMOTION AND DISEASE PREVENTION

What preventive measures can the patient take to minimize the future risk of pneumonia?

CASE STUDY 2

MR. ASPER RATION

Initial History

Mr. Ration is a 44-year-old male with a history of alcohol abuse. Paramedics brought him to the emergency department after his wife found him in a semi-conscious state. His wife stated that he had been drinking alcohol heavily for the past 3 days after being terminated from his job.

Critical Thinking Exercise 1

PRIORITIZING PATIENT CARE

How you would prioritize your assessment of this patient based on his age, history, and symptoms?

Physical examination was performed in ED with these findings: Appearance: semi-comatose, moderately obese male in mild respiratory distress at rest, poor response to painful stimuli. Height, 70 inches; weight, 235 lb.

Vital signs

HR	98/min
RR	23/min
BP	130/92
SpO$_2$	85% on RA
Temp.	38°C

HEENT	Lips are cyanotic and some vomitus is observed around the lips and nose.
Chest	
Inspection & Auscultation	Normal thoracic configuration. Course crackles in the right lung with decreased breath sounds in the left lung. Dull percussion tone over the right lower lobe.
CV	Regular rhythm, no murmurs, rubs, or gallops heard.

Extremities	Warm and moist, cyanosis noted in fingertips, no clubbing or edema, pulses normal and symmetrical.

Critical Thinking Exercise 2

MAKING INFERENCES BY CLUSTERING DATA

What inferences can you make based on the data presented?

Critical Thinking Exercise 3

DATA GATHERING TO ASSIST IN PROBLEM SOLVING

Using an evidence-based approach, what additional data would you recommend obtaining at this time? (Give a brief reason for each test or piece of data you recommend obtaining.)

The following additional tests are performed within the first hour after ED admission.

CBC	Results pending
WBC	6400/mm^3
Hgb	15.1 g/dL
Hct	44%
Electrolytes	Normal

ABG on RA	
pH	7.26
PCO$_2$	54 torr
PO$_2$	48 torr
HCO$_3^-$	24 mEq/L
BE	−4 mEq/L
SaO$_2$	88%

CASE 2 (continued)

Radiology

Portable AP Chest Film	Diffuse infiltrates throughout the right lung fields; the cardiac border is absent on the right side.

Critical Thinking Exercise 4

DECISION MAKING: ASSESSMENT OF DATA AND DEVELOPING A PLAN OF CARE

a. What types of respiratory care would you recommend at this time?

b. What (in addition to the respiratory care) would be the focus of the plan of care?

Group Critical Thinking Exercise 1

PRO AND CON DEBATE

Review Mr. Ration's clinical data and status to this point. Divide the class into two groups, instructing students to use the THINKER approach for the pro/con debate. One group will argue that Mr. Ration's status requires immediate endotracheal intubation. The group should be prepared to cite evidence and references to support its recommendation. The second group will argue that his current status does not call for immediate intubation. This group will also cite evidence and appropriate references to support a less invasive approach to management at this time. The debate can occur before the entire class. After the presentations, the class can weigh the strengths and weaknesses presented by the two sides of the debate. Was there a clear winner? Each group should give feedback regarding the verbal and nonverbal aspects of each debate team to promote the skills and traits needed for effective communication and negotiation.

At 1 hour post-arrival to the ED Mr. Ration is given mask oxygen at 8 L/min and transferred to

the medical ICU. The SpO_2 is 90% on 8 L/min of oxygen. Intravenous fluids and penicillin are started.

Two hours later Mr. Ration's vital signs are shown below.

Vital signs simple mask 8 L/min in O_2

HR	122/min
RR	33/min
BP	145/98
SpO_2	88%
Temp.	39.2°C

Critical Thinking Exercise 5

ANTICIPATING PROBLEMS AND SOLUTIONS

Based on this most recent data, what problem(s) do you anticipate and what are your recommended solutions? (Explain the rationale for your recommendations using an evidence-based approach.)

Four hours after admission to the ED, Dr. Christopher calls and requests that Mr. Ration be intubated and placed on mechanical ventilation. In addition, intravenous antibiotics are started. The physician suggests volume control ventilation at the following ventilator settings:

Mode	SIMV + PS
RR	10 b/min
VT	.75 L
PEEP	0 cm H_2O
PS	10 cm H_2O
FIO_2	.40

One hour later Mr. Ration is breathing spontaneously at a rate of 14 b/min on the above ven-

Continued

CASE 2 *(continued)*

---

tilator settings. Arterial blood gases are drawn and sent to the laboratory. Copious amounts of green secretions with solid debris have been suctioned from the endotracheal tube. Ventilator mechanics are below:

Peak inspiratory pressure	49 cm H_2O
Plateau pressure	38 cm H_2O
PEEP	0 cm H_2O

ABG FIO_2 40%

pH	7.33
PCO_2	43 torr
PO_2	68 torr
HCO_3^-	22 mEq/L
BE	–3 mEq/L
SaO_2	90%

You telephone Dr. Christopher and suggest a change to pressure control ventilation and he agrees to the following ventilator settings:

Mode	PC
RR	10 b/min
PIP	30 cm H_2O
PEEP	5 cm H_2O
FIO_2	.40

Critical Thinking Exercise 6

REFLECTING ON THE DECISION MAKING PROCESS

a. What reason(s) do you think the therapist had to suggest changing to PC mode?

b. Would it have been acceptable to leave Mr. Ration on the previous settings and not switch modes? Give reasons why or why not.

Copious amounts of secretions continue to be suctioned from the endotracheal tube. Mr Ration's color is improving.

Vital signs FIO_2 .40

HR	95/min
RR	15/min
BP	128/88
SpO_2	92%
Temp.	38.6°C

Eight hours later (14 hours after ED admission), arterial blood gases are drawn on pressure control ventilation and the results are as follows:

ABG on .40

pH	7.37
PCO_2	39 torr
PO_2	75 torr
HCO_3^-	22 mEq/L
BE	–3 mEq/L
SaO_2	93%

At 24 hours post-admission Mr. Ration becomes restless and accidentally extubates himself. He is immediately placed on oxygen by mask at 8 L/min and is noted to have an SpO_2 of 93%. Chest auscultation reveals clear breath sounds on the left side and right upper lobe and crackles in the right middle and lower lobes. Mr. Ration is coughing spontaneously and is producing green secretions.

CASE 2 *(continued)*

Critical Thinking Exercise 7

REFLECTING ON
THE DECISION MAKING PROCESS

What recommendations would you formulate while waiting for the doctor to respond to your stat page? Do you think Mr. Ration should be immediately reintubated?

a. Given the limited data above, does it favor reintubation or not? (Explain how you interpret the current data already available.)

b. What additional data would you immediately gather to aid in making your decision?

c. How important would a new ABG be to making the decision?

Forty-eight hours later (72 hours post-admission), Mr. Ration is now receiving nasal oxygen at 2 L/min and his vital signs are:

Vital signs

HR	84/min
RR	18/min
BP	128/82
SpO_2	95%
Temp.	38.1°C

Chest auscultation reveals clear breath sounds in both lungs.

The next day (96 hours post-admission), the SpO_2 is 93% on room air. Mr. Ration is switched to oral antibiotics. He is awake, alert, and is able to feed himself. His vital signs are stable. He is discharged the following day and is scheduled for a follow-up visit with his physician 1 week later.

KEY POINTS

• Despite modern antibiotic therapy, pneumonia ranks as the sixth leading cause of death in the United States and is associated with a 15% to 20% mortality rate among intensive care unit patients.[1]

• Pneumonia consists of an alveolar inflammation caused by infectious or noninfectious pathogens.

• The most prevalent type of nosocomial pneumonia is aspiration pneumonia.[4]

• Early recognition and treatment of this serious disease decreases patient morbidity and mortality.

• Most pneumonia patients can be treated as outpatients; however, in the presence of a severe infection or preexisting risk factors such as age,

underlying illness, hyperthermia, or leukopenia, the patient may be admitted to the hospital.

• Hospital-acquired pneumonia incurs an estimated cost of $4 billion per year,[10] and is the second most common nosocomial infection after urinary tract infections; however, it is the most deadly.[8]

• Pneumonia is reported to be the most common infectious cause of death in older Americans,[33,34] with a mortality rate in the elderly population estimated to be 3 to 5 times greater that that of the younger population.[11]

• Education of the patient, family, and caregiver should include instructions on recognition of the signs and symptoms that require medical intervention, especially if the patient is elderly or an infant with underlying medical conditions.

REFERENCES

1. Marrie TJ. Community-acquired pneumonia: epidemiology, etiology, treatment. *Infect Dis Clin North Am.* 1998;12:723–740.

2. Leu HS, Kaiser DL, Mori M, et al. Hospital-acquired pneumonia: attributable mortality and morbidity. *Am J Epidemiol.* 1989;129:1258–1267.

3. Finch RG, Woodhead MA. Practical considerations and guidelines for the management of community acquired pneumonia. *Drugs.* 1998;55:31–45.

4. Crouch Brewer S, Wunderink RG, Jones CB, et al. Ventilator-associated pneumonia due to *Pseudomonas aeruginosa. Chest.* 1996;109:1019–1029.

5. Crowe HM. Nosocomial pneumonia: Problems and progress. *Heart Lung.* 1996;25:418.

6. Niederman MS, Craven DE, Fein AM, et al. Pneumonia in the critically ill hospitalized patient. *Chest.* 1990;97:170–181.

7. Rello J, Ausina V, Ricart M, et al. Impact of previous antimicrobial therapy on the etiology and outcome of ventilator-associated pneumonia. *Chest.* 1993;104:1230–1235.

8. Kollef MH. New approaches to the diagnosis of VAP. *Infect Med.* 1997;14:364.

9. Cotran RS, Kumar V, Robbins SL. *Robbins' Pathological Basis of Disease.* 4th ed. Philadelphia: Saunders; 1989:778–799.

10. Bartlett JG. In: Gorbach SL, Bartlett JG, Blacklow NR, eds. *Infectious Disease.* 2nd ed. Philadelphia: Saunders; 1998:553–564.

11. Fein AM. Pneumonia in the elderly: Overview of diagnostic and therapeutic approaches. *Clin Infect Dis.* 1999;28:726–729.

12. Kollef MH, Ward S. The influence of mini-BAL cultures on patient outcomes: implications for the antibiotic management of ventilator-associated pneumonia. *Chest.* 1998;113:412–420.

13. Luna CM, Vujacich P, Niederman MS, et al. Impact of BAL data on the therapy and outcome of ventilator-associated pneumonia. *Chest.* 1997;111:676–685.

14. Rello J, Gallego M, Mariscal D, et al. The value of routine microbial investigation in ventilator-associated pneumonia. *Am J Respir Crit Care Med.* 1997;156:196–200.

15. Houston MS, Silverstein MD, Suman VJ. Risk factors for 30-day mortality in elderly patients with lower respiratory tract infection. *Arch Intern Med.* 1997;157:2190–2195.

16. Garibalde RA. Epidemiology of community-acquired respiratory tract infections in adults: Incidence, etiology, and impact. *Am J Med.* 1985; 78:32–37.

17. Pathy MSJ, ed. *Principles and Practice of Geriatric Medicine.* Vol. 1. New York: John Wiley; 1998:671.

18. Rouby JJ, Laurent P, Gosnach M, et al. Risk factors and clinical relevance of nosocomial maxillary sinusitis in the critically ill. *Am J Respir Crit Care Med.* 1994;150:776–783.

19. Craven DE, Steger KA. Epidemiology of nosocomial pneumonia: new perspectives on an old disease. *Chest.* 1995;108(Suppl):1S–16S.

20. Cook DJ, Reeve BK, Guyatt GH, et al. Stress ulcer prophylaxis in critically ill patients: resolving discordant meta-analyses. *JAMA.* 1996;275: 308–314.

21. Garrouste-Orgeas M, Chevret S, Arlet G, et al. Oropharyngeal or gastric colonization and nosocomial pneumonia in adult intensive care unit patients: a prospective study based on genomic DNA analysis. *Am J Respir Crit Care Med.* 1997; 156:1647–1655.

22. Goldman DA, Weinstein RA, Wenzel RP, et al. Strategies to prevent and control the emergence and spread of antimicrobial-resistant microorganisms in hospitals: a challenge to hospital leadership. *JAMA.* 1996;275:234–240.

23. Kollef MH, Vlasnik J, Sharpless L, et al. Scheduled change of antibiotic classes: a strategy to decrease the incidence of ventilator-associated pneumonia. *Am J Respir Crit Care Med.* 1997; 156:1040–1048.

24. Gastinne H, Wolff M, Delatour F, et al. A controlled trial in intensive care units of selective decontamination of the digestive tract with nonabsorbable antibiotics. *N Engl J Med.* 1992;326:594–599.

25. Tablan OC, Anderson LJ, Arden NH, et al. Guideline for prevention of nosocomial pneumonia: the Hospital Infection Control Advisory Committee, Centers for Disease Control and Prevention. *Infect Control Hosp Epidemiol.* 1998;19:304.

26. Prevention of bacterial infection in neutropenic patients with hematologic malignancies: a randomized multicenter trial comparing norfloxacin with ciprofloxacin: the GIMEMA Infection Program. *Ann Intern Med.* 1991;115:7–12.

27. DeRiso AJ II, Ladowski JS, Dillon TA, et al. Chlorhexidine gluconate 0.12% oral rinse reduces the incidence of total nosocomial respiratory infection and nonprophylactic systemic antibiotic use in patients undergoing heart surgery. *Chest.* 1996;109: 1556–1561.

28. Russell AD. Plasmids and bacterial resistance to biocides. *J Appl Microbiol.* 1997;83:155–165.

29. Fein MJ, et al. Efficacy of pneumococcal vaccination in adults: A meta analysis of randomized controlled trials. *Arch Intern Med.* 1994;154: 2666–2677.

30. Koivula I, et al. Clinical efficacy of pneumococcal vaccine in the elderly: A randomized, single blind population based trial. *Am J Med.* 1997;103: 281–290.

31. Sisk JE, et al. Cost effectiveness of vaccination against pneumococcal bacteremia among elderly people. *JAMA* 1997;278:1333–1339.

32. Potter J, Stott DJ, Roberts MA, et al. Influenza vaccination of health care workers in long term care hospitals reduces the mortality of elderly patients. *J Infect Dis.* 1997;175:1–6.

33. Gallo JJ, et al. Clinical aspects of aging. *Reichel's Care of the Elderly.* 5th ed. Philadelphia: Lippincott Williams & Wilkins; 1999:159–166.

34. Granton JT, Grossman RF. Community-acquired pneumonia in the elderly patient. Clinical features, epidemiology and treatment. *Clin Chest Med.* 1993; 14:537–553.

35. Fein AM, Feinsilver SH, Niederman MS. Atypical manifestations of pneumonia in the elderly. *Clin Chest Med.* 1991;12:319–336.

ACQUIRED IMMUNODEFICIENCY SYNDROME AND TUBERCULOSIS

Terry P. Lyle and Robert Tanaka

The man who never alters his opinion is like
standing water, and breeds reptiles of the mind.
WILLIAM BLAKE

LEARNING OBJECTIVES

1. Describe the incidence and routes of transmission of HIV infection, AIDS, and TB, in both the US and the world's populations.
2. List and describe the groups who are at high risk of becoming infected with HIV and TB.
3. Describe the diagnostic regimens used to rule out pulmonary complications of AIDS and active TB.
4. Discuss the pathophysiology and clinical features of the pulmonary complications of AIDS, primary TB, and reactivation TB.
5. Describe the acute care and long-term management of patients with AIDS and TB.
6. Apply specific formulas and theory to assist in clinical decision making in the patient with AIDS or TB.
7. Apply the critical thinking skills of prioritizing, anticipating, negotiating, communicating, and decision making to a case example of a patient with AIDS and TB.
8. Through performance of critical thinking exercises and group discussion of case questions, apply strategies that promote critical thinking

to the respiratory care management of a patient with AIDS and TB.

9. Use a case example to perform an initial patient assessment using a standardized system (SOAP and IPPA) and the clinical data presented.
10. Interpret clinical data from case examples, including history, physical examination, laboratory data, and radiographs to make recommendations for respiratory care management of a patient with AIDS or TB.
11. Develop a care plan for a patient with AIDS and TB, including recommendations proposed for therapy and disease management with consideration of the cost as well as ethical and quality-of-life issues.
12. Communicate facts, evidence, and arguments to support evaluations and recommendations proposed for a patient with TB and AIDS.
13. Practice the skill of negotiating to attempt to persuade acceptance of a proposed plan of care for a patient with TB or a pulmonary complication to AIDS.

14. Evaluate treatment and outcomes of interventions, giving attention to prevention, health promotion, and quality-of-life issues.
15. Describe the role of the respiratory therapist in the assessment, treatment, management, and education of the patient with active TB or with pulmonary complications associated with AIDS, as well as strategies used to prevent the transmission of HIV and TB in health care settings.

KEY WORDS

Acid-Fast Bacillus (AFB)
Active Tuberculosis
Acquired Immunodeficiency Syndrome (AIDS)
Anergy
Bacille Calmette-Guérin (BCG)
CD4+ T Lymphocytes
Human Immunodeficiency Virus (HIV)

Latent Tuberculosis
Pneumocystis carinii Pneumonia (PCP)
Primary Tuberculosis
Purified Protein Derivative (PPD)
Reactivation Tuberculosis
Seroconversion
Ziehl-Neelsen Stain

INTRODUCTION

In 1981, the Centers for Disease Control (CDC) received a series of reports from Los Angeles and New York City of cases of *Pneumocystis carinii* pneumonia (PCP) in male homosexuals. This had previously been a rare infection, which had been seen only in severely immunocompromised individuals, usually due to either genetic factors or the effects of chemotherapy. These reports, and the pattern of their appearance, led the CDC to quickly suspect that there was a new infectious agent or condition adversely affecting immunity in this patient population.

These initial reports precipitated the most heavily researched and politically charged medical events of the twentieth century. In 1984, researchers first isolated the virus, now named the human immunodeficiency virus (HIV). Since then, the acquired immunodeficiency syndrome (AIDS) has become the leading cause of death in the US in males aged 22 to 44.[1] Recently, AIDS has surpassed TB as the leading cause of death by communicable disease worldwide. The AIDS epidemic has been partly responsible for the significant increase in the incidence of TB in the US in the late 1980s and for the frightening increase in TB mortality worldwide.

It is because of the scourge these two conditions have unleashed upon the world population and their frequent coexistence that a discussion of both are included in this chapter. A brief summary of the incidence, etiology, treatment, and prevention of AIDS is presented first. Next, there is a discussion of the pulmonary complications associated with HIV infection and tuberculosis. Last, in keeping with the critical thinking focus of this text, there is a case presentation which will lead to further research and self-directed learning to expand your understanding of both HIV infection and TB.

It is important to understand that there is an ever-evolving body of knowledge about both TB and AIDS. Advances in treatment regimens will surely occur for both conditions and successful vaccines may be developed for either or both diseases in the next decade or two. Respiratory therapists should realize that it will be important to periodically review the literature to remain current on the evolving trends in the understanding, treatment, and prevention of the two greatest infectious disease killers in the world today.

CRITICAL CONTENT

INTRODUCTION

- HIV virus isolated in 1984
- AIDS and TB the number one and two infectious disease killers in the world
- HIV infection has contributed to increased incidence of TB in the US

AIDS/HIV

Definition

Researchers coined the term *acquired immunodeficiency syndrome* (AIDS) 2 years before the virus that causes the syndrome was identified. Early cases clearly indicated that for some reason, individuals had become susceptible to opportunistic infections due to a severe deficiency in their immune system. The term *acquired* was used to differentiate this new syndrome from that of patients whose immune systems had been damaged for known reasons such as the use of chemotherapeutic agents. A distinction must be made between those who have been infected with HIV and those who have been diagnosed with AIDS. In 1993, the CDC revised the definition of AIDS to include those HIV-infected individuals who have a CD4+ T lymphocyte count of less than 200/mm³ and have acquired one or more infections from a list of opportunistic infections. *HIV positive* is the term used to describe individuals who test positive for exposure to the virus, but do not exhibit the features of AIDS.

Incidence and Transmission

As of December 1999, there were a total of 733,374 cases of AIDS reported to the CDC since the epidemic began in the US in 1981.[1] Total deaths from AIDS now exceed 430,000. Worldwide, there have been an estimated 16 million persons who have died of AIDS, and an additional 34 million are currently living with AIDS.[2] Whereas globally, the disease affects both sexes fairly equally, over 80% of AIDS cases in the US have been in men. The predominantly male incidence of AIDS in the US is due to the fact that males who have sex with males (MSM) remain the highest risk group. Though this group accounts for about 60% of the AIDS cases diagnosed in 1997, the incidence of AIDS is declining most rapidly in this population. In declining order, other groups at high risk include injecting drug users (IDUs), Hispanic and African-American minorities, women who are either IDUs or who have sex with IDUs or MSMs, and children who have been infected in the perinatal period by HIV-infected mothers.[3] Hemophiliacs who received therapeutic agents made from infected concentrates of the blood supply between 1978 and 1985 and other blood recipients in this time period are also at high risk. After 1985, steps were taken to ensure that the nation's blood banks were free of HIV.

By far the highest-risk group is those between the ages of 22 and 44. Children less than 5 are the lowest risk age group, comprising only slightly more than 1% of total AIDS cases. The incidence of AIDS is declining in all age groups except in those over age 50. Since 1996, AIDS incidence and deaths have been declining in the US in all high-risk groups. This is chiefly due to great advances in drug therapy. Untreated, it takes an average of 8 years for an HIV-infected individual to deteriorate to the point that an AIDS diagnosis is made. With the new antiretroviral agents, the rate of replication of the virus is kept in check so the individual may seemingly indefinitely prolong the time from initial infection to the severe deterioration of the immune systems that leads to a diagnosis of AIDS. However, these therapies are too new to determine with certainty their long-term effectiveness.

Other therapies, such as drug regimens to prevent the occurrence of opportunistic infections such as PCP, have succeeded in decreasing mortality in those already diagnosed with AIDS. Although education programs encouraging high-risk groups to avoid risky behaviors that can lead to the transmission of AIDS have been slightly successful, the decline in cases of new HIV infection in the US has been less than 2% since 1996. Education programs to help limit transmission of the virus in the gay community have worked well. However, education has failed to have much impact in lower socioeconomic groups. For example, African-Americans are 8 times more likely to be HIV infected than the general population. At present, it is estimated that slightly more than 1 out of every 200 adults in North America between the ages of 19 and 49 is known to be HIV infected.[2]

The picture remains bleak globally. It is estimated that there were 3 million deaths due to AIDS in 1999 worldwide.[4] Not only is this a higher mortality rate than in any previous year, the annual death rate is predicted to increase worldwide for many more years. By far the region with the highest incidence is the sub-Saharan regions of Africa, where 8% of the adult population is believed to be infected. Over 95% of AIDS deaths currently occur in developing countries, and the incidence and deaths continues to inexorably increase in nearly all African countries. Though antiretroviral treatment regimens have certainly led to a rapid decline in AIDS deaths in the US, their high costs and the medical infrastructure needed to dispense them virtually preclude their adoption in developing countries.

HIV is contracted via the exchange of bodily fluids with an infected individual. This can occur via either heterosexual or homosexual sexual contact, through blood, by the sharing of contaminated needles by IDUs, or inadvertent punctures of health care workers (HCWs) with HIV-contaminated sharps. Transmission can also occur from mother to baby in the perinatal period or after birth via breast milk. There has been only one documented case of the transmission of HIV via saliva, and is not considered a possible risk for infection of HCWs. HIV cannot be transmitted via either insect bites or through casual contact.[5]

CRITICAL CONTENT

INCIDENCE AND TRANSMISSION

- 430,000 persons have died of AIDS in US since 1981.
- Worldwide, 16 million have died of AIDS to date.
- The rate of HIV infection is increasing in both the US and worldwide.
- The death rate is decreasing in the US due to improved, but costly, therapies.
- The death rate continues to increase worldwide.
- The incidence of HIV infection is still highest among MSMs in the US.
- The incidence is divided equally between men and women worldwide.
- HIV is spread by exchange of bodily fluids, especially during sexual activity.

Diagnosis and Pathophysiology

The virus replicates quickly in a new host after infection with HIV via the exchange of bodily fluids with an infected individual with a high viral load (expressed in virions/mL). This early acute infectious stage often presents few if any symptoms. If symptoms do develop during this period, usually 3 to 6 weeks after transmission, it is usually attributed to a common viral infection such as the flu or mononucleosis. Despite the frequent lack of symptoms, the viral load rises precipitously during this period. There are tests, including the reverse transcription polymerase chain reaction (PCR), that can detect the genetic material contained in both HIV-1 and HIV-2. This test is used to quantify the viral load in the blood for the purposes of monitoring the effectiveness of treatment, but it is very expensive and labor intensive, so it is not used as a routine screening test for HIV infection.[5]

Within days after exposure to HIV, the body responds by producing up to a billion CD4+ T lymphocytes and specific antibodies to ward off the invading organism. The enzyme immunoassay

(EIA), the standard screening test used to detect the presence of antibodies to HIV in the blood, can now be used to confirm the diagnosis of HIV infection. A positive test, demonstrating the presence of HIV antibodies in the blood is referred to as *seroconversion*. The mean time for seroconversion is about 3 months, and the vast majority of persons will test positive for HIV antibodies within 6 months after exposure. The Western blot test is used to confirm the diagnosis. In this period, termed the latent stage or period, the T lymphocytes are successful in limiting the viral load, though they cannot completely eliminate the virus. However, HIV has a proclivity to invade all CD4+ cells and replicates within them, destroying the CD4+ cells in the process. Over time, the unrelenting replication of new viruses overwhelms the system, and the CD4+ T lymphocytes are destroyed at a faster rate than they can be produced. When this occurs, the circulating CD4+ lymphocyte count in the blood begins to drop from its normal level of over $1000/mm^3$, thereby weakening the body's ability to ward off offending organisms. The loss of CD4+ helper T lymphocytes will severely weaken the body's cell-mediated immunity, which leaves the body vulnerable to opportunistic infections, such as TB, oral thrush, and *Pneumocystis carinii*. The suppressor CD8+ T cells are unaffected and the ratio between the suppressor T cells and the helper T cells goes up. The humoral immune system is also adversely affected and renders the body less efficient at producing specific antibodies and less capable of warding off viral and certain bacterial infections.

CRITICAL CONTENT

DIAGNOSIS AND PATHOPHYSIOLOGY

- EIA and Western blot blood tests are used to confirm HIV infection.
- HIV attacks helper T lymphocytes, leading to deficiencies in cell-mediated immunity.
- Immunosuppression leads to opportunistic infections.

Treatment

Great advances have been made in the treatment of HIV infection and AIDS since the initial reports of disease in the early 1980s, when the diagnosis of AIDS was in effect a death sentence. The development of a succession of potent antiretroviral agents, including protease inhibitors, and their use in combination has been successful in lengthening the latent period of HIV infection. In this latent stage the CD4+ T cell level remains high enough to prevent immunosuppression. Consequently, the accompanying opportunistic infections and full-blown AIDS can be delayed indefinitely. Antiretroviral therapy works by decreasing the rate of replication of HIV. Viral counts remain low enough that they do not overwhelm the host's own immune system. Antiretroviral therapy is usually administered as a multi-drug cocktail because monotherapy is associated with the quick development of resistance to each agent. Therapy is guided by frequent measurement of viral load and changing medication as viral load increases, which is indicative of resistance developing to a particular anitretroviral agent. It must be understood that antiretroviral therapy is not curative, even though the use of therapy can sometimes reduce viral loads to undetectable levels. Since tests of viral loads are not sensitive below 40 to 50 virions/mL, an undetectable level does not mean the patient is virus free. High HIV levels can be present in the lymphatics and other body tissues, even with a low or undetectable viral load in a blood sample. Viral loads usually increase substantially if antiretroviral medications are discontinued. Therefore, the use of antiretroviral medications is a lifetime therapy, not a cure.

Since protease inhibitors and multi-drug cocktails have only been in use since 1996, it is difficult to ascertain the long-term success of current treatment regimens. It is also unknown whether resistance may develop that may not be amenable to any of the current antiretroviral agents, but the initial clinical data are clearly encouraging. It may well be that HIV infection will become a chronic asymptomatic infection that can be adequately controlled, albeit not without great expense and annoying side effects, such as severe nausea, diarrhea, allergic reactions, neuropathy, and anemia.

CRITICAL CONTENT

TREATMENT

- Advances in antiretroviral therapy have been highly successful in keeping HIV viral loads in check.
- Therapy is expensive, but successfully prevents immunosuppression.
- Drug therapy is noncurative; it is a lifetime requirement.
- Side effects of antiretroviral medication can be severe.

Prevention

Prevention of AIDS has focused on educational efforts to limit the transmission of HIV. Education programs were initially directed at MSMs and IV drug users. These programs were expanded to all age groups, including teens and senior adults. Though efforts to educate everyone about the importance of practicing safe sex and avoidance of sharing contaminated needles have been successful in some high-risk groups, they have been largely unsuccessful in other groups. Increased funding for AIDS education for the CDC and the nation's public health departments has recently been approved to bolster these programs in an effort to reduce the incidence of new HIV infection.

You may recall that patient education begins with knowledge, but the ultimate goal of any health education program is to cause change in behavior. There are many issues, obstacles, challenges, and considerations to keep in mind when designing and implementing effective health education programs. Prevention of AIDS and TB presents unique challenges, especially when dealing with high-risk groups as well as risky behaviors. Community-based patient education, combined with outreach programs involving many volunteers has been shown to improve outcomes, including improved

patient compliance in following therapy regimens, incorporation of safe sex practices, and preventing the sharing of needles among IV drug users.

There is little hope that education alone will completely stop the transmission of this disease in the US. These efforts are even less successful in Third World countries in which limited economic resources and cultural practices preclude the easy availability of latex condoms and an abundant supply of sterile needles. The only real hope of significantly reducing the rate of HIV infection in these situations is the development of a vaccine. At this time it appears doubtful that there will ever be a vaccine that will completely eliminate all AIDS viruses. However, it is hoped that a vaccine will be developed that will improve the initial immunity of the new host, so that the viral load never reaches a level high enough to cause infection, or to transmit the virus via sexual contact to another person. Currently there are several ongoing HIV vaccine trials being conducted using human subjects with various vaccine preparations throughout the world.

Prevention in Health Care Workers. When the AIDS epidemic first began in the US, there was a great deal of fear that health care workers (HCWs) would be at great risk of contracting the disease. HCWs were also frightened by the legal decision allowing HIV test results to remain confidential, revealed only to the patient and the ordering physician. Early on, the CDC tried to allay these fears by instituting universal precaution guidelines in which HCWs view the body fluids of all patients as potentially infectious and adopt procedures to protect themselves from inadvertent contact.

In fact, these fears appear to have been somewhat overblown. As of June 1997, there had been only 52 HCWs who were unequivocally proven to have been infected with HIV through occupational exposure. Another 120 HCW infections were possibly due to occupational exposure, and of particular interest to the reader, only 1 respiratory therapist was potentially infected occupationally since the epidemic began.[6]

The risk of transmission of the disease is almost exclusively due to direct injection of HIV-infected blood products with a needle. It has been computed that the risk of transmission of the disease by an inadvertent needle stick from an HIV-contaminated needle or other sharp instrument is less than 1%. Mucous membrane exposure to infected bloody fluid (eg, blood splashed in an eye) has a risk of less than 1 in 1000 of transmitting the virus. The transmission of HIV from direct exposure to saliva or nonbloody mucus in a health care setting is considered virtually impossible. Furthermore, it has been found that prophylactic antiretroviral therapy immediately after an inadvertent stick may further reduce the risk of HIV infection of the HCW. Even though it is unlikely that a HCW will become infected if directly exposed to bloody secretions from an infected host, it is required that such exposures be immediately reported so that adequate surveillance and possible treatment can be initiated. Respiratory therapists must learn and practice universal precautions to prevent exposures, realizing that the risk is small to nonexistent with proper preventive strategies.

CRITICAL CONTENT

PREVENTION

- Public education has had limited success in reducing the incidence of HIV infection.
- The development of a successful vaccine is the only hope to control the worldwide AIDS epidemic.
- HIV infection acquired by HCWs on the job is quite rare.
- Following universal precautions will minimize the risk of HIV transmission in the health care setting.

Pulmonary Complications of HIV Infection

Pulmonary infections are quite common in HIV-infected individuals. Upper respiratory infections, acute bronchitis, and sinusitis will occur early in the course of the infection. Although these conditions are not uncommon in the general population, they are far more prevalent in the HIV infected.

The type and severity of pulmonary infection is related to the state of the immune system. Early in the course of HIV infection, individuals are more susceptible to common pulmonary pathogens that infect the general population. However, as the CD4+ T cell count decreases further, infections that are either rare or nonexistent in the general population become a problem (Table 17-1). In addition, there are some conditions that are considered noninfectious that will occur in severely immunocompromised individuals. What follows is a brief synopsis of the most common pulmonary complications seen in the HIV/AIDS patient.

Pneumocystis carinii Pneumonia (PCP)

Description. PCP is one of the more common pulmonary complications of HIV-infected patients whose CD4+ T cell count is less than $200/mm^3$. The incidence of PCP is approximately 7% per year in this highly immunosuppressed group if they are taking preventive drug therapy, and at least 2 to 3 three times more common if they are not taking drugs to prevent PCP.[7] PCP is caused by a very common organism found everywhere in the world. The organism was originally classified as a protozoa, but it is now thought to be

TABLE 17-1 TIMING OF OPPORTUNISTIC INFECTIONS IN HIV INFECTION

CD4+ COUNT	POSSIBLE INFECTION
>200/mm³	Sinusitis, bronchitis, common bacterial pneumonias, tuberculosis
100–200/mm³	*Pneumocystis carinii, Legionella, Pseudomonas aeruginosa,* lymphoma, Kaposi's sarcoma
50–100/mm³	Cryptococcus and other fungi
<50/mm³	Atypical mycobacteria, cytomegalovirus

a fungus. Most of the world's population have been subclinically infected with *Pneumocystis carinii* by the age of 10, but quickly develop immunity to reinfection. Those with cellular immune deficiencies lose their defenses against this organism and become easily reinfected. The source of the infection is unknown, but *P carinii* is thought to proliferate in environmental reservoirs. However, studies have demonstrated that human-to-human transmission occurs in those who are severely immunocompromised.

The typical clinical picture of PCP in an AIDS patient is fairly nonspecific. These patients are often afebrile, although temperatures of 39° to 40°C are not uncommon. Patients complain of shortness of breath and a cough that is usually nonproductive for days to weeks prior to seeking medical attention. On physical examination, they are frequently tachypneic and may have crackles on auscultation, yet most will initially have normal breath sounds. Commonly they will have a lowered Pao_2 and $Paco_2$ with an increased PAo_2-Pao_2. Infrequently, they may present with chills, weight loss, chest pain, or fatigue.

Routine lab studies are not very helpful as an aid to diagnosis. However, lactate dehydrogenase (LDH) counts are usually elevated and the degree of elevation is somewhat predictive of the severity of the disease. Hypoalbuminemia, anemia, and low lymphocyte counts are also usually present.

The classic chest radiograph presentation for advanced PCP is diffuse, bilateral interstitial or alveolar infiltrates. Early in the course of the disease, the chest film may be either normal or minimally abnormal. Atypical patterns include the presence of cysts, focal or nodular infiltrates, and hilar adenopathy. Rarely, pneumothorax or pleural effusions are also present.

The *P carinii* organism must attach to a host cell in order to proliferate. It preferentially attaches to the alveolar type I cells, which causes damage consistent with the common radiograph findings and the pulmonary function abnormalities present with this infection. Given its propensity to cause parenchymal problems, it primarily causes a restrictive pattern on pulmonary function tests (PFTs),

with a reduction in all lung volumes and a reduced diffusing capacity (D_{co}). However, a reversible obstructive pattern due to airway hyperreactivity is not uncommon in PCP.

The diagnosis of *P carinii* requires the identification of the organism in respiratory secretions. The sample usually can be obtained via sputum induction, accomplished by nebulizing a hypertonic saline solution via an ultrasonic nebulizer or other high-output device. If this technique is unsuccessful, a specimen can be obtained via bronchoscopy with bronchoalveolar lavage (BAL). Recent improvements in staining techniques have made the laboratory diagnosis of *P carinii* relatively simple.

Treatment. The preferred treatment for PCP is with trimethoprim-sulfamethoxazole (TMP-SMX), which is generally effective. However, many AIDS patients cannot tolerate the sulfonamides present in sulfamethoxazole, so trimethoprim and dapsone or IV pentamidine is substituted. Severe cases of PCP may lead to respiratory failure and acute respiratory distress syndrome (ARDS), which require mechanical ventilation. Oral or IV corticosteroids have been found to be helpful in dampening the inflammatory response seen in moderate to severe PCP. Corticosteroids are used early in the course of the disease if the PAo_2-Pao_2 gradient increases to over 35 torr. Use of corticosteroids significantly decreases the risk of respiratory failure and death in PCP.

Many studies have validated the value of prophylactic drug therapy to prevent PCP in HIV-infected individuals with low CD4+ counts. Since the advent of therapy, PCP as the cause of death in AIDS patients has dropped from 33% to 14%.[8] In the past, 300 mg of aerosolized pentamidine, given once a month via a Respirgard II™ nebulizer, was the drug of choice to prevent PCP. Due to lower costs, somewhat greater effectiveness, and fewer side effects, one daily double-strength tablet of TMP-SMZ is now recommended for HIV-infected individuals whose CD4+ counts are less than 200/mm³, or those who have an unexplained fever or oral thrush.[8] Whenever TMP-SMX is not tolerated, either dapsone can be given orally or pentamidine via inhalation.

CRITICAL CONTENT

PNEUMOCYSTIS CARINII PNEUMONIA

- It is a common cause of pneumonia in HIV-infected individuals with low CD4+ counts.
- Signs and symptoms include hypoxemia, tachypnea, and dry cough.
- Diagnosis requires identification of organisms in respiratory secretions via staining.
- It can cause respiratory failure and ARDS.
- One daily tablet of TMP-SMX can both treat and generally prevent PCP.

Tuberculosis. Tuberculosis is by far the most common opportunistic infection in the HIV-infected population worldwide. In the United States, the rate of TB in the HIV-infected population is now almost as high as the rate of PCP, and in some locations (eg, New York City) it is even higher. The incidence of TB is greater in IDUs with HIV infection than in males whose infection is associated with unprotected sex with other males. Unlike PCP, TB will occur much sooner in the course of HIV infection, when CD4+ T cell counts are still over 200/mm^3. HIV-infected individuals are susceptible to both new infections (primary TB), or can have bacteria which have been dormant in their body suddenly begin to multiply rapidly (reactivation TB). Since TB and HIV infection are so commonly coexistent, it is suggested that testing for one should ensue after diagnosing the other. The particular problems related to the diagnosis and treatment of TB in the HIV-infected is discussed later in this chapter.

Bacterial Pneumonia. Pneumonia caused by common community-acquired bacteria has replaced *P carinii* as the most common serious pulmonary complication of HIV infection. The most common organisms are *Haemophilus influenzae* and *Strepto-coccus pneumoniae*. The first bout of bacterial pneumonia will frequently occur before the diagnosis of AIDS, when the CD4+ T cell counts are still greater than 200/mm^3. These infections occur even though cellular immunity controlled by the T cells is still not seriously impaired. It has been found that the B lymphocytes controlling humoral immunity and neutrophil function are also impaired in HIV infection. Organisms causing pneumonia that are more rare and usually do not infect until the CD4+ T cell count drops to less than 200/mm^3 include *Legionella, Staphylococcus aureus,* and *Pseudomonas aeruginosa*.

The clinical pictures of bacterial pneumonias in HIV-infected patients are no different than those for the general population, and include fever, cough, and dyspnea. Unlike in PCP, the CBC will usually show an elevated white count or at least an increase in immature neutrophils. Also, in bacterial pneumonia the onset of symptoms is usually more acute than in PCP, and the LDH level is rarely as elevated as it commonly is in PCP. A diagnosis can also be elucidated by a chest radiograph, in which infiltrates are more likely to be patchy or lobar, rather than diffuse as in PCP. Sputum Gram's stains and cultures may be helpful in making a definitive diagnosis.

Treatment for bacterial pneumonia includes a course of antibiotics specific for the particular organism. Studies have indicated that the regimen of TMP-SMX used to prevent PCP is also helpful in decreasing the incidence of recurrent bacterial pneumonia in the AIDS patient.

Atypical Mycobacteria. With the successful reduction of PCP with prophylactic therapy, the incidence of infection from nontuberculous mycobacteria has increased dramatically. This infection is uncommon in the immunocompetent population and usually will not infect an AIDS patient until the CD4+ T cell count drops to less than 50/mm^3. By far the most common infectious agent in this class is *Mycobacterium avium* complex (MAC), although the infection can also be caused by *M kansasii* and other even rarer mycobacteria.

MAC is commonly found in soil nearly everywhere and in tap water in many parts of the US.

Though the disease is frequently in the lung, the organism is also disseminated throughout the body far more than is *M tuberculosis*. This disease is usually diagnosed via blood culture. It is important to note that sputum that is positive for acid-fast bacillus (AFB) can be an indication of infection with MAC as well as with *M tuberculosis*. Medication to prevent MAC infection has been successful in reducing the incidence of this opportunistic infection.

Fungal Infections. AIDS patients are susceptible to a number of serious fungal diseases endemic to their area as their CD4+ T cell counts drop to less than 100/mm^3. These infections, such as coccidoidomycosis and histoplasmosis, usually originate in the lung and will frequently disseminate to other organ systems in the severely immunocompromised host. Often their clinical presentation can be mistaken for that of TB or PCP, and diagnosis cannot be made without isolating the fungi responsible for the disease. Treatment may require the administration of amphotericin B, a highly toxic antifungal agent, although other, less toxic antifungal agents may be successful.

Cryptococcal infections are seen in approximately 7% of all AIDS patients. The fungus normally enters the body via the lung, but will cause infection only in the severely immunocompromised host. Pulmonary symptoms of cough, dyspnea, chest pain, and low-grade fever often precede the neurologic symptoms associated with cryptococcal meningitis. Fluconazole is given both for treatment and as a preventive agent for this dreaded disease.

Viral Infections. HIV itself has been found to be present in high concentrations in the lung in some cases and it can damage the alveolar macrophages. It is believed that HIV plays a role in the development of lymphoid interstitial pneumonitis (LIP), which is a fairly rare complication of AIDS.

The most common opportunistic viral agent in AIDS patients with low CD4+ T cell counts is cytomegalovirus (CMV), which is present in up to 90% of cases of advanced HIV infection. It infects other organ systems as well as the lungs. Though pulmonary CMV infections are commonly seen to coexist with PCP, CMV pneumonitis alone can lead to respiratory failure and death. Antiviral agents such as ganciclovir are of some value in both treating and preventing severe CMV infections.

Other viruses that can cause viral pneumonitis in AIDS patients are the herpes simplex virus (HSV) and varicella-zoster virus (VZV). Both can be treated and possibly prevented by acyclovir. Though the Epstein-Barr virus does not appear to cause pneumonia, its presence seems to play some role in the development of both LIP and B cell lymphoma in AIDS patients.

Malignancies and Noninfectious Pulmonary Complications. In the early years of the epidemic, many homosexual males would present with rare purplish skin lesions that were identified as Kaposi's sarcoma (KS). These are malignant lesions that often also develop on the walls of the bronchi and in the lung parenchyma. Though it is fairly common in homosexual and bisexual men who are HIV infected, it is quite rare in other high-risk groups. It has been found that Kaposi's sarcoma herpes simplex virus (KSHV) is usually present within these lesions, but whether the virus is a causative agent is unknown.

When the lesions form on the trachea or large bronchi, they can usually be identified via bronchoscopy. Parenchymal or smaller airway lesions are difficult to diagnose. Chemotherapeutic agents and radiation to treat these lesions are considered to be palliative but noncurative. Antiviral agents have been found to reduce the size of the lesions. The prognosis is poor for those with pulmonary KS lesions.

Other malignancies seen in advanced HIV infection include non-Hodgkin's lymphoma (NHL) and increased rates of lung cancer. NHL has been associated with infection with the Epstein-Barr virus and lung cancer occurs only in HIV patients with a history of smoking. Prognosis is poor in all HIV-related lung malignancies.

Noninfectious complications of HIV infection include LIP, pulmonary lymphoid hyperplasia (primarily seen in children), and nonspecific interstitial pneumonitis. As interstitial lung diseases, they are associated with decreased diffusing capacity (D_{co}), and often improve with the administration of corticosteroids.

CRITICAL CONTENT

PULMONARY INFECTIONS COMPLICATING AIDS

- AIDS patients are vulnerable to a number of opportunistic pulmonary infections.
- PCP, TB, and bacterial pneumonias are common pathogens.
- The AIDS patient is also susceptible to rare mycobacterial, fungal, and viral infections, as well as malignancies.
- The CD4+ count is useful to determine a regimen of medications to prevent the incidence of opportunistic infections in AIDS patients.
- The CD4+ count, as well as other diagnostic techniques, are all also useful in the differential diagnosis of these conditions.

TUBERCULOSIS

Unlike AIDS, tuberculosis is a disease that has afflicted mankind since ancient times. Pathologic findings consistent with TB have been found in the remains of mummies in ancient Egypt as well as in persons in South America, all of which predate European visits to the New World. A severe problem throughout recorded history, it probably reached its peak during the industrial revolution, when it is estimated that TB was the cause of death in one out of four people. As we shall see later, the high rates of TB during this era can be attributed to the causes of the disease, and this will be instructive in our understanding of how to control the transmission of TB.

Incidence

Though TB was quite common in the US at the beginning of this century, the discovery of effective antituberculosis agents in the 1940s and the implementation of public health policies of surveillance and treatment were successful in markedly reducing the incidence of TB. Indeed, by the late 1970s, many infectious disease experts felt that the virtual elimination of active TB in the US was a goal attainable by the year 2000.[9]

However, three factors contributed to an alarming increase in active TB in the US. In the mid-1980s, public health funds were siphoned away from TB surveillance and treatment programs to treat the alarming increase in AIDS cases in this country. Second, approximately one quarter of all those infected with HIV in the US also acquire active TB.[10] Third, there has been a significant increase in immigration of people from Third World countries into the US in the last two decades. Though applicants are excluded from admission into the US if they have active disease, many have been infected in their native countries and develop active TB after establishing residency here.[11] Also, in the early 1990s there were outbreaks of multidrug-resistant tuberculosis cases (MDR TB) in health care facilities, primarily in New York and New Jersey. This outbreak was caused by genetic mutation of the *M tuberculosis* organism in individuals who failed to complete the prescribed course of antituberculosis therapy and also had HIV infection, and this form of the disease had an alarmingly high mortality rate. For this reason the CDC announced stringent guidelines for the prevention of transmission of TB.[10]

The implementation of these guidelines has reduced the incidence of tuberculosis in the United States by 25% in the last 5 years. In 1998, there were approximately 18,000 cases of TB in the United States (7 cases per 100,000 of the population).[12] The incidence is not evenly distributed. The highest incidence is in the borough of Harlem, where the case rate is over 300 per 100,000, nearly 50 times greater than the incidence for the US at large. Twenty percent of the active US cases were in California and nearly 50% of the cases were in the four states with the highest immigrant population: California, New York, Texas, and Florida. Approximately 8% of these cases have been found to be resistant to isoniazid (INH), the primary anti-tuberculosis agent, and 1.3% of these cases were resistant to both INH and rifampin, and therefore qualified as MDR TB.

Unfortunately, the statistics for TB worldwide are dismal. Always common in many Third World countries, the worldwide AIDS epidemic has only made these statistics worse. The World Health Organization (WHO) estimates that approximately one in three individuals has been infected with TB. TB is the number two cause of death by communicable disease worldwide, surpassed only recently by HIV infection. It is estimated that about 2 million people die each year of TB. With proper treatment most of these deaths could be prevented. Unlike in the US, worldwide the incidence of TB has risen by approximately 16% from 1992 to 1996. Since the rate of TB infection is much higher globally than in the US, those outside the US who have been infected by HIV have a much greater risk of being exposed to *M tuberculosis*. It is estimated that approximately one out of every three HIV-infected persons in the world also acquires active TB.

The most important factors in controlling the incidence of TB in the US are the timely identification, diagnosis, isolation, and treatment of those who have active TB. It is vitally important, therefore, to understand the factors that increase the risk of contracting this disease. Those who are at high risk of acquiring active TB can be divided into two general categories: those who have come into close contact with persons with active TB and those who are immunocompromised. The most prevalent group in the first category is foreign-born individuals from areas of the world in which TB is endemic (ie, Asia, Africa, the Caribbean, Latin America, and the Pacific Islands). Approximately 39% of all TB cases in the US in 1997 were in immigrants and 22% of these patients were born in Mexico.[11] Also at high risk are family members who live with foreign-born immigrants from these areas. Although legal immigrants are screened via chest radiograph for active TB, tuberculin skin tests are not routinely done. Of course, it is impossible to screen illegal immigrants. The majority of immigrants who develop TB have most likely been infected in their native countries and have a clinical picture consistent with reactivation TB.

Other groups who are at higher risk are the homeless, blacks, American Indians, and native-born Hispanics, especially if they live in inner cities in which the prevalence of TB is high. The reasons for this are primarily socioeconomic. Those who live in crowded conditions in which ventilation is poor are more likely to inhale the TB organism. Nursing home residents and prison inmates are also at high risk for developing active TB. Prevalence of TB is high in both of these populations. The elderly in skilled nursing facilities are likely to have medical conditions described later that make it more likely for them to progress to active TB after infection. TB is common in prisons for two reasons. Overcrowded living conditions found in US prisons increase the risk of transmission of *M tuberculosis*. Second, once exposed, more will develop active TB since many prisoners are already immunocompromised secondary to prior HIV infection.

Health care workers and prison guards are also at high risk of becoming infected with TB by virtue of their increased risk of coming into contact with persons with active TB. Pulmonologists and respiratory therapists are probably at the greatest risk of TB infection since they engage in cough-inducing procedures such as bronchoscopy, intubation, and sputum induction. Since 17 HCWs have been reported to have acquired active MDR TB in the last decade, and 4 have died, it is vitally important that RTs minimize this risk by being aware of this risk and by adhering to the CDC's prevention guidelines described later.[13]

Once infected, the risk is about 10% that an individual will progress to active TB at sometime in their lives. However, as in any infectious disease, the risk is much greater in a susceptible host. Besides those infected with HIV, others at greater risk of developing active TB once infected include those on chronic oral steroid therapy, young children, chronic dialysis patients, the malnourished, insulin-dependent diabetics, and patients with silicosis. Of special importance is the role of recent infection in acquiring the active phase of disease. Approximately 75% of those infected and untreated who develop active TB will do so within 2 years after the initial infection. The risk of acquiring active TB for those who have had a positive tuberculin skin test for more than 2 years drops to less than 3%.[9]

CRITICAL CONTENT

INCIDENCE OF TB

- TB is the second leading cause of death by infectious disease worldwide.
- The relaxation of public health standards, HIV infection, and immigration of TB-positive persons caused a spike in the incidence of TB in US in the late 1980s.
- Stringent TB surveillance has led to a decline in active TB in the US since 1993.
- The current incidence of TB in the US is 7 per 100,000 in the general population.
- Immigrants and those infected with HIV are at greatest risk.
- The incidence of TB is greatest in states with large numbers of recent immigrants.
- HCWs and RTs in particular are at high risk of acquiring TB infection.
- The TB epidemic is getting worse worldwide.

Infection and Transmission

Tuberculosis is almost always caused by the inhalation of droplet nuclei 1 to 5 microns in diameter containing the *Mycobacterium tuberculosis* bacillus. Although TB may be acquired by the ingestion of *M bovis* in milk from infected cows, this mode of transmission is virtually nonexistent in the US. The likelihood of transmission from one infected person to another is dependent on a number of factors. Most important is the concentration of bacteria in the air expelled by the infected person when they cough. Individuals with either laryngeal TB or pulmonary TB with cavitation cough up the greatest concentration of bacteria aerosolized in the particle size range optimal for the transmission

of the organism to another person. Those with extrapulmonary TB (excluding the upper airway) rarely transmit their infection to others.[9] Another important factor is the length of time the organisms remain suspended in the air. The risk of transmission of the organism is greater in poorly ventilated areas. This feature explains why the incidence of TB skyrocketed in Europe during the industrial revolution, when there was a large migration of persons from the countryside to the cities to work in factories and live in close, poorly ventilated housing. It is also a reason why the incidence of TB is highest in the inner cities in the US, where the population density is highest.

The risk of infecting others is greatest from those individuals who are coughing frequently, expectorating high concentrations of TB organisms, and are unaware they have active TB. Once a diagnosis is made and a therapy regimen begun, the likelihood of infecting others diminishes considerably. This occurs because a brief course of antituberculosis medications will both reduce the number of organisms expelled and the frequency of coughing. Also, once aware, persons with active TB are more likely to cover their mouths when coughing. Although individuals are usually no longer infectious within 2 weeks of initiating standard therapy, those with MDR TB or those who are poorly compliant in taking their medications may remain infectious. The current recommendation is that at least two sputum specimens negative for acid-fast bacilli be obtained before considering the person noncontagious.

Although TB is widespread, it is not as contagious as one might think. Fewer than one in three persons in close household contact with a family member with active TB will become infected. The untreated person with active TB, on average, will infect about 10 to 15 persons over a 1-year period. The organism is usually deposited in the middle and lower lobes of the lung, where ventilation is greatest. The initial infection is usually mild and confined to a local inflammatory response, and often the person is unaware of any symptoms. The organism will spread via the lymphatic system throughout the body. Usually these organisms will be quickly subdued, though not eradicated, by a normally functioning immune system. Only 3% to 5% of persons initially infected will develop active TB within the first year after infection. Those who are most likely to do so are children and the immunocompromised (as described earlier). HIV-infected persons are 100 times more likely to develop active TB after being newly infected, and those diagnosed with AIDS are more than 300 times more likely to develop active TB.[10] If this new infection progresses to active disease and is confined to the lung, it is termed *primary TB*. The pathology is seen primarily in the middle and lower lobes, and its radiographic features will be described later.

Since TB is an aerophilic organism that grows best in areas where the Po_2 is 100 to 140 torr and the pH is slightly alkaline, it will proliferate better in the lung than in other tissues, and grows best in the apices, where the Pao_2 is the highest and the $Paco_2$ is lowest. However, active TB may occur in almost any other organ system. The more common sites for infection include the lymphatic system, the pleura, the bones and joints, the gastrointestinal system, and the urinary tract. Extrapulmonary TB, like primary pulmonary TB, has always been more common in children and the immunocompromised. With the advent of the AIDS epidemic in the US, the proportion of extrapulmonary TB has increased from 15% to 22% of all cases.[9] The worst extrapulmonary types of TB are TB meningitis and disseminated or miliary TB, both of which have a much higher mortality rate than any other form of TB.

Infected adults who are immunocompetent will usually not acquire either primary or extrapulmonary TB. However, TB organisms reproduce much more slowly than other bacteria. Further, they can become encapsulated and remain dormant for months to decades. Either spontaneously or to due to conditions in the host that render it more susceptible to infection, the TB organisms will again reactivate and proliferate. Reactivation TB will most likely occur in the upper lobes or the superior segments of the lower lobes, where conditions are the most conducive for the reproduction of TB bacteria. Cavitations are seen exclusively with reactivation TB. The characteristic radiographic findings of reactivation TB are described as "typical" (described later).

TB that is resistant to two or more common antituberculosis medications is a serious health hazard. Individuals at risk for this multidrug resistant TB (MDR TB) include those previously treated for TB who either did not comply with the treatment regimen or were improperly treated. Insufficient doses of bactericidal anti-TB drugs or the use of only one drug in active disease have led to genetic mutations of organisms that resist the bactericidal activity of the more potent anti-TB medications. Another risk factor is individuals who come into close contact with persons with MDR TB. Immigrants from southeast Asia, South America, and the Caribbean have a high incidence of MDR TB. Sixty percent of the cases of MDR TB in this country have occurred in New York and New Jersey.[14] There was a high mortality rate of patients infected with MDR TB in hospital outbreaks between 1988 and 1992. However, 90% of those who died also had coexisting HIV infection, including the 4 HCWs already mentioned. It is now thought that MDR TB in the immunocompetent host is curable, if quickly identified and properly treated.

Other mycobacteria have been found to be pathogenic to man and can produce pulmonary disease. Usually these pathogens, termed *atypical* or *nontuberculous mycobacteria*, will cause disease in immunocompromised hosts such as those with AIDS. *Mycobacterium avium-intracellulare* and *M kansasii* are the more common organisms in this class that may cause or exacerbate preexisting pulmonary disease. Unlike *M tuberculosis* these organisms do not appear to be contagious.

CRITICAL CONTENT

INFECTION AND TRANSMISSION OF TUBERCULOSIS

- Infection is caused by inhalation of droplets containing *M tuberculosis* expelled by someone with active TB.
- Initial infection is usually mild and easily controlled by a normally functioning immune system.

- Only children and immunosuppressed persons usually progress to primary TB.
- *M tuberculosis* TB can be dormant in the host for decades. Reactivation TB occurs in upper lobes when the host's defense mechanisms weaken.
- TB infections can occur in organ systems other than the lungs (extrapulmonary TB).
- MDR TB is defined as TB infections caused by organisms resistant to two or more antitubercular drugs.

Clinical Picture and Pathophysiology

A patient with active pulmonary TB may have no symptoms whatsoever or may complain only of a persistent cough that can be productive or nonproductive. Other symptoms can include fever, general malaise, dyspnea, sweats or chills, anorexia, and weight loss. Chest pain and dyspnea are sometimes seen but usually only in cases in which there is also pleural involvement. The physical examination is usually normal, but crackles or bronchial breath sounds may be heard on auscultation in some cases.

Typical laboratory findings are generally nonspecific. A mild elevation in white blood cell count may be present as well as a mild anemia, but the CBC is usually normal. Low ventilation/perfusion ratios are minimized since the area of the lung affected in reactivation TB is primarily in the upper lobes. Thus, ABGs are also usually normal, though there may be slight hypoxemia present in TB without any coexisting pathology present. Hypercalcemia and hypokalemia are the only abnormalities in blood chemistry associated with active TB, and these findings are present only infrequently.

Since the infiltrative process primarily occurs in the lung parenchyma of the upper lobes where ventilation is normally lowest, reactivation TB will cause only a mild restrictive defect with a small loss of lung volume. Primary TB, if extensive and accompanied by pleural effusion, will tend to cause a greater loss of lung volume.

The classic radiologic findings seen in TB are associated with reactivation TB, most commonly seen in the adult population. Opacities are most often seen in the upper lobes, and cavitations, sometimes with an air-fluid level, are seen in approximately 50% of cases.[10] Fibronodular lesions are also common in the upper lobes. Bronchiectasis, pleural thickening, and volume loss, though less frequent, may also be seen in reactivation TB. Though radiograph findings are never considered diagnostic, upper lobe opacities, especially when cavitation is present, are often considered presumptive of active TB when accompanied by a positive tuberculin skin test.

Children and HIV-infected patients are more likely to have the atypical radiologic findings seen in primary TB. These findings are less specific and can be seen in many other pulmonary abnormalities. Atelectasis and consolidation are seen more often in the lower lobes. Lymphadenopathy is a common finding in children (96%) and is also seen 46% of the time in adults with primary TB. Pleural effusions and diffuse miliary lesions (tiny densities that look like seeds) are infrequently present.

CRITICAL CONTENT

CLINICAL PICTURE AND PATHOPHYSIOLOGY OF TB

- Symptoms and physical findings of active TB are nonspecific. The most common symptoms include cough and crackles over the affected area.
- Classic chest radiograph findings are seen in reactivation TB only and include upper lobe infiltrates and cavity formation.
- Atypical chest radiograph findings are seen in primary TB.

Diagnosis

The key to prevention of the spread of TB is the quick identification, diagnosis, isolation, and treatment of individuals with active TB. Unfortunately, the diagnosis of TB is multifaceted and often problematic.

The first step in the diagnosis of TB is careful history taking, to identify patients who have a high risk of active TB. One should have a high degree of suspicion for individuals with pulmonary symptoms whose country of origin, socioeconomic status, residence (eg, nursing home or correctional facility), and occupation (eg, health care worker or prison guard) increase the likelihood of active TB.

Tuberculin Skin Test. A tuberculin skin test is administered to persons at high risk or those with a chest radiograph consistent with reactivation TB. A small amount of inert purified protein derivative (PPD) of M tuberculosis is injected intracutaneously (Mantoux method) into the forearm. If the individual has specific antibodies to TB, a delayed hypersensitivity reaction will be seen within 48 to 72 hours after injection. A positive reaction is usually an induration or hardening of the skin of greater than 10 to 15 mm in diameter. Reactions of 5 to 10 mm are considered positive in a person with HIV infection.

It must be understood that a positive PPD is only indicative of latent TB infection. It is of no help in determining whether an individual has active TB. Furthermore, there are cases in which a patient may have active TB, but will have a negative tuberculin skin test. Coexisting HIV infection can make the diagnosis of tuberculosis a bit more problematic. A positive skin test for TB relies on an intact cellular immune system. A false negative PPD is seen in 10% to 25% of all persons with active TB and over 50% of severely immunocompromised patients such as HIV-infected individuals with a CD4+ count of less than 200.[10] AIDS patients will often not react to any skin antigen test (anergy), and those with coexisting TB will often have a false negative or a minimally reactive skin test. The elderly and those who have had many TB skin tests may have what has been called the booster reaction and may not react at all to the first TB skin test, but will react positively if reinjected with tuberculin 7 days after the first injection.

A false positive reaction can be seen in those who have been inoculated with the bacille Calmette-Guérin (BCG) vaccine. The BCG vaccine is used in countries in which M tuberculosis is epidemic, where it seems to limit the incidence of extrapulmonary TB in children and reduces somewhat the conversion from latent to active TB in some individuals. However, since BCG is not a very effective vaccine and because it causes difficulty in interpreting a TB skin test, it has never been used extensively in the US. Other false positive reactions can occur in those who have been exposed to some non-TB mycobacterium (such as M avium) or to improper administration of the Mantoux skin test. Because of the ambiguities in the interpretation of the tuberculin skin test, research has been done on the use of a blood test to screen for active TB. To date, no blood test has been developed that is sufficiently sensitive and specific to merit the increased costs a change to this method of screening would bring.

Chest X-Ray. The next step in the diagnosis of TB is a chest radiograph. A normal chest film in the presence of a positive PPD test rules out active TB. These individuals are considered to have latent TB infection only. Future TB skin tests on these individuals are unnecessary and will require follow-up x-rays only if they develop symptoms suggestive of active TB. An abnormal chest radiograph alone is never diagnostic for active TB. Characteristic radiographic findings (described earlier) are a useful aid in the diagnosis of reactivation TB, but tend to be too nonspecific to be of much use in diagnosing primary TB. Since a person who has once been treated for active TB will have residual radiographic abnormalities, it is difficult to rule out active TB via chest radiograph in those who have been successfully treated previously for TB.

Sputum Sample. A sputum sample will next be collected, either spontaneously or via induced sputum or bronchoscopy, on individuals with an abnormal chest radiograph having a positive skin test, or those with a negative test if suspicion is high that they have active TB (ie, HIV-infected individuals with low CD4+ counts). The sputum sample for acid-fast bacillus (AFB) is stained with the Ziehl-Neelsen stain. The advantages of this test are that the results of a positive stain can be obtained are almost immediately, and it has a specificity for *M tuberculosis* of 80% or more.[10] However, a positive test will also occur due to infection with atypical mycobacteria. The disadvantage is that a sample usually requires a large number of organisms in order to test positive. Patients with laryngeal TB or reactivation TB with cavitations are the most likely to test AFB positive. Of course, these are the very patients who are most likely to spread TB. However, the sputum culture will be negative about half the time in patients who subsequently are diagnosed as having active TB. Further, a positive AFB result is seen less than 40% of the time in children and those who are HIV positive. Both children and HIV-positive cases with coexistent active TB are unlikely to have cavitary TB and thus are unlikely to yield positive results. To increase the odds of detection, sputum collection for AFB is usually done once a day for 3 successive days. A new technique for the initial screen, called a fluorescent antibody test, is currently being used at larger institutions with a high number of TB cases to supplement the information obtained via the standard acid-fast technique.

Since a negative AFB does not rule out TB and a positive AFB may result from the presence of a non-TB mycobacterium, a more definitive diagnosis must await the outcome of an actual culture. Unfortunately, until recently this took a minimum of 3 to 8 weeks. Furthermore, it takes additional time to find out whether the organism cultured is resistant to two or more of the common antituberculous drugs (indicative of MDR TB). In 1998, new radiometric broth and molecular probe techniques were perfected that will lead to definitive identification of *M tuberculosis* in an average of 9 days, and the drug susceptibility study can be obtained 5 days after its identification.[15] Also, a great deal of research is currently being conducted in this area and tests have been developed employing PCR technology (such as BACTEC and MTD), which have reduced the time needed for identification of TB to as little 5 hours. Unfortunately these tests are expensive and may actually be too sensitive. Positive tests for genetic sequences peculiar to TB may be found in individuals who had been

infected but never had, and do not currently have, active TB. The chief value of these new tests may be that they will quickly differentiate between the AFB-positive smears caused by *M tuberculosis* and those caused by some atypical mycobacterium.

CRITICAL CONTENT

DIAGNOSIS OF TB

- A positive PPD skin test only documents exposure to TB, not active infection.
- The chest x-ray is the next diagnostic tool. If it is abnormal, a sputum specimen is obtained.
- Acid-fast staining of sputum to identify mycobacterium is next. Other non-TB mycobacteria can also stain AFB positive. Sputum AFB testing is done three times to increase the likelihood of identification.
- Culture of TB in sputum is definitive of diagnosis and now takes an average of 9 days, with drug sensitivity testing taking 5 more days.

Treatment

With the discovery of streptomycin in the 1940s, the incidence and morbidity of TB began to drop precipitously in the US. However, it was soon discovered that TB bacilli could quickly develop resistance to this drug as well as any other chemotherapeutic agent. Like HIV infection, a multiple drug strategy had been found to be essential in the successful treatment of active TB.

The risk of developing active TB is approximately 10% over the lifetime of a person who has recently developed a positive PPD skin test but does not have active TB. Consequently, a 6- to 12-month regimen of isoniazid (INH) is usually prescribed when a positive PPD is found. However, INH therapy is not without risks, the most serious of which is that it may cause hepatitis. The risk of INH-induced hepatitis is less than 1% in the general population. The risk increases with alcohol use and

PART II • PATIENT PROBLEMS IN RESPIRATORY CARE

with increasing age. INH hepatitis has a 10% mortality rate. Other side effects include peripheral neuropathy, anemia, and gastrointestinal complaints. For this reason, guidelines have been developed to aid the prescribing physician in determining the cost/benefit analysis of INH therapy. Liver function tests are done at the outset of therapy and periodically during the course of therapy. In general, INH is recommended regardless of age for recent PPD skin converters and for all PPD-positive HIV-infected patients, as well as those who are PPD negative but have had close contact with an active case. INH is also recommended for PPD-positive individuals younger than 35 who were born in a country with a high incidence of TB, even when the time of skin conversion is unknown. Prophylactic INH therapy is also recommended in all PPD-positive cases in persons whose medical condition (ie, silicosis or long-term steroid therapy) will likely increase their risk of contracting active TB.

Preventive INH therapy is very effective, especially if taken for 12 months. Yet therapy does not completely eliminate the risk of contracting active TB, and its value diminishes with time. Although a course of therapy may virtually eliminate the risk of active disease for the subsequent decade, it is conceivable that some TB organisms, long dormant, may cause reactivation TB much later in life. In cases in which the organism is INH-resistant, INH will have no value whatsoever. With recent converters, efforts should be made to determine the likely person who passed on the organism and whether the sputum culture in that case was resistant to INH. A 6- to 9-month course of rifampin seems to be an effective preventive therapy for an INH-resistant, latent TB infection. In the small percentage of cases that have been infected with an organism that is resistant to both INH and rifampin, a multidrug regimen is necessary for effective prophylaxis.

For the HIV infected, the CDC also recommends that TB preventive therapy with INH be taken at least 3 months longer than is recommended for the general population by those with a positive PPD skin test. The CDC also recommends INH therapy for those anergic AIDS patients who have had a high risk of exposure to TB. A three- to four-drug regimen is recommended for 2 months for preventive treatment of those in whom there is a high index of suspicion that the patient may have been exposed to INH-resistant TB.

Active TB, even MDR TB, is amenable to successful chemotherapeutic treatment if care is taken to prescribe the right group of drugs, careful surveillance to ensure therapeutic response is carried out, and monitoring is done to ensure that the patient is compliant in taking all medications. Treatment can generally be done in an outpatient setting unless the case is severe or there are complicating factors that require hospitalization. The usual strategy is to give high doses initially of at least three medications for 2 to 3 months. This strategy should quickly decrease the population of bacteria, thereby decreasing coughing and improving the radiographic appearance of tubercular lesions. The strategy is then to continue the therapy for a total of 6 to 12 months, perhaps with lower dosages or different drugs, to kill bacteria that had been dormant or encapsulated and thus had eluded the initial therapy regimen.

The most common drugs first prescribed are isoniazid (INH), rifampin, and pyrazinamide. The CDC recommends that drug sensitivity testing be done on all cultures and the drug regimen adjusted if the results indicate resistance to one or more of the preparations. Other first-line drugs that can be prescribed initially because of their bactericidal activity include streptomycin and ethambutol.

For the HIV infected, it is recommended that a four-, rather than the standard three-drug regimen be instituted. Treatment regimens often must be longer for HIV-infected patients to prevent a relapse of the infection. Rifampin is contraindicated for AIDS patients who are also taking protease inhibitors and the drug rifabutin is commonly substituted.[16] HIV-infected patients are much more likely to suffer adverse reactions to the standard antituberculosis medications. During therapy one must watch for adverse reactions. In addition to those previously described, others include flu-like symptoms caused by hypersensitivity to one or more of the medications, nausea, vomiting, and anorexia.

Treatment failures occur due to poor patient compliance with taking the prescribed course of medication, failure to order a proper regimen of antituberculosis medications, and failure to properly monitor whether the prescribed medications are effective. The first problem has been rectified in many parts of the US by the use of directly observed therapy (DOT). Patients are required to take their medication in front of a health care worker. These programs are administered by county public health departments, which send workers to the home to dispense and observe that the medication is actually taken. Those who fail to comply are subject to arrest and imprisonment in some locales in the US. The last two problems can be rectified by referring patients with active TB to specialists who are familiar with the latest guidelines published by the CDC and the American Thoracic Society. This is especially important in areas where there is a high incidence of MDR TB. It is also important for patients who are also HIV infected. For reasons that are not entirely clear, HIV-infected individuals are more likely to be infected with TB organisms that are resistant to the common antituberculosis medications. It is therefore recommended that drug sensitivity testing be done to ensure that the medications ordered are effective. In these cases it is important to start with at least a four- and sometimes a six-drug regimen. Treatment for MDR TB includes the use of second-line TB drugs not listed above.

Treatment regimens can last as long as 24 months. In treating active TB, it is also important to get sputum for culture at monthly intervals to ensure that cultures remain negative. It is also recommended that sputum be obtained every 3 months for 9 months after the completion of therapy to ensure that relapse has not occurred.

CRITICAL CONTENT

TREATMENT

- Isoniazid (INH) is given to a recent PPD converter (latent TB).
- Multidrug therapy is given for both active TB and MDR TB.
- Periodic AFB sputum smears are done to ensure effectiveness of the drug regimen.
- Directly observed therapy (DOT) is instituted to ensure that the patient actually takes all medications.

Prevention

After the significant increase in active TB in the US from 1986 to 1992, the CDC, in concert with the nation's public health departments, implemented a number of policies that have been responsible for the 25% decrease in the incidence of active TB from 1992 to 1997. Once again there is some optimism that the US may reach the goal established by the Advisory Council for the Elimination of Tuberculosis (ACET), that of virtually eliminating TB as a public health hazard by the year 2010.

Chief among these efforts are policies to limit the rate of active TB among those born outside the US who acquire active TB after entering this country. Immigrants account for nearly 40% of the new active TB cases in the US each year. The evidence indicates that the majority of these cases are believed to be cases of reactivation TB. Though no one is admitted legally into this country without first having a negative chest film for active TB, little follow-up is done upon admission to those who have radiographic evidence of scar tissue consistent with prior TB infection. Further, the incidence of MDR TB is higher among the immigrant population than in native born persons with active TB.[11] DNA testing of isolates of the TB culture has shown that most immigrants with active TB were infected in their native country, many with multidrug-resistant organisms. The CDC has recently published recommendations for prevention and control of TB in the immigrant population.[11] These guidelines call for increased surveillance of the foreign born who have evidence of TB infection without active TB in order to determine if they acquire active TB after entering the country.

After declines in public funding for the control of TB in the 1970s and early 1980s, the US has recently nearly doubled its budgetary allocations to public health departments. The role of public health is to ensure that those with active TB actually take the full course of chemotherapeutic agents prescribed. The method used for this is DOT, which was described earlier. Public health workers also investigate those who have been in close contact with individuals with active TB, screen for latent infection, and ensure, when appropriate, that prophylactic therapy is begun. The added vigilance by the CDC and public health departments has not only been effective in decreasing the total incidence of TB; policies to control the incidence of TB in the HIV-infected population have also been successful. Even though the number of individuals living with AIDS has increased, the total number of these patients with active TB has actually decreased.

Prevention in Health Care Facilities. More important to the RT are the recommendations of the CDC on how to prevent the transmission of TB to both HCWs and to patients in the hospital.[17] These guidelines arose due to the alarming rate of transmission of TB to HIV-infected individuals and to HCWs in the late 1980s. By far the most important guideline is the early identification, isolation, and prompt treatment of those with active TB. RTs should assist by maintaining a high index of suspicion of a patient with pulmonary symptoms who is in a group with a high risk for TB. Questions to ask are whether they are from a geographic area known to be at high risk, or if they have come into contact with someone with TB. These patients should be kept in well-ventilated areas and away from immunocompromised individuals until they are evaluated for TB. If the chest film reveals abnormalities that may be consistent with TB, the patient should be isolated *before* a sputum sample for AFB is obtained. At minimum, a high-risk patient with pulmonary symptoms should be asked to wear a surgical mask until he or she can be isolated.

The level of suspicion of possible TB one might have for a patient with pulmonary symptoms is also related to the type of facility at which the therapist is employed. Each health care facility should systematically assess its risk of caring for persons with active TB. A risk assessment should be done, using the CDC guidelines, to determine the risk level of the entire facility, particularly that of patient care areas such as the ER and bronchoscopy room, and of particular occupational groups. (Respiratory care is one of the highest-risk occupations in a health care facility). The results of that risk assessment will dictate what areas of the hospital need to be modified and what workers need to be closely monitored for recent infection.

Since the risk of transmission of TB is directly related to the concentration of droplet nuclei containing the bacteria in the air, the CDC has recommended the adoption of various engineering controls to limit and contain the bacteria dispersed in the hospital environment. Areas such as the ICU, ER, pulmonary function labs, and bronchoscopy and isolation rooms should be modified to increase the rate of ventilation in the room from a minimum of 6 to an optimum of 12 complete air exchanges per hour. Exhaust from these rooms should either be vented outside or cleansed using HEPA filters. Negative air pressure is recommended in these high-risk areas to improve the rate of fresh air ventilation and also to ensure that contaminated air from these rooms will not escape to other patient care areas. Closed, hooded systems with exhaust captured by HEPA filters can be used for sputum induction procedures for outpatients.

In areas where improving the rate of ventilation to the recommended levels is not feasible, the use of ultraviolet lighting in ventilation ducts and at the top of the room is recommended. Ultraviolet radiation emitted by these lamps will kill many of the bacteria dispersed in the air. However, care must be taken to prevent irradiating the air space of the patients and health care workers. Since TB bacteria can remain suspended in the air for long periods of time, it is imperative that the doors to isolation rooms remain closed when a patient with active pulmonary or laryngeal TB is being treated there.

Perhaps the most controversial of the CDC recommendations for the prevention of transmission of TB in health care facilities is their insistence that HCWs wear highly efficient masks when treating patients with suspected or confirmed active TB.[18] The common surgical mask is too porous to be an effective barrier to prevent droplets from being inhaled. The CDC originally recommended that masks used by HCWs to provide protection in active TB cases should meet the following criteria: (1) they must be HEPA-type masks than can filter particles down to 1 micron in size; and (2) a fit testing program was to be instituted to ensure that the mask size selected was actually an effective barrier with minimal leakage. These guidelines were perhaps too stringent, especially the last criterion. Many health care workers complained that these filters significantly increased the work of breathing. Subsequently, OSHA relaxed its standards to certify three types of masks with three levels of filtering efficiency. The lowest level, the N-95 mask, which must filter at least 95% of respirable particulates larger than 1 micron, has become the most common mask used in isolation rooms. However, it is still recommended to wear the higher quality R and P series masks that filter 99% and 99.97% of respirable particulates for bronchoscopy and other cough-inducing procedures.

The RT should assist other health care personnel in ensuring that the patient understands the risk of infecting others and the importance of complying with the therapeutic regimen. At minimum, the patient must be instructed to keep the door of his isolation room closed at all times and to wear a simple surgical mask if he must leave the room. After he leaves the hospital he must be impressed with the importance of covering his mouth when coughing.

CRITICAL CONTENT

TB PREVENTION

- Prevention efforts include identifying and treating patients in high-risk groups (especially foreign-born and HIV-positive individuals).

- Ensure that DOT is implemented in all active TB cases.
- To prevent transmission of infection in health care facilities, efforts should be made to identify and isolate high-risk individuals with abnormal chest radiographs, even before AFB sputum cultures are obtained.
- Well-ventilated and negative pressure rooms should be used for high-risk patients and HCWs should wear HEPA masks when in patient rooms.

Summary

The guidelines and changes in US public health policies discussed previously have been very effective in reducing the incidence of TB. Assuming successful implementation of the new guidelines to increase surveillance of the foreign born who have been infected prior to admission to this country, it is reasonable to think the US might succeed in virtually eliminating TB in the first two decades of the new millennium. However, the outlook worldwide is much less favorable. WHO predicts that more people will come down with active TB in the year 2000 than at any other time in the history of the world. WHO declared in 1993 that the TB epidemic was a global emergency and has issued a number of recommendations to fight this scourge, including the universal use of DOT. Unfortunately, less than half of the world's nations have the financial resources or the political will to fight this epidemic. In test nations that have implemented WHO policies, the cure rate for active TB has been 95%. Despite these efforts, it is estimated that the number of new cases of TB has actually increased by 16% worldwide over the last 4 years. As in the US, the AIDS epidemic is a significant factor in the increase in the number of TB cases. It is likely that TB will not be controlled until a successful vaccine for *M tuberculosis* is discovered and administered worldwide.

SITE- AND AGE-SPECIFIC CONSIDERATIONS

The incidence of TB among children in the US is slightly lower than in the general population. Extrapulmonary TB is seen more frequently, comprising about 30% of cases in children with active TB. Children are less likely to suffer from pulmonary cavitation and are thus generally less contagious than adults with active TB. Children are also less likely to produce sputum that will be positive for acid-fast bacilli, even when they have active pulmonary TB. Since cultures may be negative, a diagnosis of active TB in a child can be made if he or she has been in close contact with another person with active TB, has a positive TB skin test, and chest radiograph abnormalities consistent with TB.

The incidence of HIV among adults over 50 is increasing. In fact, it is the only age group in the US in which the rate of new AIDS cases is increasing. The route of transmission is primarily via heterosexual contact. The reasons for this increase are that older age groups are the least likely to use safe sex precautions. Programs are being implemented to educate persons in this age group on ways to prevent the transmission of the disease.

There has been one major success story in the efforts to prevent the transmission of HIV. Children who are HIV infected generally acquire the virus perinatally from their mothers. The route of transmission can be either the transfer of the virus at the placenta or via breast milk. It has been found that antiretroviral therapy given to the mother during pregnancy and labor, and to the infant for 6 weeks after birth can reduce the perinatal transmission of the virus by nearly 70%. Unfortunately, the cost of this prophylactic therapy is prohibitively high for use in Third World countries. WHO sponsored studies were done to determine if a cheaper, streamlined, alternative of chemoprophylactic therapy could be successful in preventing perinatally-acquired HIV in sub-Saharan nations. These studies were roundly criticized for allowing a control group of women to receive a placebo. However, the studies indicated that antiretroviral therapy during labor alone could reduce the infection rate by about one third.

CONSIDERATION OF COSTS AND ETHICAL ISSUES

The most effective way to limit the sometimes prohibitive costs of treating both TB and HIV infection is to employ effective strategies to prevent their transmission. In the case of TB, the judicious use of prophylactic therapy is much cheaper than treating the actual disease. WHO estimates that the average cost for the treatment of active TB is between $2000 and $3000 per person in industrialized nations. This cost includes the use of directly observed therapy (DOT). However, if the medication regimen is not followed judiciously, the bacteria can become multidrug resistant. The cost of treating a case of MDR TB can rise to nearly a quarter of a million dollars in the US.

WHO estimates that the cost of drug therapy in poorer countries is less than $20 per person and DOT programs could be implemented that would bring the average cost of treating each active TB case in these countries to between $100 and $200. WHO suggests these minimal investments worldwide would be effective and decrease both the incidence and mortality from TB.

The costs of treating the HIV infected are much higher. In the US, it is estimated that advances in antiretroviral and preventive therapy for opportunistic infections has lengthened life expectancy, but has also significantly increased the costs of care. It is estimated that the lifetime cost of care for a single HIV/AIDS patient is approximately a quarter of a million dollars. The monthly cost of drug therapy and clinic visits for a person with a CD4+ count less than $200/mm^3$ is now over $3000. Clearly, these costs for patient care are far beyond the reach of developing nations. Many countries cannot even afford the moderate cost of the standard regimen of antiretroviral therapy for preventing perinatal transmission of HIV from mother to infant. It is for this reason that studies were designed to test the efficacy of treatment regimens to prevent perinatal transmission that these countries could more easily afford.

Despite the World Health Organization's belief in DOT, the CDC remains skeptical that developing countries can afford the sustained investments necessary to make this program work. They feel that the only way in which the incidence and deaths from these two diseases can be controlled worldwide is through the successful development of vaccines for both HIV and TB infection.

These staggering costs for the treatment of HIV infection could raise sensitive ethical issues in the future. Health care economists estimate that if the US adheres to the current standards of medical practice, health care costs will increase dramatically in view of our graying population. Unless changes are made in the allocation of resources, the US will expend 25% of its gross domestic product on health care by 2025. Most expect that the country's economic well-being cannot be sustained with

those kinds of health care expenditures. Rationing care could increasingly become the new reality.

Already rationing is occurring in the care of the HIV infected. Since this disease disproportionately affects minorities and the poor, most of the costs for their care must be borne by the state. In some states, lottery systems are already in place to determine who will receive the full antiretroviral therapy regimen. In others, capitated systems have limited the use of the costly protease inhibitors. In an environment in which health care costs are increasingly scrutinized, AIDS care and research has been aided by the advocacy of the wealthy, educated, homosexual community. However, as the incidence of this infection increases in the less politically powerful poor and minority communities, will the funding for AIDS care decrease? Will the common arguments that the acquisition of this infection is due to inappropriate high-risk "immoral" behavior such as indiscriminate sex and IV drug abuse begin to have a greater impact on public policy decisions?

CASE STUDY 1

MR. IVEY DRUGGERA

Presentation

Mr. Druggera, a 36-year-old, 5 foot 11 inch, 70-kg Hispanic male presents to the emergency department with complaints of weakness and a recent 10-lb weight loss. A chronic cough, productive of small amounts of blood-streaked sputum, has been present for the past several weeks. Night sweats and a low-grade fever were also present.

Critical Thinking Exercise 1

PRIORITIZING PATIENT CARE

You are asked to perform an initial evaluation of this gentleman.

a. List some of the initial questions you would ask Mr. Druggera.

b. What data would you obtain in your initial physical assessment?

Additional historical data obtained indicate that he was born in Haiti and came to New York City in his early twenties. He has lived in New York for 10 years and admitted to having been an IV drug abuser. He states that he has worked in many jobs, primarily as a manual laborer, and has moved frequently in the past 4 years. He has a 20 pack-year smoking history. He also stated that he had been treated for TB before. His initial vital signs and auscultatory findings are as follows:

CASE STUDY 1 *(continued)*

Vital signs

HR	100/min
RR	18/min
BP	110/70
SpO_2	92%
Temperature	38.5°C

Breath sounds were decreased in upper lung fields with mild expiratory wheezes.

Critical Thinking Exercise 2

MAKING INFERENCES BY CLUSTERING DATA

Identify the elements obtained from his history and initial physical assessment that would lead you to the inference that he is at risk of TB and HIV infection.

Two hours later Mr. Druggera is admitted for a full diagnostic work-up and initial therapy. Sputum results are AFB positive. Culture results for *M tuberculosis* are pending. HIV test results are also positive with a CD4+ count of 275/mm³. The CBC reveals a mild anemia and a white cell count of 12,000 (90% polys). His liver enzymes were fairly normal though his LDH level of 200 mU/mL was slightly elevated. (See Figure 17-1 for the chest x-ray results taken at this time.)

Critical Thinking Exercise 3

DECISION MAKING

a. What therapeutic regimen should be instituted for Mr. Druggera? Why?

b. What respiratory therapy modalities would you suggest? Why?

c. How would you monitor the patient to assess the response to each therapy you listed above?

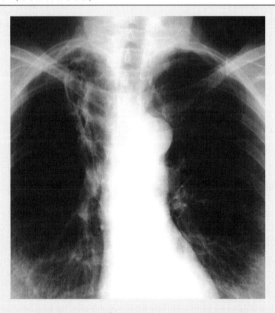

FIGURE 17-1 Radiograph of apical right upper lobe infiltrate with cavity formation visible. Minimal left upper lobe infiltrate is also faintly seen.

Mr. Druggera's hospital course was uneventful and he was discharged 5 days later. The infection control department of the hospital decided to perform tuberculin skin tests on all HCWs who had come into contact with this patient in the ED prior to institution of isolation procedures. These tests were performed within a week after the patient was discharged and all came back negative.

Group Critical Thinking Exercise 1

DECISION MAKING: DEVELOPING A LONG-TERM CARE PLAN

a. Describe what drugs will be prescribed and the rationale for each choice.

b. List the types of follow-up care Mr. Druggera will require.

CASE STUDY 1 *(continued)*

c. Describe in detail what instructions will have to be given to Mr. Druggera regarding his long-term therapy.

d. What specific advice must Mr. Druggera be given to minimize the risk of transferring his infections to others?

The patient was compliant with TB therapy for 6 months. The culture and sensitivity eventually revealed that the organism was *M tuberculosis* that was resistant to INH but sensitive to other antituberculosis medications. However, he suffered side effects from his antiretroviral therapy and took them only intermittently and developed a rash while taking TMP-SMX and also discontinued this medication. Twelve months later he presented to the ED cachetic and complaining of severe shortness of breath and a cough productive of scant amounts of mucoid sputum. Vital signs at that time were as follows:

Vital signs

BW	65 kg
HR	120/min
RR	26/min
BP	N/A
SpO_2	85%
Temperature	39°C

Critical Thinking Exercise 4

PRIORITIZING PATIENT CARE

You are asked to do the initial physical assessment on Mr. Druggera. List the following items in the order that you would perform them:

a. All the elements of the physical assessment

b. All diagnostic tests, and

c. Any immediate treatment modalities you feel he may require.

Upon admission, the following lab data were obtained:

ABG 21%

pH	7.44
Pco_2	28
Po_2	48
HCO_3^-	19.0
BE	−3
Sao_2	82%

Other lab tests were as follows:

Labs	WBCs 6000 (80% polys and 11% lymphocytes)
	CD4+ count was 6/mm^3
	He now has a viral load of 1.5 million HIV viral copies per milliliter of blood.

Critical Thinking Exercise 5

MAKING INFERENCES BY CLUSTERING DATA

a. What inferences can you draw given your knowledge of Mr. Druggera's history and the physical assessment and lab data above?

b. Practice clustering data to make these inferences.

c. Given your inferences, what other data will need to be obtained?

That afternoon Mr. Druggera underwent a bronchoscopy. The bronchoalveolar lavage (BAL) for Mr. Druggera revealed organisms consistent with *Pneumocystis carinii* pneumonia (PCP). Despite antibiotic therapy for PCP and antibiotics

CASE STUDY 1 (*continued*)

for a suspected coexistent community-acquired pneumonia, Mr. Druggera deteriorated over the next 24 hours. (See Figure 17-2 for chest x-ray taken at this time.) ABGs drawn while the patient was on a nonrebreather mask and breathing 36 times a minute revealed:

ABG nonreb mask

pH	7.36
P_{CO_2}	36
P_{O_2}	52
HCO_3^-	20.0
BE	−4
Sa_{O_2}	86%

Despite instituting CMV with conventional volume ventilation at the settings you recommended, the Pa_{O_2} fails to improve over the next 2 hours. Peak inspiratory pressures are 50 cm H_2O and plateau pressures are 45 cm H_2O. His minute ventilation on these settings is now 18 liters a minute, yet his Pa_{CO_2} is 44 torr.

Critical Thinking Exercise 6

PROBLEM SOLVING AND DECISION MAKING

a. Why is Mr. Druggera's Pa_{O_2} so low?

b. Why is his minute ventilation so high?

c. Why are the peak pressures so high?

d. What would you recommend now?

Group Critical Thinking Exercise 2

BECOMING A PROFESSIONAL (DECISION MAKING, COMMUNICATION, AND NEGOTIATION)

a. As a group, come to agreement as to the recommendations you would make to the physician regarding Mr. Druggera's care.

b. The physician is unfamiliar with the literature or the rationale that supports your recommendation. How would you convince him to accept your recommendations?

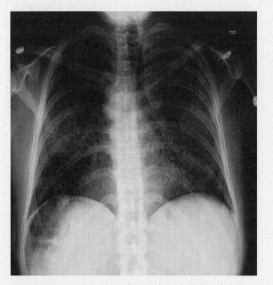

FIGURE 17-2 Radiograph with diffuse bilateral reticulonodular infiltrates and bilateral air bronchograms visible.

CASE STUDY 1 *(continued)*

Group Critical Thinking Exercise 3

PRO-CON DEBATE

The scourge of the AIDS/HIV epidemic in sub-Saharan Africa has been well-publicized. Groups on both sides of this debate need to scour the Internet (suggest at minimum the WHO and CDC web sites) and come up with the latest figures regarding the magnitude of the problem and some suggestions as to how to solve it. One side of the debate should take the minimalist position and argue that there is little the industrialized countries can do to treat those who are already infected. Describe what limited steps these countries can take to combat the epidemic. The other side will argue that the industrialized countries need to do a great deal more to prevent the spread of disease and treat those infected with HIV. Develop the moral, economic, and medical reasons to support each position.

Group Critical Thinking Exercise 4

PRO-CON DEBATE

Your instructor will assign two groups to perform this exercise. Mr. Druggera has never let it be known what his wishes are should it become impossible to improve his condition with continued treatment. There are advocates who take the position that in cases in which the patient has not expressed his or her wishes, the medical staff should not have to continue extraordinary medical care when the point of futility has been reached. Both groups should first investigate whether this patient's case has now become hopeless. Next one group should argue in support of withdrawing care for Mr. Druggera now that he is in severe ARDS. The other group should take the opposite position and give reasons why it should never be up to the medical staff to withdraw care without express instructions from the family unless the patient is legally dead. The presentation may be made in front of another group (the balance of the class) who can discuss and judge the effectiveness of the arguments.

KEY POINTS

- AIDS, a relatively new communicable disease, and tuberculosis (TB), a scourge since ancient times, are the number one and two infectious disease killers in the world.

- It is important to make the distinction between infection with the human immunodeficiency virus (HIV) and *Mycobacterium tuberculosis* and the diseases caused by these infections.

- Since untreated HIV infection will almost inexorably lead to immunocompromise, the AIDS epidemic in the US in the 1980s contributed to an increased incidence of TB in this country during that time.

- The enzyme immunoassay (EIA) is the standard screening test used to detect the presence of antibodies to HIV in the blood, and can now be used to confirm the diagnosis of HIV infection.

- 430,000 have died of AIDS in US since 1981 while 16 million have died of AIDS worldwide to date.

- The rate of HIV infection is increasing in both the US and the world.

- The death rate due to AIDS continues to increase worldwide.

- Though the incidence of HIV infection has not decreased in the United States, the incidence of AIDS has diminished due to the advent of effective, though expensive, antiretroviral therapy.

- Drug therapy is noncurative, it is a lifetime commitment.

- When helper T-cell counts reach precariously low levels due to the ravages of HIV infection, a patient becomes susceptible to a number of opportunistic infections, including recurrent bacterial pneumonias, TB, and PCP.

- Since HIV is contracted by exchange of bodily fluids, especially during sexual activity, HCWs have little risk of becoming infected with HIV on the job if they follow Standard Precautions.

- *M tuberculosis* is airborne and nosocomial transmission of the organism to HCWs, especially respiratory therapists, is a real problem unless the early identification and effective isolation of active TB patients and the proper use of HEPA masks and other engineering controls are implemented.

- Preventive INH therapy is effective in preventing those with latent TB infection from progressing to active TB either within months (primary TB) or years later (reactivation TB).

- Active TB, even multidrug resistant TB (MDR TB), can be effectively treated with a combination of antituberculosis medications given for a period of up to 2 years.

- It is extremely important that those with active disease be carefully monitored to ensure that they comply with the therapeutic regimen of anti-TB medications, to ensure that they do not become re-infected with multidrug resistant TB, and thus present with an even more dire public health hazard.

- Through public education, the marshalling of public health resources, and advances in preventive therapy have decreased the incidence of AIDS in the US, the cost and sophistication will mean there is little impact in controlling these diseases in developing countries.

- The only hope in eradicating these disease in the US, and achieving significant inroads worldwide, is for the development of effective vaccines for both.

SUGGESTED RESOURCES: WEB SITES

http://www.hopkins-tb.org
Johns Hopkins Center for Tuberculosis Research. Good site with information on emerging trends, epidemiology, and treatment of TB.

http://www.cdc.gov/nchstp/hiv_aids/stats/hasr1101.pdf
Latest CDC surveillance report.

http://www.cdc.gov/hiv/dhap.htm
CDC site for AIDS/HIV prevention. CDC site for HIV infection and TB. Gives good explanations of AIDS and TB. On HIV/AIDS section, visit Morbidity and Mortality Weekly Report (MMWR) sites for latest information on AIDS reported by the CDC.

http://www.cdcnpin.org/cgi-bin/webic.exe?conffile =np_srch.wi&template=d_srchmn.wi
CDC search site for HIV and TB information.

http://vh.radiology.uiowa.edu/Providers/TeachingFiles/ PulmonaryCoreCurric/HIVLungDisease/HIVLung Disease.html
Case study for a patient with AIDS. May be helpful to see how pulmonary disease is diagnosed in an AIDS patient.

http://hivinsite.ucsf.edu/
University of California, San Francisco (UCSF) HIV site. Easy-to-use site where you can get basic information as well as the latest research on HIV. Visit the case study section (use site guide). The patient who presents with cough and fatigue is very similar to the case in this text and contains an excellent discussion on the differential diagnosis of possible pulmonary complications of AIDS.

http://www.niaid.nih.gov/publications/tb.htm
Tuberculosis site from the National Institute of Allergy and Infectious Diseases (NIAID), National Institutes of Health. Links to fact sheets and a review of the NIAID tuberculosis research program, including updates on novel treatments and therapeutic strategies.

http://www.cdc.gov/search.htm
CDC web search (use to search CDC for info on AIDS and TB).

http://www.ncbi.nlm.nih.gov/PubMed/
PUB MED. Search engine for peer reviewed journals on AIDS and TB.

http://respiratorycare.medscape.com/Home/Topics/ RespiratoryCare/RespiratoryCare.html
Medscape Respiratory Care Section. Has good links for all respiratory care. Designed for pulmonary specialists.

http://www.unaids.org/
UNAIDS web site. Good place to check world AIDS statistics as well as status of the worldwide epidemic.

REFERENCES

1. Centers for Disease Control. HIV/AIDS Surveillance Report. December 1999.

2. UNAIDS Joint United Nations Programme of HIV/AIDS, AIDS epidemic update: December 1999:1–9.

3. CDC diagnosis and reporting of HIV and AIDS in states with integrated HIV and AIDS surveillance-United States, January 1994-June 1997. *MMWR*. 1998;47:309, 319–320.

4. UNAIDS. Joint United Nations Programme of HIV/AIDS. AIDS Epidemic, December 1999. http://www.unaids.org.

5. Centers for Disease Control and Prevention. Public health service guidelines for the management of health care worker exposures to HIV and recommendations for post-exposure prophylaxis. *MMWR*. 1998;47(RR-71):1–6.

6. Centers for Disease Control, 1999 USPH/ISDA guidelines for the prevention of opportunistic infection in persons infected with HIV: US Public Health Service and Infectious Diseases Society of America. *MMWR*. 1999;48(RR-10):1–66.

7. Centers for Disease Control and Prevention. Prevention and treatment of tuberculosis among patients infected with human immunodeficiency virus: principles of therapy and revised recommendations. *MMWR*. 1998;47(RR-20):1–66.

8. 1997 guidelines for the prevention of opportunistic infection in persons infected with HIV: disease specific recommendations. *Clin Infect Dis*. 1997;(suppl 3)(25):S299–312.

9. McDermott L, Glassroth J, Mehta J, et al. Tuberculosis. Part 1. *Disease-a-Month*. 1997 Mar;43(3): 113–180.

10. LaBue P, Catanzaro A, Dutt A, et al. Tuberculosis. Part 2. *Disease-a-Month*. 1997 Apr;43(4):187–274.

11. Centers for Disease Control and Prevention. Recommendations for prevention and control of tuberculosis among foreign born persons. *MMWR*. 1998;47(RR-16):1.

12. Centers for Disease Control and Prevention. Tuberculosis Morbidity—United States. *MMWR*. 1998;47(13):253–257.

13. Davis Y, McRay E, Simone P. Hospital infection control practices for tuberculosis. *Clin Chest Med*. 1997;18:19–33.

14. Rattan A, Kalia A, Ahmad N. Multidrug-resistant Mycobacterium tuberculosis: Molecular perspectives. *Emerg Infect Dis*. 1998;4:195–209.

15. Saubolle M. The Clinical Microbiology Laboratory in the Diagnosis and Monitoring of Opportunistic Infections in HIV-Infected Persons. Conference on the Laboratory Science of HIV. 1998:141–151.

16. Centers for Disease Control and Prevention. Prevention and treatment of tuberculosis among patients infected with human immunodeficiency virus: principles of therapy and revised recommendations. *MMWR*. 1998;47(RR-20):1–57.

17. Centers for Disease Control and Prevention. Guidelines for preventing the transmission of Mycobacterium tuberculosis in health-care facilities. *MMWR*. 1994;43(RR-13):1–132.

18. Fennelly K. Personal respiratory protection against Mycobacterium tuberculosis. *Clin Chest Med*. 1997; 18:1–17.

18

CONGESTIVE HEART FAILURE WITH PULMONARY EDEMA

Terry S. LeGrand and Robert Wayne Lawson

*Do not go where the path may lead, go instead
where there is no path and leave a trail.*
—RALPH WALDO EMERSON
(1803–1882)

LEARNING OBJECTIVES

1. Describe facts, descriptions, and definitions related to congestive heart failure (CHF), including CHF that is complicated by pulmonary edema.

2. Discuss the etiology, pathophysiology, and clinical features of the patient with CHF with pulmonary edema.

3. Describe the acute care and long-term management of patients with CHF.

4. Apply the critical thinking skills of prioritizing, anticipating, negotiating, communicating, and decision making to a case example of CHF with pulmonary edema.

5. Through performance of critical thinking exercises and group discussion of the case in question, apply strategies that promote critical thinking in the respiratory care management of a patient with CHF presenting with acute pulmonary edema.

6. Use a case example to perform an initial patient assessment using a standardized system and the clinical data presented.

7. Interpret clinical data from case examples including history, physical examination, lab data, and radiographs to make a differential diagnosis and recommendations for respiratory care management.

8. Develop a care plan for a patient with CHF and pulmonary edema, including recommendations for therapy and disease management, with consideration of the cost as well as ethical and quality-of-life issues.

9. Communicate facts, evidence, and arguments to support evaluations and recommendations proposed for the care of a patient with CHF complicated by pulmonary edema.

10. Practice the skill of negotiating to attempt to gain acceptance of a proposed plan of care for a patient with CHF and pulmonary edema.

11. Evaluate treatment and outcomes of interventions, giving attention to health promotion and quality-of-life issues.

12. Describe the role of the respiratory therapist in the assessment, treatment, management, and education of the patient with CHF complicated by pulmonary edema.

INTRODUCTION

Heart failure has been defined as the inability of the heart to pump an adequate amount of oxygenated blood to meet the metabolic demands of the tissues.[1] The syndrome of congestive heart failure (CHF) manifests clinically as peripheral venous or pulmonary congestion or both. Heart failure is the result of primary heart muscle pathology, or secondary pathology such as ischemic or valvular disease.

To gain a better understanding of the nature of cardiac failure, it is helpful to view the heart as being composed of two sides separated by a wall called the *septum.* The right side of the heart receives venous blood, termed *preload,* from the peripheral circulation and pumps it to the lungs for oxygenation. The left side receives oxygenated blood from the lungs and pumps it to the systemic circulation. The degree of resistance against which the volume of blood is pumped from the heart is termed *afterload.* Valves separating the atria (the upper chambers) from the ventricles (the lower chambers) maintain one-way flow through the heart.

Cardiac output (CO) is determined by the product of left ventricle stroke volume (SV) and heart rate (HR) (ie, $CO = SV \times HR$). Stroke volume is determined by the relationship between filling volume (preload), contractility of the myocardium, and outflow resistance (afterload). When thinking about origins of cardiac failure, compensatory mechanisms, and even treatment of cardiac failure, it is useful to keep these relationships in mind.

CRITICAL CONTENT

THE HEART AS A PUMP

- The volume of blood filling the heart is called preload.
- The resistance the heart pumps against is called afterload.
- Stroke volume is the amount of blood pumped with each beat, and is a function of preload, afterload, and myocardial contractility.
- Cardiac output is stroke volume times heart rate.

ETIOLOGY

There is a large number of underlying causes of heart failure, including myocardial weakness and inflammation, coronary artery disease, loss of muscle cells with scarring (cardiomyopathy), decreased blood flow (ischemia) with consequent lack of oxygen delivery, acute myocardial infarction (MI), and diastolic dysfunction (ventricular hypertrophy). Other underlying causes include hypertension, increased resistance to ejection, congenital heart disease, and increased stroke volume, as well as valvular abnormalities, such as aortic, mitral, or tricuspid insufficiency.

Precipitating causes of heart failure, when there is underlying pathology like that identified in the preceding paragraph, include hypoxemia, increased salt intake, medication noncompliance, arrhythmia, infection (eg, pneumonia), myocardial depressant drugs, and high-output states (eg, sepsis, anemia, hyperthyroidism, pregnancy, or renal failure). These precipitating events push the already diseased heart into a situation in which more cardiac output is being demanded by the body systems, but the heart is not able to respond and fails to produce the required increased output.

Hypertensive patients comprise a significant portion of those at risk for heart failure. In such patients, there are two key mechanisms that result in heart failure. One mechanism, increased afterload, causes a hypertrophy-dilation effect that produces a reduction in coronary artery flow reserve, leading to cardiac dysfunction and failure. The other mechanism involves diseased coronary vasculature due to atherosclerosis and/or microangiopathy, causing increased coronary artery resistance and impaired oxygen supply. This condition can lead to myocardial ischemia or infarction, resulting in heart failure.[2] See Table 18-1 for a list of typical causes of CHF.

Recognition of underlying pathology as well as precipitating factors is necessary to appropriately treat CHF. This is particularly true for those patients who present with pulmonary edema.[1] Many of the described causes of CHF can be viewed as factors or diseases that reduce ventricular stroke volume. This reduction in stroke volume is often the result of a reduction of preload and/or contractility, or imposition of increased ventricular afterload. Therapeutic approaches to treatment of CHF, directed at improving one or more of these elements controlling ventricular stroke volume, is discussed later in this chapter.

TABLE 18-1   CAUSES OF CONGESTIVE HEART FAILURE

Myocardial weakness, inflammation, failure
　　Coronary artery disease
　　Cardiomyopathy
　　Ischemia
　　Acute myocardial infarction
　　Myocarditis
　　Diastolic dysfunction
Hemodynamic overload
　　Valvular stenosis or regurgitation
　　Hypertension
　　Increased afterload
　　Congenital heart disease

PATHOPHYSIOLOGY

The heart is equipped with compensatory mechanisms that enable it to adapt to normal and abnormal changes in load. Chronic cardiac overload activates these mechanisms, but can ultimately result in the syndrome of heart failure. One compensatory mechanism involves the Frank-Starling relationship, which states that performance of the heart muscle relates to the length (amount of stretching) of the myocardial fibers; thus the more the fibers stretch, the greater the force of contraction, *within limits*. This mechanism works by attempting to increase CO by increasing SV. The volume in the left ventricle at the end of diastole (LVEDV) represents the length of the myocardial fibers. Volume is difficult to measure clinically, so left ventricular end-diastolic pressure (LVEDP) is used to approximate LVEDV. Clinically, pulmonary artery diastolic (PAD) pressure or pulmonary capillary wedge pressure (PCWP) substitutes for LVEDP. Many factors can interfere with the accuracy of the preceding assumptions and estimations (eg, mitral valve disease, the effect of pleural pressure on transmural filling pressure of the LV, etc.) so the student should refer to a more comprehensive discussion of this subject for a complete explanation. Contraction or shortening of myocardial fibers, on the other hand, can be represented by measures of left ventricular performance, such as cardiac output and stroke volume.[3]

Figure 18-1 shows cardiac function curves representing stroke volumes produced by LVEDP under normal conditions and under conditions of enhanced and reduced contractility. In the normal heart (B), it can be seen that a given increase in LVEDP produces a comparable increase in stroke volume. The upper curve (A) represents enhanced contractility (the ability of the heart to eject blood), in which relatively small increases in LVEDP produce significant increases in stroke volume. Sympathetic nervous system stimulation, elevated circulating catecholamines, or inotropic drugs can cause enhanced contractility. Increased contractil-

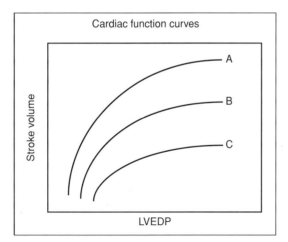

FIGURE 18-1 Cardiac function curves. Stroke volume as a function of left ventricular end-diastolic pressure in: (A) the hyperdynamic heart, (B) the normal heart, and (C) the failing heart.

ity can also result from increased heart rate, which increases the amount of calcium available to contractile proteins in the cardiac myocytes. The lower curve (C) represents reduced contractility and a failing heart. Higher end-diastolic volume (dilatation) initially increases pump function on this curve, but this increased volume leads to higher diastolic pressures, left atrial hypertension, and pulmonary congestion.[1]

The second compensatory mechanism also depends upon the relationship between stroke volume, heart rate, and cardiac output. Thus, increasing HR can enhance left ventricular output, because CO is a function of left ventricular SV and HR. Patients with CHF often increase their heart rate in an attempt to compensate for the decreased SV, and thus tend to be tachycardic. However, because of an increase in cardiac work that often accompanies the increased rate, the benefit from increasing HR is negated in patients with CHF.[1]

The third compensatory mechanism employed by the heart in the face of chronic overload is activation of neurohumoral systems. Such activation includes sympathetic nervous system stimulation,

elevated catecholamine levels, an activated renin-angiotensin system, and elevated atrial natriuretic peptide levels. These changes help to maintain blood pressure and perfusion, but can result in salt and water retention, which worsens circulatory congestion.[4,5]

CHF results from chronic overload of the previously described compensatory mechanisms. It may be due to increased preload, valvular regurgitation or shunting, decreased contractility, or increased afterload. Increased afterload can be caused by hypertension or outflow obstruction (eg, aortic stenosis). Conversely, the failing heart muscle, which exhibits poor contractility, may experience an excessive burden from normal preload and afterload. Also, generalized hypervolemia, such as during renal failure, can result in circulatory congestion with only mild cardiac dysfunction.[1]

CRITICAL CONTENT

COMPENSATORY MECHANISMS THAT ALLOW THE HEART TO ADAPT TO CHANGES IN LOAD

- The amount of blood the heart ejects is related to how much the muscle fibers are stretched by preload (Frank-Starling mechanism).
- If stroke volume remains constant, cardiac output can be enhanced by increasing heart rate.
- Chronic volume overload evokes a neurohumoral response in the heart to increase heart rate and/or contractility.

Note: CHF results from chronic use of these compensatory mechanisms.

Pulmonary edema results from elevated atrial and venous pressures only when normal mechanisms for maintaining the fluid integrity of the intravascular space have been overwhelmed (Fig.

18-2). Pressure inside blood vessels (hydrostatic pressure) tends to move fluid from the vessels to the interstitium. It is counteracted by plasma osmotic pressure created by proteins in blood and selective permeability of the capillary walls. Plasma osmotic pressure tends to pull fluid from the interstitium into the blood vessels. When the heart muscle fails to pump blood efficiently into the systemic circulation, an increase in pulmonary capillary hydrostatic pressure occurs, and cardiogenic pulmonary edema results (Fig. 18-3).

Left atrial pressures, usually approximated by measurement of the pulmonary capillary wedge

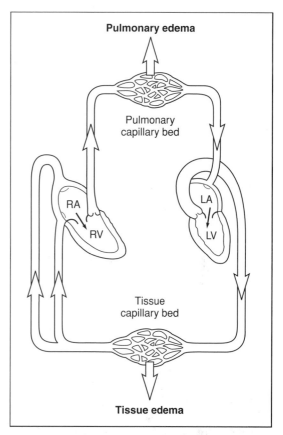

FIGURE 18-3   Mechanism of pulmonary and tissue edema. In the case of pulmonary edema, the failing heart muscle is unable to efficiently pump blood around the vascular circuit, resulting in fluid flux into the interstitium and alveoli of the lungs.

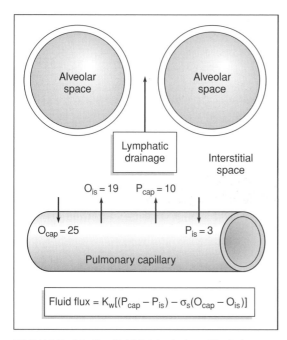

FIGURE 18-2   Fluid flux in the lung. The balance between hydrostatic pressure and plasma osmotic pressures creates a net movement of fluid from the vascular compartment to the interstitium. O_{cap} = plasma oncotic pressure; P_{cap} = capillary hydrostatic pressure; O_{is} = interstitial fluid oncotic pressure; P_{is} = interstitial hydrostatic pressure; K_w = capillary filtration coefficient (describes capillary fluid permeability characteristics); (σ_{is} = reflection coefficient (relating how easily the capillary endothelium prevents passage of solute particles).

pressure (PCWP), that are greater than 20 to 25 mm Hg are associated with pulmonary edema.[1] The left atrial pressure at which pulmonary edema develops is a function of time. A moderate, acute elevation may cause pulmonary edema, while the same elevation, if chronic, may be well tolerated without significant congestion.[6] Pulmonary edema can also be caused by noncardiac factors—conditions that lower plasma osmotic pressure or increase capillary permeability—and is termed *noncardiogenic pulmonary edema* (see Chapter 22). The focus of this chapter is CHF resulting in cardiogenic pulmonary edema.

Systemic hypertension, coronary artery disease, or aortic insufficiency are common causes of left-sided heart failure. The term congestive heart failure is often used synonymously with left ventricular failure. It is characterized by specific symptoms, including exertional dyspnea (from pulmonary venous congestion with a decrease in lung compliance) and fatigue. Dyspnea tends to worsen in the supine position due to increasing pulmonary vascular engorgement, causing paroxysmal nocturnal dyspnea, often associated with a dry cough. Nocturia may result from excretion of edema fluid, especially as kidney perfusion increases in the recumbent position, from decreased work of the heart at rest, or the delayed effect of daytime diuretics. Angina pectoris will be present if coronary artery disease exists. It is important to differentiate dyspnea due to left ventricular failure from that caused by other disorders (eg, chronic lung disease, obesity, severe anemia, ascites, or abdominal distention).[1]

Although it is generally recognized that CHF is most often associated with left ventricular failure, right ventricular failure can eventually lead to excess work, and ultimately failure of the left ventricle. The most common causes of right-sided heart failure are left heart failure, mitral valvular stenosis, pulmonary vascular hypertension, pulmonic valvular stenosis, and right ventricular MI.

Anorexia, bloating, and right upper abdominal pain reflecting hepatic and visceral congestion secondary to elevated venous pressure characterize right heart failure. Jugular venous distention (JVD) may also be present, indicative of elevated pressure in the circulation returning to the right heart. Other characteristics are hepatomegaly and tenderness, dependent edema that subsides overnight in the early stages but persists in later stages, and right-sided pleural effusion. In addition, patients may exhibit coolness of their extremities and peripheral cyanosis due to reduced peripheral blood flow. Sinus tachycardia and a right ventricular S_3 heart sound are also common findings. Overload to the right side of the heart causes elevated right ventricular diastolic and right atrial pressures. High pressure is transmitted back into the systemic venous circulation causing fluid to leak out of the systemic capillaries, leading to peripheral edema. Ascites and hepatic congestion can occur if right atrial pressures become severely elevated for a prolonged period.[1]

DIAGNOSIS AND MANAGEMENT

The clinical syndrome of CHF can be similar among patients with very different etiologies. However, the diagnostic and therapeutic approach may be different, depending on the specific cause. It is important to establish the presence of heart failure as the cause of the patient's signs and symptoms before implementation of a treatment plan, since other disease processes may cause similar symptoms.

There are three major manifestations of circulatory congestion syndrome. They include pulmonary congestion, manifesting as shortness of breath (SOB) and/or respiratory failure; peripheral congestion, evidenced by the presence of JVD, enlarged liver, ascites, and lower extremity edema; and low-output state, presenting with hypotension, lethargy, or low urine output. The most common manifestation of circulatory congestion syndrome is pulmonary edema.[1]

CRITICAL CONTENT

MAJOR MANIFESTATIONS OF CIRCULATORY CONGESTION SYNDROME

- Pulmonary congestion (pulmonary edema and SOB)
- Peripheral congestion (JVD, hepatomegaly, ascites, extremity edema)
- Low-output state (hypotension, lethargy, reduced renal output)

Early recognition of pulmonary edema is critical to its successful management. Pulmonary edema should be suspected when a patient presents in acute respiratory distress. Such patients can deteriorate rapidly, therefore it is crucial to use a logical, systematic approach to prevent misdiagnosis and provide effective treatment. It is important to obtain an accurate history from the patient or, if necessary, from a family member. Establishing the presence of known potential causes of heart failure, such as prior myocardial infarction, angina, or hypertension will be helpful in accurately detecting pulmonary edema. If the patient presents with a history of dyspnea on exertion (DOE), orthopnea, or paroxysmal nocturnal dyspnea (PND), cardiac etiology is suggested, but noncardiogenic pulmonary edema needs to be ruled out.

It is important to question the patient about any recent increase in salt intake or noncompliance with drugs. Determine if he or she has experienced palpitations, lightheadedness, or syncope, all of which are suggestive of arrhythmia. Recent onset of fever, cough, and sputum production, on the other hand, suggests pneumonia, which is common among the elderly. A complete history should also determine the presence of coexisting disorders that may exacerbate cardiac conditions (eg, anemia, thyroid disease, or pregnancy). If the patient is sitting straight upright, exhibits diaphoresis, tachycardia, and hypertension, as well as crackles and wheezes on auscultation, then severe left-heart failure is suggested. Further evidence for significant left ventricular dysfunction is pulsus alternans (beat-to-beat variation in systolic pressure). Mild to moderate pulmonary congestion is usually associated with crackles as well, but often only at the bases or to midlung fields. Mild tachycardia may be present with normal or slightly elevated blood pressure. Cardiogenic shock usually exists when systolic hypotension (<80 mm Hg) and pulmonary edema present together, a dire situation with a high mortality that requires immediate, aggressive therapy.[1]

If the apical impulse is increased in strength and exhibits a leftward and downward displacement, and if an S_3 gallop is present, reflecting valvu-

lar dysfunction, there is a strong presumption of pulmonary congestion of cardiac origin. JVD, hepatomegaly, ascites, and peripheral edema suggest right-heart failure. The most common cause of right-heart failure is left-heart failure, thus its presence tends to confirm cardiogenic pulmonary edema.[1]

ECG findings can help detect precipitating factors, such as ischemia (ST segment depression), acute MI (ST segment elevation), prior MI (pathologic Q waves), left atrial enlargement, and arrhythmias, especially atrial and ventricular tachycardia. The chest radiograph provides evidence of pulmonary congestion and can help differentiate between pneumonia and interstitial lung disease. Specific radiographic signs of pulmonary congestion are upper zone flow redistribution, as well as interstitial and alveolar edema and the presence of Kerley B lines. Bilateral pleural effusions may also be present, especially with severe left-sided failure. Cardiomegaly (cardiothoracic ratio >0.5) confirms the findings suggested by the patient's history, physical examination, and ECG. Absence of cardiomegaly does not exclude pulmonary edema of cardiogenic origin, however. Left ventricular hypertrophy may not be present if heart failure is due to acute MI or arrhythmia.[1]

A definitive diagnosis of pulmonary edema can be made only with a pulmonary artery catheter and measurement of PCWP, an estimate of left atrial pressure. Low to normal PCWP suggests noncardiogenic pulmonary edema. A markedly elevated wedge pressure (>20 to 25 mm Hg) confirms cardiogenic pulmonary edema.[1] An intermediate reading suggests the need for further diagnosis.

CRITICAL CONTENT

ASSESSMENT OF CARDIOGENIC PULMONARY EDEMA

- Obtain history to establish causes of heart failure, such as MI, angina, or hypertension.
- Question patient about recent noncompliance with diet or drug regimen.

- Perform physical assessment to identify signs and symptoms.
- Obtain an ECG to detect precipitating factors, such as ischemia, acute MI, or left atrial enlargement, as well as to provide evidence of pulmonary congestion.
- Definitive diagnosis is possible only with a pulmonary artery catheter.
- PCWP >20 to 25 mm Hg plus signs and symptoms confirms cardiogenic pulmonary edema.

Therapy should begin with general measures to treat pulmonary congestion. Primary treatment of acute pulmonary edema includes reduction of myocardial workload, increasing contractility, and reducing fluid retention. Reduction of myocardial workload means rest, supplemental oxygen, and perhaps vasodilators (to reduce ventricular afterload). Contractility can be increased with digitalis, and fluid retention can be reduced with diuretics (eg, furosemide). This initial approach can be applied to all patients, regardless of the origin of the edema. Such measures should be applied rapidly in conjunction with continuing diagnostic evaluation. Resuscitate the patient if necessary, and maintain a systolic pressure greater than 95 mm Hg. If cardiogenic shock is present, pressor agents will be necessary.

General goals of initial management include improving oxygenation, reducing anxiety, decreasing venous return, decreasing afterload, and treatment of precipitating factors. For evaluation and treatment, place the patient in an upright position, give supplemental oxygen therapy, and secure IV access, preferably a central line if pressors are needed. Vital signs should be monitored frequently while history is obtained and a physical examination is performed. A complete blood count (CBC) should be obtained to check for anemia and elevated white blood cell count, and serum electrolytes should be evaluated.

It is important to rule out recent or ongoing MI, thus cardiac enzymes and biomarkers can be measured for this purpose. Traditional enzyme tests used for diagnosis of MI include creatine kinase (CK), aspartate aminotransferase (AST) (formerly known as serum glutamic-oxaloacetic transmaminase, SGOT), and lactate dehydrogenase (LDH). A more specific marker of MI has become available recently, troponin I, found only in cardiac muscle.[7–9] Like CK, this biomarker becomes positive about 4 to 8 hours after an MI occurs, but unlike CK, troponin I levels remain elevated for 5 to 9 days after the event, permitting late diagnosis of MI. This information may be critical in determining the cause of heart failure in a patient presenting with cardiogenic pulmonary edema. An arterial blood gas should be ordered and repeated to assess improvement in acidosis, hypercarbia, and hypoxemia as treatment progresses. Pulse oximetry can be used to track oxygenation, but it should be used with caution in a patient with poor peripheral perfusion. Obtain a 12-lead ECG to evaluate for acute MI or ongoing ischemia, which necessitates the use of thrombolytic therapy or nitroglycerin.

If the patient is adequately ventilating and has a systolic blood pressure greater than 95 to 100 mm Hg, therapy may be continued with morphine sulfate. Monitor the patient for lethargy, respiratory depression, and hypotension. Morphine increases venous capacitance, reducing preload and right atrial pressure. It also reduces afterload and anxiety.

Nitrates have a primary venous dilatory effect, so they will reduce venous return, but have less effect on afterload, since they dilate arteries less than veins.[1] Nitroglycerin should be given only if blood pressure is maintained. It may be given sublingually or as nitropaste. Intravenous infusion provides an easily controllable route of administration. Dosage should be titrated to systolic blood pressure.

Intravenous diuretics are used in all patients with pulmonary edema. Furosemide, a rapidly acting loop diuretic, and bumetanide are used most often. Diuretics should be used with caution in patients with low blood pressure, or those with suspected MI or aortic stenosis. It is important to avoid hypotension in such patients, thus the patient should be observed for overdiuresis and resultant hypotension. Furosemide's action peaks at 15 to 30 minutes, but it appears to work sooner, presumably due to vasodilatory properties of the drug.[1] It is important to monitor the patient for hypokalemia, a side effect of furosemide, due to the risk of ventricular arrhythmias. Persistent acidosis and hypoxemia despite implementation of the preceding measures indicate a possible need for intubation and mechanical ventilation. Positive end-expiratory pressure (PEEP) may be beneficial, though it should be used with caution due to its potential to decrease cardiac output.

While most patients require reduction of venous return, some also require afterload reduction. Such patients should be identified using echocardiography by assessing ventricular systolic/diastolic function. Afterload reduction is appropriate if systolic dysfunction is the primary problem causing the heart failure. Angiotensin-converting enzyme (ACE) inhibitors such as captopril may be used in conjunction with diuretics. Observe the patient closely for systemic hypotension, especially after the initial dose; titrate subsequent doses to achieve a systolic blood pressure of 100 mm Hg.[1]

If the patient is experiencing pulmonary edema with hypotension, venous return and afterload should *not* be decreased. Instead, IV catecholamine pressor agents should be used to support systemic blood pressure and enhance organ perfusion. Dobutamine may be used for mild to moderate hypotension (80 to 100 mm Hg systolic pressure); however, invasive hemodynamic monitoring is required to assess the efficacy of this therapy. Dopamine in low doses may be required for more severe hypotension with signs of decreased tissue perfusion (lethargy, peripheral vasoconstriction, decreased urine output) to maintain renal and splanchnic perfusion. Dopamine may precipitate sinus, ventricular, or atrial tachycardia, so the patient requires careful monitoring. Norepinephrine has greater alpha-adrenergic effects at low doses and may be used as an alternative to dopamine. Systemic hypertensive crisis may require the use of IV nitroprusside.[1]

Circulatory assist devices such as an intraaortic balloon pump (IABP) can be used to support function in the failing left ventricle.[10] In addition, in recent years a variety of mechanical left ventricular assist devices and other forms of temporary mechanical hearts have been developed that can externally assist cardiac output while the patient awaits cardiac transplantation. The device with the longest track record, the IABP, has a polyurethane membrane mounted on a vascular catheter and is positioned in the descending thoracic aorta distal to the left subclavian artery. The balloon inflates and deflates in concert with the mechanical cardiac cycle. When the balloon inflates at the onset of diastole, it causes proximal and distal displacement of blood in the aorta. This displacement creates increased pressures that increase coronary artery and systemic perfusion. The balloon deflates just prior to the onset of the next systole, resulting in reduced systolic pressure (reduced afterload) and decreased myocardial oxygen demand. The primary effects of IABP therapy are increased myocardial oxygen supply and decreased myocardial oxygen demand. The combined effect of the balloon's inflation and deflation is improved myocardial oxygenation, increased cardiac output, increased systemic perfusion, and of crucial importance to the patient with heart failure, a reduction in left ventricular workload.[10]

As shown in Fig. 18-2, two forces regulate intravascular fluid balance in the lung: hydrostatic and plasma osmotic pressures. Net fluid movement under normal circumstances is from the intravascular space to the interstitium, where fluid is continually drained and returned to the systemic circulation by the lymphatic system. If the lymphatic system is overwhelmed, interstitial and alveolar edema may result.

The addition of PEEP to normal ventilating pressures causes intravascular hydrostatic pressures in alveolar vessels and pressures around the interstitial space to increase, but there is no net change in the pressure gradient across perialveolar vessels.[11] Interstitial pressure surrounding vessels not adjacent to alveoli (extraalveolar vessels, ie, pre- and postcapillary and larger vessels) decreases as PEEP increases. Radial tension on these vessels is produced by the expanding lung structure, causing the vessels to enlarge. This tension lowers resistance to blood flow. If cardiac output remains the same, hydrostatic pressure stays the same or increases with PEEP. Constant internal pressure and decreasing interstitial pressure would be expected to cause fluid to move out of these vessels, increasing lung edema in the interstitial space in the extraalveolar area.[12] However, clinical observation of patients with cardiogenic pulmonary edema indicates that positive pressure ventilation appears to reduce the appearance of thin, pink, frothy secretions and improves the cardiovascular status of these patients. Cardiac output and systemic blood pressure may increase with increases in intrathoracic pressure in CHF patients. Such increases are most likely to occur where venous engorgement is sufficient to prevent great vessel collapse with increased intrapleural pressures. Blood pooling outside the thorax plus decreased filling of the right ventricle permits the heart to be more efficient and effective. Thus PEEP may improve patients with CHF by decreasing preload and reducing afterload.[13]

Studies have been conducted to determine the mechanism by which the application of PEEP reduces extravascular lung water, but these studies have produced conflicting results.[14–17] One study noted that an increase in lymphatic flow through the thoracic duct was associated with application of PEEP,[17] but this increase was thought to account for no more than 10% to 15% of lung water clearance.[18]

More radical measures such as heart transplantation and use of mechanical hearts and left ventricular assist devices (LVADs) are options to consider in the patient with a failing heart. Mechanical hearts and LVADs are used until a suitable donor is located and a heart transplant is scheduled. In some cases patients may wait as long as 1 year, remaining hospitalized on heart support until a donor heart becomes available. These more drastic measures generate numerous cost and ethical issues that must be resolved by society and medical institutions as well as individual patients and their families.

In summary, management of CHF presenting with acute pulmonary edema involves improving oxygenation, reducing the patient's anxiety, decreasing venous return to the heart, increasing myocardial contractility, decreasing afterload, and of course

treatment of precipitating factors. Diuresis, improvement in cardiac function, and maintenance of systolic blood pressure are critical factors in the management of the patient with cardiogenic pulmonary edema. Selected patients may also be candidates for heart transplantation.

CRITICAL CONTENT

MANAGEMENT OF CHF WITH PULMONARY EDEMA

- Improve oxygenation
- Reduce anxiety
- Decrease venous return to the heart
- Increase myocardial contractility
- Decrease afterload
- Treat precipitating factors

SITE- AND AGE-SPECIFIC CONSIDERATIONS

Congestive heart failure is a significant health problem in the United States because of its increasing prevalence in the older adult population, as well as its impact on health care costs. More than 75% of CHF patients are over age 65, and this disease is the leading cause of hospitalization in this age group.[19] In addition, large numbers of elderly persons are receiving care for chronic CHF at alternate sites, often following hospitalization for the acute episode(s). Age-specific considerations have been found to exist regarding diagnosis and treatment of CHF,[20] specifically due to a higher incidence of adverse effects and complications among the elderly compared to younger patients.

A major cause for decompensation leading to hospitalization among the elderly population appears to be insufficient compliance with regard to lifestyle changes and medications.[20] This finding suggests that the older patient may find it more difficult to change habits that contribute to CHF.

Moreover, compliance with a complex drug regimen poses a problem for many older patients due to the sheer number of medications they may be required to take. Respiratory therapists should be aware of such critical patient education and behavior issues and do their part in reinforcing the need for compliance with medication regimens. See Chapter 9 for a more detailed discussion of patient education.

CONSIDERATION OF COSTS AND ETHICAL ISSUES

Congestive heart failure is estimated to account for more than $10 billion annually in health care costs.[19] In one study, the median length of hospital stay was 8 days, with a range of 5 to 12 days, and the median cost per person was estimated at $6275, with a range of $3468 to $12,366 per person.[21] While the majority of patients survive their initial hospitalization for CHF,[21] many of them are discharged to other facilities where they continue to incur health care costs, such as skilled nursing facilities, hospice programs, rehabilitation hospitals, or other acute care hospitals.

The end of life for patients with severe CHF is frequently characterized by repeated hospitalizations and declining quality of life. However most patients, including those with poor prognoses, usually receive maximal medical therapy until death.[22] Physicians tend to discuss resuscitation issues with this patient population less often than with patients who have other terminal illnesses such as cancer or AIDS.[22] One study indicated that 25% of patients with severe CHF express a preference not to be resuscitated during a hospital stay, but that less than 5% of patient charts contain such documentation.[22] Data from this study indicate that this discrepancy appears to be the result of differences between physicians' perceptions of their patients' wishes regarding resuscitation and the actual wishes of the patients. Sixty-nine percent of patients interviewed stated they did not want to be resuscitated in the event of cardiopulmonary arrest, but only

18% of their physicians believed their patients did not want to be resuscitated.[22]

It is incumbent upon all health care workers, including respiratory therapists, to listen closely to what patients say to them. If you find a patient expressing concerns over the intensity of the care being provided, you should immediately bring this to the attention of the other members of the patient care team. Patients have the right and expectation that their decisions regarding extraordinary care will be followed.

HEALTH PROMOTION AND QUALITY-OF-LIFE ISSUES

Patients who are hospitalized for acute exacerbation of severe CHF tend to have a poor 6-month survival rate.[21] Those who survive, however, usually retain relatively good functional status and have good health perceptions. One study indicated that patients are less likely to require hospital readmission in the future if they feel that their quality of life is good following CHF exacerbation.[23]

While CHF continues to be a burdensome and costly illness, creative strategies for outpatient management continue to be explored.[24] Disease management programs conducted in collaboration with physicians, nurse-practitioners, and clinical pharmacists are expected to contribute to successful development and implementation of multidisciplinary clinics for outpatient management of CHF.[24] Such programs should result in decreased health care expenditures as well as increased quality of life for patients.

INTRODUCTION TO CASE STUDIES

Now you proceed with the most exciting part of this chapter, that of working through two hypothetical cases. Your instructors will assign you to work on specific critical thinking exercises and group critical thinking exercises, depending on the available time, types of patients you are likely to encounter during your clinical rotations, and available resources.

Please check with your instructors to verify which case(s) and exercises you should complete, working individually or in groups. Your instructors may also direct you to develop learning issues as part of your problem-based learning (PBL) process or assign specific, predetermined learning issues developed for this chapter. Please check with your program faculty before proceeding with the following case(s).

CASE STUDY 1

MRS. MINNIE KRACKLE

Initial Case Scenario

Mrs. Krackle is a 75-year-old female who is brought to the emergency department at 9:00 AM by her husband. She has experienced nausea and vomiting since the evening before and feels as though "something is pressing on my chest." Her respirations appear rapid and shallow. After arrival at the ED, Mrs. Krackle begins to complain of pain in her chest radiating to the neck and left arm.

Critical Thinking Exercise 1

PRIORITIZING PATIENT CARE

Describe how you would evaluate this patient, explaining appropriate assessment and treatment that should occur during the first minutes in the ED.

CLINICAL DATA ON ED ADMISSION

Vital signs

HR	127/min
RR	18/min
BP	137/88
SpO_2 %	N/A
Temp.	98.2°F

Auscultation Bilateral crackles at bases.

CV ECG findings include sinus tachycardia with occasional PVCs and ST segment elevation.

The respiratory therapist attempts to obtain a pulse oximetry reading, but the patient's extremities are cold, and the pulseoximeter probe fails to read her oxygen saturation.

Critical Thinking Exercise 2

TROUBLESHOOTING THE PULSE OXIMETER

a. Why do you think the respiratory therapist is unable to obtain a reading?

b. Discuss applications and limitations of pulse oximetry.

c. What steps should be taken next (in regards to the oximeter)?

Additional Data from the ED

The patient's husband confirms she has a history of coronary heart disease. She began experiencing the present symptoms the evening before, and states that she noticed a feeling of pressure in her chest. Mrs. Krackle reports that she had a heart attack 15 years earlier and was on medication for hypertension several years ago, but has not taken it in recent months. The patient is observed in the ED for 2 hours. Her lips begin to appear cyanotic, and she is becoming increasingly short of breath. Her current chest radiograph can be seen in Fig. 18-4.

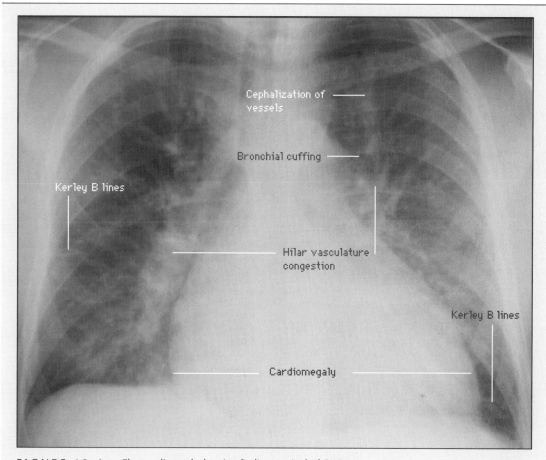

Cephalization of vessels

Bronchial cuffing

Kerley B lines

Hilar vasculature congestion

Kerley B lines

Cardiomegaly

FIGURE 18-4 Chest radiograph showing findings typical of CHF.

Critical Thinking Exercise 3

MAKING INFERENCES BY CLUSTERING DATA

There are a number of pieces of data that all point toward a similar conclusion.

a. What are the pieces of data that point toward this common inference?

b. What inference would you make about Mrs. Krackle's likely diagnosis from this cluster of data?

Critical Thinking Exercise 4

REFLECTING ON THE PROCESS OF MAKING INFERENCES

Go back now and carefully consider how you came to the inference you made in the previous exercise. Answering the following will help you reflect on how you came to the conclusion(s) you did.

a. Which of the above pieces of data were very persuasive in guiding you to the inference you drew?

b. Which pieces of data were only suggestive, but not conclusive, as to what inference you should come up with?

c. What do you think was the main point of doing this particular exercise?

Critical Thinking Exercise 5

DECISION MAKING

a. What would be the next immediate steps in management of this patient?

b. What additional diagnostic tests would be appropriate?

c. What would you monitor to assess the patient's response to treatment?

Ms. Krackle is admitted to the ICU and the following data are obtained 4 hours after admission.

Vital signs

HR	145/min
RR	30/min
BP	148/85
SpO_2	81%
Temp.	N/A

ABG 2 L/M NC

pH	7.19
Pco_2	81
Po_2	33
HCO_3^-	30.0
BE	−1
Sao_2	78%

General Mrs. Krackle is increasingly distressed and unable to breathe comfortably except in the upright position. Her mental status appears to be deteriorating.

Auscultation Crackles throughout lung fields.

CXR Chest radiograph shows dense, fluffy infiltrates.

Group Critical Thinking Exercise 1

ASSESSMENT AND DECISION MAKING/MODIFICATION OF CARE PLAN

Have the group discuss this patient's current status. Given the patient's current condition, have your group propose at least two different forms of intervention. Present your group's alternatives to the full class (or alternately to a faculty member). Include:

a. Your assessment of Mrs. Krackle's current condition.

b. The pros and cons of each of the interventions you would consider, and any further diagnostic tests that may be of value.

It is now 5 hours after admission. Mrs. Krackle has been given digitalis and furosemide. BiPAP is started with IPAP = 15 cm H_2O and EPAP = 5 cm H_2O.

Critical Thinking Exercise 6

ANTICIPATING POTENTIAL PROBLEMS

a. What are the potential problems likely to be encountered initiating this form of therapy at this time?

b. How will you make use of your knowledge that these problems may present themselves?

The following are the patient's latest data 3 hours following initiation of NPPV.

ABG est. 50%

pH	7.38
Pco_2	48
Po_2	79
HCO_3^-	29.0
BE	+3
Sao_2	94%

General	The patient's color is improved and she answers questions appropriately. Urine output is 1050 mL over the last 2½ hours.
Auscultation	Crackles remain audible in the lung bases.

Findings from a bedside echocardiogram the following day indicate that the septal and lateral left ventricular walls are hypokinetic and her ejection fraction is 40%. She is weaned off of NPPV after about 18 hours of use. After 2 days with close monitoring and supportive care, Mrs. Krackle is stabilized and discharged home.

 Critical Thinking Exercise 7:

COMMUNICATION

a. What sort of predischarge education would be appropriate for Mrs. Krackle?

b. How would you address the problem she demonstrated with compliance with her medication?

CASE STUDY 2

MR. WILLIAM NEWHART

Initial History

Mr. Newhart, who works as a stockbroker, is a 55-year-old Caucasian male with a diagnosis of congestive heart failure secondary to cardiomyopathy. Eight months ago, he developed a moderately severe upper respiratory infection, which progressed into an acute febrile illness with hepatic, renal, and cardiac symptoms. At the time, he was diagnosed with viral myocarditis, for which he was treated with azathioprine and prednisone. Since that time, he has experienced progressive dyspnea with four hospitalizations for treatment of CHF, and remains in the hospital at this time. After a thorough diagnostic work-up that included an endomyocardial biopsy, he was diagnosed with dilated cardiomyopathy secondary to the previous bout of viral myocarditis. His ejection fraction has progressively fallen during the past 4 months and is now 21%. The patient is unable to perform even the most basic activities of daily living. Due to his rapidly deteriorating condition, he remains in the medical ICU awaiting a donor heart for transplantation. A pulmonary artery catheter (PAC) was placed to monitor hemodynamic changes and to guide therapy. The patient also has an arterial line placed in the left radial artery.

CASE STUDY 2 *(continued)*

Critical Thinking Exercise 1

PRIORITIZING PATIENT CARE

Explain how you would prioritize your assessment of this patient based on his presenting symptoms.

PHYSICAL EXAMINATION DATA ON ADMISSION

Vital signs

HR	132/min
RR	28/min
BP	110/60
SpO_2 %	N/A
Temp.	36.8°C

Appearance	A cachectic-appearing 55-year-old Caucasian male, height 6 feet 1 inch, weight 135 pounds, in moderate respiratory distress, conscious, alert, oriented to time, place, and person, but very anxious.
HEENT	Normal in appearance, pupils equal, round, and reactive to light and accommodation (PERRLA), cranial nerves intact.
Neck	Trachea in the midline with noticeable jugular venous distention, bilateral carotid pulses with no bruits.
Chest	
Inspection	Normal thoracic configuration.
Palpation	Pulsus alternans is also noted. The PMI is displaced laterally.
Auscultation	Bibasilar crackles heard on inspiration and exhalation.

CV	S_1 and S_2 heart sounds are heard diffusely along with S_3 and S_4 gallop.
Abdomen	Slightly distended with evidence of hepatomegaly and a positive hepatojugular reflex.
Extremities	Cool and clammy with some nailbed cyanosis and capillary refill time of 10 seconds.

Critical Thinking Exercise 2

MAKING INFERENCES BY CLUSTERING DATA

a. What inference can you make about the potential for this patient to develop both pulmonary and dependent edema, and why?

b. Practice clustering data by identifying all the data that lead you to make the above inference.

Critical Thinking Exercise 3

ANTICIPATING FINDINGS

a. What additional data would you obtain for your assessment of this patient in the ICU?

b. Why would you look for and collect specific findings?

c. What specific findings do you anticipate and how would they guide you in management of this patient?

CASE STUDY 2 *(continued)*

Mr. Newhart's clinical, laboratory, and hemodynamic data 1 hour after admission:

Vital signs

HR	132/min
RR	26/min
BP	90/60
SpO_2	N/A
Temp.	37.1°C

ABG 6 L/min

pH	7.21
PCO_2	49
PO_2	54
HCO_3^-	19.0
BE	−9
SaO_2	87%

Auscultation	Bibasilar inspiratory and expiratory crackles.
Chest x-ray	Nine rib inspiration, bilateral interstitial infiltrates spreading out from the hila consistent with interstitial edema, cardiomegaly, with a cardiothoracic index of 0.70.

Hemodynamic data

Cardiac output (CO)	2.9 L/min
Cardiac index (CI)	1.9 L/min/m²
Central venous pressure (CVP)	14 mm Hg
PCWP	22 mm Hg
Systemic vascular resistance (SVR)	1544 dynes sec/cm⁵
Pulmonary vascular resistance (PVR)	303 dynes sec/cm⁵
Mean arterial pressure (MAP)	70 mm Hg
Pulmonary artery pressure (PAP)	50/24 mm Hg
$P\bar{v}O_2$	29 mm Hg

CBC

WBC	7000/mm³
Hgb	13.8 g/dL
Hct	40%
RBC	4.4 million/mm³
Electrolytes	normal
Neutrophils	66%
Bands	3%
Lymphocytes	18%
Monocytes	8%
Eosinophils	4%
Basophils	1%

Critical Thinking Exercise 4

PROBLEM SOLVING USING CLINICAL DATA

What does the clinical, lab, and hemodynamic data suggest about this patient's condition? Explain the rationale for your interpretation.

Critical Thinking Exercise 5

ANTICIPATING PROBLEMS AND SOLUTIONS

a. How will you determine how this patient's condition is progressing?

b. What problems would you anticipate?

c. What possible solutions might be appropriate?

Due to the patient's deteriorating cardiovascular status and his most recent ABGs indicating respiratory failure, the patient is electively intubated, and mechanical ventilation is initiated.

CASE STUDY 2 *(continued)*

The dosage of dobutamine is increased from 6 to 10 mg/kg/min and a 40 mg bolus of furosemide is administered by IV push.

Mr. Newhart's clinical data 2 hours post-intubation:

Vital signs

HR	112/min
RR	18/min
BP	110/70
SpO_2	N/A
Temp.	37.1°C

ABG 50% +5 PEEP

pH	7.36
Pco_2	36
Po_2	76
HCO_3^-	20.0
BE	−5
Sao_2	94%

Auscultation	Diminished bilaterally with scattered inspiratory and expiratory crackles.
Chest x-ray	Eight rib inspiration, improvement in bilateral interstitial infiltrates, cardiomegaly again noted.

Hemodynamic data		Ventilator settings	
CO	3.6 L/min	Mode	SIMV
CI	2.4 L/min/m²	VT	700 mL
CVP	10 mm Hg	SIMV f	12 b/min
PCWP	19 mm Hg	Total f	18 b/min
SVR	1622 dynes-sec/cm⁵	FIO_2	0.50
PVR	177 dynes-sec/cm⁵	PEEP	5 cm H_2O

MAP	83 mm Hg	Other data	
PAP	38/22 mm Hg	Urine output	35 mL/h
$P\bar{v}O_2$	38. mm Hg		

The patient was maintained with supportive measures including mechanical ventilation and appropriate pharmacologic agents. A donor heart was located, and the transplant was successfully completed. Postoperatively, the patient was maintained on cyclosporine and azathioprine to prevent rejection of the donor heart. He was educated about lifestyle changes and proper nutrition and started on a directed exercise program. He was discharged 2 weeks after surgery with the addition of prednisone to his regimen of immunosuppressive drugs, which were tapered to maintenance levels. He was followed as an outpatient twice a week for the first 8 weeks, and then monthly. Nine months out, the patient had returned to most of his activities of daily living including work, and showed no signs of transplant rejection.

 Group Critical Thinking Exercise 1

HEALTH CARE COSTS AND ETHICS

Mr. Newhart had excellent health care coverage, but many people do not. Form two groups to research and then debate the following statement:

a. All health care insurance plans should be mandated to include coverage for heart transplants.

One group should research the supporting position and the other the contrary position. The debate should be presented to a group of students and/or a faculty member in your educational program. Teams need to cite specific evidence and reasons for their positions.

CASE STUDY 2 *(continued)*

Group Critical Thinking Exercise 2

THE PRO/CON TEAM DEBATE

Use the second case study to present arguments for and against the position that Mr. Newhart needs a heart transplant. Provide data, evidence, and reasons to support your group's recommendation. Explicitly state the special circumstances, needs, and considerations at this point in case management. Be sure to explain why this decision is the best one at the time and what could happen if there are any further delays. Have one team (three to five students) prepare this recommendation in support of heart transplantation and have a different team prepare the contrary recommendation. The contrary team uses the same case information and data to develop the argument that Mr. Newhart should not be a candidate for heart transplantation at this point in his care. Again the team should provide data, evidence, and reasons to support their recommendation. The instructor acts as the discussion facilitator, keeping the discussion focused, but not supporting either position. The debate can be presented to a third group if the class is large enough. This group can serve as judges and express their opinion on the persuasiveness of the arguments presented by the two sides debating the issue. After the exercise, as a single group the entire class can discuss which team appeared to make the more persuasive case. How and why was their case made more effectively?

Group Critical Thinking Exercise 3

PROBLEM SOLVING AND REFLECTION

Reflect on the decision to place a PAC in this patient. Given the current controversy surrounding the use of the PAC as a monitoring technique, was it appropriate to perform this invasive procedure on this critically ill patient? According to the most recent consensus conference on the use of PACs, what are the indications for PAC monitoring? What are the hazards and complications? Do the potential benefits outweigh the risks for this patient?

KEY POINTS

- Heart failure has been defined as the inability of the heart to pump an adequate amount of oxygenated blood to meet the metabolic demands of the tissues.

- Heart failure is the result of primary heart muscle pathology, or secondary pathology such as ischemic or valvular disease.

- Cardiac output (CO) is determined by the product of left ventricle stroke volume (SV) and heart rate (HR), i.e., CO = SV × HR.

- Stroke volume is determined by the relationship between filling volume (preload), contractility of the myocardium, and outflow resistance (afterload).

- There are a large number of underlying causes of heart failure, including myocardial weakness and inflammation, CAD, loss of muscle cells with scarring (cardiomyopathy), decreased blood flow (ischemia), AMI, hypertension, increased resistance to ejection, congenital heart disease, as well as valvular abnormalities, such as aortic, mitral, or tricuspid insufficiency.

- Precipitating causes of heart failure include hypoxemia, increased salt intake, medication noncompliance, arrhythmia, infection, (e.g., pneumonia), myocardial depressant drugs, and high-output states (e.g., sepsis, anemia, hyperthyroidism, pregnancy, or renal failure).

- Many of the causes of CHF can be viewed as factors or diseases that reduce ventricular stroke volume, often the result of a reduction of preload and/or contractility, or imposition of increased ventricular afterload.

- CHF results from chronic use of the compensatory mechanisms that allow the heart to adapt to changes in load (e.g., Frank-Starling mechanism, increased heart rate, neurohumoral response).

- PCWP that are greater than 20–25 mm Hg are associated with pulmonary edema.

- The term congestive heart failure is often used synonymously with left ventricular failure.

- There are three major manifestations of circulatory congestion syndrome:

  a. Pulmonary congestion (pulmonary edema/SOB)

  b. Peripheral congestion (JVD, hepatomegaly, ascites, extremity edema)

  c. Low-output state (hypotension, lethargy, reduced renal output)

- PCWP > 20–25 mmHG + signs/symptoms confirms cardiogenic pulmonary edema.

- Primary treatment of acute pulmonary edema includes reduction of myocardial workload, increasing contractility, and reducing fluid retention.

- General goals of initial management include improving oxygenation, reducing anxiety, decreasing venous return, decreasing afterload, and treatment of precipitating factors.

- PEEP may improve patients with CHF by decreasing preload and reducing afterload.

- Management of CHF presenting with acute pulmonary edema involves improving oxygenation, reducing the patient's anxiety, decreasing venous return to the heart, increasing myocardial contractility, decreasing afterload, and treatment of precipitating factors.

- More than 75% of CHF patients are over age 65, and CHF is the leading cause of hospitalization in this age group.

- A major cause for decompensation leading to hospitalization among the elderly population appears to be insufficient compliance with regard to lifestyle changes and medication.

- Congestive heart failure is estimated to account for more than $10 billion annually in health care costs.

SUGGESTED RESOURCES—WEB SITES

http://www.americanheart.org/
The American Heart Association

http://www.lungusa.org/
The American Lung Association

http://info.med.yale.edu/intmed/cardio/imaging/contents.html
Yale University School of Medicine cardiothoracic imaging site

---

REFERENCES

1. Roth SL. Congestive heart failure. In: Dantzker DR, MacIntyre NR, Bakow ED, eds. *Comprehensive Respiratory Care.* Philadelphia: Saunders; 1995: 714–725.

2. Iriarte M, Olea JP, Sagastagoitia D, et al. Congestive heart failure due to hypertensive ventricular diastolic dysfunction. *Am J Cardiol.* 1995; 76:43D–47D.

3. Braunwald E. Assessment of cardiac function. In: Braunwald E, ed. *Heart Disease: A Textbook of Cardiovascular Medicine.* 4th ed. Philadelphia: Saunders; 1992:419–443.

4. Just H. Peripheral adaptations in congestive heart failure: A review. *Am J Med.* 1991;90:235.

5. Packer M. Neurohumoral interaction and adaptations in congestive heart failure. *Circulation* 1988; 77:721.

6. Braunwald E. Clinical aspects of heart failure. In: Braunwald E, ed. *Heart Disease: A Textbook of Cardiovascular Medicine.* 4th ed. Philadelphia: Saunders; 1992:444–463.

7. Adams J E, Bodor GS, Davila-Roman VG, et al. Troponin I. A marker with high specificity for cardiac injury. *Circulation* 1993;88:101–106.

8. Adams J E, Sicard GA, Allen BT, et al. Diagnosis of perioperative myocardial infarction with measurement of cardiac troponin I. *N Engl J Med.* 1994; 330:670–674.

9. Antman EM, Tanasijevia MJ, Thompson B, et al. Cardiac specific troponin I levels predict the risk of mortality in patients with acute coronary syndromes. *N Engl J Med.* 1996;335:1342–1349.

10. Kahn JK. *Intra-Aortic Balloon Pumping: Theory and Clinical Applications.* Princeton Junction, NJ: Communications Media for Education, Inc.; 1992: 1–20.

11. Pilbeam SP. Methods to improve oxygenation. In: Russell J, ed. *Mechanical Ventilation: Physiological and Clinical Applications.* 3rd ed. St. Louis: Mosby-Year Book; 1998:262–290.

12. Helmholz HF. Static total compliance and "best PEEP." *Respir Care.* 1981;26:637.

13. Guyatt GH. Positive pressure ventilation as a mechanism of reduction of left ventricular afterload. *Can Med Assoc J.* 1982;126:1310.

14. Kirahawa A, Sakamoto H, Shimizu R. Effect of positive end-expiratory pressure on extravascular lung water and cardiopulmonary function in dogs with experimental severe hydrostatic pulmonary edema. *J Vet Med Sci.* 1996;58:349–354.

15. Kato M, Otsuki M, Wang LQ, et al. Effect of positive end-expiratory pressure on respiration and hemodynamics in dogs with pulmonary edema caused by increased membrane permeability. *Masui-Japanese J Anesthesiol.* 1998;47:9–21.

16. Colmenero-Ruiz M, Fernandez-Mondejar E, Fernandez- Sacristan MA, et al. PEEP and low tidal volume ventilation reduced lung water in porcine pulmonary edema. *Am J Resp Crit Care Med.* 1997; 155: 964–970.

17. Mondejar E F, Mata GV, Cardenas A, et al. Ventilation with positive end-expiratory pressure reduces extravascular lung water and increases lymphatic flow in hydrostatic pulmonary edema. *Crit Care Med.* 1996;24:1562–1567.

18. Kambara K, Longworth KE, Serikov VB, et al. Effect of interstitial edema on lung lymph flow in goats in the absence of filtration. *J Appl Physiol.* 1992;72:1142–1148.

19. Rich MW. Epidemiology, pathophysiology, and etiology of congestive heart failure in older adults. *J Am Geriatr Soc.* 1997;45:968–974.

20. Hunziker P, Bertel O. Heart failure in the elderly. *Schweizerische Rundschau fur Medizin Praxis.* 1995;84:1272–1276.

21. Jaagosild P, Dawson NV, Thomas C, et al. Outcomes of acute exacerbation of severe congestive heart failure: quality of life, resource use, and survival. *Arch Intern Med.* 1998;158:1081–1089.

22. Krumholz HM, Phillips RS, Hamel MB, et al. Resuscitation preferences among patients with severe congestive heart failure: results from the SUPPORT project. *Circulation.* 1998;98:648–655.

23. Candlish P, Watts P, Redman S, et al. Elderly patients with heart failure: a study of satisfaction with care and quality of life. *Int J Quality Health Care.* 1998;10:141–146.

24. Paul S. Implementing an outpatient congestive heart failure clinic: the nurse practitioner role. *Heart Lung.* 1997;26:486–491.

MULTIPLE TRAUMA WITH PULMONARY EMBOLISM

Charles R. Hall, Sr., and R. Randall Baker

For the things we have to learn
before we can do them, we learn by doing them.
ARISTOTLE
384–322 B.C.

LEARNING OBJECTIVES

1. State facts, descriptions, and definitions related to multiple trauma and pulmonary embolism.
2. Discuss the etiology, pathophysiology, and clinical features of a patient with multiple trauma and pulmonary emboli.
3. Discuss the acute and long-term management of patients with multiple trauma and pulmonary emboli.
4. Apply the critical thinking skills of prioritizing, anticipating, negotiating, communicating, and decision making to a case example of a patient with multiple trauma and pulmonary emboli.
5. Use case examples to perform assessments using a standardized system.
6. Interpret clinical data from case examples including history, physical examination, lab data, and radiographs to make recommendations for respiratory care management.
7. Develop a care plan for a patient with multiple trauma and pulmonary emboli, including rec-

ommendations for therapy and disease management with consideration of the cost as well as ethical and quality-of-life issues.
8. Communicate facts, evidence, and arguments to support evaluations and recommendations proposed for the care of a patient with multiple trauma and pulmonary emboli.
9. Evaluate treatment and outcomes of interventions, giving attention to health promotion and quality-of-life issues.
10. Describe the role of the respiratory therapist in the assessment, treatment, management, and education of the patient with multiple trauma and pulmonary emboli.
11. Through performance of critical thinking exercises and group discussion of case questions, apply strategies that promote critical thinking in the respiratory care management of a patient with multiple trauma and pulmonary emboli.

KEY WORDS

Anticoagulant
Cardiac Tamponade
Chest Wall Splinting
D-Dimer
Deep Vein Thrombosis (DVT)
Flail Chest

Glasgow Coma Scale
Hampton's Hump
Hemothorax
International Normalized Ratio (INR)
Paradoxical Abdominal Breathing

Paradoxical Chest Wall Movement
Pneumomediastinum
Pneumothorax
Pulmonary Contusion
Pulmonary Emboli
Subcutaneous Emphysema

Thrombolytic
Traumatic Diaphragmatic Rupture
Trauma
Triage
Westermark's Sign

INTRODUCTION

In the United States, significant costs are associated with traumatic injury, in terms of both lives and health care dollars. Approximately 1 of 4 Americans are injured each year.[1] In 1997, accidents and their adverse effects were the number one cause of death in children and adults aged 1 through 34 years, and were one of the 8 leading causes of death in all other age groups.[2] Injuries from accidents and violence are a major cause of disability and impair quality of life. The years of potential life lost due to unintentional injury is greater than that of cancer or heart disease. When deaths from suicides and homicides are included, the potential years of life lost approximately doubles.[3] Annual medical spending on injury in the United States is over $70 billion,[1] and some individual hospitals estimate their costs to hospitalize and care for youths injured by violence are over $2.5 million per year.[4]

Most injuries treated in the emergency department (ED) are not considered trauma (ie, a life-threatening injury). In the ED and in the field, victims of traumatic injury are triaged based on the seriousness of their injuries. Trauma victims can suffer from immediately life-threatening injuries that often require the resources of highly specialized medical teams. Many of these life-threatening injuries are associated with ventilation and gas exchange. A respiratory therapist is frequently a vital part of the trauma team, and thus is directly

CRITICAL CONTENT

MORBIDITY AND MORTALITY FROM INJURY IS A SERIOUS PROBLEM
- One of four Americans are injured each year.
- Injury is the leading cause of death in young people.
- Injuries from accidents and violence are a major cause of disability and impaired quality of life.
- Medical expenditures in the United States due to injuries total more than $70 billion per year.

---

involved in the initial evaluation and care of the trauma victim. Respiratory therapists must use sound critical thinking skills in their initial assessment and management. To help decrease morbidity and mortality, respiratory therapists are also needed during the recuperation phase to assess and treat respiratory complications that may arise.

The initial traumatic injury and associated complications make trauma management very complex. The approach of this chapter is to try to simplify this subject by using a systematic head-to-toe review of several trauma-related problems associated with ventilation and gas exchange, including the posttrauma complication of pulmonary embolism.

The chapter also focuses on a few of the vital critical thinking skills that respiratory therapists must possess in their immediate and long-term management of a trauma patient.

CRITICAL CONTENT

**LIFE-THREATENING AIRWAY INJURIES
ARE COMMON IN TRAUMA VICTIMS
AND REQUIRE SKILLFUL MANAGEMENT**

- Respiratory therapists must possess sound critical thinking skills in trauma assessment and management.
- Respiratory therapists are a vital part of the health care team and can use their expertise to decrease morbidity and mortality.

ETIOLOGY

The mechanisms of injury are diverse. The nature and extent of an injury depend upon 1) the velocity of the impact, 2) the site of impact, and 3) the materials that impact with the body. Contributing factors that result in trauma include motor vehicle accidents (MVAs), falls, burns, industrial accidents, drownings, sports-related injury, suicide attempts, and acts of violence and nature. Confounding factors include the victim's age and/or underlying physical condition. Injuries are often associated with alcohol and drug abuse or other high-risk behaviors. Three general classifications of trauma are blunt, penetrating, and multiple trauma.

CRITICAL CONTENT

The nature and extent of an injury depends upon:
- The velocity of the impact;
- The site of impact; and
- The materials that impact upon the body.

Blunt trauma, in which there is no penetration of the body, is usually caused by high-velocity impacts or crushing events. Industrial accidents and MVAs are common causes of blunt trauma. Penetrating trauma is a potentially life-threatening situation in which an object passes through the skin and into an organ or one of the body cavities such as the skull, thorax, or abdomen. This is different from a laceration, which is a ragged, mangled tearing of the flesh, although penetration may accompany a severe laceration. Stabbings, gunshots, falls, and MVAs are common causes of penetrating trauma. Many victims arriving in the ED have sustained major trauma to multiple organ systems, and associated injuries can pose severe consequences if overlooked. Multiple trauma is sometimes referred to as combined, mixed, or polytrauma and can involve both blunt and penetrating injuries.

Life-threatening injuries associated with either blunt or penetrating trauma include head and upper airway injury, traumatic brain injury (TBI), spinal cord injury (SCI), chest injury, abdominal injury, and severe bone fractures. Complications associated with chest injury result from rib fracture, pulmonary contusion, pneumothorax (and its various subtypes), hemothorax, pericardial tamponade, flail chest, or great vessel disruption. These injuries may lead to unconsciousness, arrhythmias, hypotension, organ injury, severe external and internal bleeding, and respiratory failure.

CRITICAL CONTENT

Multiple trauma victims are at high risk for morbidity and mortality from significant injury to more than one organ system and the complications associated with these injuries.

Some posttrauma problems associated with increased morbidity and mortality in multiple trauma victims include infection, pneumonia, deep vein thrombosis (DVT), pulmonary embolism (PE), and acute respiratory distress syndrome (ARDS). Pneumonia and ARDS are discussed elsewhere in this textbook. Deep vein thrombosis (ie, release of blood clots) is a major complication in orthopedic surgical patients and is frequently linked to PE.[5] Additional types of emboli found in trauma patients include air, tissue, bone, and fat. It is estimated that over 600,000 cases of PE occur annually and that the associated mortality is approximately 10%.[6] There is an increased risk for DVT and PE, including fatal PE, in patients undergoing abdominal surgery, with the highest risk in patients undergoing major trauma or orthopedic surgery, including pelvic and long bone fractures.[7]

CRITICAL CONTENT

Common posttrauma complications include:
- Infection
- Pneumonia
- Deep vein thrombosis
- Pulmonary embolism
- Acute respiratory distress syndrome

ASSESSMENT OF THE TRAUMA PATIENT

Role of the Respiratory Therapist

If not assessed and treated properly, significant injuries may have profoundly devastating effects for the victim, including long-term disability or death. Emergency department assessment of a trauma patient is a difficult task and is most often carried out in a coordinated manner by a designated trauma team. The team leader, usually the most senior physician, is in charge of the treatment process and acts as the team coordinator. Respiratory therapists are core team members and assist in this initial assessment process. These high-stress emergency situations are handled much better if the respiratory therapist is familiar with the surroundings, their role, and the roles of each member of the trauma team.

The respiratory therapist in the ED must quickly recognize and treat situations that may lead to life-threatening respiratory failure, and their primary role is to assess, establish, and maintain the airway. This is always the respiratory therapist's *first* major priority in a case of trauma. Inadequate ventilation and gas exchange in a trauma patient can exacerbate concurrent traumatic injuries and rapidly lead to irreversible anoxic brain injury or death.

CRITICAL CONTENT

THE RESPIRATORY THERAPIST'S ROLE IN INITIAL ASSESSMENT IS IMPORTANT!

- The respiratory therapist in the ED must quickly recognize and treat situations that may lead to life-threatening respiratory failure.
- The respiratory therapist's *first* major priority in a trauma is to assess, establish, and maintain the airway.

Assessment Overview

In general, primary assessment of a trauma patient involves a primary and secondary **ABCD** survey. The respiratory therapist should place the highest priority on the primary **ABCD** survey. Is the **A**irway open? Is the patient **B**reathing? Is there adequate **C**irculation? Is there a heart rhythm indicating the need for **D**efibrillation? The following are areas the respiratory therapist should prioritize in the secondary **ABCD** survey. Is intubation of the **A**irway indicated? Is **B**reathing effective with adequate ventilation? In **C**irculation, has IV access been obtained and what drugs have been used? What would be included in the differential **D**iagnosis?[8] The acronym **ABCD** is common and can mean different things when used as an assessment tool. One method, which changes the **D** and includes an additional parameter **E**, is **A**irway, **B**reathing, **C**irculation, **D**isability (level of consciousness), and **E**xposure (removal of the victim's clothes for complete assessment).

Once the patient's airway and ventilation are stabilized, the respiratory therapist may assist other team members as they complete a head-to-toe evaluation, commonly referred to as the secondary assessment. Part of the secondary assessment in the ED is to gather pertinent patient history. **AMPLE** is one acronym used to guide this process. History about known drug **A**llergies and current **M**edications should be obtained, if possible. Other pertinent information is the **P**ast medical history, time of **L**ast meal, and **E**vents leading up to the injury. Vital signs are obtained and the order of the head-to-toe assessment usually proceeds through head, ear, eyes, nose, and throat (HEENT); neck; chest; cardiovascular (CV); abdomen; back; genitourinary (GU); rectal; and extremities.

CRITICAL CONTENT

Primary assessment of a trauma patient involves primary and secondary **ABCD** surveys:
- The respiratory therapist places highest priority on the primary **ABCD** survey: **A**irway, **B**reathing, **C**irculation, and **D**efibrillation.
- The next highest priority is on the secondary **ABCD** survey: Is it necessary to intubate the **A**irway? During **B**reathing, is ventilation effective? In **C**irculation, has IV access been obtained and what drugs have been used? What is the differential **D**iagnosis?

As previously stated, problems with ventilation and gas exchange can exacerbate concurrent traumatic injuries and rapidly lead to irreversible anoxic brain injury or death. Therefore respiratory therapists must be able to quickly gather subjective and objective data to know when to provide respiratory support. Subjective data can include patient comments about pain or difficulty breathing. Objective data can include the actual quality of the patient's speech, the amount of effort

needed to speak, or the presence of facial injuries. Other routine objective data include pulse oximetry, blood gases, and vital signs. Both the objective and subjective data collected by the therapist during the primary and secondary surveys should guide the need for respiratory support that includes 1) ensuring a patent airway, 2) providing supplemental oxygen, and 3) instituting positive pressure ventilation when spontaneous ventilation is absent. The next few sections of this chapter cover the typical pathophysiology, clinical features, treatment, and management of trauma-related conditions.

CRITICAL CONTENT

Objective and subjective data should guide respiratory support that includes:
- Ensuring a patent airway
- Providing supplemental oxygen
- Instituting positive pressure ventilation when spontaneous ventilation is absent

PATHOPHYSIOLOGY

Various pathophysiologic changes are associated with trauma and will vary with the severity of injury. Significant injuries are often unseen and require sound assessment skills to determine their presence. To understand and treat the diverse nature of trauma-related injuries, respiratory therapists must have knowledge of these conditions and their impact on patient management. A systematic approach should be used when first assessing a trauma patient, as discussed in the previous section. During the primary survey, the respiratory therapist must be on the lookout for conditions that are life-threatening and could lead to respiratory failure (eg, airway obstruction or tension pneumothorax).

The development of respiratory failure is one of the most common life-threatening problems associated with traumatic injuries. Respiratory failure affects all age groups and is a major cause of morbidity and mortality. The respiratory therapist must be able to both assess trauma victims for the presence of respiratory failure and be aware of the types of injuries that can lead to respiratory failure. Furthermore, the respiratory therapist must understand the nature of the patient's pathologies in order to rapidly implement effective assessment and management techniques.

This section will emphasize injuries that may lead to hypercapnic respiratory failure by either decreasing minute ventilation or causing significant ventilation-perfusion mismatch. The respiratory therapist must understand that the first gas exchange abnormality observed with intrinsic lung dysfunction is hypoxemia rather than hypercapnia. Respiratory failure may present as hypoxemia alone or hypoxemia with hypercapnia. While there is considerable overlap, hypoxemic respiratory failure is frequently associated with ARDS, which is covered in detail in Chapter 22. Although the classification is arbitrary, it can help the therapist by grouping injuries that may seem extremely diverse into conditions with similar pathogenesis and therapeutic approaches.

CRITICAL CONTENT

The development of respiratory failure is one of the most common life-threatening problems associated with traumatic injuries. Respiratory therapists must:

• Be able to both assess trauma victims for the presence of respiratory failure and be aware of the types of injuries that can lead to respiratory failure.

• Understand the nature of the patient's pathologies in order to rapidly implement effective assessment and management techniques.

• Understand that the first gas exchange abnormality observed with intrinsic lung dysfunction is hypoxemia rather than hypercapnia.

Blood CO_2 is determined by the balance between CO_2 production and CO_2 elimination by the lungs. Increased CO_2 production rarely results in hypercapnia due to the feedback mechanisms that are part of the central control of ventilation that increase alveolar ventilation to improve CO_2 removal. The more likely cause of hypercapnia is a decrease in alveolar ventilation. Alveolar hypoventilation results from either an absolute decrease in minute ventilation without a change in deadspace ventilation or ventilation-perfusion mismatch in the lungs with normal or elevated minute ventilation. Deadspace ventilation is increased in this latter situation.

Hypercapnic respiratory failure is due to conditions that either decrease minute ventilation or create ventilation-perfusion mismatch. These two pathogenetic mechanisms can be differentiated by the alveolar-arterial oxygen difference ($P_{AO_2} - Pa_{O_2}$). A normal $P_{AO_2} - Pa_{O_2}$ (≤ 20 mm Hg) in the presence of hypercapnia and hypoxemia indicates hypoventilation (ie, a decrease in alveolar ventilation). The extent of hypoxemia is dependent upon the level of hypercapnia.

Ventilation-perfusion mismatch is normally present when the $P_{AO_2} - Pa_{O_2}$ is greater than 20 mm Hg, and is accompanied by hypercapnia only when the mismatch is severe. The number of effective alveolar-capillary (A-C) units is decreased during a mismatch of ventilation and perfusion. Hypoxemia results when there is an increase in the relative number of underventilated A-C units. Then stimulation of peripheral chemoreceptors usually results in an increase in overall ventilation. Normal A-C units are then overventilated, initially resulting in a lower arterial P_{CO_2}. When the number of underventilated A-C units reaches a critical level, and minute ventilation is not further increased to compensate for this, the lung's ability to excrete CO_2 is impaired and arterial P_{CO_2} is increased.

Decreased alveolar ventilation may be secondary to central respiratory depression, airway obstruction, thoracic or abdominal pain, or increases in deadspace. Central respiratory depression can result from head or spinal cord injury or from the administration of narcotics or sedatives. Alteration in spontaneous respiration occurs in 60% of

CRITICAL CONTENT

Hypercapnic respiratory failure is due to conditions that either decrease minute ventilation or create significant ventilation-perfusion mismatch.
- A normal $P_{AO_2} - P_{aO_2}$ ($\leq$20 mm Hg) in the presence of hypercapnia and hypoxemia indicates hypoventilation (ie, a decrease in alveolar ventilation).
- Ventilation-perfusion mismatch is normally present when the $P_{AO_2} - P_{aO_2}$ is greater than 20 mm Hg, and is accompanied by hypercapnia only when the mismatch is severe.

patients with traumatic brain injury (TBI).[9] The posttraumatic changes in spontaneous respiration include apnea, Cheyne-Stokes respiration, irregular breathing, and tachypnea.[9] Injury to the cervical spinal cord (C3-C5) can cause partial or complete loss of diaphragmatic innervation, which impairs ventilation.

Hypoventilation may also result from airway obstruction. Airway obstruction may be due to changes in the oropharyngeal soft tissue or mechanical blockage. Soft tissue obstruction may result from loss of consciousness following TBI or direct injury to the face or neck. Mechanical barriers to ventilation include foreign body aspiration (eg, teeth, food, gravel, vomitus, and blood) and uncleared airway secretions. Airway obstruction may also result in ventilation-perfusion mismatch. In this case, hypercapnia will be present only when the ventilation-perfusion abnormality is severe.

Splinting from thoracic or abdominal pain can result in decreased alveolar ventilation. This cause of hypoventilation should be suspected in the presence of fractured ribs. Increased physiologic deadspace from hypovolemia and shock can also result in decreased alveolar ventilation. This occurs as the result of inadequate perfusion of parts of the lung during severe hypovolemia/shock, which causes significant increases in ventilated, but not perfused (deadspace), A-C units. When increased deadspace

is the cause of alveolar hypoventilation, hypercapnia will usually be present only when the patient is unable to increase their minute ventilation in the presence of central respiratory depression from either the trauma or sedation.

CRITICAL CONTENT

Decreased alveolar ventilation may be secondary to:
- Central respiratory depression
- Airway obstruction
- Thoracic or abdominal pain
- Increases in deadspace without corresponding increases in overall ventilation

Traumatic injuries to the chest wall, pleural space, lung parenchyma, and mediastinum can result in both decreased alveolar ventilation and ventilation-perfusion mismatch. Direct injury to the chest wall may lead to flail chest, pneumothorax, hemothorax, pulmonary contusion, tracheobronchial disruption, and diaphragmatic disruption.

Flail chest occurs when fractures of three or more ribs in two places are present on the same side of the chest, or on either side of the sternum. This injury reduces chest wall stability, increases work of breathing, and results in paradoxical chest wall movement in the affected area. There is controversy regarding the cause of the hypoxemia and hypercapnia observed in flail chest.[10] The "pendelluft" phenomenon, in which paradoxical chest wall movement causes air to move from the damaged to the normal lung upon inspiration and in the opposite direction during expiration, was previously offered as an explanation for inadequate ventilation and gas exchange.[11] However, more recent studies indicate that ventilation and oxygen uptake are greater in the lung on the side with the flail segment.[12, 13] The hypoxemia and hypercapnia may be caused by underlying injury, such as pulmonary contusion, and hypoventilation from splinting.[10] Continued splinting may lead to atelectasis and pneumonia, causing further disruptions in gas exchange.[10] The force required to cause flail chest injuries often results in underlying injuries to the lung, with mortality rates of 10% to 50%.[14–16]

Blunt or penetrating trauma to the chest wall that allows air into the pleural space results in pneumothoraces. In blunt trauma, a pneumothorax can result from tearing of pleural membranes by sharp rib fractures, tracheobronchial disruption, or alveolar rupture. The air can enter through the chest wall and parietal pleura in penetrating trauma. The pathophysiology associated with a pneumothorax varies from none to cardiovascular collapse, depending on the amount of air within the pleural space and whether the air is under positive pressure (tension pneumothorax). Decreased compliance and hypoxemia are associated with pneumothoraces greater than 20%. Cardiovascular collapse is associated with tension pneumothoraces in which the positive pressure within the pleural space causes shifting of the mediastinum, complete collapse of the affected lung, decreased venous return, hypoxemia, hypotension, and decreased cardiac output. It is unclear whether the cardiovascular changes seen in tension pneumothorax are due to inhibition of venous return caused by increased intrathoracic pressure or are due to severe alterations in gas exchange. Regardless of the mechanism, tension pneumothoraces are life threatening and must be recognized and treated immediately.

CRITICAL CONTENT

Pathophysiologies associated with pneumothorax vary from none to cardiovascular collapse.

- Decreased compliance and hypoxemia are associated with pneumothoraces greater than 20%.
- Cardiovascular collapse is associated with tension pneumothoraces.

Hemothorax is another insult to the pleural space that may result from penetrating or blunt trauma to the chest wall, lung, or mediastinal blood vessels. The patient's status will depend on the amount of blood that has accumulated in the pleural space. Gas exchange may be compromised through compression of lung tissue and mediastinal shift can occur. Decreased venous return and cardiac output with hypotension can result due to hypovolemia from a large hemothorax. Similar compression of lung tissue may occur following diaphragmatic rupture and invasion of abdominal contents into the thoracic space. If sufficient alveolar surface is compromised, hypercapnia and hypoxemia will result. Disruption of the diaphragm may impair respiratory mechanics as well as gas exchange.

Injury to lung parenchyma following penetrating or blunt trauma or rapid deceleration of the lung against the chest wall can result in pulmonary contusion, hematoma, or laceration. Pulmonary contusions consist of ruptured alveoli and pulmonary capillaries, hemorrhage, edema, and increased pulmonary vascular permeability.[10] The parenchymal injuries associated with pulmonary contusions can lead to progressive respiratory failure. Ruptured blood vessels and increased vascular permeability leads to edema and associated disruption of gas exchange.

Pulmonary embolism results in occlusion of pulmonary arteries. Most commonly, pulmonary emboli result from blood clots that form in the deep veins of the legs above the knees. These clots break off, flow back to the right heart, and are pumped into the pulmonary artery. The clots move down the arterial tree until they reach vessels with a diameter too small for them to pass. Clinical risk factors for development of pulmonary embolism are venous stasis, injury to blood vessel walls, and increased coagulability.

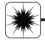

CRITICAL CONTENT

CLINICAL RISK FACTORS FOR PULMONARY EMBOLISM

- Venous stasis
- Injury to blood vessel walls
- Increased coagulability

Major trauma increases the short-term risk for both venous thrombosis and pulmonary emboli a hundredfold.[17] Tissue injury as a result of trauma may directly injure blood vessel walls and increase coagulability.[18] In addition, patients recovering from trauma may have increased venous stasis during prolonged confinement to a bed, limb immobilization, and localized vascular damage.

Patients recovering from trauma are also subject to conditions that can directly create emboli from sources other than blood clots. Traumatic fractures of the pelvis or long bones in the legs may result in mobilization of fat or tissue emboli. In addition, injuries to the pulmonary hilum and lung parenchyma may lead to the generation of air emboli.

CRITICAL CONTENT

Major trauma increases the short-term risk for both venous thrombosis and pulmonary emboli a hundredfold.

- Traumatic fractures of the pelvis or long bones in the legs may result in mobilization of fat or tissue emboli.
- Injuries to the pulmonary hilum and lung parenchyma may lead to the generation of air emboli.

A major pathophysiologic feature of PE is the development of alveolar deadspace. This mismatch of ventilation and perfusion occurs when occlusion of a pulmonary arteriole diminishes blood flow in pulmonary capillaries and ventilation to the alveoli in that region continues. An increase in deadspace decreases alveolar ventilation and CO_2 removal. However, after a PE, patients routinely increase minute ventilation and exhibit hyperventilation and hypocapnia. Measuring minute ventilation shows that arterial CO_2 is not decreased as much as it should be for a given increase in ventilation due to increased alveolar deadspace.

The hypoxemia associated with PE is thought to be due to bronchoconstriction that results from release of chemical mediators from thrombi, including histamine, serotonin, and prostaglandins. These mediators circulate from areas of the lung with emboli and can act on uninvolved bronchi, creating low ventilation-perfusion ratios (ie, shunt-like effects) and hypoxemia.

Pulmonary vascular resistance can increase due to occlusion of the pulmonary vessels. However, the vascular bed within the lungs is capable of both recruitment and distention and significant increases in resistance are only noted when 50% to 70% of the pulmonary vessels are occluded. Severe PE and release of the previously mentioned vasoactive mediators can, however, cause syncope or hypotensive shock. When the pulmonary vascular resistance is severe enough to lead to acute right heart failure, jugular venous distention (JVD) and increased systemic blood pressure may be noted.

Finally, atelectasis may result following PE due to several mechanisms. First, mediator-related bronchoconstriction can lead to volume loss in the lung. Secondary bronchoconstriction from hypocapnia in the overventilated, deadspace regions of the lung results in further volume loss. Finally, decreased blood flow and oxygenation of several lung regions decreases surfactant synthesis in the affected areas. The decreased compliance decreases lung volume and may precipitate alveolar collapse and fluid leakage into intact alveoli.

CRITICAL CONTENT

DEADSPACE IS A MAJOR PATHOPHYSIOLOGIC FEATURE OF PULMONARY EMBOLISM

- After a PE, patients routinely increase minute ventilation and exhibit hyperventilation and hypocapnia.
- Measuring minute ventilation demonstrates that arterial CO_2 is not decreased as much as it should be for a given increase in ventilation, due to increased alveolar deadspace.

CLINICAL INJURY FEATURES ASSOCIATED WITH RESPIRATORY FAILURE

Clinical features that may result in respiratory failure greatly depend on the mechanism and severity of the injury. Generally, a conscious trauma victim that has anxiety, dyspnea, increased work of breathing (WOB), and possibly cyanosis, may have impending respiratory failure. Increased WOB may be demonstrated by diaphoresis, complaints of shortness of breath (dyspnea), accessory muscle use, and nasal flaring, as well as intercostal and supraclavicular retractions. Tachycardia and tachypnea resulting from hypoxemia may also be present. For the respiratory therapist, basic clinical observation in the ED should focus on those problems that adversely impact ventilation and/or the process of gas exchange. Following is a brief overview of clinical features associated with some of the more common types of injuries faced by a respiratory therapist that may lead to respiratory failure.

CRITICAL CONTENT

Respiratory therapists must focus in emergency care on those problems that:
- Adversely impact ventilation
- Impair the process of gas exchange

Traumatic Brain Injury

Victims may present with severe or mild traumatic brain injuries (TBI) that lead to problems with ventilation. The most important clinical observation is any change in the state of consciousness since the time of the injury. A hallmark of brain injury is alteration of consciousness. A presenting TBI victim can have significant cognitive, physical, and psychological deficits, and thus should be assessed for alertness and orientation. A common method of assessing orientation is to focus on person, place, time, and event. For example, you can ask patients their name, where they are, the date, and what happened to them.

The respiratory therapist should look for a lack of verbal response to questioning or the absence of purposeful movements. The RT should also look for obvious bleeding, contusions, or deformities in the head area. Someone on the trauma team should be assigned to assess the patient's rating on the Glasgow Coma Scale (GCS) and should assess the eyes to see if the pupils are equal, round, reactive to light, and have normal accommodation (PERRLA). Accommodation is a normal adjustment reflex of the eye for viewing objects at various distances. Moving an object such as a pen toward the eye and then away from the eye should elicit reflex lens movement. Fixed and dilated pupils or pupils that react to neither light nor accommodation usually indicate brain death. However, drugs can cause either abnormal dilation (mydriasis) or constriction (miosis). Pinpoint pupils or pupils that are severely constricted are usually associated with drugs or lesions of the pons. Abnormal dilation of the pupils is common in cases of deep coma.

Cognitive deficits in language and communication, information processing, memory, and perception skills can occur following traumatic injury to the head. The respiratory therapist should look for memory loss of items such as date, address, or occupation. Deficits may also be found in strength, fine motor skills, endurance, balance, and coordination. *Mild* TBI may result in a brief loss of consciousness (BLOC), loss of memory immediately before or after the injury, an alteration in the mental state at the time of an accident, or other focal neurological deficits. *Severe* TBI may lead to disordered breathing patterns such as apnea or hyperpnea, or Biot's or Cheyne-Stokes breathing.

Spinal Cord Injury

Spinal cord injuries (SCI) are often associated with head injuries. Decreased or absent muscle movement due to a SCI contributes to ventilation and oxygenation problems. It is extremely important for the respiratory therapist to be aware of this possibility, particularly in injuries to the cervical vertebrae. The diaphragm is innervated by nerves exiting the spinal cord at levels C3 to C5. Severing of the spinal cord above this level will result in total

CRITICAL CONTENT

TRAUMATIC BRAIN INJURY (TBI)

- A hallmark of brain injury is alteration of consciousness.
- TBI can cause cognitive, physical, and psychological deficits.
- Mild TBI may result in a brief loss of consciousness.
- Severe TBI may lead to disordered breathing patterns

respiratory muscle paralysis and death. Injuries in the C3 to C5 region can cause a decrease in respiratory strength due to effects on the diaphragm. Diaphragmatic weakness may be demonstrated by paradoxical abdominal breathing. The respiratory therapist in the ED should look for tachypnea (a rapid, shallow breathing pattern) as well as the use of accessory muscles. A loss of bladder and bowel sphincter control is consistent with cervical injuries as well. Improper or lack of neck or back stabilization can compound SCI and significantly affect the morbidity and mortality of a trauma victim.

CRITICAL CONTENT

The level of a spinal cord lesion determines the clinical picture:

- Damage to the spinal cord above C5 results in total respiratory muscle paralysis that may lead to apnea and death.
- Injuries in the C3 to C5 region can cause a decrease in respiratory strength due to effects on the diaphragm.
- Clinical respiratory signs that might indicate spinal cord injury include apnea, rapid and shallow breathing, paradoxical abdominal breathing, and accessory muscle use.
- If spinal cord injury is suspected, the patient's neck and back must be stabilized.

Consequently, health care personnel must ensure special handling of the airway of a patient with suspected or possible head and neck injury.

Airway Injury

Upper airway injuries are a possible cause of upper airway obstruction, which can significantly alter ventilation. Injuries to the face or neck region can be manifested by external and internal swelling, which can lead to partial or complete airway obstruction. Even subtle areas of bruising or swelling could lead to a complicating injury. Examination of the face, oral cavity, nares, and neck by observation and palpation is critical. The victim may have obvious bleeding, broken teeth, or obstructing material (including dentures) in the oropharynx. Unstable mandible and maxillary bones should be noted by the respiratory therapist since these injuries make emergency intubation difficult. Examination of the neck may reveal soft tissue damage, bruising, or air in the soft tissues (subcutaneous emphysema). Subcutaneous emphysema may be present when crepitus (a crackling tactile sensation or sound) is palpated. Often, severe injuries may not be noted until restraints to immobilize the head and neck are removed. Laryngeal injuries may present with stridor, hoarseness, cough, neck pain, hemoptysis, dysphonia, aphasia, or dysphasia.

Lower airway injuries in trauma victims can quickly lead to respiratory failure from either ventilation problems, gas exchange problems, or both. Common problems include chest wall contusion, pulmonary contusion, rib fractures, flail chest, traumatic diaphragmatic rupture, and great vessel injury. Inadequate ventilation following lower airway injury is commonly due to splinting associated with pain or chest wall instability. Pain alone can decrease ventilation, vital capacity, and the clearing of secretions. In the ED, typical signs of pain include tachycardia, tachypnea, increased blood pressure, sweaty palms, and anxiety, as well as moaning, crying, or yelling. The patient may also wince or grimace when touched or moved. Rib fractures, the most common injury in blunt trauma victims, are a common cause of pain, as are pneumo- and hemothoraces. Victims with broken ribs must also be assessed for abdominal injuries such as a torn diaphragm, lacerated liver, or ruptured spleen.

Any significant bleeding may result in hypovolemic or hemorrhagic shock. Shock is usually indicated by marked paleness of the skin, cold clammy extremities, cyanosis, a weak and tachycardic pulse, shallow rapid breathing, and decreased or unobtainable blood pressure.

CRITICAL CONTENT

RESPIRATORY THERAPISTS MUST ALWAYS BE ALERT WHEN A PATIENT PRESENTS WITH A POSSIBLE AIRWAY INJURY!

- Upper and lower airway injuries may cause complete or partial airway obstruction.
- Lower airway injuries can quickly lead to respiratory failure from ventilation and/or gas exchange problems.

Chest Problems

Lower airway and internal chest problems can significantly impact gas exchange. An ECG may show dysrhythmias that could indicate a myocardial contusion. Clinically, if a contusion is noted on the external chest, there might be severe underlying injuries, which can include pulmonary contusion, disruption or rupture of great vessels, or injury to other intrathoracic structures. Internal chest injuries may also exist if a contusion is found only in the abdominal area. After a pulmonary contusion injury, hemorrhage into areas of the lung typically worsens over the first 24 to 48 hours. Hypoxemia and hypercarbia are usually maximal during the initial 72 hours. Unless the patient develops a clinical course that leads to a pulmonary infection or ARDS, the contusion generally resolves over 7 days.[19] The presence of hemoptysis or hematemesis may indicate an esophageal or airway injury. It is important for the RT to know and be able to differentiate between

TABLE 19-1 COMMON CLINICAL FEATURES OF PNEUMOTHORAX

WITHOUT TENSION[a]	WITH TENSION[a]
• Distress • Dyspnea or increased WOB • Labored respirations (if significant) • Diaphoresis may be present • Tachycardia • Tachypnea • Chest pain • Asymmetric chest wall movement that is decreased on the affected side • Decreased or distant breath sounds on the affected side • Increased resonance to percussion on the affected side	All the signs and symptoms found without without tension, plus: • Progressive cyanosis • Tracheal shift upon palpation • Cardiac compromise, decreased blood pressure • JVD

[a]Other clinical presentations could be diminished tactile fremitus, coughing, wheezing, fatigue, or decreased level of consciousness.

Chest radiograph: May visualize the edge of the visceral pleura displaced from the chest wall because of the trapped gas in the pleural space. The space between the visceral pleura and internal chest is radiolucent (black) with vascular markings absent. In a tension pneumothorax, the pressure of the gas in the space between the chest wall and the lung is sufficient to shift the lung and mediastinal structures to the opposite side.

TABLE 19-2 COMMON CLINICAL FEATURES OF HEMOTHORAX

• Distress	• Decreased resonance to percussion depending on patient's position and area percussed
• Dyspnea	
• Labored respirations if significant	• Tachycardia and tachypnea may be present if significant
• Diaphoresis may be present	
• Asymmetric chest wall movement that is decreased on affected side with possible bulging	• Tracheal shift upon palpation if tension is present
• Lung sounds usually decreased depending on patient's position	• May be cardiac compromise due to hypovolemia or tension
• Pleuritic or dull chest wall pain	• Usually no JVD due to the hypovolemia

Chest radiograph: May present with blunting of the costophrenic angle if the patient is positioned upright and fluid layer may be seen in lateral film. Blood may spread out throughout the hemithorax in the supine position and appear as an increased opacity or haziness of one lung field.

the clinical features of common chest problems caused by trauma, including pneumothorax (Table 19-1), hemothorax (Table 19-2), cardiac tamponade (Table 19-3), traumatic diaphragmatic rupture (Table 19-4), and flail chest (Table 19-5).

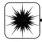

CRITICAL CONTENT

Common chest problems associated with trauma include:
- Pneumothorax
- Hemothorax
- Cardiac tamponade
- Traumatic diaphragmatic rupture
- Flail chest

Pulmonary Embolism

As the respiratory therapist, you must know the clinical features of PE, since traumatic injury may result in the mobilization of air, blood, fat, or tissue emboli to the lungs. Evaluation of a patient suspected of PE depends on the local availability of equipment and expertise. Typically, evaluation begins with a thorough physical examination and

TABLE 19-3 COMMON CLINICAL FEATURES OF CARDIAC TAMPONADE

SLOW ONSET[a]	ACUTE ONSET[b]
• Dyspnea	Same manifestations found in slow onset plus:
• Orthopnea	
• Hepatic engorgement	
• JVD	• Muffled or distant heart sounds
• Paradoxical pulse	• Rising or elevated venous pressure
• Reductions in amplitude of QRS complexes	• A falling or absent blood pressure

[a]Resembles clinical manifestations of heart failure.

[b]Within minutes.

Chest radiograph: In the case of acute onset, the chest radiograph is of limited value as the amount of fluid causing deadly tamponade may be too small to cause any noticeable changes in the size and contour of the cardiac shadow. In case of the slow onset, look for changes in heart size, especially in the absence of radiographic signs of congestive heart failure (especially with clear lungs). Fluid may obliterate the angles and recesses that demarcate the various segments of the cardiac contour and there may be straightening of the upper left heart border combined with prominent rounding of the left and right heart borders.

T A B L E   1 9 - 4   COMMON CLINICAL FEATURES OF TRAUMATIC DIAPHRAGMATIC RUPTURE

- Most commonly seen on the left
- Most common organs herniated are the stomach and bowels. Less common are the spleen and omentum
- May be asymptomatic
- Most common complaint is dyspnea
- Respiratory distress
- Tenderness in left upper quadrant
- Left thoracic or shoulder pain may occur (significant sign if herniation is large, but vague if small)
- Respiratory and circulatory compromise if herniation is large enough to create a mediastinal shift
- Only signs of small herniations would be developing signs of visceral strangulation, GI tract obstruction, or atelectasis days to weeks after injury

Chest radiograph: The single best diagnostic test. Look for elevation, irregularity, or obscurity of any part of the hemidiaphragm. While bowel loops in the chest are an obvious sign, small herniations are more subtle. Radiographic findings to look for are atelectasis, mediastinal shift, pleural fluid, or an air-fluid level above the diaphragm. Traumatic diaphragmatic rupture is often associated with lower rib fractures, pneumothorax, and hemothorax.

history taking. This evaluation guides the choice of diagnostic studies. A patient with focal leg pain, tenderness, and swelling, who has known risk factors for deep vein thrombosis (DVT), is considered to have the highest probability of embolism.[20] Pelvic and long bone fractures also place a patient in a high-risk category.[21]

T A B L E   1 9 - 5   COMMON CLINICAL FEATURES OF FLAIL CHEST

- Pain
- Dyspnea
- Tachycardia
- Tachypnea
- Hypoxemia
- Paradoxical chest wall movement
- Chest wall splinting*

*May support chest wall initially, thereby masking paradoxical chest wall movement.

Chest radiograph: May be difficult to note specific broken ribs to suggest flail without the physical clinical presentation. Large number of ribs broken in one area of the chest should increase the suspicion of flail. Look for anterior or lateral rib breaks that correspond to posterior breaks of the same rib.

The classic clinical features found in patients with both minor and major PE are 1) acute onset dyspnea, 2) pleuritic chest pain (aggravated by inspiration), and 3) hemoptysis. When a PE is minor, the clinical features are often nonspecific and may be caused by other conditions, such as viral or bacterial pulmonary infections and acute bronchitis. Patients with a major (massive) embolus may have the classic clinical features along with one or more of the following: syncope, apprehension, diaphoresis, tachypnea, tachycardia, hypotension, right ventricular overload (acute cor pulmonale), JVD, and mental confusion.[5] Chest signs and symptoms are nonspecific and may even be normal. Chest findings may include dull chest pain, decreased breath sounds, crackles, wheezes, pleural rub, or pleural effusion.[5] The ECG may be normal and nonspecific or show inverted T waves and a depressed ST segment referred to as $S_1Q_3T_3$.[21] There may also be an increased P_2 (second heart sound) heard upon auscultation.[22]

The V/Q scan is the diagnostic procedure of choice and is used in most facilities when PE is suspected. Other diagnostic procedures are useful to reduce the number of missed diagnoses. These procedures include chest radiography, electrocardiography, pulmonary angiography, computed tomography

(CT), impedance plethysmography, ultrasound, and magnetic resonance imaging.[20, 21, 23] It is important to note, however, that the chest radiograph is often not very useful in diagnosing a PE. This will be discussed in more detail later in this chapter.

Specific laboratory analyses that have shown some benefit include arterial blood gases and the D-dimer assay. The D-dimer assay is a blood test that helps determine the clinical risk for DVT. D-dimer is a specific degradation product of cross-linked fibrin, and it is elevated in patients with a thrombus formation.[23] One recommended diagnostic strategy is to assess the patient's clinical probability from the history, physical examination, ECG, and chest radiograph. If the patient falls into a low- or inter-mediate-risk category, a D-dimer assay is performed. An abnormal D-dimer assay would dictate a V/Q scan. A normal D-dimer in a low- or interme-diate-risk patient would require clinical follow-up and further evaluation with additional diagnostic studies. Patients categorized as high risk should immediately receive a V/Q scan without receiving a D-dimer assay.[21]

CRITICAL CONTENT

CLINICAL FEATURES OF PULMONARY EMBOLISM

- Classic clinical features of minor or major PE: acute onset of dyspnea, pleuritic chest pain (aggravated by inspiration), and hemoptysis.
- Other signs and symptoms vary depending on the severity of the embolus and include syncope, apprehension, diaphoresis, tachypnea, tachycardia, hypotension, right ventricular overload (acute cor pulmonale), JVD, and mental confusion.

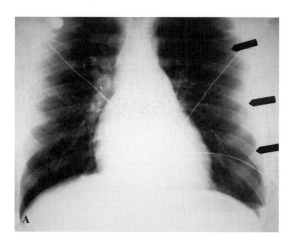

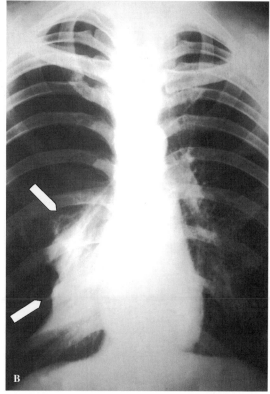

FIGURE 19-1 *A:* This chest radiograph shows a left-sided pneumothorax (arrows). *B:* This chest radiograph shows an approximately 95% pneumothorax on the right side which occurred following a stab wound. Notice the lack of lung vessels peripherally on the right (arrows). The collapsed lung has almost no air in it, and thus is seen as a soft tissue density next to the heart. This pneumothorax is under tension as manifested by some depression of the right hemidiaphragm, increased width of the intercostal spaces on the right side, and virtually complete collapse of the right lung. Only minimal, if any, shift of the medi-astinum to the left is present.

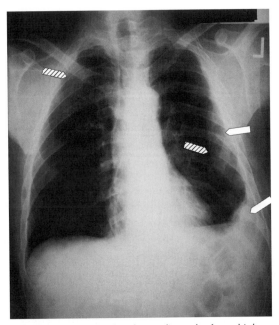

FIGURE 19-2 This chest radiograph of a multiple trauma victim shows multiple rib fractures on the right and left (shaded arrows) as well as a significant radiolucency on the left consistent with a pulmonary contusion (top white arrow). Note that the contusion is in the same area as multiple rib fractures. There is also a hemothorax that is noted by the increased radiolucency and blunting of the left costophrenic angle (bottom white arrow).

Common Radiographic Features

Respiratory therapists should have the ability to quickly assess the chest radiograph for obvious problems, including pneumothorax (Fig. 19-1), rib fractures (Fig. 19-2), pulmonary contusion (Fig. 19-2), hemothorax (Fig. 19-2), cardiac tamponade (Fig. 19-3), traumatic diaphragmatic rupture (Fig. 19-4), pneumomediastinum (Fig. 19-5), and subcutaneous emphysema (Fig. 19-5).

Rib fractures that are not displaced are often difficult to detect on a standard radiograph, making it difficult to determine the severity of the injury. If the first radiograph is taken while the patient is still on a backboard (Fig. 19-6), it may be difficult to note small but significant findings because of the backboard's silhouette. A pulmonary contusion may appear as an opaque consolidation

without localization to segmental boundaries. A pulmonary contusion may also be difficult to detect when there is a significant hemothorax, and it may not show up immediately.

A pneumomediastinum is identified radiographically by the presence of one or more vertical linear hyperlucent streaks in the mediastinal region. Unless the pneumomediastinum is significant, it is often subtle and frequently missed. However, the air collected in the mediastinum may pass upward into the soft tissues of the neck and thoracic wall and result in subcutaneous emphysema, which will present radiographically with dark areas (radiolucency) of air in tissue. You may find the air in the neck, lateral chest, or axillary areas. A pneumomediastinum should be considered when subcutaneous emphy-

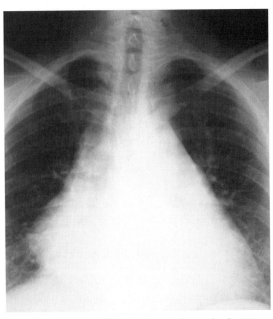

FIGURE 19-3 This is a chest radiograph of a 50-year-old white male with cardiac tamponade secondary to chronic pericardial effusion. There is marked obliteration of the retrocardiac and retrosternal clear spaces. The radiograph also demonstrates straightening of the upper left heart border combined with prominent rounding of a grossly enlarged right heart border. There is marked nonspecific cardiac enlargement. Although there is some increase in pulmonary vasculature, in general the lungs are relatively clear.

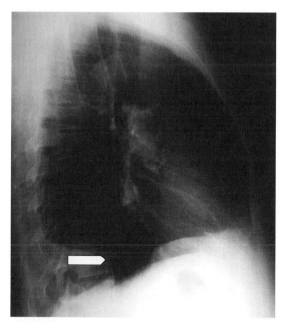

FIGURE 19-4 This lateral chest radiograph is of a 39-year-old male victim of a pedestrian versus automobile accident. A traumatic diaphragmatic rupture is noted by the loss of the diaphragmatic contour in the area of the rupture (arrow).

sema is present and other potential sources of air (eg, pneumothorax or penetrating chest trauma) are absent. You may also see areas of radiolucency in the tissue around penetration sites such as the area of a chest tube insertion, needle insertion, or stab wound.

The radiographic presentation of cardiac tamponade varies based on whether the onset is fast or slow. When onset is acute, the chest radiograph is of limited value because the amount of fluid in the tamponade may be too small to cause any noticeable changes in the size and contour of the cardiac shadow. With slower onset, look for heart size changes in the absence of radiographic signs of congestive heart failure (CHF) (especially with clear lungs). Fluid may obliterate the angles and recesses that demarcate the various segments of the cardiac contour, and there may be straightening of the upper left heart border combined with prominent rounding of the left and right heart borders.

A radiograph is the single best diagnostic tool when looking for traumatic rupture of the dia-

phragm. Look for elevation, irregularity, or obscurity of any part of the hemidiaphragm. While bowel loops in the chest are an obvious sign, small herniations are more subtle and are often missed. Radiographic findings to look for are: atelectasis, mediastinal shift, pleural fluid, or an air-fluid level above the diaphragm. Traumatic diaphragmatic rupture is often associated with lower rib fractures, pneumothorax, and hemothorax.

The chest radiograph is of limited value in confirming the diagnosis of PE. Its best use is in suggesting alternative diagnoses such as pneumonia,

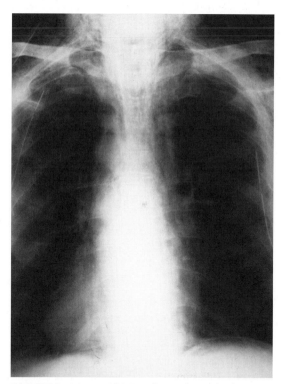

FIGURE 19-5 This is a chest radiograph of a 63-year-old white male with COPD who had reconstructive surgery for trauma to the face. The radiograph shows a pneumomediastinum, bilateral pneumothoraces, and subcutaneous emphysema, which extends to the anterior, posterior, and lateral chest walls as well as to the peritoneum. Some neck musculature is outlined by air and the right pectoralis major muscle is especially well seen. Insertion of chest tubes resolved the pneumothoraces by day 3, with complete resolution of the subcutaneous emphysema by day 8.

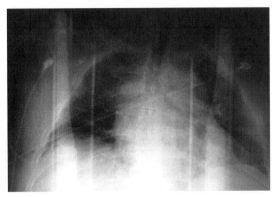

FIGURE 19-6 This is an initial AP chest radiograph of a 29-year-old black male motor vehicle accident victim who was brought to the ED. The spine board has not been removed from behind the victim. Note the typical radiolucency of the board, including the outlines of the handle openings. Care should be taken when assessing peripheral chest structures. This patient had broken ribs on the left as well as a cervical fracture.

cancer, or CHF. Forty percent of patients with a PE will have a normal chest radiograph.[21] The classic abnormalities that may be associated with PE include: evidence of central pulmonary artery occlusion with increased lucency of the peripheral lung field (Westermark's sign), atelectasis, small pleural effusions, and a pleural-based, wedge-shaped density of pulmonary infarction (Hampton's hump).[21]

CRITICAL CONTENT

Common radiographic presentations that are associated with trauma include:
- Pneumothorax
- Hemothorax
- Rib fractures
- Pulmonary contusion
- Pneumomediastinum
- Subcutaneous emphysema
- Cardiac tamponade
- Traumatic diaphragmatic rupture
- Pulmonary embolism

TREATMENT AND MANAGEMENT

High-stress emergency situations will be handled much better if the respiratory therapist is comfortable and at ease. Make sure the roles of the other members of the trauma team are well understood. Treatment and management of the injured patient should focus on restoring ventilation and gas exchange. You will be stationed at the head of the bed, so just relax and focus on **your** job.

Respiratory Support Considerations

As the respiratory therapist, your initial treatment must focus first on life-threatening situations involving the airway. *The Textbook of Advanced Cardiac Life Support* (ACLS) gives a solid foundation for airway care as well as special resuscitation procedures.[8] Respiratory therapists who work in the ED and ICU should be trained ACLS providers at a minimum, and preferably ACLS instructors. Respiratory support includes ensuring a patent airway, providing supplemental oxygen, and instituting positive pressure ventilation when spontaneous ventilation is absent. Respiratory therapists should be familiar with different airway appliances, the benefits and limitations of each, their indications and contraindications, and their use. Respiratory therapists should also know when to initiate and recommend endotracheal intubation. Indications

CRITICAL CONTENT

Indications for intubation include:
- Cardiac arrest with ongoing chest compressions
- Inability of a conscious patient to ventilate adequately
- Inability of the patient to protect the airway
- The inability of the rescuer to ventilate the unconscious patient with noninvasive conventional methods

for intubation include cardiac arrest with ongoing chest compressions, inability of a conscious patient to ventilate adequately, inability of the patient to protect the airway, and the inability of the rescuer to ventilate the unconscious patient with noninvasive conventional methods.[8]

The ACLS textbook also covers airway control in trauma victims and the approach to cardiac arrest associated with injuries. If there is a known or suspected cervical spine injury, excessive movement of the spine, which may produce or exacerbate spinal cord injury, must be avoided. Know when in-line stabilization techniques of the neck should be used. As the respiratory therapist, you may need assistance or may assist someone else in this process. You should presume a cervical spine injury is present in any victim with head injury, facial injury, or other multiple injuries until proper evaluations have ruled it out.[8]

CRITICAL CONTENT

CERVICAL STABILIZATION IN A TRAUMA VICTIM IS IMPORTANT!

- Avoid excessive movement of the spine in a known or suspected cervical spine injury.
- Know when in-line stabilization techniques of the neck should be used.
- Presume a cervical spine injury is present in any victim with head injury, facial injury, or other multiple injuries until proper evaluations have ruled it out.

Cardiac Support Considerations

Once the airway is established and secured and you are ventilating and oxygenating the trauma victim, focus should be shifted to cardiac support. There is controversy over the value of chest compressions in victims of trauma-associated cardiac arrest.[8] You should initiate chest compressions in pulseless trauma victims only after airway control and defibrillation are provided. Resuscitative efforts on

victims that have deteriorated to asystole and are normothermic are generally considered futile,[8] yet many trauma teams refuse to give up. It is the responsibility of the person in charge of the situation, a physician, to end the resuscitative efforts.

Other Emergent Considerations

Other members of the trauma team carry out most treatments other than airway control in emergent situations, while the RT maintains ventilation and oxygenation. If you are the only therapist, let someone else do compressions; maintain focus on the airway. Examples of emergent treatments include pericardiocentesis to treat cardiac tamponade and tube thoracostomy for pneumo- or hemothorax. More aggressive interventions in the ED include surgical procedures such as emergent thoracotomy for direct massage of the heart or clamping of large hemorrhaging vessels such as the aorta. Severe head trauma victims who are rapidly deteriorating or already in a coma require immediate airway control and ventilation followed by a diagnostic CT scan once stabilized.

Thromboembolic Complications

Trauma victims are at risk of developing long-term venous thromboembolic complications, including pulmonary embolism, therefore an important task for the health care team is to prevent DVT and its complications. Currently, there are regional variations in the delineation of risk groups, the proportion of patients receiving prophylaxis, and the prophylactic method chosen.[7] The recommendations for the prevention of thromboembolism range from early ambulation or intermittent pneumatic compression (IPC) in low-risk patients to significant pharmacologic therapy, including use of low molecular weight heparin (LMWH), low-dose unfractionated heparin, aspirin, and warfarin in moderate- to high-risk patients. Patients with DVT or PE should be treated with anticoagulant therapy that includes intravenous heparin or adjusted-dose subcutaneous heparin sufficient to prolong the activated partial prothrombin time (APTT) or international normalized ratio (INR) to a therapeutic range. Long-term anticoagulant therapy can be continued for up to 3 months using oral anticoagulants. In certain situations where high-risk patients have contraindications or complications of anticoagulant therapy, an inferior vena cava (IVC) filter may be placed.[7] These devices are designed to filter and trap thrombi that could cause a PE. Their design allows filtering to occur without blockage of venous return. Filters are most often positioned in an infrarenal vena cava position to trap thrombi arising from the lower extremities. This positioning helps avoid potential occlusion of the renal veins. Various brands of permanent caval filters are available in the United States, including the Greenfield filter (most common), Gianturco-Roehm filter, and Simon-Nitinol filter.[7]

CRITICAL CONTENT

Prevention and treatment for PE is primarily centered on:

- Prevention of thromboembolism
- Early ambulation
- Intermittent pneumatic compression (IPC)
- Significant pharmacologic therapy in moderate- to high-risk patients

SITE- AND AGE-SPECIFIC CONSIDERATIONS

Trauma injury can happen to anyone, anywhere, at any age. In general, family violence accounts for 8% of all trauma events in the United States and 23% of victims are acquainted with the perpetrator.[4] There is a higher per capita death rate in rural versus urban populations.[24] In rural areas, survivability varies depending on the victim's proximity to a formal trauma center. Patients who die at the scene usually are older and less severely injured. Associated reasons for increased mortality in the older, less injured rural victims are the lack of access, delayed

discovery, and transport difficulties.[24] In urban areas, trauma patients are more likely to be young adults aged 17 to 30 years old and their problems are more likely to be of longer duration.[25] Also in urban areas, gang-related situations, including drive-by shootings, account for 15% of injuries[4] and homicide is the sixth leading cause of death in adults aged 25 to 44 years.[26] Violent trauma victims at one large metropolitan trauma center had a mean age of 20 and 90% were male. Firearms were involved in 44% of the injuries, stab wounds in 30%, and assaults in 26%. Drug use was found in 27% and alcohol use was found in 43%.[4]

Both the young and old are subject to increased morbidity and mortality from complications associated with trauma, including ARDS, DVT, and PE. Unintentional injuries and their adverse effects are the leading cause of death in those aged 1 to 24; even in infants less than 1 year old, trauma is the eighth leading cause of death.[2] While young people are more likely to die immediately from a significant injury, trauma victims 65 years of age or older that survive an injury initially are 2 to 3 times more likely to die from complications.[24] Deep vein thrombosis is an unpredictable hazard in all trauma populations, but is related to age, length of hospital stay, or the presence of spinal fracture. The rate of DVT is around 5% even with the use of standard prophylaxis. Those at highest risk include the elderly, particularly those over 40, patients with spinal fractures, and patients with prolonged hospitalization.[27]

CONSIDERATIONS OF COSTS AND ETHICAL ISSUES

Traumatic injuries are very costly to the health care community. Studies have estimated that yearly medical spending on injury is over $70 billion.[1,28] Much of the increased injury severity and cost is associated with victims exhibiting high-risk behavior. Many persons injured by trauma are intoxicated or under the influence of drugs, and many were driving under the influence of these agents. In one study of youths less than 25 years old, 16% had a prior injury related to a gunshot wound (GSW), assault, or stabbing. Of the 16%, 94% had suffered the injury within the previous 5 years.[29] The cost of firearm violence to society has been estimated at more than $3 billion per year for acute care and lost productivity.[4] In one large hospital, the estimated cost over a 3-year period for hospitalizing youths involved in high-risk behavior was $4,000,000.[4] The estimated mean cost range for each injury was $10,000 to $18,000 per GSW, $4,000 to $5,000 per stab wound, and $5,000 to $7,000 per assault. In 93% of the admissions, the taxpayer paid for the youth's injury. Trauma victims in large urban-suburban communities who exhibit high-risk behavior generate enormous trauma costs, most of which is borne by public agencies.[29]

The costs to diagnose and treat complications of trauma are high. In a cost survey of one hospital, it cost over $313,000 to detect only 17 clinically unsuspected DVTs.[27] This represents a charge of over $18,000 per DVT. For the elderly, the average cost of care in 1994 during the initial hospitalization for hip fracture was about $7,000 per patient. Additional costs of care for the 4 months after the initial hospitalization was $8,000.[30] Another study estimated the total cost for a hip fracture at approximately $40,000.[31] An injury and resultant complications can be extremely expensive.

CRITICAL CONTENT

TRAUMA IS COSTLY TO THE HEALTH CARE SYSTEM

- Yearly medical spending on injury is over $70 billion.
- Injury severity and cost of treatments are increased in victims exhibiting high-risk behavior.
- The cost of firearm violence to society is estimated at more than $3 billion per year for acute care and lost productivity.
- The costs for diagnosis and treatment of complications such as PE are high.

PATIENT EDUCATION, HEALTH PROMOTION, AND QUALITY-OF-LIFE ISSUES

Injuries continue to be a significant public health problem and place a heavy burden on individuals, families, and society.[32] Education, prevention, control, treatment, and rehabilitation are required to reduce the number of deaths and nonfatal injuries as well as the associated high costs.[33] Everyone would agree that is it difficult to stop high-risk behavior or to prevent the ongoing crisis our nation has with gun violence. At best, these are issues that present major social challenges, and at worst it is often out of our control. However, outside of the hospital, respiratory therapists can take an active role in community outreach programs, including organizations such as the Boys and Girls Clubs of America or Mothers Against Drunk Drivers (MADD). If the opportunity arises to talk to parents, schools, or youth associations, respiratory therapists should take advantage of the opportunity to share with these groups what they know as health professionals about the impact trauma from high-risk behaviors can have on the individuals involved and society at large.

Within the hospital, respiratory therapists are frequently educating trauma patients. Unfortunately at that time it is too late to provide the preventive education that might have prevented the injury. During recovery from a major injury, patients are usually not very receptive to receiving a lecture on how to avoid the injury in the first place. The focus of the therapists' patient education at that point is usually centered around teaching self-care. This might involve showing them how to use a metered dose inhaler or proper use of an incentive spirometer. Respiratory therapists may teach the family how to change a trach or how to perform suction.

Injuries, even those that do not require hospitalization, can significantly affect an individual's quality of life. Hospitalized patients and even patients with injuries not requiring hospitalization such as back strains and dislocations can average more than five outpatient visits per case to physician offices or other health care providers.[1] If the patient is socioeconomically disadvantaged and/or has no medical insurance, additional costs, if not paid by public funding sources, can negatively impact their life. Over 50% of the hospitalized injured incur prescription costs which can average over $100 per case.[1] Even the fear of crime victimization is shown to affect some older adults' quality of life and will tend to dictate their daily routine, particularly in urban areas.[34] This fear can limit their participation in activities outside the home as well as their use of and access to routine health care.[35]

CRITICAL CONTENT

INJURIES AS A PUBLIC HEALTH PROBLEM

- Prevention, control, treatment, and rehabilitation are required to reduce the number of deaths and nonfatal injuries as well as their associated high costs.
- Injury and complications place a heavy burden on individuals, families, and society.
- The incidence of certain types of high-risk behavior is significantly greater in patients relying on public funding sources.

The case studies that follow are additional examples of patients a respiratory therapist will deal with every day. By all means be a lifelong learner yourself. This chapter demonstrates two things you can count on as a respiratory therapy professional: 1) people will always get injured and, 2) you will always be needed to help.

INTRODUCTION TO CASE STUDIES

The following two cases are incorporated into this chapter so that students can apply their understanding of multiple trauma and pulmonary embolism to the diagnosis, treatment, and long-term management of patients. The cases challenge the learner to evaluate the age-specific considerations, patient education needs, health care costs and ethical concerns of trauma and pulmonary embolism management. Whenever possible, the cases will prompt more than one recommendation for patient care to allow comparisons of the advantages, disadvantages, and limitations of various therapeutic approaches.

Please check with your instructor to verify which cases and critical thinking exercises you should complete. The exercises may be done individually or within groups. In addition, your instructor may ask you to research and present leaning issues as part of your PBL process. Learning issues may be assigned by the instructor or developed during group discussion.

CASE STUDY 1

TOM TRAVICT

Initial Case Scenario

You are one of two respiratory therapists on call for trauma in your 300-bed hospital in upstate Michigan. Your hospital is classified as a level 2 trauma facility. Suddenly, at 1320, a blunt stable trauma call is displayed on your emergency room pager. As you and the other respiratory therapist arrive in the emergency department (ED), a nurse tells you that an individual is in transport after being involved in a snowmobile accident; esti-

mated time of arrival (ETA) is 3 minutes. No other information is available.

You don your personal protective equipment (PPE) while the other respiratory therapist double checks the supplies for airway management. You take your position at the head of the bed. At 1335, a middle-aged man, white, male in moderate distress is triaged to your room. You notice that he is on a backboard his neck is in a C-collar, his head is immobilized by a strap to the blackboard, and he

CASE STUDY 1 *(continued)*

is wearing medical anti-shock trousers (MAST). You also note an IV line.

Critical Thinking Exercise 1

ANTICIPATING PROBLEMS AND SOLUTIONS

a. What problems would you anticipate based on the information known thus far?

b. What problems would you anticipate if Mr. Travict had been classified as a blunt unstable trauma victim?

c. What further information about an accident would assist the ED health care team in the assessment of a victim?

The emergency medical technician (EMT) tells you that the victim and a passenger, his 12-year-old son, were riding a snowmobile that lost control, hit another snowmobile, and subsequently hit a tree. The 12-year-old boy was deceased at the scene. The female driver of the other snowmobile, the man's sister, is in transit. The EMT also states that the victim was responsive upon arrival to the scene and through transport; there is a suspicion of a left femur fracture. The patient's Glasgow coma score (GCS) upon arrival at the scene was E3V4M5. However, he states that civilian first responders confirm a BLOC immediately after the accident. Vital signs at the scene were RR 28, BP 100/65, and HR 110. The EMT further states that significant blood staining of the snow was noted at the scene and an odor of alcohol was noted on the victim's breath. Also, the victim stated his last meal was around noon and that he has no allergies to any medications.

Critical Thinking Exercise 2

PRIORITIZING PATIENT CARE

How would you prioritize your patient assessment and treatment during the first few minutes of Mr. Travict's time in the ED?

The Primary Assessment

The victim groans loudly as you assist moving him off the transport stretcher. He appears confused and disoriented. A hospital social worker states that his driver's license lists his name as Tom Travict, age 38, weight 228 pounds, and height 5′ 7″.

Critical Thinking Exercise 3

ANTICIPATING PHYSICAL EXAMINATION FINDINGS

Based on the information obtained:

a. What general signs and symptoms would you be looking for in an accident victim?

b. What specific signs of respiratory distress should one look for?

c. What abnormalities would you anticipate in oxygenation and ventilation?

d. As the respiratory therapist, what immediate actions would you anticipate based on your initial assessment?

At 1338, the following is noted with the primary survey.

Airway: Mr. Travict is on a simple oxygen mask and his SpO_2 is 90%. He appears to have trouble breathing. He mumbles in choppy, barely audible sentences. His nose is patent with no apparent bleeding and his midface is stable. A contusion and approximately 4-cm laceration is noted above the left orbit. Upon oral examination, you find that a left lower incisor is loose with slight bleeding around the base. You also see a loose partial denture and remove it from the upper palate. You suction out a small amount of blood from the oropharynx.

Breathing: The patient is breathing spontaneously. Respiratory rate is 32/min with moderate work to breathe as noted by nasal flaring, choppy speech, and chest effort to inhale. Due to the C-collar, it is difficult to note significant accessory muscle use or

CASE STUDY 1 (*continued*)

jugular venous distention (JVD) in the neck. Just after the MAST and Mr. Travict's upper clothes are removed, you note a large bruise over the left chest appearing to extend under the C-collar. Clear breath sounds are auscultated on the right, but decreased breath sounds on the left anterior and lateral chest wall. Asymmetric chest wall movement is noted. Slight supraclavicular retractions are noted on inspiration. The trachea is midline. Marked tenderness over the left breast area noted upon palpation. Crepitations are heard over a deformed area of the left chest between ribs 6 and 9 with slight paradoxical chest movement in the same area. No subcutaneous emphysema is noted.

Circulation: No apparent gross bleeding is noted by any team member. Heart rate via monitor is 115/min. Blood pressure is 110/70.

Defibrillation/Disability: Sinus tachycardia is noted on ECG. While Mr. Travict appeared disoriented upon arrival, he responds appropriately to person, place, and time. His GCS is E3V4M5. Pupils are equal and reactive to light and accommodation (PERRLA).

Exposure: While performing the above assessments, a nurse cut off the remainder of Mr. Travict's clothes. Mr. Travict is log rolled and the backboard removed. Without interfering with assessment, the patient is covered as much as possible with warm blankets.

Critical Thinking Exercise 4

MAKING INFERENCES BY CLUSTERING DATA

a. What inferences can you make about the information obtained from Mr. Travict's primary ABCDE assessment?

b. What inferences can you make overall about his general condition?

c. Practice clustering data that leads you to these inferences.

At 1405, all appropriate radiographs are taken and blood work, including blood gas, is drawn. Ten minutes later the following radiology and ABG results are available:

Radiology

Cervical	Clear: C-collar removed.
Spine	Clear: spine board removed.
KUB	Clear.
AP Chest	Multiple rib fractures on the right and left; diffuse hazy opacity throughout right and left hemithorax; specific area of opacity consistent with contusion in left hemithorax; blunting of the left costophrenic angle; normal mediastinal width. (See Fig. 19-2.)
Bone	Left leg: Femoral fracture. Pelvis: Posterior dislocation of left femoral head; left acetabular fracture.

ABG mask 8 L/min

pH	7.25
P_{CO_2}	64
P_{CO_2}	59
HCO_3^-	27.5
BE	−1.5
Sa_{O_2}	84%

The Complication

You place Mr. Travict on a nonrebreather and the Sp_{O_2} increases to 91%. Suddenly, alarms sound! You note the patient's blood pressure has dropped to 88/56, heart rate has increased to 132, respiratory rate has decreased to 12 and Sp_{O_2} has decreased to 72%. Mr. Travict is no longer responsive to commands with GCS E2V1M3. The other respiratory therapist begins to bag Mr. Travict. You note rapid abdominal distention as she continues to ventilate. The physician agrees with your recommendation to intubate. With assistance from the other respiratory therapist, you intubate Mr. Travict and verify proper tube placement with a CO_2 detector. No frank bleeding is noted in the tube. Upon auscultation, you note good aeration in the right lung and decreased sounds on the left. You pull the ETT back 2 cm without any change. The other therapist states, "It's difficult to squeeze the bag." Mr. Travict's heart rate has decreased to 72 and his blood pressure is now 80/52. You note a reduction in chest wall movement on the left, marked JVD, and cyanosis. Palpation reveals a right shift of the trachea, and percussion reveals increased resonance on the left.

Critical Thinking Exercise 5

ASSESSMENT AND DECISION MAKING

a. What is your assessment of the likely cause of this continued deterioration? Cite your reasons for your assessment.

b. What immediate action appears to be indicated at this time?

The physician immediately performs a needle aspiration in an appropriate site with immediate improvement in vital signs. After you assist the other respiratory therapist in securing the endotracheal tube, the physician asks for your assistance with placement of a chest tube, while the other respiratory therapist places Mr. Travict on the ventilator. Upon placement of the chest tube, approximately 300 mL of blood was collected in the chest tube drainage system. You are then asked to put on a lead apron and help immobilize the patient's head and neck as radiology obtains a chest x-ray. Blood is also obtained for further laboratory analysis to include another ABG. A nurse called for CT and OR availability.

The Secondary Assessment

At 1510, once Mr. Travict is stabilized, the secondary assessment begins. Following are the results:

History obtained from victim

Allergies	NKDA
Medications	Unable to obtain
Past medical	Unable to obtain
Last meal	Approximately 3 hours ago
Events preceding injury	Unable to obtain

Vital signs

HR	105
RR	14 via ventilator
BP	90/58
SpO_2	96%
Temp.	36.9°C

HEENT	Normocephalic with small contusion and approximately 4-cm laceration over the left orbit; PERRLA; extraocular motions intact; sclerae clear; tympanic membranes clear bilaterally.
Neck	Slight tracheal deviation is still noted to the right of midline; noticeable JVD with patient supine and flat; no obvious injuries or penetrations are noted.
Chest	Slight asymmetry of chest wall noted even after chest tube placement. A large contusion is noted on the left anterior chest extending to the left posterior axillary region. Decreased breath sounds on left anterior and lateral chest wall; clear on the right. Slight increased resonance to percussion on the left upper chest as compared to the right.

CASE STUDY 1 (continued)

Heart	Regular rate and rhythm without murmurs, gallops, or rubs.
Abdomen	Obese, soft, nondistended, nontender, no organomegaly palpable. Bowel sounds auscultated.
Back	Atraumatic and nontender upon palpation.
GU	Foley catheter in place; urine clear.
Rectal	Heme negative with normal sphincter tone.
Extremities	Upper extremities atraumatic with movement; right lower extremity atraumatic; a distortion of the left femur is noted; marked left thigh and hip tenderness with pain upon palpation; left knee contusion noted with abrasions; no noted cyanosis, clubbing, or edema.

As you prepare Mr. Travict for transport to CT, the following results are available:

CLINICAL LAB DATA
ABG while on 100% FIO_2 via mechanical ventilator

pH	7.35
PCO_2	38
PO_2	80
HCO_3	20.7
BE	−4
SaO_2	99%

SMA -7

Na	137
Cl	110
BUN	14
Glucose	90
K	5.3
TCO_2	24
Creatinine	0.6

CBC

WBC	12.4
Hgb	10.8
Hct	33.3
Platelets	140
RBC	4.24

Other labs

PT/PTT	15.1/29.8
ETOH	negative

Mr. Travict is given 2 units of blood and medicated for pain. He is transported to CT and then to the OR.

Postsurgery

Five days later, while checking Mr. Travict's chart prior to performing a nebulizer and CPT treatment, the nurse tells you that he has been angry today and refuses to take his medication. She states, "He cries at the drop of a hat." You note in the chart that he is having problems grasping with his right hand and that he is also having problems with short-term memory. His leg has been set and is in traction.

When you go into his room to do his treatment, Mr. Travict appears agitated. He states, "I'm tired of it hurting to breathe! I don't want to live anymore without my son. It's all my fault." He begins to cry intensely. It was noted that the patient was very agitated during the following ABG draw:

ABG NC 4 L/min

pH	7.50
PCO_2	31
PO_2	57
HCO_3^-	24
BE	+1
SaO_2	91%

CASE STUDY 1 (continued)

Signs and symptoms

Breathing uneven and labored.

RR   40/min

HR   135/min

Crackles and wheezes noted in right base.

Old contusion area still noted over the left chest.

Appears to be splinting left side.

You note a swollen area supraclavicularly.
Palpation demonstrates a crunchy, crackling feeling as you depress the area. You also note a slight swelling of the skin around the chest tube insertion site with similar results after palpation.

Critical Thinking Exercise 6

ANTICIPATING PROBLEMS AND SOLUTIONS

a. What problems would you anticipate based on the above information?

b. What actions would you anticipate at this time or in the immediate future?

Just as you begin to call the physician, she walks up to the nursing station where you are. She states that she has ordered a sedative and more pain medication. She then enters Mr. Travict's room to talk to him. Thirty minutes later, you are able to complete the treatment. Later that day, the physician tells you she has requested a neurological and psychological consult. The discharge plans are to send Mr. Travict to the local rehab center in 2 days for extensive rehabilitation.

Critical Thinking Exercise 7

REFLECTION ON YOUR DECISIONS AND ACTIONS TO IMPROVE CLINICAL DECISION MAKING

Describe why and how you would reflect on this case in order to figure out retrospectively what worked or did not work. How would you use this information to manage cases in the future?

Group Critical Thinking Exercise 1

THE PRO/CON DEBATE

The pro group presents the argument that conventional intubation and mechanical ventilation is the choice therapy for a severe flail chest injury, and the con group makes the same argument for noninvasive positive pressure ventilation (NPPV). Provide data, evidence, and reasons to support your group's recommendations. Each group explains how their therapy would improve clinical outcomes over the other. One variation of this exercise is to have each group switch and argue the opposite point of view. Critical thinking can be enhanced when persons are required to debate both the pro and then the con points of view.

Group Critical Thinking Exercise 2

THE PRO/CON DEBATE

The pro group will present the argument that hyperventilation therapy is the best treatment method for emergent treatment of the closed head injury patient. The con group will present the argument that hyperventilation therapy is dangerous and has no place in emergent treatment of closed head injury. The con group will provide alternate treatment strategies. Again, the groups can be switched for a variation.

CASE STUDY 1 *(continued)*

Group Critical Thinking Exercise 3

COMMUNICATION AND NEGOTIATION

Describe how you would communicate and negotiate with other members of the trauma team in the initial treatment of a trauma victim.

If you were in a small trauma hospital, how would you approach the determination of each person's role? How would this differ if you were in a large regional trauma center? Discuss what you would do if your recommendations during ED assessment and treatment were not accepted.

CASE STUDY 2

KATHLEEN KLOTT

Initial Case Scenario

You are the respiratory therapist performing patient assessment consults in your 300-bed hospital in upstate Michigan. You are paged to the third floor at 0200 hours. Upon arrival, you are directed to evaluate Ms. Klott, a 47-year-old female patient with radiating pain and respiratory difficulty. After a quick review of the chart, you remember treating Ms. Klott in the ED a few days earlier after she was involved in a snowmobile accident and suffered pelvic and long bone fractures.

Critical Thinking Exercise 1

PRIORITIZING PATIENT CARE

How would you prioritize your patient assessment during the first few minutes after arrival to Ms. Klott's room?

First Visit

Upon arrival to the room, you find Ms. Klott attempting to sit up in bed. She appears to be anxious and in moderate respiratory distress. She is crying and complains that it hurts sometimes in her left shoulder but mostly when she breathes. She also states, "My poor nephew is dead, it's all my fault. I never should have made him go snowmobiling with us." Ms. Klott is on an aerosol mask at a FIO_2 of 40%. Her vital signs are as follows:

Vital signs

HR	132
RR	40/min
BP	122/59
Spo_2 %	N/A
Temp.	38°C

You draw an ABG and analyze it. After posting the results, you contact Ms. Klott's physician. She asks that you perform an ECG and write a verbal order for a stat chest x-ray. You also suggest getting a minute ventilation; she agrees. Following are the results:

ABG aerosol mask 40%

pH	7.45
Pco_2	34
Po_2	79
HCO_3^-	23.3
BE	0
Sao_2	95%

CASE STUDY 2 (continued)

Minute ventilation	Obtained 9.6L. Predicted 4.7 L.
Radiology	Parenchymal and pleural opacities in the left base. Hampton's hump in the periphery of the left lung base.
ECG	Demonstrates a $S_1Q_3T_3$ pattern

Critical Thinking Exercise 2

CLINICAL ASSESSMENT AND DECISION MAKING

Interpret Ms Klott's ABG with aerosol mask 40% (above). Note any abnormalities and include a discussion of possible causes. Include a discussion of the significance of the results to the patient's ventilatory and oxygenation status.

After discussion of the data with Ms. Klott's attending physician, you are requested to help prepare and accompany her to nuclear imaging for a ventilation/perfusion scan. The next day, during a chart review, you notice the results of the V/Q scan. The report read as follows: *A matched ventilation and perfusion defect corresponding to the similar-sized defect on the CXR was seen in the left lower lobe lateral segment. However, the scan does not fall into the high probability category and is, therefore, nondiagnostic.* Later, during rounds, it is stated by the physician that Ms. Klott is classified as high-risk for PE. While discussing options for further diagnostic testing, an emergency call comes from Ms. Klott's room. You and the physician proceed to the room.

Second Visit

Upon entering Ms. Klott's room, you find her attempting to sit upright. She is diaphoretic and restless. She is on an aerosol mask with a FiO_2 of 40% that is dangling around her neck. As you reposition the mask, she states "I can't get enough air; my chest feels tight." She then says that her difficulty breathing has been going on "for about 30 minutes." Her SpO_2 is 86%. You adjust the current aerosol nebulizer to the 100% setting with no change in SpO_2. After changing out the equipment to a more appropriate device, Ms. Klott's SpO_2 increases to 90%.

Critical Thinking Exercise 3

TROUBLESHOOTING

a. Can you give an explanation as to why Ms. Klott's SpO_2 did not increase when the oxygen was increased to 100%?

b. Why was the device changed out?

c. What could be a reason the SpO_2 didn't increase more than it did once the new equipment was set up?

You convince her to keep the mask on while you draw an ABG. Her physician is called. Blood is also drawn for a CBC and a portable check x-ray and 12-lead EDG are ordered. You return with the ABG results, when suddenly the alarms sound on her pulse oximeter and you notice that SpO_2 has dropped from 90% to 80%. Below are the results of the ABG:

ABG aerosol mask 100%

pH	7.40
P_{CO_2}	43
P_{O_2}	27
HCO_3^-	26
BE	+1
SaO_2	55%

Clinical findings

RR	36
HR	110
SpO_2	80%–84%

CASE STUDY 2 *(continued)*

Per the attending physician, you help transport Ms. Klott to the ICU based on her current status. In the unit, you set up her oxygen device and make sure all monitoring equipment is functioning. You insert an arterial line per physician order and draw an ABG. The following are the current data:

Vital signs

HR	120
RR	34/min
BP	140/55
Spo_2	92%
Temp.	N/A

ABG aerosol mask 100%

pH	7.56
Pco_2	25
Po_2	61
HCO_3^-	22.5
BE	+2
Sao_2	95%

Radiology AP chest

Diffuse interstitial opacities are present bilaterally; airspace opacity is present in the left lung both centrally and in the left base.

Critical Thinking Exercise 4

CLINICAL DECISION MAKING

Can you give an explanation as to the difference between the previous ABG that was drawn on Ms. Klott as compared to the ABG that was obtained after insertion of the arterial line?

Anticoagulant therapy is started and Ms. Klott is scheduled for placement of an IVC filter. Later that day, the IVC was successfully placed in an infrarenal position. The surgical report stated that no clots were observed in the IVC at the time of the procedure and that the INR was maintained between 2.3 and 3.5. During rounds, thrombolytic therapy is discussed as an option and pulmonary angiography is scheduled.

Day 15 in Course of Stay

Ms. Klott has been discharged to the floor. Her leg and hip are healing well and she is scheduled to be discharged the next day.

KEY POINTS

- One of four of Americans are injured each year and injury is the leading cause of death in young people.

- Trauma can happen to anyone, anywhere, at any age, at any time.

- Injuries from accidents and violence are a major cause of disability and poor quality of life, contributing to a significant public health problem.

- The nature and extent of an injury depends upon: the velocity of the impact, the site of impact, and the materials that impact on the body.

- Multiple trauma victims are at high risk for mortality and morbidity from significant injury to more than one organ system and the complications associated with these injuries.

- Common posttrauma complications include: infection, pneumonia, deep vein thrombosis, pulmonary embolism, and adult respiratory distress syndrome.

- Major trauma increases the short-term risk of both venous thrombosis and PE a hundredfold.

- Spinal cord injury above C5 results in total respiratory muscle paralysis that may lead to respiratory failure and even death.

- Health care personnel should presume a cervical spine injury is present in any victim with head injury, facial injury, or other multiple injuries until proper evaluations have ruled it out.

- Respiratory therapists must be able to distinguish the clinical features of common chest problems associated with trauma, which include pneumothorax, hemothorax, cardiac tamponade, and traumatic diaphragmatic rupture or paralysis.

- The respiratory therapist in the ED must quickly recognize and treat situations that would lead to life-threatening respiratory failure.

- Examples of emergent treatments in trauma victims include intubation, mechanical ventilation, pericardiocentesis, thoracostomy, direct massage of the heart, or direct internal clamping of large vessels.

- The respiratory therapist's first major priority in a trauma is to assess, establish, and maintain the airway!

- Indications for intubation include cardiac arrest with ongoing chest compressions, the inability of a conscious patient to ventilate adequately, the inability of the patient to protect the airway, and the inability of the rescuer to ventilate the unconscious patient with conventional methods.

- Respiratory support includes ensuring a patent airway, providing supplemental oxygen, and instituting positive pressure ventilation when spontaneous ventilation is absent.

- Respiratory therapists in emergency care must focus on those problems that impact ventilation and impair the process of gas exchange.

- Respiratory therapists must be able to both assess trauma victims for the presence of respiratory failure and anticipate injuries that could lead to respiratory failure.

- Respiratory therapists must possess sound critical thinking skills in trauma assessment and management.

- Prevention, control, treatment, and rehabilitation are required to reduce the number of deaths and nonfatal injuries as well as their associated high costs.

- Injury and its complications place a heavy burden on individuals, families, and society.

SUGGESTED RESOURCES

http://www.uhrad.com
http://www.heartinfo.com
http://www.trauma.org
http://www.virtualhospital.org

REFERENCES

1. Miller TR, Lestina DC. Patterns in US medical expenditures and utilization for injury, 1987. *Am J Public Health*. 1996;86:89–93.

2. National Center for Health Statistics Vital Statistics System: 10 leading causes of death. 1997.

3. National Center for Health Statistics Vital Statistics System: Years of potential life lost before age 65 by cause of death. 1995.

4. Tellez M, Mackersie RC, Morabito D, Shaugoury C, Heye C, et al. Risks, costs, and the expected complications of re-injury. *Am J Surg*. 1995;170: 660–664.

5. Hirsh J, Hoak J. Management of deep vein thrombosis and pulmonary embolism: A statement for healthcare professionals. *AHA Sci Council*. 1996; 93:2212–2245.

6. Rubenstein I, Murray D, Hoffstein V. Fatal pulmonary emboli in hospitalized patients: an autopsy study. *Arch Intern Med*. 1988;148:1425–1426.

7. Bick RL, Haas SK. International consensus recommendations: summary statement and additional suggested guidelines. *Med Clin North Am*. 1998; 82:613–633.

8. The Textbook of Advanced Cardiac Life Support. Dallas, Texas: American Heart Association; 1994.

9. Baigelman W, O'Brien JC. Pulmonary effects of head trauma. *Neurosurgery*. 1981;9:729.

10. Domino K. Pulmonary function and dysfunction in the traumatized patient. *Anesthesiol Clin North Am*. 1996;14:59–84.

11. Maloney JV, Schmutzer KJ, Raschke E. Paradoxical respiration and "pendelluft." *J Thorac Cardiovasc Surg*. 1961;41:291.

12. Jackson J. Management of thoracoabdominal injuries. In: Capan LM, Miller SM, Turndorf H, eds. *Trauma: Anesthesia and Intensive Care*. Philadelphia: Lippincott; 1991:481.

13. Stene JK, Grande CM, Bernhard WN, et al. Perioperative anesthetic management of the trauma patient: Thoracoabdominal and orthopedic injuries. In: Stene JK, Grande CM, eds. *Trauma Anesthesia*. Baltimore: Williams & Wilkins; 1991:177.

14. Campbell DB. Trauma to the chest wall, lung, and major airways. *Semin Thorac Cardiovasc Surg*. 1992;4:234.

15. Relihan M, Litwin MS. Morbidity and mortality associated with flail chest injury: A review of 85 cases. *J Trauma*. 1973;13:663.

16. Schaal MA, Fischer RP, Perry JF. The unchanged mortality of flail chest injuries. *J Trauma*. 1979; 19:492.

17. Geerts WH, Code KI, Jay RM, et al. A prospective study of venous thromboembolism after major trauma. *N Engl J Med*. 1994;331:1601.

18. Prendergast TJ, Ruoss SJ. Pulmonary disease. In: McPhee S, et al, eds. *Pathophysiology of Disease*. 2nd ed. Stamford, Conn: Appleton & Lange; 1997.

19. Cohn SM. Pulmonary contusion: Review of the clinical entity. *J Trauma Injury Infect Crit Care*. 1997;42:973–979.

20. Opinions regarding the diagnosis and management of venous thromboembolic disease. ACCP consensus conference committee on pulmonary embolism. *Chest*. 1998;113:499–504.

21. Baker WF. Diagnosis of deep venous thrombosis and pulmonary embolism. *Med Clin North Am*. 1998;82:459–476.

22. Goldhaber SZ. Pulmonary embolism. *Med Prog*. 1998;339:93–104.

23. Traill ZC, Gleeson FV. Venous thromboembolic disease. *Br J Radiol*. 1998;71:129–134.

24. Rogers FB, Shackford SR, Hoyt DB, et al. Trauma deaths in a mature urban vs. rural trauma system: a comparison. *Arch Surg*. 1997;132:376–382.

25. Dale J, Green J, Reid F, et al. Primary care in the accident and emergency department: I. Prospective identification of patients. *Br Med J*. 1995;31:423–426.

26. Peters KD, Kochanek KD, Murphy SL. Deaths: final data for 1996. *Natl Vital Stat Rep*. 1998;47: 1–100.

27. Piotrowski JJ, Alexander JJ, Brandt CP, et al. Is deep vein thrombosis surveillance warranted in high-risk trauma patients? *Am J Surg*. 1996;172:210–213.

28. Malek M, Chang B-H, Gallagher SS, et al. The cost of medical care for injuries to children. *Ann Emerg Med*. 1991;20:997–1005.

29. Mackersie RC, Davis JW, Hoyt DB, et al. High-risk behavior and the public burden for funding the costs of acute injury. *Arch Surg*. 1995;130:844–851.

30. Cook PJ, Lawrence BA, Ludwig J, et al. The medical costs of gunshot injuries in the United States. *JAMA*. 1999;282:447–454.

31. Zethaerus N, Stromberg L, Jonsson B, et al. The cost of hip fractures. *Acta Orthop Scand*. 1997;68: 13–17.

32. Rice DP, Max W: Annotation: the high cost of injuries in the United States. *Am J Pub Health*. 1996;86:14–15.

33. Healthy people 2000 review, 1994. Hyattsville, Md: National Center for Health Statistics; 1995. [DHHS Publication PHS 95-1256-1.]

34. Ross CE. Fear of victimization and health. *J Quant Criminol*. 1993;9:159–175.

35. Joseph J. Fear of crime among black elderly. *J Black Studies*. 1997;27:698–717.

20

MANAGEMENT OF THE PULMONARY PATIENT WITH BURN INJURY

Timothy B. Op't Holt

*It has always been our ambition to get inside
that white space and now we are there,
so the space can no longer be blank.*
CAPTAIN ROBERT FALCON SCOTT of HMS *Discovery*,
November 25, 1902;
referring to crossing beyond 80°S latitude, beyond which all maps were blank.
We strive in our own ambitions to get into that "white space."

LEARNING OBJECTIVES

1. Describe facts, descriptions, and definitions related to skin and inhalation burn injuries.
2. Discuss the etiology, pathophysiology, and clinical features of a patient with inhalation and/or skin burns.
3. Discuss the ventilatory management of patients with burns
4. Apply the Siemens Servo 900C and 300 ventilators in the treatment of patients with burns.
5. Apply the critical thinking skills of prioritizing, anticipating, negotiating, communicating, decision making, and reflection by completing exercises and a case example of a burned patient.
6. Apply strategies to promote critical thinking in the respiratory care management of patients who are burned through completion of chapter exercises and group discussion.
7. Use the clinical case example in the chapter to perform an initial patient assessment, using the SOAP format and the clinical data presented.
8. Interpret clinical data from the case example including history, physical examination, lab-

oratory data, hemodynamic data, and radiographic data to make recommendations for respiratory care management.
9. Develop a care plan for the patient in the case, including recommendations for therapy and disease management, with consideration of the cost, ethical, and quality-of-life issues.
10. Communicate facts, evidence, and arguments to support evaluations and recommendations proposed in the respiratory care plan for the patient with burns.
11. Evaluate treatment and outcomes of interventions to propose changes in the care plan.
12. Describe the use of positive end-expiratory pressure (PEEP), pressure control ventilation, permissive hypercapnia, and the open-lung technique in the ventilatory management of the patient who has been burned.
13. Describe the airway care of the patient with burns.
14. Describe the infection control practices necessary in the care of patients with burns.

Members of nearly every department of the hospital are included on the burn team. Communication and cooperation among team members is essential to reach the goal of successful management of the burned patient. The respiratory therapist is involved because the patient is usually subjected to inhalation injury, prolonged bed rest, fluid shifts, and the threat of pneumonia. Therapists evaluate pulmonary mechanics, perform therapy to facilitate breathing, and closely monitor the status of the patient's respiratory functioning. It is these roles that will be examined in this chapter.

INTRODUCTION

Burn injury has for years been one of the most feared injuries, due to the pain, deformity, and death associated with the injury and its attendant therapy. While there are many patients who do not survive their burns or the sepsis that often follows, the number of survivors has increased more than twofold in the period between 1952 and 1993. For example, patients aged 15 to 44 in 1952 could be burned over 46% of their total body surface area (TBSA) and expect a 50% mortality rate. By 1993 the TBSA yielding a 50% mortality rate had increased to 72%.[1] Clearly, advances in therapy of the airway and lungs and of the burn itself, improvements in fluid management, nutritional support, and in the treatment of sequela such as sepsis, have dramatically decreased burn mortality. Although there have been advances in care, a burn remains a traumatic and painful incident for both the patient and family.

The costs to society of fire and burns are staggering. Figures from 1991 indicate that 60,000 to 80,000 people annually require in-hospital care for burns. The average cost per patient at that time was $36,000 to $117,000. The cost of a fire-related death in 1991 was estimated at between $250,000 and $1.5 million, including loss of future productivity.[2]

ETIOLOGY

The National Center for Injury Prevention and Control maintains a database on death due to burns. Fire and burn deaths occur with greatest frequency in residential fires, especially in multifamily dwellings and in low income census tracts. Other causes of burn injury and death include playing with matches and other ignition devices, careless smoking, drug and alcohol intoxication, arson, use of poorly functioning heating devices, hot liquids, fuels, open flames, structural fires, explosives, motor vehicle crashes, chemicals, self-inflicted burns, welding, and sunburn. Approximately 12 individuals die in fires each day. In 1995, 4345 persons died as a result of fire and burns. Victims are usually the very young and very old, due to their difficulty escaping and decreased agility. House fire death rates are highest in the southeast, occurring most often in the cold winter months when heating devices are in use. The death rate for males remains nearly twice that of females. Fortunately, age-adjusted death rates for fire decreased 33%, from 2.1 to 1.4 deaths/100,000 persons, during the period from 1985 to 1995.[3] This is due to improved building design, increased use of smoke and fire detectors, and use of safer appliances and heating devices.

CRITICAL CONTENT

INTRODUCTION AND ETIOLOGY

- Burn survival has increased in recent years.
- Treatment of burn injury requires the involvement of the respiratory therapist.
- Fire and burn deaths occur with greatest frequency in residential fires.
- Each day 12 individuals die in fires.
- Death rates from fire for males is twice that of females.

PREHOSPITAL MANAGEMENT

In the prehospital management of the burned patient, once the victim has been removed from the ignition or chemical source, the burn must be stopped; burning clothing must be extinguished and removed and chemical burns must be copiously lavaged with gallons of water. All personnel must practice universal precautions, including gown, gloves, masks, and protective eyewear. Initial management includes care of the airway, attention to breathing and circulation, and cervical spine immobilization.

Exposure to heated gases and smoke results in damage to the respiratory tract. Direct exposure of the upper airway to heat may result in upper airway edema, which may cause airway obstruction. Initially, 100% humidified oxygen should be given to all patients, even if there are no signs of respiratory distress. As edema progresses, the patient may become progressively more hoarse, which indicates impending airway closure and the need for intubation.

In burn patients, intubation is indicated by unconsciousness or acute respiratory distress. Because of the likelihood of impending airway problems, intubation is also indicated for burns of the face or neck. Signs of impending airway edema include singed nasal hairs and expectoration of car-

bonaceous sputum. Airway edema is characterized by a brassy cough, stridor, and hoarseness. Once the airway is established, the chest must be assessed for adequate expansion. Chest expansion may be impeded by burn eschar. The patient must then be adequately ventilated to overcome the effects of smoke inhalation and/or carbon monoxide poisoning. Cardiopulmonary resuscitation is begun if indicated. The type of burn is assessed (second or third degree), and the size of the burned area is calculated using a body surface area illustration in order to calculate intravenous fluid administration. The weight of the victim in kilograms is estimated. The 24-hour fluid load is calculated according to the Parkland Formula as follows:

$$(4.0 \text{ cc})(\text{weight in kg})(\% \text{ body surface area burned}) = \text{total fluid for 24 hours}$$

One half of this amount is administered in the first 8 hours after the time of injury, using lactated Ringer's. The burns are covered with a clean dressing or sheet, and the patient is transported to the hospital.

Once at the hospital, treatment continues as in the field, with additional diagnostic studies including CBC, electrolytes, glucose, blood urea nitrogen, creatinine, arterial blood gases, chest radiograph, and carboxyhemoglobin. Escharotomy may be needed to eliminate constriction of extremities if pulses are weak or absent.

High-volume fluid administration is needed due to the excessive evaporative loss that occurs with burns. The adequacy of fluid infusion is monitored by watching urine output, which should be at least 1 mL/kg/hr. If urine output falls, additional fluid is administered. Other indicators of adequate resuscitation include clear sensorium, absence of nausea, and a normal temperature and blood pressure. Inadequate fluid administration results in inadequate perfusion of renal and mesenteric vascular beds, which may result in organ failure. Unfortunately, this massive fluid administration often results in a greatly increased capillary hydrostatic pressure in the lungs, with resultant pulmonary edema. This results in increased intrapulmonary shunting, and the requirement for high levels of positive end-expiratory pressure (PEEP) during mechanical ventilation.[4]

CRITICAL CONTENT

INITIAL MANAGEMENT

- The patient must be removed from the source of ignition or chemical burning and the burning stopped.
- All personnel must practice universal precautions.
- Ensure a patent airway, and assess breathing, circulation, and perform cervical spine immobilization.
- All patients receive 100% humidified oxygen.
- Assess for signs of impending airway edema. If present, intubation is imperative!
- Fluid replacement is critical; maintain urine output of at least 1 mL/kg/hr.
- Burns are covered with a clean dressing or sheet before transport to hospital.

PARKLAND FORMULA (24-HOUR FLUID LOAD)

(4.0 cc)(weight in kg)(% body surface area burned) = total fluid for 24 hours

(one half of this given in the first 8 hours postburn)

PATHOPHYSIOLOGY OF BURN SHOCK AND BURN EDEMA

Burn shock is the derangement of cardiovascular function that accompanies burns of greater than 35% to 40% TBSA. Following a burn, fluid, protein, and electrolytes translocate from the vasculature into burned and nonburned tissues, resulting in an increased hematocrit and hypovolemic shock. This forms the basis for fluid resuscitation of the burn victim. In addition to the loss of fluids, there

is a massive release of mediators into the blood, which contributes to the shock. Even if the hypovolemia is corrected, the presence of these mediators perpetuates the shock. Increases in pulmonary (PVR) and systemic vascular resistance (SVR), together with myocardial depression occur despite adequate volume and preload support, exacerbating organ dysfunction.

Since burns quickly lead to hypovolemia, the hemodynamic changes are predictable. These include decreased plasma volume, cardiac output, and urine output, and an increased SVR, all of which lead to a decrease in peripheral blood flow. Following a burn, it is not unusual that edema forms in both burned and nonburned tissues, requiring massive fluid administration. This edema formation continues until 24 hours postburn. Edema formation occurs in two phases; the first phase occurs within the first hour postburn. The second continues from 12 to 24 hours postburn. The extent of this second phase is dependent upon the type and extent of burn injury and whether fluid resuscitation is given.[5]

Fluid transport across the capillary membrane is governed by the Landis-Starling equation:

$$J_v = K_f[P_c - P_{if}] - Coeff_o(P_p - P_{if})$$

where J_v is the volume of fluid that crosses the capillary membrane; K_f is the capillary filtration coefficient, which is the product of the capillary surface area and the hydraulic conductivity; P_c is the capillary hydrostatic pressure; P_{if} is the interstitial fluid hydrostatic pressure; $Coeff_o$ is the osmotic reflection coefficient; P_p is the colloid osmotic pressure of plasma; and P_{if} is the colloid osmotic pressure of interstitial fluid. Normally, J_v is ~6 mm Hg out of the capillary, and the resultant fluid is reabsorbed at the venule end of the capillary, and/or eliminated by the lymphatics (J_L) (Fig. 20-1). However, in burn injury this filtration rate is greatly increased, which overwhelms the lymphatics, resulting in edema. Edema may be the result of an increase in the capillary filtration coefficient, the capillary hydrostatic pressure, or the colloid osmotic pressure of interstitial fluid. Likewise, edema formation is favored by decreases in the reflection coefficient, interstitial fluid hydrostatic pressure, or the colloid osmotic pressure of plasma. In burns, all of these factors react to promote edema formation. The most important factors in development of burn edema are a highly negative interstitial fluid hydrostatic pressure and an increased capillary hydrostatic pressure. It has been proposed that the generation of this negative interstitial fluid hydrostatic pressure may be due to the denaturation of collagen.

As previously mentioned, local and circulating mediators that contribute to burn shock are present after burn injury. These mediators include histamine, prostaglandins, thromboxane, kinins, serotonin, catecholamines, oxygen radicals, platelet aggregation factor, angiotensin II, vasopressin, and corticotropin-releasing factor. Many mediators increase vascular permeability, thereby contributing

CRITICAL CONTENT

BURN SHOCK

- Accompanies burns of >35% TBSA
- Is due to fluid, protein, and electrolyte translocation from the vasculature into the interstitial space of burned and nonburned tissue
- Filtration overwhelms the lymphatics, resulting in edema
- Is associated with local and circulating mediators
- Translocation forms the basis for fluid resuscitation
- Fluid transport is governed by the Landis-Starling equation

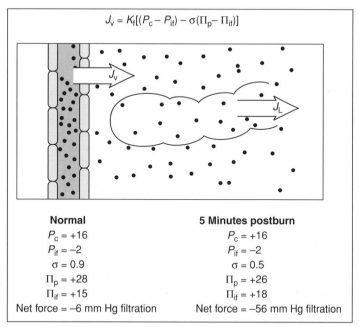

$$J_v = K_f[(P_c - P_{if}) - \sigma(\Pi_p - \Pi_{if})]$$

Normal	5 Minutes postburn
$P_c = +16$	$P_c = +16$
$P_{if} = -2$	$P_{if} = -2$
$\sigma = 0.9$	$\sigma = 0.5$
$\Pi_p = +28$	$\Pi_p = +26$
$\Pi_{if} = +15$	$\Pi_{if} = +18$
Net force = −6 mm Hg filtration	Net force = −56 mm Hg filtration

FIGURE 20-1 The normal pressures of the Starling equation for skin result in a slight imbalance favoring filtration with lymph flow (J_V) exactly equal to fluid filtration (J_L). In burned skin, all Starling factors are increased, creating a large net filtration which exceeds lymph flow and causes rapid edema. Data shown represent filtration forces in skin before and after burn injury.

to edema. Therefore, if inhibitors of these mediators were available, some aspects of burn edema could be pharmacologically limited. There is ongoing research into the use of mediator inhibition.

HEMODYNAMIC CONSEQUENCES OF ACUTE BURNS

Cardiac output (CO) decreases in the immediate postburn period, presumably due to the release of mediators into the blood. This is believed to be the case because CO decreases even before there is a decrease in plasma volume; it is therefore not caused by decreased preload. However, once the plasma volume decreases, hypovolemia and decreased venous return (decreased preload) probably play a major role in the continuation of CO depression. Even after restoration of the circulating volume, CO remains decreased. This is attributed to the myocardial depressant factor released from the wounds and a resultant decrease in contractility. CO remains decreased in the postresuscitative phase, and this is believed to be due to increased afterload of the left and right heart as a result of increased PVR and SVR.

Sympathetic stimulation and hypovolemia result in the release of mediators, causing vasoconstriction and a resultant increase in SVR. SVR is also increased as a result of increased blood viscosity as plasma leaks from the capillaries. This increase in SVR partially accounts for the depression of cardiac output.

PVR also increases with the release of mediators and loss of circulating blood volume. Fluid resuscitation contributes to the circulating blood volume, which, when it encounters pulmonary venule constriction, leads to an increased pulmonary capillary wedge pressure (PCWP), and pulmonary edema. The previously discussed myocardial depression also contributes to the rise in PCWP and edema. An additional factor that causes pulmonary edema is the developing hypoproteinemia. This reduces the capillary colloid osmotic pressure, thereby favoring fluid shift into the inter-

stitium. Pulmonary edema causes an intrapulmonary shunt that is refractory to ambient oxygen therapy, necessitating the use of PEEP to restore functional residual capacity (FRC).

In summary, following a burn, a cascade of physical and chemical factors result in a fluid shift into the interstitium, causing significant hypovolemia, hypotension, and edema in both burned and nonburned tissues. These phenomena are collectively referred to as burn shock and burn edema. They are accompanied by myocardial depression and pulmonary edema, which complicate management of the ventilated burn patient.

CRITICAL CONTENT

BURN HEMODYNAMICS

- Cardiac output decreases in the immediate postburn period.
- Hypovolemia (decreased preload) and mediator release contribute to cardiac output depression.
- Cardiac output remains decreased due to increased PVR and SVR.
- Pulmonary edema increases intrapulmonary shunt, necessitating the use of PEEP.

FLUID RESUSCITATION

Resuscitation from burn shock focuses on replacing the intravascular volume lost due to fluid shifts into the intracellular and interstitial spaces. It is interesting to note that the total body water may not change in a burn; it is only redistributed. There is no consensus about the exact type of fluid to use during resuscitation; however, there is consensus that the least amount of fluid necessary to maintain adequate organ perfusion should be given; the volume used should avoid over- or underresuscitation; and that the replacement of extracellular salt lost into the burned tissue and into the cells is essential for resuscitation.[6]

While a number of formulas exist to calculate fluid replacement, the Parkland formula is used in the case that is presented at the end of this chapter. The Parkland formula utilizes the crystalloid lactated Ringer's solution, which has a sodium concentration of 130 mEq/L. Crystalloid is preferred over colloid (albumin) because it is less expensive and because protein can leak across capillaries in thermal injuries. The Parkland formula that was previously described recommends 4 mL IV fluid/kg body weight times the percentage of TBSA burned be given in the first 24 hours, with one half that amount administered in the first 8 hours postburn. The end point of fluid resuscitation is 1.0 mL/kg/hr of urine output. Burn shock resuscitation has been completed when there is no further accumulation of edema fluid, which is usually 18 to 30 hours postburn. This is because the leaking capillaries eventually seal. In the case example presented in this chapter the patient required over twice the usual amount, perhaps because of the magnitude of his burns. Resuscitation fluid is infused until the volume of fluid needed to maintain adequate urine volume equals the maintenance fluid volume, which is the patient's normal maintenance volume plus insensible loss.

INHALATION INJURY

Inhalation injury includes thermal damage to the respiratory tract, as well as the chemical injuries that accompany the inhalation of the toxic byproducts of combustion of materials in a fire. Inhalation injury is the factor responsible for 80% of the mortality seen in thermally-injured patients. The extent of injury depends upon the ignition source, temperature, concentration, and solubility of the toxic gases generated, therefore it is important to know what materials were consumed in the fire. Nearly every flammable material in a house or automobile when burned produces a toxic byproduct such as aldehyde, acrolein, hydrogen cya-

nide, or sulfur dioxide. Caustic materials such as acroline and aldehydes produce an inflammatory reaction in the bronchi and physically damage the airways. In contrast, inhalation of carbon monoxide or hydrogen cyanide does not damage the airways, but does alter gas exchange.[7]

Carbon monoxide (CO) is often a significant factor in the injuries sustained by fire victims, and it is one of the most frequent causes of death following inhalation injury. Three mechanisms contribute to morbidity and mortality in CO poisoning. First, an inhaled carbon monoxide fraction of 0.1% can, given adequate exposure time, result in a carboxyhemoglobin level of 50%. This is due to the very high affinity carbon monoxide has for hemoglobin, some 200 to 250 times that of oxygen. Second, CO poisoning shifts the oxyhemoglobin curve to the left, tightly binding oxygen to hemoglobin, potentially resulting in decreased tissue oxygen delivery. Third, competitive inhibition with cytochrome oxidase enzyme systems results in the inability of cellular systems to utilize oxygen, resulting in tissue hypoxia.

The symptoms of CO poisoning vary with carboxyhemoglobin (CoHb) level. Up to 10%, there are no symptoms. At 10% to 30% CoHb, there is headache. At 30% to 40% CoHb, there is severe headache, dizziness, nausea, vomiting, and collapse. Beyond 40% CoHb, there are convulsions, syncope, and tachycardia. Death occurs within minutes to hours when CoHb exceeds 70%. The exhaled CO level can be measured by a CO detection device. CoHb levels in blood are measured by a cooximeter.

Arterial Pao_2, Spo_2, and calculated oxyhemoglobin values may be normal, and should therefore not be relied upon to determine the presence of carbon monoxide. Only cooximetry can measure carboxyhemoglobin. Therefore, cooximetry should be performed on all patients suspected of inhalation injury. Repeat measurements are used to guide oxygen therapy. Since there will be a metabolic acidosis in conjunction with tissue hypoxia, $P\bar{v}o_2$, pH, and plasma lactate may be measured to evaluate therapeutic response. The presence of mental disorientation is an important clue to CO poisoning.

Since the half life of carboxyhemoglobin is 250 minutes in room air, it is imperative that victims be placed on 100% oxygen as soon as possible. While the nonrebreather mask does not usually deliver 100%, it is typically the best device available for initial oxygen delivery and for transportation purposes. CoHb half life at 100% oxygen is 40 to 60 minutes. If the victim is unconscious or cannot maintain the airway, they must be intubated and ventilated with 100% oxygen. Some authorities recommend hyperbaric oxygen therapy, wherein oxygen at 3 atmospheres (atm) may be administered. This therapy reduces CoHb half life to 30 minutes.

Hydrogen cyanide is produced by the combustion of nitrogen-containing polymers. The toxicity of hydrogen cyanide is produced by the inhibition of cellular oxygenation, with resultant tissue anoxia, caused by reversible inhibition of cytochrome oxidase (Fe^{3+}) by cyanide. Diagnosis at the scene is difficult, but the odor of bitter almonds should arouse suspicion. Symptoms include lethargy, nausea, headache, weakness, and coma. Treatment at the site includes intravenous administration of sodium thiosulfate, hydroxycobalamin, and 100% oxygen.

Regardless of the toxin inhaled, fire personnel will evaluate the ABCs and administer oxygen. The respiratory therapist at the hospital will further evaluate the respiratory status and initiate any other indicated definitive therapy. The first priority will be evaluation of the patient's airway for the presence of thermal injury.

Thermal injury to the oropharynx follows the same pathway as with cutaneous burns, with regard to edema formation. Important clues to the possibility of thermal injury of the airway are findings such as evidence of heat damage to mouth/nose area (redness, swelling, etc), and singed nasal hairs or eyebrows. The massive edema of the face and oropharynx is extremely dangerous, potentially leading to complete airway obstruction. This is why tracheal intubation should be considered as soon as the signs and symptoms of inhalation injury are realized.

Actual thermal injury to the lower airways is rare because the upper airway is an efficient cooling mechanism. Injury to the lower airway is only caused by the inhalation of hot particles or steam. When the lower airways are damaged, there is separation of the basement membrane from the ciliated epithelium, followed by edema that is visible on bronchoscopy. This is followed by the formation of an exudate and large airway narrowing, that increases the susceptibility to pneumonia, sepsis, and death.

Following the inhalation of a toxic substance, pulmonary microvascular changes occur due to the release of inflammatory mediators. This leads to adherence of neutrophils to the capillary endothelium, which is followed by release of oxygen free radicals and proteases by neutrophils. Subsequently, there is an increase in extravascular lung water and lung lymph flow. Pulmonary artery pressure, PCWP, and PVR increase within 4 to 12 hours after the injury, all of which are consistent with an increase in pulmonary vascular permeability. The resultant pulmonary edema decreases lung compliance and reduces the FRC. This has important implications for the mechanical ventilation of the patient that will be discussed later in this chapter.

CRITICAL CONTENT

INHALATION INJURY

- First priority is evaluation of the airway for presence of thermal injury.
- It is responsible for 80% of the mortality in thermally injured patients.
- Carbon monoxide is one of the most frequent causes of death.
- CoHb must be measured by cooximetry, because pulse oximetry is inaccurate.
- Toxic by-products of combustion frequently cause the actual lung damage.
- Thermal injury to the lower airways is rare.
- Toxic substances cause pulmonary edema and decreased FRC.
- Plugging of airways causes atelectasis, hypoxemia, and increased pneumonia risk.

Within the airways, the mucociliary escalator is damaged, so the sloughed pulmonary epithelium is not effectively cleared. Add to that the presence of serous exudate, blood cells, and mucus, and the result is plugging and partial plugging of the airways, causing atelectasis, shunting, decreased ventilation/perfusion ratios, hypoxemia, and an increased risk of pneumonia.

RESPIRATORY MANAGEMENT OF INHALATION INJURIES

Initial management consists of assuring a patent airway. Oxygen by nonrebreather mask or manual resuscitation bag is provided as a precaution, assuming exposure to carbon monoxide. In the hospital, the airway is assured and observed for the presence of edema. Maximal edema and peak airway narrowing occurs at 24 hours postinjury. Therefore, in a nonintubated patient, airway patency must be carefully monitored for at least the first 24 hours. A baseline arterial blood gas with cooximetry is obtained, as is a chest radiograph. For those patients exposed to asphyxiants (CO, methane, NO_2), but have no evidence of airway injury, supportive care is given in the form of oxygen therapy, unless ventilatory failure has occurred, in which case mechanical ventilation is indicated. Patients should receive 100% oxygen until their carboxyhemoglobin level is zero.

The use of hyperbaric oxygen (HBO) in patients with carbon monoxide poisoning is controversial. The half life of CoHb at 3 atm of 100% oxygen is 30 minutes, which would make HBO the logical choice for CO poisoning. However, the half life of CoHb while breathing 100% oxygen at atmospheric pressure is 40 to 50 minutes, so there may not be a definite advantage to HBO in those patients who receive 100% oxygen at the scene. Complications of HBO include cardiac arrest, seizures, cardiac dysrhythmias, and patient isolation. Advocates of HBO say that it is indicated in those patients with a very high CoHb level who are symptomatic (coma, seizures, or respiratory failure).

Those patients who sustain airway injury may suffer a variety of abnormalities, including hypoxemia, retained secretions, bronchospasm, and respiratory failure. Treatment guidelines are included in Table 20-1. General care includes raising the head of the bed 30°, which helps decrease airway edema and keeps abdominal contents from pushing on the diaphragm, making ventilation more difficult and restricting lung expansion. In those patients who have circumferential burns, chest wall escharotomy may be necessary to increase chest wall compliance when edema has restricted chest wall movement.

Most burn patients have arterial hypoxemia. This is treated by either high- or low-flow oxygen therapy, depending on the extent of the hypoxemia and the goal of therapy. Patients with an inhalation injury and an increased likelihood of shunting will need a high concentration of oxygen and some form of positive pressure. However, patients with a thermal injury to the face and upper airway may

TABLE 20-1 GUIDELINES FOR THE TREATMENT OF RESPIRATORY COMPLICATIONS SECONDARY TO BURNS

AIRWAY COMPROMISE	INTUBATION
Hypoxemia	100% oxygen initially until CoHb is 0%, thereafter titrate oxygen so SpO_2 is >93%
Retained secretions	Coughing exercises, incentive spirometry, intrapulmonary percussive ventilation treatments, suctioning, chest physical therapy, adequate humidification, PEP or flutter valve therapy
Bronchospasm	Bronchodilators, beta$_2$ agonists, anticholinergics
Respiratory failure	Pressure-controlled mechanical ventilation

not tolerate a face mask or face tent, and the airway may rapidly close due to edema, so intubation is often necessary for the initiation of continuous positive airway pressure (CPAP) for the treatment of shunting. If both hypoxemic and hypercapnic ventilatory failure are present, mechanical ventilation with PEEP will be necessary.

Retained secretions are removed by a variety of methods, including coughing, suctioning, postural drainage and percussion (chest physiotherapy; CPT), intrapulmonary percussive ventilation (IPV), and bronchoscopy. Retained secretions are indicated by the presence of coarse crackles, dry sputum, and consolidation or atelectasis on the chest radiograph.

Patients who are not intubated must be encouraged to cough and deep breathe to clear secretions. All patients must be adequately hydrated to avoid inspissation of secretions. Whether a patient is intubated or not, chest physiotherapy maneuvers may assist those patients who have >30 mL of sputum/day. It is most important during CPT that appropriate positioning be performed. Often the presence of a burn wound may preclude percussion. However, proper postural drainage is just as effective as postural drainage and percussion in patients who are adequately hydrated. If the patient is able to cooperate, you may try positive expiratory pressure (PEP) or flutter valve therapy as an alternative.

Incentive spirometry, while not a direct method for removing secretions, is effective in treating atelectasis and encouraging deep breathing, which assists in secretion removal. Intrapulmonary percussive ventilation is a method of internal chest vibration that encourages secretions to flow up the airways where they can be expectorated or suctioned. Anecdotal reports of burned patients with atelectasis have recounted significant relief from secretions and atelectasis with this method. Controlled clinical studies in selected populations are needed to validate these anecdotal reports.

Acetylcysteine instilled or via aerosol may assist in the breakdown of retained secretions, although there is no convincing evidence of this. It is known that direct instillation of acetylcysteine to mucus plugs during bronchoscopy can break down the plug. It may be that current practice of aerosolizing or instilling a 1 to 2 mL dose of 10% to 20% acetylcysteine is simply not enough to effect a response. It is also widely known that acetylcysteine is irritating and causes bronchospasm. For this reason, if acetylcysteine is administered, it should be combined with a bronchodilator.

Narrowing of the airways is the result of two factors: airway edema from the inhalation injury, and actual bronchospasm as a result of smooth muscle contraction. In the first case, bronchodilators are of little use. However, in the event of smooth muscle spasm, $beta_2$ adrenergic (eg, albuterol) and anticholinergic (eg, ipratropium bromide) bronchodilators are effective when given to the spontaneously breathing patient or to those who are mechanically ventilated. When using a metered dose inhaler (MDI), proper technique is of paramount importance. When using an MDI, therapy is more effective when a spacer is utilized.[8]

VENTILATORY MANAGEMENT

Mechanical ventilation of the burned patient is indicated in hypoxemic and/or hypercapnic ventilatory failure. Hypercapnic ventilatory failure may be precipitated by a variety of factors, including thermal injury superimposed on preexisting chronic obstructive pulmonary disease (COPD), the administration of analgesics and neuromuscular blockers, or the massive increased production of carbon dioxide caused by the hypermetabolic response to burn injury. Acute hypercapnic ventilatory failure can be diagnosed by noting a $Paco_2$ >50 mm Hg and a pH <7.30.

Hypoxemic ventilatory failure occurs as a result of the interstitial and alveolar edema resulting from the massive fluid resuscitation and inhalation of irritant gases that increase the permeability of the alveolar wall. Subsequently, the interstitium and alveoli are flooded, leading to alveolar collapse and fluid filling. Wound infection and subsequent sepsis also lead to further leaking of the capillaries and alveolar wall, and the acute respiratory distress syndrome (ARDS). The current definition of ARDS includes bilateral pulmonary infiltrates, an inciting incident, a PCWP <18 cm H_2O, and a PaO_2 to FIO_2 ratio of <200. These criteria are often met in the burned patient. See Chapter 22 for a review of ARDS.

Several approaches have been used to limit the peak and plateau pressures imposed by mechanical ventilation in order to avoid barotrauma or volutrauma. These conditions may occur in traditional volume-controlled ventilation with tidal volumes (VTs) of 10 to 12 mL/kg body weight. Pressure- and volume-limiting approaches include high-frequency ventilation, lower tidal volume ventilation (eg, 6 to 8 mL/kg), and pressure-controlled ventilation.

Although various approaches may be used successfully, described here is one approach that would be considered reasonable. Ventilation may be initiated in a volume-controlled mode, usually synchronized intermittent mandatory ventilation (SIMV) with pressure support (if the patient is spontaneously initiating breaths) or just volume control (if the patient is to be paralyzed and sedated). Ventilator settings are maintained to achieve a normal pH, $PaCO_2$, and PaO_2. VT is usually set to 8 to 10 mL/kg. Fraction of inspired oxygen (FIO_2) is usually begun at 1.0, and kept there until the CoHb is 0%, then weaned to ≤0.5.

If FIO_2 cannot be subsequently weaned to ≤0.5, PEEP is increased until that can be accomplished. This may necessitate PEEP levels of 30 to 50 cm H_2O. A level of PEEP that allows a decrease in the FIO_2 to ≤0.5 is probably the PEEP level that is at, or just above, the lower inflexion point. The lower inflexion point is that point on the lung compliance curve where the compliance takes a sudden vertical turn, indicating alveolar recruitment and restoration of the FRC. This is the essence of what has been referred to as the "open lung" technique. Once the lung is open, the FIO_2 can be reduced to a safe level (≤0.5). See Chapter 22 for more discussion on this topic.

In the event that a high FIO_2 and PEEP are inadequate to maintain PaO_2 ≤60 mm Hg, the patient can be put on pressure control ventilation

(PCV) and the inspiratory time gradually increased, to achieve an inspiratory:expiratory (I:E) ratio of up to 1.5:1. This is the institution of pressure-controlled inverse ratio ventilation (PC-IRV). Others have increased the I:E to as much as 4:1, but there is probably a higher risk of cardiovascular decompensation at such high I:E ratios. Transient desaturations are managed by increasing FIO_2, then decreasing it while watching the SpO_2.

Peak and plateau pressures are closely monitored. If peak pressure exceeds 40 cm H_2O or plateau pressure exceeds 35 cm H_2O, barotrauma or volutrauma are more likely. If this is the case, pressure control ventilation is suggested to maintain the existing tidal volume. If this does not sufficiently lower the ventilator pressures, the VT may be reduced to as low as 6 mL/kg. A ventilatory method specific to opening alveoli and maintaining lung volume while providing adequate alveolar ventilation at 6 to 8 mL/kg will decrease mortality and decrease the number of days mechanical ventilation is needed.[9] A compliance-sensitive mode, such as pressure regulated volume control (PRVC), is useful because this mode monitors the tidal volume and changes the inspiratory pressure to achieve the desired tidal volume as compliance changes.

Hypercapnia is the result of reduced minute volume secondary to decreasing the tidal volume, whether this reduction is the result of volume or pressure control. When hypercapnia is allowed to exist in order to protect the lung, it is referred to as permissive hypercapnia. In the event of permissive hypercapnia, clinicians should monitor renal function to assure that adequate compensation occurs so the pH remains >7.25. $PaCO_2$ is then controlled by changes in mandatory rate.[10]

Tracheostomy in the burn victim is considered if prolonged ventilatory failure is expected, if the patient is not tolerating the endotracheal tube, or if pulmonary toilet is difficult. Tracheostomy tubes are easier to care for, are more comfortable for the patient, do not have adverse effects on the vocal cords, and enhance bronchopulmonary hygiene. However, the tracheostomy site is a portal for infection, and thus requires meticulous care.

WEANING

When the patient no longer requires sedation and paralysis (if PC-IRV or PRVC were required), the mode may be changed to SIMV-pressure control plus pressure support. The decision to change to SIMV-volume control mode is made once the peak pressure is ≤40 cm H_2O. The level of pressure support should be titrated to achieve a VT of 6 to 8 mL/kg. Once the mandatory breath pressure level has been titrated to achieve a VT of 8 to 10 mL/kg, ventilation is controlled by changing the mandatory rate. The mandatory ventilatory rate is often weaned to 1 to 4 breaths/min, provided that the patient's total rate is <30 breaths/min.

As the patient's Pao_2 improves, PEEP is decreased in increments of 3 to 5 cm H_2O. The minimum PEEP level should be 5 cm H_2O. Once a PEEP of 5 cm H_2O is reached at an Fio_2 ≤0.5, mandatory ventilator rate is 1 to 4 breaths/min, pressure support is ≤10 cm H_2O, and arterial blood gases are within normal limits, withdrawal of the ventilator is usually considered.

CRITICAL CONTENT

MECHANICAL VENTILATION

- Indicated in hypoxemic and/or hypercapnic respiratory failure
- Limit pressures by using VTs of 6 to 8 mL/kg if plateau pressure is >35 cm H_2O
- PEEP is implemented to allow an Fio_2 ≤0.5; use enough to exceed the lower inflection point on the lung pressure-volume curve if possible
- PRVC or IRV may be used to maintain VT and increase mean airway pressure
- Tracheostomy may be indicated for prolonged airway maintenance
- Weaning progresses as tolerated once the massive fluid shift has been reabsorbed

Three methods may be used: a trial of continuous positive airway pressure (CPAP), a trial using a T-adapter, or a trial using a tracheostomy collar. There is no clear evidence that one method is superior. The best one for a given patient is that which is best tolerated. If the patient has acceptable spontaneous ventilatory parameters and arterial blood gases, the trial is continued. If the patient meets criteria for extubation or removal of the tracheostomy tube, this is also indicated. Following removal of the airway, the patient is observed for signs of respiratory distress. Therapy is then preventive (incentive spirometry, intermittent positive-pressure breathing [IPPB], etc) and therapeutic (oxygen, bronchodilators, bronchial hygiene).

COMPLICATIONS OF INHALATION INJURY

Complications are divided into those that occur early and those that manifest late. Early complications include barotrauma (for those on mechanical ventilation) and infection. Barotrauma is manifested in various forms: pneumothorax, pneumomediastinum, pneumoperitoneum, or subcutaneous emphysema. Efforts to minimize airway pressures (described earlier) will help prevent these complications. The incidence of infection, notably pneumonia, is 38%. Risk factors include the actual inhalation injury, intubation and resultant colonization of the lower airway, aspiration, and oropharyngeal colonization with pathogenic organisms.

Infection is prevented by paying rigorous attention to hand washing, and the use of protective barriers (gown, gloves, mask, and hair covering). Ventilator-associated pneumonia is prevented by changing the ventilator circuit no more frequently than every 48 hours, meticulous oral hygiene, cuff management to minimize aspiration, and the use of closed suction systems. All items brought into the patient's room should be disinfected (ventilator, monitors, percussor) or dedicated to single-patient use (ventilator circuit, nebulizers, tubing, and accessories).

Late complications include damage to the airway, continued inflammation, and ARDS. Late airway complications include erosion of the oral mucosa, tracheoesophageal (T-E) fistula, and tracheal stenosis, all of which are avoided by careful endotracheal tube and cuff maintenance. Careful attention to airway pressure and FIO_2 may help attenuate the inflammatory process which, if unchecked, can lead to ARDS.

CRITICAL CONTENT

COMPLICATIONS OF INHALATION INJURY

- Early: barotrauma (if receiving mechanical ventilation); infection
- Late: airway damage (mucosal erosion, T-E fistula, tracheal stenosis); continued inflammation; ARDS

SITE- AND AGE-SPECIFIC CONSIDERATIONS, COSTS, ETHICAL, HEALTH PROMOTION, AND QUALITY-OF-LIFE ISSUES

There are site- and age-specific considerations that were discussed earlier at the beginning of the chapter. These topics, as well as those related to costs, ethical issues, health promotion, and quality of life are summarized in Table 20-2.

TABLE 20-2 SITE- AND AGE-SPECIFIC CONSIDERATIONS, COSTS, ETHICAL, HEALTH PROMOTION, AND QUALITY-OF-LIFE ISSUES

SITE- AND AGE-SPECIFIC CONSIDERATIONS	CONSIDERATION OF COSTS AND ETHICAL ISSUES	HEALTH PROMOTION AND QUALITY-OF-LIFE ISSUES
• Burned patients are best cared for in a designated burn unit, by a burn team. • Respiratory therapists are included as members of the team, and should have special training to appreciate the needs of the burn victim. • Individuals of all ages are subject to burn injury, but there is a greater incidence in the very young and very old. • Burns have a greater incidence in the southeast US. • Statistics are available on the types of burn injury by age group (ie, scald injury in children, combustible fuel injury in adults).	• Burn therapy is very expensive. • The bill for the patient in the case study in this chapter was approximately $1.5 million for 5 months of care. • A social worker is included on the burn team to help with social and economic issues. • All burn victims are fluid resuscitated regardless of severity. • Initial resuscitative efforts are not withheld even in the most severely burned patients.	• Burn teams include rehabilitative specialists such as physical and occupational therapists. • Innovations in burn treatment have led to a remarkable rate of return to active life. • Most burns are preventable, therefore public awareness campaigns are crucial to burn prevention.

INTRODUCTION TO CASE STUDY

Now you proceed to the most exciting part of this chapter, that of working your way through a hypothetical case. Your instructor will assign you to work on specific critical thinking exercises, and potentially group critical thinking exercises, depending on the available time, types of patients you are likely to encounter in your clinical rota-

tions, and resources available. Please check with your instructor to verify which exercises you are to work on. Your instructor may assign you to develop the learning issues as part of your problem-based learning (PBL) process, or you may be assigned specific predetermined learning issues that have been developed for this chapter. Please check with your program faculty before proceeding to the following case.

CASE STUDY 1

MR. BILL BURNS

Initial Case Scenario

2/24 day 1: Bill Burns, a 35-year-old man, is brought to the medical center by helicopter from an outlying hospital after suffering a burn injury.

Critical Thinking Exercise 1

PRIORITIZING PATIENT CARE

Explain how you would prioritize your patient assessment and treatment during the first few minutes of Mr. Burns' arrival to the emergency department.

History of Present Illness

Mr. Burns was transferred to the medical center via helicopter from an outlying hospital. He was the driver of a car that was struck from behind by a semi-tractor trailer traveling at a high rate of speed. The victim's car was engulfed in flames, but the victim's friends who had been in the car with him were able to extricate him. At the outlying hospital, it was noted that his face was badly burned, including singed nasal hairs, and that he had carbonaceous sputum. He was subsequently intubated on the scene with an 8 mm ID endotracheal tube and ventilated with a resuscitation bag. Upon arrival at the medical center, ventilation was begun with a Siemens Servo 900C ventilator.

Past Medical History

It is unknown if he has had previous illnesses. However, he takes no medicines, has no known drug allergies, and has had no surgeries. He lives in Bagdad, Florida, with his wife and two children. His wife reported that her husband does not smoke, drink alcohol, or use illicit drugs.

Critical Thinking Exercise 2

MAKING INFERENCES BY CLUSTERING DATA

a. What inference can you make about Mr. Burns' respiratory status?

b. Practice clustering data that leads you to this inference. Briefly explain how each piece of data points toward your inference.

Critical Thinking Exercise 3

ANTICIPATING PHYSICAL EXAMINATION FINDINGS

a. What physical findings do you need to determine if there is a cardiorespiratory problem?

b. What laboratory studies are needed to determine the patient's respiratory therapy needs?

c. What symptoms is the respiratory therapist looking for in this patient?

The following clinical and laboratory data are obtained at the time of admission:

ABG 18:25 100% bag mask

pH	6.90
Pco_2	78
Po_2	56
HCO_3^-	14.5
BE	−24
Sao_2	80%

PHYSICAL EXAMINATION RESULTS

Subjective N/A (patient sedated, paralyzed, and ventilated on a Servo 900C ventilator)

Objective Vital signs: temperature 96.4°F; heart rate 120 beats/min; ventilatory rate 16/min; BP 90/60 mm Hg; weight approximately 200 lb (90 kg)

HEENT: Intubated; face appears to have partial-thickness burns. Nasal hairs are singed.

Neck: no collar on arrival.

Lungs: equal bilateral breath sounds with bilateral coarse crackles

Cardiovascular: regular rate and rhythm

Abdomen: Soft and nontender

Extremities: Full-thickness burns to both upper extremities, anterior and posterior torso, circumferential deep burn to left upper extremity, decreased right radial pulse. Vessels in both upper extremities are thrombosed.

Chest radiograph #1: Diffuse bilateral infiltrates. Endotracheal tube in position. (See Fig. 20-2).

Assessment S/P MVA with 55% TBSA burn, mostly full-thickness.

Plan
1. Trauma consult
2. Escharotomy left upper extremity
3. May need bronchoscopy to facilitate gas exchange
4. To burn unit for aggressive wound care
5. Continue paralysis and sedation
6. Aggressive fluid resuscitation
7. C-collar
8. Log roll
9. Nutritional consult

Initial ventilator settings: Siemens Servo 900C: SIMV, Fio_2 1.0, Vt 900 mL, mandatory rate 12 breaths/min, PEEP +5 cm H_2O, PS +8 cm H_2O.

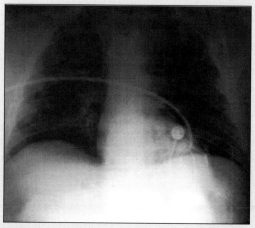

FIGURE 20-2 Mr. Burns chest radiograph #1, showing interstitial infiltrates, endotracheal tube in position.

CASE STUDY 1 *(continued)*

 Critical Thinking Exercise 4

ANTICIPATING PROBLEMS AND SOLUTIONS

a. What should constitute the respiratory care plan for this patient?

b. Prioritize the respiratory care plan.

c. What else should constitute the plan of care for this patient?

d. What hypotheses do you have regarding this patient's prospective respiratory problems?

At 1945 hr the respiratory therapist noted gradually-increasing peak inspiratory pressure (PIP). Current PIP at 40 cm H_2O with a plateau pressure of 36 cm H_2O.

 Critical Thinking Exercise 5

ANTICIPATING PROBLEMS AND SOLUTIONS

a. What ventilator setting change(s) would seem reasonable at this time?

b. Cite your rationale.

The physician asks the respiratory therapist to suggest ventilator adjustments. Upon the therapist's recommendation, pressure-controlled ventilation is instituted at 2030 with the following parameters: FiO_2 1.0, f 12, PEEP +18, PC 14 (target VT 800 mL).

ABG at 2100 hr 100% PCV

pH	7.11
PcO_2	56
PO_2	478
HCO_3^-	17.8
BE	−13.5
SaO_2	99%

 Critical Thinking Exercise 6

ASSESSMENT AND DECISION MAKING

a. Describe the patient's acid-base and oxygenation status.

b. What ventilator parameter changes are indicated at this time?

c. What is your rationale for the changes you specified?

At 2200 hr, the ventilator settings are changed as follows: FiO_2 0.6, f 18, PEEP +18, PC 20 (target VT 1000 mL).

 Critical Thinking Exercise 7

REFLECTION ON YOUR DECISION MAKING

a. Examine the decision-making process you use when you are asked to propose ventilator adjustments. List the steps you take, step-by-step.

b. What are important considerations beyond arterial blood gases when making ventilator adjustments or recommendations?

ABG at 2300 hr 60% PCV

pH	7.22
PcO_2	39
PO_2	118
HCO_3^-	16.0
BE	−11
SaO_2	97.8%

CASE STUDY 1 *(continued)*

Critical Thinking Exercise 8

INFORMATION GATHERING AND DECISION MAKING

a. Describe the patient's acid-base and oxygenation status.

b. What ventilator parameter changes are indicated at this time?

c. What is your rationale for the changes you specified?

d. What additional information would you like to know about the patient's condition?

2/25 (day 2): The day therapist reads the following physician note while making morning rounds. Burn resident progress notes:

Subjective   N/A (patient sedated, paralyzed, and ventilated on a Servo 900C ventilator).

Objective   Vital signs: HR 116 to 124 beats/ min; systolic blood pressure 80s to 90s mm Hg. Intake 25.0 L/ 2.4 L output. Breath sounds with bilateral crackles. Admitting chest radiograph shows interstitial infiltrates (see Fig. 20-2).

Assessment   The patient has received massive amounts of fluid, twice that required by the Parkland formula. Receiving mechanical ventilation via Siemens Servo 900C. Not tolerating tube feeds yet. Patient is manifesting a severe inhalation injury super- imposed on a deep 55% TBSA burn.

Plan   1. ABG at 1000 hr
   2. Monitor fluid intake/urine output closely
   3. Pulmonary artery catheter

ABGs are obtained at 1010 hr with Mr. Burns on the following ventilator settings: FIO_2 0.6, f 18, PEEP +25, PC 20 (target VT 1000 mL).

ABG at 1010 hr 60% PCV

pH	7.28
PCO_2	40
PO_2	68
HCO_3^-	18.5
BE	−7.5
SaO_2	91%

Critical Thinking Exercise 9

ASSESSMENT AND DECISION MAKING

a. Based on the most recent data, what ventilator setting changes are indicated?

b. Cite your rationale.

Group Critical Thinking Exercise 1

PRO/CON DEBATE: MEDICAL ETHICS

In two groups, address this issue: This patient may be left with crippling injuries and a lifetime of expenses. Should we try to save this patient? One group should be assigned to present the pro argument, the other the con. Although at first glance the argument may seem to be heavily weighted on one side of this issue, a critical thinker should be able to present salient points on either side of this debate. If possible, the pre- sentations should be made before a larger group (the full class) with discussion from the audience after the presentations.

2/26 (day 3): On rounds the next day, the day shift respiratory therapist notes the following: Burn attending physician's progress notes:

Subjective	N/A (patient sedated, paralyzed, and ventilated on a Servo 900C ventilator)
Objective	T_{max} 101.7°F, other vital signs stable. Cardiac output 24 L/min.
Assessment	Patient took ~70 L of lactated Ringer's to seal leak.
Plan	Decrease IV fluids.

2/28 (day 5): On day 5 of Mr. Burns' ICU specialized burn unit stay, the respiratory therapist reads the following attending physician's note:

Subjective	Patient paralyzed and sedated.
Objective	PCWP 26 mm Hg on dobutamine 10 (μg/kg/hr. Cardiac output 9.8 L/min. $S\bar{v}o_2$ 65%. Tolerating tube feeding.
	Chest radiograph: Infiltrates and subcutaneous emphysema. Endotracheal tube and Swan-Ganz catheter in place (see Fig. 20-3).
A/P	Hemodynamics now stable, continue ventilatory support, wean dobutrex.

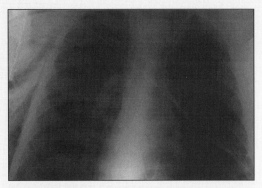

F I G U R E 2 0 - 3   Mr. Burns chest radiograph #2, showing infiltrates and subcutaneous emphysema, endotracheal tube and Swan-Ganz catheter in place.

The respiratory therapist charts this information after the assessment: Ventilator settings are Fio_2 0.4, f 20, PEEP +35, PC 25 (target V_T 1000 mL). Breath sounds diminished with crackles. No secretions with suctioning. Spo_2 100%, $S\bar{v}o_2$ 70%.

Critical Thinking Exercise 10

TROUBLESHOOTING

If the high airway pressure alarm sounds, what would be the specific sequence of steps the respiratory therapist should follow to identify and then resolve the problem?

3/1 (day 6): The respiratory therapist reads the following information during the evening rounds from the burn resident progress notes:

Subjective	Patient paralyzed and sedated.
Objective	Ventilator settings: Fio_2 0.4, f 20, PEEP +35, PC 30 (target V_T 1000 mL).
	ABGs: pH 7.49, $Paco_2$ 38 mm Hg, Pao_2 181 mm Hg.
	T_{max} 101.5°F, on ceftazidime and vancomycin.
	Cardiovascular: heart rate 124–140 beats/min, blood pressure 103/55–146/102 mm Hg, cardiac index 4.5 L/min/m^2, SVR 635 RU, $S\bar{v}o_2$ 65%, PCWP 24–28 mm Hg.
	Hematology: WBC 12, Hb 8.2, HCT 25.4, PLT 63,000.
	Electrolytes: K 3.9, Na 146, Cl 114, CO_2 27, BUN 20, creatinine 1.8, glucose 188.
A/P	1. Continue sedation and paralysis.
	2. Begin weaning PEEP today.

CASE STUDY 1 *(continued)*

Critical Thinking Exercise 11

ASSESSMENT AND TROUBLESHOOTING

a. What therapy is indicated based on the laboratory data above?

b. What is your assessment of the cardiac index? Given this CI, what is your explanation for the most likely cause of the current $S\bar{v}O_2$?

c. What actions should the respiratory therapist take when the low minute volume alarm sounds on the ventilator?

3/3 (day 8): Attending physician notes 2 days later:

Subjective	Patient waking up.
Objective	Pulmonary: PEEP successfully weaned to +25 cm H_2O in 2–3 cm H_2O increments throughout the day.
	Cardiovascular: Heart rate 106–127 beats/min, blood pressure 98/48–189/62 mm Hg. $S\bar{v}O_2$ 75–78%, CI 2.6 L/min/m², PCWP 20–26 mm Hg. Hematology: WBCs 15.4, Hb 9.8, Hct 30.3, PLT 105,000. T_{max} 102°F.
Assessment	1. Stable hemodynamics.
	2. Tolerating tube feedings.
Plan	1. Discontinue paralytics.
	2. Continue weaning PEEP.

3/4 (day 9): During the course of the day the PEEP was successfully weaned to +13 cm H_2O in 2–3 cm H_2O increments. ABGs on FIO_2 0.4, f 20, PEEP +13, PC 35 cm H_2O (target VT 1000 mL) are obtained and are seen as follows:

ABG 40% PCV

pH	7.46
PCO_2	40
PO_2	119
HCO_3^-	28
BE	+4
SaO_2	98%

Later that evening, Mr. Burns is transported to the OR for excision of burns on his back and placement of Integra (2300 cm²).

3/5 (day 10): The respiratory therapist reports the following information: Cs 48–52 cc/cm H_2O, spontaneous ventilatory rate of 5 breaths/min. Breath sounds decreased.

Critical Thinking Exercise 12

ASSESSMENT AND DECISION MAKING

Does this patient have acute respiratory distress syndrome or acute lung injury? How are these entities differentiated?

3/6 (day 11): PEEP weaned slowly to 8 cm H_2O, with subsequent decrease in SpO_2 to 94%. A decision is made to change Mr. Burns from a Servo 900C ventilator to a Servo 300. The mode is changed to SIMV (PC) + PS with the following settings: FIO_2 0.4, f 4, PEEP +8, PS +8, PC 28 (target VT 1000 mL).

CASE STUDY 1 *(continued)*

Group Critical Thinking Exercise 2

PRO/CON DEBATE:
CHOICE OF VENTILATORS

Your instructor will assign two groups to debate the merits of the decision in this case to switch the patient from his current ventilator (Servo 900C) to a Servo 300. The groups should present their arguments in front of the full class, where a discussion of the debate can occur after its conclusion. Was there a clear winner of this debate? Was one side more persuasive than the other? If so, what made their argument appear to be stronger?

3/7 (day 12): ABGs on these ventilator settings: Servo 300: FIO$_2$ 0.4, f 4, PEEP +8, PS 8, PC 30 (target VT 1000 mL):

ABG 40% PCV

pH	7.44
PCO$_2$	44
PO$_2$	86
HCO$_3^-$	30.3
BE	+5
SaO$_2$	97%

Later, the respiratory therapist notes a spontaneous rate of 36 breaths/min and Cs of 50 cc/cm H$_2$O. Breath sounds are decreased with crackles. In addition, a physician order error was noted. The mode was subsequently changed to SIMV(VC) + PS at the same settings to be in agreement with the specific mode ordered. Secretions are thin and yellow. When confirming the ventilator orders with the physician, she states that they are planning to do a bronchoscopy in the morning. Burn resident physician notes:

Subjective	Arousable.
Objective	Pulmonary, as above.
	Cardiovascular: heart rate 110–138 beats/min; blood pressure 115/60–150/68 mm Hg, T$_{max}$ 105°F. PCWP 11–18 mm Hg.
	Hematology: WBCs 9.8, Hb 11.3, Hct 33.2, PLT 164,000.
	Electrolytes: Na 143, K 4, Cl 111, CO$_2$ 29, BUN 29, creatinine 0.9, glucose 157.
Assessment	Pulmonary: good oxygenation and ventilation. CV: hemodynamics stable.
Plan	Neuro: wean sedation, ID: continue antibiotics.

Critical Thinking Exercise 13

ASSESSMENT AND
DECISION MAKING

a. What ventilator setting changes are indicated? Cite your rationale.
b. What should be done when there is a discrepancy between the written physician's order and what is actually set on the ventilator?
c. What is the most likely rationale for performing a bronchoscopy on Mr. Burns at this time?

3/8 (day 13): The bronchoscopy was performed, revealing tracheal and mainstem bronchi scarring. Mode switched back to SIMV(PC).

3/10 (day 15): The following information is reviewed by the respiratory therapist: Burn resident physician notes:

CASE STUDY 1 *(continued)*

Subjective	Sedated.
Objective	Pulmonary: FIO_2 0.4, f 20, PEEP +12, PS 8, PC 25 (target VT 1000 mL) with ABG of pH 7.45, $PaCO_2$ 45 mm Hg, PaO_2 101 mm Hg. Temp. of 104.9°F.
	Cardiovascular: heart rate 115–127 beats/min; ventilatory rate 20–28 breaths/min, blood pressure 104/43–156/57 mm Hg. CVP 17–24 cm H_2O.
	Hematology: WBCs 16.4, Hb 9.2, Hct 28.3, PLT 255,000.
Assessment	CV: hemodynamics stable, tolerates tube feeding.
	On triple antibiotic therapy and amphotericin B for *Candida*.
Plan	Wean PEEP and rate, continue antibiotics.

Later that day: ventilator settings: FIO_2 0.4, f 20, PEEP +10, PS 8, PC 23 (target VT 1000 mL). The respiratory therapist reports VT of 300–700 mL with PS. Spontaneous ventilatory rate of 10–18 breaths/min. Total ventilatory rate of 29–45 breaths/min. Thick yellow secretions are noted. There is significant wheezing upon auscultation.

 Critical Thinking Exercise 14

ASSESSMENT AND DECISION MAKING

a. What therapy is indicated?

b. How does the therapist know to make this recommendation?

c. How important is antibiotic therapy for burn patients? Why?

After consultation with Mr. Burns' physician, an order for 3 puffs albuterol Q4 hr via MDI was obtained by the respiratory therapist.

3/12 (day 17): Burn resident physician notes:

Subjective	Sedated.
Objective	Cardiovascular: heart rate 110–141, blood pressure 102/40–151/42 mm Hg. CVP 12–18 cm H_2O.
	Hematology: T_{max} 104.8°F. WBCs 11.8, Hb 9.3, Hct 27.8, PLT 287,000. Electrolytes: BUN 90, creatinine 1.0.
	Wound cultures growing gram-negative rods, pseudomonas, and staph.
Assessment	CV: hemodynamics stable Renal: BUN increased probably due to amphotericin B.
Plan	Continue current therapy. Bronchoscopy today.

While administering the bronchodilator treatments, the respiratory therapist reports frequent, moderate amounts of thick, yellow, blood-tinged secretions while suctioning, necessitating bagging and normal saline lavage. SpO_2 decreased to 89% during bagging and suctioning. Mr. Burns continues to run a high-grade fever and produce large amounts of thick, yellow, blood-tinged secretions in spite of aggressive therapy with vancomycin. The physician asks the therapist to assist with therapeutic bronchoscopy later that afternoon.

3/16 (day 21, four days later): ABGs at 0230 hr on ventilator settings of FIO_2 0.4, f 6, PEEP +5, PS 8, PC 25 (target VT 1000 mL).

CASE STUDY 1 (*continued*)

ABG 40% SIMV (PC) + PS	
pH	7.40
P_{CO_2}	55
P_{O_2}	72
HCO_3^-	34
BE	+7
Sa_{O_2}	93.8%

PEEP was increased to +10 cm H_2O. Subsequent Pa_{O_2} was 174 mm Hg, then over the next couple of hours it went down to 75 mm Hg. Respiratory therapist reports suctioning clear-yellow thin secretions. Continue albuterol treatments. Burn resident physician note:

Subjective	Up in chair for 4 hr yesterday.
Objective	Pulmonary as above. CV: heart rate 116–141 beats/min, blood pressure 113/44–180/83 mm Hg.
	Hematology: T_{max} 102.7°F, WBCs 17.4.
Assessment	Pulmonary: working towards extubation, CV stable, tolerating tube feedings.
Plan	ID: continue antibiotics, wean SIMV f.

3/17 (day 22): The respiratory therapist charts the following information in the medical record: Ventilator settings: F_{IO_2} 0.4, f 2, PEEP +10, PS 8, PC 25 (target V_T 1000 mL). Spontaneous ventilatory rate is 37 breaths/min. PS V_T is 450–550 mL. Suctioning clear-yellow thin secretions, continuing albuterol. Cuff pressure reported to be 40–60 cm H_2O. Burn resident physician note:

Subjective	Waking up.
Objective	Pulmonary as above. CV: heart rate 112–144 beats/min, blood pressure 128/40–154/53 mm Hg.
	Temp. spiked to104.4°F. WBCs 23, BUN 64, creatinine 1.2.

Assessment	CV stable. Nutrition: prealbumin up to 21.
Plan	Pulmonary: will continue weaning. Begin tobramycin and ceftazidime for pneumonia.

Group Critical Thinking Exercise 3

PRO/CON DEBATE: IS IT TIME TO TRACH MR. BURNS?

Your instructor will assign two groups to research and prepare arguments for and against having a tracheostomy performed on Mr. Burns at this point in his ventilatory management. Be sure to cite as many reasons as possible to support your side of the argument. This debate may be performed in front of the class, with other students rating the effectiveness of arguments on each side of the issue.

3/18 (day 23): The next morning, the Sp_{O_2} is 93%–95%, with decreased spontaneous rate. During the night shift the ventilator rate was increased to 20 breaths/min and the PEEP was increased to +14 cm H_2O. The night shift staff report these changes were made by the on-call physician because the patient "appeared to be in distress." Thereafter, the patient's spontaneous ventilatory rate was 0–9 breaths/min. The respiratory therapist reports crackles on auscultation, albuterol continued Q4 hr, suctioning yielded a small amount of thick yellow-white secretions. Acetylcysteine lavage with albuterol treatments are begun.

Critical Thinking Exercise 15

PROBLEM SOLVING AND DECISION MAKING

Analyze the recent ventilator adjustments and then answer the following question.

a. Is this the optimal method of liberating the patient from the ventilator? How is this determined?

CASE STUDY 1 *(continued)*

Burn resident physician notes:

Subjective   Waking up.

Objective   Pulmonary: night on-call physician increased ventilatory support, patient had apparent respiratory distress episode; chest radiograph shows right lower lobe infiltrate.

CV: heart rate 120–130, blood pressure 111/48–154/54 mm Hg.

Hematology: T_{max} 104.4°F, WBCs 21.7. Electrolytes: Na 149, K 3.8, Cl 111, CO_2 31; BUN 68, creatinine 1.4.

Assessment   Pneumonia, cultures pending with tobramycin and ceftazidime. CV stable. Tolerating tube feedings.

Plan   Renal: BUN and creatinine rising slowly, Na down, continue hydration.

3/19 (day 24): The ventilator rate is decreased to 6 breaths/min. Ventilator settings are now: FIO_2 0.4, f 6, PEEP +14, PS 8, PC 25 (target V_T 1000 mL). Subsequent ABGs are:

ABG 40% SIMV (PC) + PS	
pH	7.36
PCO_2	54
PO_2	118
HCO_3^-	30.7
BE	+3.5
SaO_2	98.3%

The respiratory therapist reports PS V_T between 680 and 880 mL, PIPs in the 30s, and Cs 50 cc/cm H_2O. A few crackles are heard on auscultation, suctioning yields a small amount of white/yellow secretions. Acetylcysteine lavage and CPT following albuterol treatments.

Subjective   Arousable at times, otherwise sedated and quiet most of time.

Objective   VS: temperature 104.6°F, heart rate 114–136, blood pressure 112/48–147/54 mm Hg. Lab: WBCs 17.8, BUN 90, creatinine 1.9.

Assessment/ Plan
1. Pulmonary: pneumonia, continue tobramycin and ceftazidime.
2. CV stable.
3. Renal: BUN and creatinine increased, 2 more days of amphotericin B.

 Critical Thinking Exercise 16

ANTICIPATING PROBLEMS AND SOLUTIONS

a. What data are presented that would predict success at weaning the patient from the ventilator at this time?

b. What data are presented here that may predict failure to be weaned at this time?

c. What approach to weaning would you advocate at this time (if any)?

3/23 (day 28): Mr. Burns is successfully weaned off the ventilator over the last few days. Weaning continued with a CPAP trial at 0630 hr: FIO_2 0.28, CPAP +5 cm H_2O. Spontaneous rate is 25 breaths/min. Maximum inspiratory pressure is −50 cm H_2O and V_T is 712 mL. Minute ventilation is 17.8 L/min. Suctioning yields small to large amounts of yellow secretions. Chest radiograph #3: Right lower lobe and small left lower lobe infiltrates. Endotracheal tube and CVP catheter in place (see Fig. 20-4). The patient is extubated to 40% aerosol face mask at 0720 hr. Albuterol, acetylcysteine, and CPT are continued Q4 hr.

CASE STUDY 1 *(continued)*

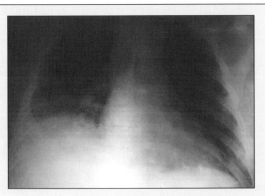

FIGURE 20-4   Mr. Burns chest radiograph #3, showing right lower lobe and small left lower lobe infiltrates, and endotracheal tube and CVP catheter in place.

3/24-3/30 (days 29-35): Mr. Burns remained off the ventilator for the next 3 days. He was receiving oxygen via nasal cannula with a stable ventilatory status and arterial saturations in the 90s. He continued to receive albuterol, acetylcysteine and CPT Q4 hr. However, at 1530 hr on the third day postextubation, Mr. Burns went into respiratory arrest, presumably due to mucus plugging. The patient was reintubated with a 7.0 mm ETT and ventilated for 3 more days. Therapy included albuterol, acetylcysteine lavage, and CPT Q4 hr. The patient was successfully extubated on 3/30. Aerosol albuterol was continued, and the patient was transferred to the floor. He remains in rehabilitation for his extensive burns.

KEY POINTS

- Annually, 60,000 to 80,000 persons are hospitalized for burn injuries. Of those, 4300 persons die (6.5%). The death rate of males from fire is twice that of females.

- Due to fire prevention efforts, the mortality rate is steadily decreasing.

- Initial management of the burn victim includes assuring an airway, ventilation, circulation, and spinal immobilization.

- All victims receive 100% oxygen to eliminate carboxyhemoglobin in the blood.

- Signs of impending airway edema indicating the need for intubation include singed nasal hairs and carbonaceous sputum.

- Due to fluid shifting from the vasculature to the interstitial space, hypotension occurs, necessitating massive fluid infusion.

- Massive fluid infusion often leads to pulmonary edema. Inhalation of noxious gases may cause

acute respiratory distress syndrome. Regardless of the cause, in the event of respiratory failure, the victim will require mechanical ventilation.

- Oxygenation is initially managed by a high FIO_2. Positive end-expiratory pressure is then increased until the FIO_2 can be decreased to ≤0.5.

- Ventilation may be managed in a volume-controlled mode until plateau pressure exceeds 35 cm H_2O, at which time a pressure-controlled mode is used to achieve a tidal volume of 6 to 8 mL/kg ideal body weight. This may necessitate sedation and paralysis.

- A low tidal volume may result in permissive hypercapnia, as long as the pH does not drop below 7.20. If it does, alveolar ventilation may be increased by increasing the ventilatory rate.

- Mucous plugging is a significant factor that is managed with adequate hydration and tracheobronchial hygiene (suctioning, aerosol therapy, and chest physiotherapy).

- Nosocomial pneumonia is a significant hazard, avoided by strict adherence to infection control protocol and changing ventilator circuits no more often than every 48 hours.

- Weaning is accomplished by allowing the patient to wake up and begin triggering the ventilator.
- Pressure support will be necessary to accomplish tidal volumes of 5 mL/kg. The mode may be changed to volume control SIMV as tolerated, followed by pressure support with PEEP.
- Prolonged mechanical ventilation may necessitate tracheostomy. However, the tracheostomy is a port of infection.
- Burn victims are best cared for by a burn team.
- Burn therapy is very expensive.

SUGGESTED RESOURCES

Internet resources: Over 300,000 sites were located by searching Netscape under "burn injury." Sites included specific burn centers, statistics, help groups, lawyers, prevention organizations, and medical information.
Integra web site: www.integra-ls.com/bus-skin_product.shmtl
Branson RD, Hess DR, Chatburn RL. *Respiratory Care Equipment*. 2nd ed. Philadelphia: Lippincott;1999.
White GC. *Basic Clinical Lab Competencies for Respiratory Care*. 3rd ed. Albany, NY: Delmar;1998.
Pilbeam SP. *Mechanical Ventilation: Physiological and Clinical Application*. 3rd ed. St. Louis: Mosby;1998.

REFERENCES

1. Herndon DN, Muller MJ, Blakeney PE. Teamwork for total burn care. In: Herndon DN, ed. *Total Burn Care*. Philadelphia: Saunders; 1996:1.

2. Pruitt BA, Mason AD. Epidemiological, demographic and outcome characteristics of burn injury. In: Herndon DN, ed. *Total Burn Care*. Philadelphia: Saunders; 1996:5–15.

3. Fingerhut LA, Warner M. Injury chartbook. Health, United States, 1996-97. Hyattsville, Md: National Center for Health Statistics, 1997.

4. Mlcak RP, Dimick AR, Mlcak G. Pre-hospital management, transportation and emergency care. In: Herndon DN, ed. *Total Burn Care*. Philadelphia: Saunders; 1996:33–43.

5. Kramer GC, Nguyen TT. Pathophysiology of burn shock and burn edema. In: Herndon DN, ed. *Total Burn Care*. Philadelphia: Saunders; 1996:44–52.

6. Warden GD. Fluid resuscitation and early management. In: Herndon DN, ed. *Total Burn Care*. Philadelphia: Saunders; 1996:53–60.

7. Traber DL, Pollard V. Pathophysiology of inhalation injury. In: Herndon DN, ed. *Total Burn Care*. Philadelphia: Saunders; 1996:175–183.

8. Dhand R, Tobin MJ. Inhaled bronchodilator therapy in mechanically ventilated patients. *Am J Resp Crit Care Med*. 1997;156:3–10.

9. The Acute Respiratory Distress Syndrome Network. Ventilation with lower tidal volumes as compared with traditional tidal volumes for acute lung injury and the acute respiratory distress syndrome. *N Engl J Med*. 2000;342:1301–1308.

10. Hirvela ER. Advances in the management of acute respiratory distress syndrome: Protective ventilation. *Arch Surg*. 2000;135:126–135.

NEUROMUSCULAR DISORDERS

Robert Wayne Lawson

The important thing is not to stop questioning.
Curiosity has its own reason for existing.
One cannot help but be in awe
when he contemplates the mysteries of eternity,
of life, of the marvelous structure of reality.
It is enough if one tries merely to comprehend
a little of this mystery every day.
Never lose a holy curiosity.

ALBERT EINSTEIN
(1875–1955)

LEARNING OBJECTIVES

1. Describe the pulmonary function findings associated with neuromuscular disorders.
2. Describe the primary pathophysiological finding in neuromuscular disease and the arterial blood gas pattern associated with it.
3. Identify four pulmonary complications associated with neuromuscular disease and explain the clinical implications of each.
4. List the four anatomic sites that are abnormally affected in patients with neuromuscular disease.
5. Explain the interaction of the respiratory centers, receptors, motor neurons, and ventilatory musculature in the maintenance of normal ventilation.
6. Describe the monitoring of a patient with a progressing neuromuscular disorder and develop a respiratory care plan based on specific patient data.
7. Discuss the etiology, pathophysiology, clinical features, and management of a patient with Duchenne's dystrophy.

8. Explain the three pathophysiological mechanisms responsible for disorders of the neuromuscular junction.
9. Discuss the etiology, pathophysiology, clinical features, diagnosis, and management of the patient with myasthenia gravis.
10. Describe one feature that distinguishes Lambert-Eaton myasthenic syndrome from myasthenia gravis.
11. Explain the pathophysiology of botulism poisoning and tetanus and apply this information to patient care management.
12. Discuss the etiology, pathophysiology, clinical features, diagnosis, and management of the patient with Guillain-Barré syndrome.
13. Describe the clinical features and management of the patient with postpolio syndrome and apply this information to patient care management.
14. Explain the etiology, pathophysiology, clinical features, and management of a patient with amyotrophic lateral sclerosis.

15. Discuss the management of a patient with a spinal cord injury above the level of C6, above the level of C5, above the level of C4, and above the level of C3.
16. Describe the evaluation of a patient admitted to the emergency room with a diagnosis of heroin overdose.
17. Apply the critical thinking skills of prioritizing, anticipating, negotiating, communicating, decision making, and reflection by completing exercises and case examples with neuromuscular disease.
18. Describe the role of the respiratory therapist in the diagnosis, treatment, and management of the patient with neuromuscular disease.
19. Use clinical case examples in this chapter to perform an initial patient assessment, using a standardized system (SOAP notes and IPPA) and the clinical data presented.
20. Interpret clinical data from the case examples, including history, physical examination, lab data, and radiographic data to make recommendations for respiratory care management.
21. Develop a care plan for patients in each case, including recommendations for therapy and disease management, with consideration of cost, ethical, and quality-of-life issues.
22. Communicate facts, evidence, and arguments to support evaluations and recommendations proposed in the care plan for patients with neuromuscular disease.
23. Practice the skill of negotiating in an attempt to gain acceptance of your proposed care plan for each patient case with neuromuscular disease.
24. Evaluate treatment and outcomes of interventions to propose changes in the care plan.
25. Apply strategies to promote critical thinking in the respiratory care management of patients with neuromuscular disease through completion of chapter exercises and group discussion.

KEY WORDS

Acetylcholine
Acute Anterior
   Poliomyelitis
Acute Inflammatory
   Demyelinating
   Polyneuropathy
Acute Respiratory
   Failure
Amyotrophic Lateral
   Sclerosis
Aortic Body
   Chemoreceptors
Apneustic Center
Aspiration
Atelectasis
Axon Terminal
Becker's Dystrophy

Bronchopulmonary
   Stretch Receptors
Carotid Body
   Chemoreceptors
Central
   Chemoreceptor
C-Fiber Receptors
Cholinergic Crisis
Chronic Respiratory
   Failure
Clostridium botulinum
Clostridium tetani
Dorsal Respiratory
   Group
Duchenne's Dystrophy
Guillain-Barré
   Syndrome

Irritant Receptors
Juxtapulmonary
   Capillary Receptors
Lambert-Eaton
   Myasthenic Syndrome
Lower Airway Infection
Medullary Center
Motor End Plate
Motor Neurons
Muscle Spindles
Myasthenia Gravis
Myasthenic Crisis
Myotonic Dystrophy
Neuromuscular
Neuromuscular
   Junction
Opisthotonos
Paresthesia

Peripheral
   Chemoreceptors
Plasmapheresis
Pneumotaxic Center
Poliomyelitis
Polymyositis-
   Dermatomyositis
Postpolio Syndrome
Presynaptic Terminal
Secretion Retention
Spinal Cord Injury
Spinal Interneuron
Subneural Cleft
Synaptic Cleft
Synaptic Trough
Trismus
Ventral Respiratory
   Group

INTRODUCTION

Neuromuscular disease comprises a group of disorders in which the primary pathophysiological manifestation is ultimately failure of the ventilatory pump to adequately move air into the lungs. Because all neuromuscular disorders affecting ventilation inhibit inspiratory volume resulting in a reduced total lung capacity (TLC), they are by definition considered to be restrictive diseases, as demonstrated by pulmonary function testing. Most lung volumes and capacities are reduced as are maximal inspiratory and expiratory pressures as well as thoracic wall compliance. The primary clinical manifestation is hypoventilation, resulting in hypercapnia, hypoxemia, and acidosis. Long-term clinical manifestations vary with the disorder, but can include secretion accumulation, atelectasis, and lower airway infection. Neuromuscular disorders can be categorized into four basic groups according to which component of the ventilatory pump is affected: 1) disorders of the muscles, 2) disorders of the neuromuscular junction, 3) disorders of the peripheral motor nerves, and 4) disorders of the central nervous system, which includes the cerebrum or brain, and the spinal cord.

CRITICAL CONTENT

Categories of neuromuscular diseases affecting the ventilatory pump:

- Disorders of the muscles
- Disorders of the neuromuscular junction
- Disorders of the peripheral motor nerves
- Disorders of the central nervous system, including the brain and spinal cord

The respiratory system is composed of two primary elements, the gas exchange organs (the lungs), and the ventilatory pump, which drives the system. The ventilatory pump is a system of four integrated components: 1) the respiratory centers located in the brain, where the origin of rhythmic breathing is found, 2) receptors, that respond to chemical and physical stimulation, 3) motor neurons, that receive input from the respiratory centers and pass it to the ventilatory musculature, and 4) the ventilatory musculature, which provides the mechanical energy to move air into and out of the lungs (Fig. 21-1).

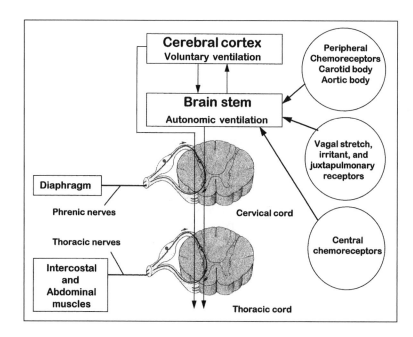

FIGURE 21-1 Origins of innervation of the ventilatory musculature that provides the mechanical energy to move air into and out of the lungs.

COMPONENTS OF THE VENTILATORY PUMP

• The respiratory centers, located in the brain
• Receptors, that respond to chemical and physical stimulation
• Motor neurons, that receive input from the respiratory centers and pass it to the ventilatory musculature
• The ventilatory muscles, which provide the mechanical energy to move air into and out of the lungs

NEUROMUSCULAR PHYSIOLOGY AND VENTILATION

Control of breathing is provided by the *medullary center* in the brain stem, which is thought to be the origin of rhythmic breathing. It is comprised of two groups of respiratory neurons, the *dorsal respiratory group* and the *ventral respiratory group*. Signals from the medullary center to the muscles of ventilation are modified by afferent impulses from a number of areas in the brain. The medullary chemoreceptors and two groups of respiratory neurons in the pontine area, the *apneustic center* and the *pneumotaxic center,* serve to further adjust medullary output. In certain situations, cortical input can override automatic control and provide voluntary control of breathing.

CENTRAL NERVOUS SYSTEM COMPONENTS FOR CONTROL OF BREATHING

• Medullary respiratory center
• Apneustic center
• Pneumotaxic center

The Receptors

Two groups of chemoreceptors provide input to the medullary center: the *central chemoreceptors* and the *peripheral chemoreceptors.* The central chemoreceptors are located ventrolaterally immediately beneath the floor of the fourth ventricle in the brain stem and are thus in close proximity to the cerebrospinal fluid (CSF). These receptors are sensitive to the hydrogen ion concentration [H^+] of the CSF, which is very closely related to the arterial carbon dioxide gas tension (Pa_{CO_2}). CO_2 diffuses from the blood into the CSF, causing a change in the CSF [H^+]. Because the CSF buffering capacity is much lower than that of blood, small changes in CSF P_{CO_2} result in significant changes in [H^+]. Increases in the Pa_{CO_2} produce increases in CSF [H^+], resulting in increased minute ventilation, while decreasing Pa_{CO_2} causes a decrease in minute volume. Input from these receptors is most closely associated with the moment-to-moment control of ventilation.

There are two groups of peripheral chemoreceptors: the *carotid body chemoreceptors,* located at the bifurcation of the common carotid artery into internal and external branches, and the *aortic body chemoreceptors,* located along the arch of the aorta. Afferent neurons from the carotid bodies are part of the carotid sinus nerve which joins with the glossopharyngeal nerve (IX; ninth cranial nerve), while afferent neurons from the aortic bodies join the vagus nerve (X; tenth cranial nerve). Both these nerves provide input to the medullary center. The peripheral chemoreceptors are stimulated by decreasing arterial oxygen gas tension (Pa_{O_2}), increasing Pa_{CO_2}, and increasing blood [H^+]. They serve as the primary response to hypoxemia, they respond to abrupt changes in Pa_{CO_2}, and as a primary response to increasing [H^+] associated with metabolic acidosis.

A number of mechanoreceptors are found in the chest wall and lungs. Chest wall mechanoreceptors monitor and respond to inspiratory effort. The most important of these, the *muscle spindles,* found in all skeletal muscle including the muscles of ventilation, provide an ongoing feedback loop to help maintain adequate tidal volumes against differing ventilatory loads.

Three types of vagally-mediated sensory receptors are found in the lungs: 1) the *irritant receptors,* 2) the *bronchopulmonary stretch receptors,* and 3) the *C-fiber receptors.* These three receptors provide input to the medullary center. Located in the epithelial lining of the bronchi are the irritant receptors, which respond to mechanical, chemical, and physiological stimuli, resulting in hyperpnea, bronchoconstriction, increased secretion production, coughing, and glottic closure. Bronchopulmonary stretch receptors, found primarily in the airway smooth muscle of the extrapulmonary airways (trachea and mainstem bronchi), respond to changes in lung volume and are thought to help modulate the depth of tidal volume in various circumstances, with the Hering-Breuer reflex limiting inspiratory volume, and Head's paradoxical reflex stimulating further inspiratory volume. Located in the interstitium at the alveolar level, juxtaposed to the pulmonary capillaries, are the *pulmonary C-fiber receptors,* termed the *juxtacapillary or J receptors,* while a second group, the *bronchial C-fiber receptors,* are located within the walls of bronchi.[1,2]

CRITICAL CONTENT

RECEPTORS INVOLVED IN THE CONTROL OF VENTILATION

- Chemoreceptors
- Central chemoreceptors
- Peripheral chemoreceptors
- Carotid body chemoreceptors
- Aortic body chemoreceptors
- Mechanoreceptors
- Muscle spindles
- Irritant receptors
- Bronchopulmonary stretch receptors
- Pulmonary C-fiber receptors
- Bronchial C-fiber receptors

These receptors respond to lung volume changes, mechanical deformation caused by increased interstitial volume, and to various chemical stimuli. Stimulation of these receptors causes rapid, shallow breathing, bronchoconstriction, and increased mucus secretion.[1,2]

Motor Neurons

Output from the respiratory control centers in the brain descend to the anterior horn cells of the spinal column. Axons for autonomic control of breathing descend from the medullary respiratory center along bulbospinal tracts, while axons for voluntary control of breathing descend from the cortex along corticospinal tracts, thus allowing for separation of autonomic and voluntary control of breathing. The anterior horn cells are comprised of the alpha and gamma motor neurons that innervate skeletal muscle, including the muscles of ventilation.

Alpha motor neurons innervate skeletal muscle fibers, and are responsible for initiating muscle contraction, while gamma motor neurons innervate the intrafusal muscle fibers of the muscle spindles. Muscle spindles are mechanoreceptors found within all skeletal muscle, and are responsible for adjusting muscle tension against differing loads. Each alpha motor neuron branches at its end point and comes into contact with anywhere from three to several hundred muscle fibers, depending on the muscle group, at a point termed the *neuromuscular junction,* also termed the *motor end plate* (Fig. 21-2).

The neuromuscular junction is composed of a nerve ending called a *presynaptic terminal,* the muscle fiber plasma membrane, which it overlies, and the space separating the two, called the *synaptic cleft.* The presynaptic terminals of motor neurons are the sites of production, storage, and release of the excitatory neurotransmitter substance *acetylcholine* (ACh). The invagination in the muscle fiber plasma membrane in which the presynaptic terminal sits is termed the *synaptic trough* (Fig. 21-2C). At the bottom of the trough, numerous small folds called *subneural clefts* are found on the muscle fiber plasma membrane. Numerous acetylcholine

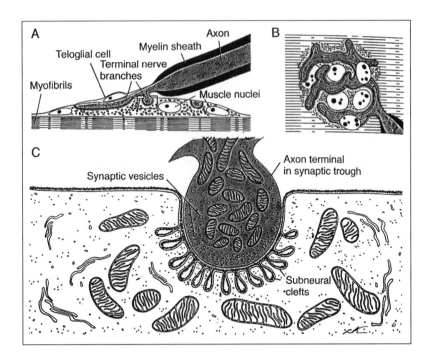

FIGURE 21-2
Schematic representations of the motor end plates as seen by light and electron microscopy. **A.** End plate as seen in histological sections in the long axis of the muscle fiber. **B.** As seen in surface view with the light microscope. **C.** As seen in an electron micrograph of an area such as that in the rectangle on A. (From Fawcett as modified from R. Couteaux: Bloom and Fawcett: A Textbook of Histology. Arnold Publishers; 1986.)

receptors (AChRs) are found on the subneural clefts. An action potential in the nerve causes the rapid influx of calcium into the presynaptic terminal, which in turn causes the release of ACh from vesicles stored in the terminal. ACh moves rapidly across the synaptic cleft, binding to AChRs, causing depolarization and subsequent contraction of the muscle fiber. Within a few milliseconds of its release, the ACh is then hydrolyzed by the enzyme *acetylcholinesterase*, allowing the muscle to relax.

CRITICAL CONTENT

The neuromuscular junction (motor end plate)—"where the action is":

1. Alpha motor neurons innervate skeletal muscle, ending in the motor end plate.
2. Acetylcholine (ACh) is released at the motor end plate, resulting in muscle contraction.
3. ACh is hydrolyzed by acetylcholinesterase, causing the muscle to relax.

Ventilatory Musculature

The muscles of ventilation include the *diaphragm,* the *external and internal intercostals,* the muscles of the *anterior abdominal wall* and the *accessory muscles* of ventilation (Fig. 21-3). The primary muscle of inspiration is the diaphragm, accounting for the majority of work done during quiet breathing. The diaphragm is innervated bilaterally by the phrenic nerves, which have their origin in cervical nerves C3, C4, and C5. As inspiratory work increases, the other primary muscles of inspiration, the external intercostals, innervated by intercostal nerves arising from thoracic nerves T1 through T12, become active. As inspiratory work increases still further, the accessory muscles of inspiration become active. These include the sternocleidomastoids, innervated by the spinal branch of the accessory nerve (XI), and the scalenes, innervated by branches of cervical nerves C4 through C8. The muscles of exhalation include two groups, the first of which are the internal intercostals, innervated by intercostal nerves arising from thoracic nerves T1 through T12. The second group, those of the ante-

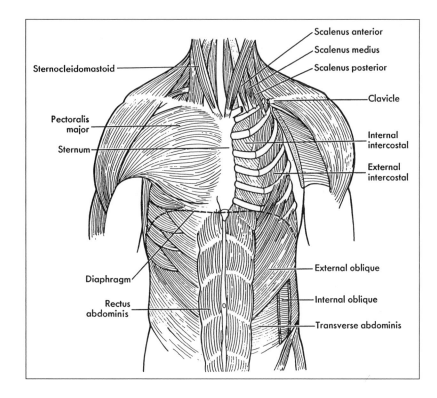

- Sternocleidomastoid
- Pectoralis major
- Sternum
- Diaphragm
- Rectus abdominis
- Scalenus anterior
- Scalenus medius
- Scalenus posterior
- Clavicle
- Internal intercostal
- External intercostal
- External oblique
- Internal oblique
- Transverse abdominis

FIGURE 21-3
The muscles of ventilation.

rior abdominal wall, include the rectus abdominis, the external and internal obliques, and the transverse abdominis, innervated by branches of thoracic and lumbar nerves T7 through L1.

CRITICAL CONTENT

MUSCLES OF VENTILATION AND THEIR INNERVATION

- Diaphragm: phrenic nerves
- External intercostals: intercostal nerves
- Internal intercostals: intercostal nerves
- Muscles of the anterior abdominal wall:
  External oblique: thoracic and lumbar nerves
  Internal oblique: thoracic and lumbar nerves
  Transverse abdominis: thoracic and lumbar nerves
  Rectus abdominis: thoracic and lumbar nerves

DISORDERS OF THE MUSCLES

A disorder of the muscle not related to a change in the innervation of the muscle is termed a *myopathy,* and is characterized by progressive weakness, many times leading to respiratory failure. The term *dystrophy* refers to the destruction and regeneration of muscle fibers, and the eventual replacement of the muscle fibers by fibrous and fatty connective tissue.

Muscular Dystrophy (Duchenne's and Becker's Dystrophies)

The most frequently encountered muscular dystrophy (MD) is *Duchenne's dystrophy.* It is an inherited X-linked recessive trait primarily affecting males, and is seen in roughly 1 in 3300 male births.[3] Discovered in the late 1980s, a mutation in the dystrophin gene and its protein product dystrophin, leading to a deficiency in that protein, form the pathogenetic basis for muscular dystrophy. Duchenne's dystrophy and Becker's dystrophy are the two most common forms of the disease.[4,5] Usually beginning early in life, these dystrophies are characterized by painless weakness, most prominently in the pelvic girdle and thighs, less prominently in the shoulders, and least often in the distal extremities.

Duchenne's dystrophy usually becomes apparent when the child first begins to walk, and by adolescence the patient is usually confined to a wheelchair. Inevitable involvement of the muscles of ventilation leads to progressive hypoxemia, followed by hypercapnia. Common complications include scoliosis secondary to wasting of the spinal support muscles, and recurrent lower airway infections secondary to loss of an adequate cough reflex. Until respiratory care procedures became commonplace, patients seldom lived to reach 20 years of age. Patients usually succumbed to pneumonia and other complications associated with chronic ventilatory failure. However, with the advent of mechanical ventilatory support techniques, both invasive and noninvasive, coupled with aggressive bronchial hygiene procedures, antibiotic therapy, and techniques to prevent or slow the progress of scoliosis, patients are now living well into their third decade of life.

Becker's dystrophy is another type of X-linked muscular dystrophy, with an incidence of 1 in 20,000 male births,[3] but this form of MD has a later onset and a slower and more variable course. Patients frequently live into their sixth decade of life. Becker's dystrophy is now recognized as a milder variant of Duchenne's dystrophy. *Myotonic dystrophy* is another, more rare disorder characterized by muscular weakness accompanied by difficulty in relaxing contracted muscles. Ultimately, management of these disorders mirrors that of Duchenne's dystrophy.

Polymyositis-Dermatomyositis

Polymyositis-dermatomyositis is a rare disease of the muscles, falling into the broad category of idio-

CRITICAL CONTENT

CHARACTERISTICS OF DUCHENNE'S AND BECKER'S DYSTROPHIES

- Painless weakness, most prominently in the pelvic girdle and thighs, and less prominently in the shoulders
- Inevitable involvement of the muscles of ventilation leads to progressive hypoxemia followed by hypercapnia
- Becker's is a milder variant with slower onset and variable progression

pathic inflammatory myopathies. Its etiology is undetermined, but it is suspected to be autoimmune in nature. It has also been associated with several viral infections including hepatitis C.[6] Polymyositis-dermatomyositis usually manifests itself either in the first or the fifth to sixth decades of life, and is twice as common in females as in males. It is characterized by symmetrical weakness and atrophy of proximal muscle groups, including those of the neck and pharynx, accompanied by a variety of dermatologic symptoms. The prognosis is variable from complete recovery to chronic and progressive symptoms lasting for years. One study demonstrated pulmonary involvement in 40% of patients studied.[7]

Complications include respiratory failure secondary to ventilatory muscle weakness, as well as pulmonary parenchymal abnormalities, including interstitial pneumonitis and aspiration pneumonia. In the majority of cases with pulmonary involvement, the disease is progressive, ultimately leading to pulmonary fibrosis and cor pulmonale. Standard treatment includes immunosuppressive therapy, including corticosteroids. In patients resistant to conventional therapy, intravenous immunoglobulin (IVIG) has been shown to be effective.[8,9] Pulmonary complications are treated with bronchial hygiene procedures and mechanical ventilatory support as indicated.

CRITICAL CONTENT

CHARACTERISTICS OF POLYMYOSITIS-DERMATOMYOSITIS

- Symmetrical weakness
- Atrophy of proximal muscle groups: neck and pharynx
- A variety of dermatologic symptoms
- Pulmonary involvement can include fibrosis

CRITICAL CONTENT

CHARACTERISTICS OF MYASTHENIA GRAVIS

- It is an acquired antigen-specific autoimmune disease.
- Weakness and fatigability occurs that is exacerbated with repetitive effort.
- It is caused by circulating antibodies that damage the ACh receptors that lie within the muscle fiber plasma membrane.

DISORDERS OF THE NEUROMUSCULAR JUNCTION

Disorders of the neuromuscular junction are caused by three basic pathophysiological mechanisms: 1) impaired postsynaptic membrane receptor mechanisms, 2) a deficiency in neurotransmitter synthesis and/or release, and 3) depolarizing or nondepolarizing blockade of ACh binding sites by drugs or toxins.

Myasthenia Gravis

Myasthenia gravis (MG) is an acquired antigen-specific autoimmune disease.[10] MG is characterized by weakness and fatigability that is exacerbated with repetitive effort. The thymus is thought to be the primary site of autosensitization.[11] MG is associated with pathologic alterations of the thymus in roughly 80% of cases—65% of patients with hyperplasia of the thymus and 15% with thymoma.[3,12] Clinical classification of patients with MG is based on the distribution and severity of symptoms. It has an annual incidence of 2 to 5 per 1,000,000 persons, and affects both sexes with a male:female ratio of 3:2.[3] While it may occur at any age, it has peak incidence in women in the third decade of life, and in men in the sixth decade of life. MG is caused by circulating antibodies that damage the ACh receptors that lie within the muscle fiber plasma membrane. This results in both a qualitative and quantitative deficiency in their function.

Diagnosis is made on the basis of clinical history, the presence of circulating AChR antibodies, electromyographic findings, and the results of anticholinesterase testing. Clinically, cranial nerve involvement is seen early on, with 40% of patients experiencing diplopia and ptosis secondary to extraocular muscle weakness as their only symptoms.[3] Further progression of MG can involve the facial muscles, causing loss of facial expression, as well as glossopharyngeal, hypopharyngeal, and laryngeal muscle weakness, leading to dysphagia and dysphonia. The muscles of the extremities are usually the next muscle groups to become involved, and finally the ventilatory musculature degenerates, leading to acute respiratory failure. In 40% of cases initial weakness may also be generalized.[3]

Symptoms are exacerbated with exercise and improve with rest, and may vary from hour to hour or from day to day. Circulating ACh receptor antibodies are found in 80% to 90% of patients with MG. Electromyography demonstrates a characteristic degradation of amplitude of the evoked muscle action potential. Diagnosis is made by testing with the quick-response, short-acting anticholinesterase drug, edrophonium chloride. A total of 2 to 10 mg are injected intravenously and the patient is observed for signs of returning strength. A response is usually seen within 30 seconds, lasts for several minutes, and is considered diagnostic for MG.[3]

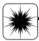

CRITICAL CONTENT

DIAGNOSIS OF MYASTHENIA GRAVIS

- Clinical history
- The presence of circulating ACh receptor antibodies
- Electromyographic findings
- Results of anticholinesterase testing

Primary treatment of the patient with MG includes anticholinesterases, corticosteroids, azathioprine, plasmapheresis, and thymectomy. Anticholinesterase therapy helps to restore muscle strength, while alternate-day corticosteroid therapy suppresses ACh antibody production. Azathioprine, an immunosuppressive drug used to prevent transplant rejection, is also effective at reducing symptoms and inducing remission. However, azathioprine requires careful monitoring during treatment because of potential bone marrow and liver toxicity.

Myasthenic crisis refers to an acute episode of muscular weakness brought on by circulating antibodies that attack ACh receptors. Symptoms of myasthenic crisis include weakness and fatigue that is exacerbated with repetitive effort. *Cholinergic crisis* refers to acute muscular weakness caused by excessive ACh secondary to overmedication with an antiacetylcholinesterase drug. Symptoms of cholinergic crisis include progressive weakness, as well as muscarinic effects. These muscarinic effects include bradycardia, diaphoresis, excessive lacrimation, increased bronchial secretions, miosis, abdominal cramps, nausea, vomiting, and diarrhea.

Plasmapheresis lowers ACh antibody titers, resulting in measurable improvement, but is very expensive and does not offer greater long-term protection than immunosuppressive drugs. For patients with generalized disease not responding to the above therapies, thymectomy increases remission and reduces symptomatology over time. Treatment of pulmonary symptoms includes assisted ventilation, hyperinflation techniques, and bronchial hygiene procedures as indicated.

CRITICAL CONTENT

TREATMENT OF MYASTHENIA GRAVIS

- Anticholinesterase therapy
- Corticosteroids
- Azathioprine
- Plasmapheresis
- Thymectomy
- Respiratory care as needed

Lambert-Eaton Myasthenic Syndrome

Lambert-Eaton myasthenic syndrome (LEMS) is an acquired autoimmune disorder in which circulating autoantibodies cause a deficiency in voltage-sensitive calcium channels on the axon terminal plasma membranes. Calcium ingress during nerve depolarization is necessary for ACh release. The deficiency in calcium channels results in a smaller-than-normal number of ACh vesicles being released, which causes a weak response by the muscle. A characteristic of this disorder is that with repeated stimulation, ACh builds up in the synaptic cleft, thus briefly increasing evoked potentials to a more normal amplitude. In other words, repeated stimulation of the muscle causes it to briefly grow stronger rather than weaker as in MG. This finding is diagnostic of the disorder. LEMS is strongly associated with small-cell carcinoma of the lung.[13]

CRITICAL CONTENT

CHARACTERISTICS OF LAMBERT-EATON MYASTHENIC SYNDROME

- Acquired autoimmune disorder
- Repeated stimulation of the muscle causes it to briefly grow stronger rather than weaker, and this is diagnostic of the disorder
- Strongly associated with small-cell carcinoma of the lung

Patients have weakness and fatigability of proximal limb and torso muscles and dry mouth; men have impotence with minimal involvement of the cranial nerve musculature.

Treatment includes therapies aimed at the malignancy (if present), along with corticosteroid therapy for non-neoplastic cases. Treatment of pulmonary symptomatology (if present) includes bronchial hygiene procedures, hyperinflation techniques, and assisted ventilation as indicated.

Botulism

Botulism is a neuroparalytic disorder caused by a neurotoxin produced by the anaerobic gram-positive spore-forming bacterium *Clostridium botulinum.* The organism is found throughout the environment, including in soil, water, and agricultural products. Botulism is characterized by a symmetric, descending, flaccid paralysis of motor and autonomic nerves, usually beginning with the cranial nerves. While there are eight antigenically-distinct botulinal toxins, only three commonly produce disease in humans. The toxin produced by *C botulinum* is one of the most potent microbial protein neurotoxins known, with an estimated lethal dose of 10^{-9} mg/kg body weight.

While the most common route of transmission is ingestion of the toxin in contaminated, improperly canned food, wound infection is also documented as a source. Since 1994, there has been a dramatic rise in botulism poisoning associated with black tar heroin use.[14] Recently, the potential use of botulinum toxin by terrorists has become a worldwide concern.[15]

Once introduced into the body, the toxin spreads hematogenously to cholinergic neuromuscular junctions throughout the body where it binds to axon terminals, thus inhibiting the release of ACh. Clinical symptoms usually begin within 12 to 24 hours of ingestion, with gastrointestinal symptoms including nausea, vomiting, and abdominal pain. Cranial nerve musculature is affected first, causing diplopia, dysarthria, dysphagia, and dysphonia. Cholinergic autonomic involvement causes dry mouth and sore throat. The descending paralysis spreads to motor neurons of the peripheral musculature, including those that supply the muscles of ventilation.

Diagnosis of botulism poisoning is made on the basis of history, symptomatology, speed of onset and progression, electromyographic testing, and the presence of a normal CSF protein level. Treatment includes administration of a trivalent equine antitoxin obtained from the Centers for Disease Control and Prevention (CDC) through an emergency distribution system, elimination of residual toxin from the gastrointestinal tract, and mechanical ventilatory support as indicated and general supportive measures. The prognosis for this disorder if treated promptly is full recovery. While outbreaks of botulism poisoning are rare, when they do occur, they constitute a public health emergency requiring rapid recognition, both for treatment of affected patients, and for prevention of additional cases.

CRITICAL CONTENT

CHARACTERISTICS OF BOTULISM POISONING

- Caused by a neurotoxin produced by the bacterium *Clostridium botulinum*
- Causes a symmetric, descending, flaccid paralysis of motor and autonomic nerves
- Diagnosed by history, symptoms, electromyographic testing, and a normal CSF protein level
- Treated with antitoxin and mechanical ventilatory and general supportive measures

Tetanus

Tetanus is a neurologic syndrome caused by a neurotoxin produced by the anaerobic gram-positive spore-forming bacterium *Clostridium tetani.* The organism is found in soil, the stool of many animals, and house dust. When accidentally introduced into a wound, the spores germinate into the vegetative form. The bacterium then multiplies, releasing the toxin tetanospasmin, which parallels botulism toxin in its potency. The toxin binds to axon terminals of spinal inhibitory interneurons, preventing the release of the inhibitory neurotransmitter substances glycine and γ-aminobutyric acid. This loss of inhibitory influence on motor neurons results in their unchecked firing with sustained muscular contraction, producing the classic tonic muscle contractions associated with tetanus. While rare in the population as a cause of disease, the mortality rate among victims remains high. The elderly are particularly susceptible to its effects and complications.[16]

The most common clinical picture of tetanus is the generalized form of the disease. After an incubation period varying up to 14 days, trismus appears as the most common presenting symptom. Opisthotonos and respiratory and extremity muscle spasm are common. Spasms and even convulsions occur spontaneously and with auditory and tactile stimuli. Autonomic problems are also common. Diagnosis is made largely on the basis of the clinical picture.

Treatment includes initial stabilization of the patient, wound debridement if possible, antibiotic therapy, administration of human tetanus immune globulin, and muscle relaxants. Supportive care includes maintenance of a protected, patent airway, mechanical ventilation if acute respiratory failure ensues, and general supportive measures. With appropriate care, full recovery usually occurs within 3 to 6 weeks.

Effective vaccines against tetanus have been available since the 1940s and confer a very high level of immunity in the vast majority of vaccinees. Of the 124 cases of tetanus infection reported in the period from 1995 to 1997, only 13% of those patients reported having received a primary series of tetanus toxoid before disease onset.[17] The Immunization Practices Advisory Committee of the United States Public Health Service recommends active immunization of infants and children with diphtheria and tetanus toxoids and pertussis adsorbed (DPT) at 2 months, 4 months, 6 months, 15 months, and 4 to 6 years, and after that every 10

years.[3,17,18] Repeated active immunization is necessary because the antibody titers decrease over time. All patient contacts with the health care system should be used to review and update vaccination status as necessary.[17]

CRITICAL CONTENT

CHARACTERISTICS OF TETANUS

- Caused by a neurotoxin produced by the bacterium Clostridium tetani
- Characterized by severe sustained muscle spasms
- Treated with stabilization, wound debridement, antibiotic therapy, human tetanus immune globulin, muscle relaxants, and airway and respiratory care as needed
- Repeated active immunization is necessary

DISORDERS OF THE PERIPHERAL MOTOR NERVES

Diseases of the peripheral motor nerves affect one or more of the three basic components of a peripheral motor neuron: 1) the neuron cell body, 2) the axon, and 3) the Schwann cell or its product, the myelin sheath.

Guillain-Barré Syndrome

Guillain-Barré syndrome (GBS), also called acute inflammatory demyelinating polyneuropathy, is a disorder characterized by acute, ascending symmetrical flaccid paralysis of voluntary musculature, including those supplied by the cranial nerves and those controlling ventilation, with associated loss of deep tendon reflexes and increased CSF protein. While the neurological deficits are primarily motor, sensory and autonomic deficits are frequently seen as well. It is an immune-mediated disorder that is preceded by an infectious disorder several weeks prior to the onset of neurologic symptoms in roughly 60% of cases.[3] It is now known that infection with the bacterium *Campylobacter jejuni* is responsible for up to 40% of GBS cases, and is often associated with a more severe form of the disease with prolonged disability.[19,20]

GBS is caused by lymphocytic infiltration of spinal roots and peripheral nerves accompanied by macrophage-mediated demyelination of those nerves, and in severe cases, some axonal degeneration. With an annual incidence of roughly 3/100,000 in the population, GBS is the most common cause of flaccid paralysis in the world.[3,21–23] According to a national hospital discharge database compiled by the Commission on Professional and Hospital Activities, in the US the age-specific incidence increases with age from 1.5/100,000 in persons <15 years old to 8.6/100,000 in persons 70 to 79 years old.[23] While GBS has no ethnic preference, there are conflicting data in the literature with regard to seasonal and gender preference.

CRITICAL CONTENT

CHARACTERISTICS OF GUILLAIN-BARRÉ SYNDROME

- Immune-mediated, preceded by infectious disorder in 60% of cases
- Infection with *Campylobacter jejuni* responsible for up to 40% of cases
- Causes acute ascending symmetrical flaccid paralysis of voluntary musculature
- The most common cause of flaccid paralysis in the world
- Abnormally high CSF protein concentration

With respect to clinical manifestations, paresthesia of the feet is a common initial symptom. Within hours to a few days of the first symptoms, weakness is noted, most often in the feet, progressing upward to affect the trunk, arms, and face, but it may begin instead in the arms, head, and neck. Autonomic dysfunction is frequently seen, including cardiac rate and rhythm disturbances as well as hypotension and hypertension. Autonomic dysfunction and cranial nerve involvement are associated with increased length of stay in both acute care and inpatient rehabilitation facilities.

Weakness and paralysis may be mild or severe, and progress to a maximum level of deficit within 14 to 30 days, remaining unchanged for a variable period of time, usually not more than 2 to 4 weeks. This is followed by a course of recovery lasting for weeks to months, with 15% to 20% of patients having some remaining motor deficit at 1 year. Severe cases may progress to paralysis of all voluntary musculature within a matter of a few hours to a few days.

Loss of ventilatory function and gag reflex, dysphagia, autonomic dysfunction, and the sometimes frightening speed of their onset make GBS a potentially life-threatening illness and it should be treated accordingly. A review of the literature shows that about 20% to 30% of patients with GBS require mechanical ventilation, with an average of 4 to 6 weeks on the ventilator.[21,22] Diagnosis is usually made on the basis of history, clinical progression, and abnormally high CSF protein concentration. Electrodiagnostic testing is also useful but not usually necessary for diagnosis.

Management of GBS should include admission to the intensive care unit with careful monitoring of vital signs, arterial oxygen saturation, and bedside spirometry, including vital capacity (VC) and maximum inspiratory pressure (MIP). Frequent monitoring of these two bedside spirometric parameters is the single most important technique for assessing the progress of GBS, and their importance cannot be overstated. An arterial blood gas (ABG) should be obtained upon admission to serve as a baseline. Repeat ABG analysis should occur if any significant change is noted in the patient's cardiopulmonary or mental status.

Heart rate and rhythm, as well as pulse oximetry saturation (Spo_2) should be monitored continuously, and blood pressure and bedside spirometry should be measured at least every 4 hours. Loss of pharyngeal and hypopharyngeal reflexes along with dysphagia and a weak cough predispose these patients to airway compromise. Accordingly, early intervention to protect the airway should be considered, even in the absence of obvious ventilatory impairment. A VC ≤10 to 15 mL/kg and/or MIP ≤20 to 30 cm H_2O, along with the clinical indicators of airway compromise mentioned above, mandate intubation with mechanical ventilatory support.

Treatment is largely supportive, and along with mechanical ventilation should include vigilant airway care and fluid and nutritional support, as well as prophylactic anticoagulant therapy to prevent venous thrombosis and resultant pulmonary embolism. In addition, rotating bed care to prevent decubitus ulcers and physical therapy (PT) to keep joints mobile and prevent muscle contractures should be employed.

While physical rehabilitation is crucial to functional recovery, care should be exercised not to overfatigue motor units, because this is associated with paradoxical weakening. Plasmapheresis, especially if begun early, has been shown to decrease recovery time and time on mechanical ventilation. Infusion of high doses of human immunoglobulin has also been shown to be of benefit.[3] Up to 40% of patients with GBS will require admission to an inpatient rehabilitation unit.[21] The necessity for ventilatory support prior to rehabilitation is associated with an extended length of stay in an inpatient rehabilitation facility.[22]

Complications of GBS include aspiration, lower airway infection, pulmonary embolism, atelectasis, gastrointestinal bleeding, and cardiac problems secondary to autonomic dysfunction.

CRITICAL CONTENT

MANAGEMENT OF GUILLAIN-BARRÉ SYNDROME
- Monitoring of vital signs, SpO_2
- Frequent monitoring of vital capacity and maximum inspiratory pressure
- Baseline arterial blood gases
- Early intervention to protect the airway
- Mechanical ventilatory support for ventilatory failure
- Plasmapheresis
- General supportive measures

With advances in modern medicine, the mortality rate of GBS has fallen dramatically and according to most studies is now between 2% and 5%.[3]

DISORDERS OF THE CENTRAL NERVOUS SYSTEM

Disorders of the central nervous system include those originating in the cerebrum or brain, as well as those originating in the extracranial extension of the brain, termed the spinal cord. Disorders of the brain interfere with the central drive to ventilate, while disorders of the spinal cord interfere with transmission of ventilatory impulses from the medullary respiratory center and cerebral cortex to the muscles of ventilation.

Poliomyelitis

Poliomyelitis or *acute anterior poliomyelitis* is an acute illness that selectively invades and kills motor neurons of the brain stem and spinal cord, resulting in asymmetric flaccid paralysis. Caused by one of three strains of poliovirus from the genus Enterovirus of the family Picornaviridae, its importance has become largely historical because of the development of a polio vaccine by Jonas Salk. While still a problem in underdeveloped countries, widespread vaccination programs since the 1950s have all but eliminated the disease in the developed world. The polio epidemic of the early to mid twentieth century was largely responsible for the development of mechanical ventilation. Furthermore, the development of mechanical ventilation is largely responsible for the origins of the respiratory care profession.

The virus is contracted orally and replicates in the oropharynx and lower gastrointestinal tract. From there, the polio virus spreads hematogenously to the central nervous system, where it attacks motor neurons of the brain stem and spinal cord. It is spread from host to host by saliva and feces and is most commonly seen today in association with poor hygiene. Paralytic poliomyelitis is also an extremely rare complication of polio vaccination.[24] Neurologic symptoms including paralysis are rare complications of poliovirus infection, occurring in only 1% to 2% of infected persons.[3] Advancing age, recent strenuous exercise, tonsillectomy, pregnancy, and immune deficiency, especially B lymphocyte impairment, are associated with an increased incidence of paralysis.[3]

For the very small percentage of patients who become symptomatic with infection, after an incubation period of 4 to 10 days flu-like symptoms develop. These include fever, malaise, headache, nausea, and vomiting, followed several days later by back and neck stiffness. Paralysis usually develops within 5 days of the headache. While the disease preferentially attacks large motor neurons of the peripheral musculature, any motor neuron may be involved, including those controlling pharyngeal and ventilatory musculature. Poliomyelitis is rarely seen in the United States, and thus can be difficult to diagnose. It can be differentiated from other acute motor polyneuropathies because no other acute disease produces the headaches, stiff back and neck, and fever along with asymmetric flaccid paralysis without sensory deficits and increased white cell count in the CSF.

Treatment during the acute phase is largely supportive, including assisted ventilation for respiratory failure, physical therapy to maintain joint mobility and to prevent contractures and bone loss, along with measures to prevent decubitus ulcers. Most patients who survive the acute phase recover a majority of their motor functions. In 1988, the World Health Assembly adopted the goal of eradicating poliomyelitis by the year 2000. According to data from the World Health Organization (WHO), substantial progress toward this goal has been made in many areas of the world.[25]

Postpolio Syndrome

Some patients, who back in the 1950s had an episode of acute anterior poliomyelitis with weakness and paralysis, are now presenting with a new onset of slow progressive weakness and fatigue. This new onset adds to the weakness already existing in previously-affected muscles. The term for this poorly-understood phenomenon is *postpolio syndrome*. It may be accompanied by fasciculations

CRITICAL CONTENT

CHARACTERISTICS OF POLIOMYELITIS

- Acute viral illness that selectively invades and kills motor neurons of the brain stem and spinal cord, resulting in asymmetric flaccid paralysis
- The Salk vaccine assists in WHO eradication efforts
- Treatment during the acute phase is largely supportive, including:
    Assisted ventilation for respiratory failure
    PT to maintain joint mobility and to
        prevent contractures and bone loss
    Measures to prevent decubitus ulcers

and further muscle atrophy. Postpolio syndrome is thought to be related to accelerated aging of motor units secondary to the initial infection. Treatment is only supportive. Patients that required assisted ventilation during the acute phase in the 1950s may require it again with the onset of postpolio syndrome. A recent study done on 17 postpolio subjects indicated that a structured endurance training program can result in increased strength in some muscle groups and in improved work performance.[26]

Amyotrophic Lateral Sclerosis

Amyotrophic lateral sclerosis (ALS) is a fatal degenerative disorder of the anterior horn cells and corticospinal tract of the spinal column. It is characterized by slow, progressive paralysis of voluntary musculature, with an annual incidence of 1 to 2.5 cases per 100,000 population.[27] While the etiology remains unknown, the existence of small geographical pockets of increased prevalence point to exogenous factors. The vast majority of cases in the United States are random, but a small percentage of families (5% to 10%) have more than one member with ALS, suggesting a genetic risk factor.[27] Males are affected slightly more often than females. Evidence now exists that a mutation in the gene that codes for Cu/Zn superoxide dismutase may be implicated.[28–30] This superoxide dismutase is an endogenously produced free radical scavenger, resulting in free radical toxicity. Abnormalities in the excitatory neurotransmitter glutamate that lead to excitotoxicity are now thought to play a crucial role in neuronal cell death.[31] Also, exposure to electromagnetic fields, various exogenous toxins, and certain trace elements have been implicated as possible etiologic agents.[32,33]

The onset of ALS is insidious, with weakness occurring in the limbs, trunk (including the muscles of ventilation), and pharynx. This weakness may be symmetric or asymmetric, with upper or lower motor neuron involvement predominating. The muscle weakness is accompanied by wasting, fasciculations, and cramps. Spasticity and reflex hyperactivity of the legs is common. The average survival time after diagnosis is 3 years, but a small number of patients may survive for as long as 10 years.[3]

Diagnosis is made on the basis of clinical and electrodiagnostic findings. Treatment is supportive and includes mechanical ventilation as indicated. The use of mechanical ventilation in the care of the patient with ALS, along with strong family support, can greatly prolong their life.

CRITICAL CONTENT

CHARACTERISTICS OF AMYOTROPHIC LATERAL SCLEROSIS

- Fatal degenerative disorder of the anterior horn cells and corticospinal tract of the spinal column
- Causes slow, progressive paralysis of voluntary musculature
- Diagnosis is made on the basis of clinical and electrodiagnostic findings
- Treatment is supportive, and includes mechanical ventilation

Spinal Cord Injury (SCI)

Trauma results in approximately 35 spinal cord injuries per 1,000,000 population in the United States each year.[3] Please refer to Chapter 14 for additional information on SCIs. The extent of neurologic deficit depends on the extent and location of the injury to the spinal cord. Roughly half of the injuries are at the cervical level and about half of those result in quadriplegia. These injuries occur from direct trauma, cord compression, and/or ischemia. Transection of the cord above the level of C3 results in the loss of all ventilatory muscle function and requires permanent mechanical ventilation, while injury to the cord between C3 and C5 preserves some diaphragmatic function. Transection of the spinal cord at the level of C5 results in the loss of most intercostal muscle function, both inspiratory and expiratory, along with the loss of function of all anterior abdominal wall musculature. Even if diaphragmatic function is spared in such an injury, ventilation will not be normal. Effective ventilation will depend entirely on diaphragmatic activity. Loss of intercostal muscle function results in loss of the ability to expand the thoracic cage, as well as a reduction in FRC secondary to loss of intercostal muscle tone. Because an effective cough depends on both anterior abdominal wall and internal intercostal muscle function, this primary pulmonary defense mechanism is largely obliterated, though with time flaccidity of the intercostal muscles is replaced by spasticity, resulting in improvement of spontaneous cough. These patients are susceptible to accumulation of secretions, atelectasis, and lower airway infection.

CRITICAL CONTENT

CHARACTERISTICS OF SPINAL CORD INJURY

- Injury above the level of C3 results in the loss of all ventilatory muscle function
- Injury to the cord between C3 and C5 preserves some diaphragmatic function
- Injury at the C5 level results in problems due to loss of use of intercostal and abdominal muscles

Initial treatment of SCI includes ensuring adequate ventilation, preventing shock, and immobilizing the neck to prevent further cord damage. If intubation is required, nasotracheal intubation is the preferred route. Because tracheostomy procedures also put pressure on the vertebral column, they should be avoided if possible during initial treatment. Even when diaphragmatic function is spared, these patients may initially present in acute respiratory failure and temporarily require mechanical ventilatory support. Hospital care includes aggressive bronchial hygiene procedures, including medication aerosol therapy, chest physiotherapy and suctioning to prevent pulmonary complications, rotating bed therapy to reduce decubitus ulcer formation, maintenance of fluid-electrolyte and nutritional status, and measures to prevent venous thrombosis.

CRITICAL CONTENT

HOSPITAL CARE FOR THE SPINAL CORD INJURY PATIENT

- Aggressive bronchial hygiene procedures
- Rotating bed therapy
- Maintenance of fluid-electrolyte and nutritional status
- Measures to prevent venous thrombosis
- Nasotracheal intubation preferred if intubation is required

Drug Overdose

A variety of drugs such as narcotics, hypnotics, and sedatives have the ability to directly suppress the medullary respiratory center, resulting in hypoventilation. The decision to intubate and mechanically ventilate these patients is governed by clinical findings. Indications for intubation of the drug overdose patient include depressed ventilation as indicated by ABG findings of acute respiratory failure, hemodynamic instability as demonstrated by cardiac dysrhythmias and hypotension, and poor mentation as measured by a standardized reference

such as the Glasgow coma scale. Poor mentation is an indicator of the patient's possible inability to adequately protect their airway, and should be considered an indication for intubation even in the presence of a normal ABG and good cardiovascular function. Unless complications develop, airway and ventilatory support of these patients is generally short-term and can be withdrawn as the drug is eliminated from the body.

Complications include concomitant cardiopulmonary disease, aspiration secondary to the presence of the drug overdose, and the development of acute lung injury (ALI) secondary to the drug, heroin being an example of a drug known to cause ALI.

CRITICAL CONTENT

CHARACTERISTICS OF DRUG OVERDOSE

- Poor mentation should be considered an indication for intubation
- Airway and ventilatory support of these patients is generally short-term and can be withdrawn as the drug is eliminated from the body
- Aspiration and ALI are pulmonary risks

RESPIRATORY CARE OF PATIENTS WITH NEUROMUSCULAR DISEASE

Despite the number and variety of diseases and disorders that result in weakness and paralysis of the muscles of ventilation, many similarities exist in their management. Muscular weakness and paralysis predispose the patient to complications, including acute and chronic respiratory failure, secretion retention, atelectasis, aspiration, lower airway infection, parenchymal scarring, and fibrosis. Because these complications are associated with increased morbidity and mortality, patients with neuromuscular disorders require aggressive and meticulous respiratory care. These problems are treated with some combination of supplemental oxygen therapy, bronchial hygiene procedures, hyper-inflation techniques, assisted ventilation, long-term ventilation, and pulmonary rehabilitation.

Patient Assessment

The reader should refer to Chapter 7 for a comprehensive discussion of patient assessment. Along with chest physical examination findings and the patient's own description of their disorder, assessment and monitoring of muscular ability is of prime concern in patients with compromised neuromuscular status. Bedside spirometry is ideal for this purpose. VC, MIP, and maximum expiratory pressure (MEP) are useful measures of ventilatory muscle strength. A MEP of ≥40 cm H_2O is necessary for an effective cough to clear pulmonary secretions. VC ≤10 mL/kg and MIP <−20 to −30 cm H_2O are associated with impending ventilatory failure and the need for ventilatory support. Spontaneous tidal volume (VT) and respiratory rate (f) are useful measures of ventilatory efficiency and work of breathing (WOB). Respiratory rates in excess of 30/min coupled with VT less than 5 mL/kg are associated with increased WOB, ventilatory muscle fatigue, and the development of ventilatory failure. A rapid shallow breathing index (f/VT) of >105 is associated with difficulty in maintaining effective spontaneous ventilation. Changes in the progress of the disorder and response to therapeutic interventions can be evaluated with serial monitoring of these parameters. Though not often used at the bedside, maximum voluntary ventilation can be used to assess ventilatory reserve. Patients who are able to double their minute volume on command generally have sufficient ventilatory reserve for adequate spontaneous ventilation.

Arterial blood gas analysis remains the gold standard for assessment of acid-base status and the prime indicator of the adequacy of alveolar ventilation, while pulse oximetry is a useful tool in monitoring oxygenation status. It should be noted, however, that the decision to commit a patient to mechanical ventilation should not be based on blood gases alone. The entire clinical picture must always be taken into account, including knowledge of the disease process and its typical progression.

For example, patients with Guillain-Barré syndrome often experience a progressive decline in VC and MIP. A normal vital capacity is about 70 mL/kg. As VC decreases, initially there is a decline in cough effectiveness, and increased potential for the development of atelectasis. ABGs, however, may be normal at this stage. As the VC continues to decline, a mild hypoxemia may develop. Often, the decision to intubate and mechanically ventilate the patient is made when MIP declines to ≤−30 cm H_2O and VC falls to ≤10 to 15 mL/kg or ≤1.0 L, independent of blood gas findings. This allows the clinician to intervene in an elective fashion, prior to the development of acute ventilatory failure and the corresponding acidemia.

CRITICAL CONTENT

PATIENT ASSESSMENT IN NEUROMUSCULAR DISEASE

- VC, MIP, and MEP are useful measures of ventilatory muscle strength
- MEP of ≥40 cm H_2O is necessary for an effective cough
- VC ≤10 mL/kg and MIP <−20 to −30 cm H_2O are associated with the need for ventilatory support
- Spontaneous VT and f are useful measures of ventilatory efficiency and WOB
- An f >30/min coupled with VT <5 mL/kg are associated with increased WOB, ventilatory muscle fatigue, and ventilatory failure
- A rapid shallow breathing index (f/VT) of >105 is associated with difficulty in maintaining effective spontaneous ventilation

Treatment

Management of the patient with a neuromuscular disorder should be focused on the potential for complications, by maintaining and protecting the airway, ensuring adequate ventilation, mobilizing secretions, and treating and preventing further atelectasis. Figure 21-4 relates the approximate decrease in vital capacity to the expected patho-

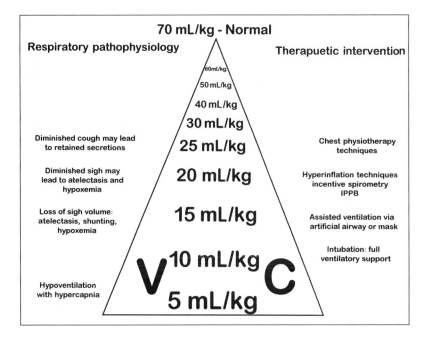

70 mL/kg - Normal

Respiratory pathophysiology

Therapuetic intervention

60ml/kg

50 mL/kg

40 mL/kg

30 mL/kg

25 mL/kg

20 mL/kg

15 mL/kg

10 mL/kg

5 mL/kg

V C

Diminished cough may lead to retained secretions

Diminished sigh may lead to atelectasis and hypoxemia

Loss of sigh volume: atelectasis, shunting, hypoxemia

Hypoventilation with hypercapnia

Chest physiotherapy techniques

Hyperinflation techniques incentive spirometry IPPB

Assisted ventilation via artificial airway or mask

Intubation: full ventilatory support

FIGURE 21-4 The approximate decrease in vital capacity in relation to the expected pathophysiologic result and the appropriate therapeutic intervention.

physiologic result and the appropriate therapeutic intervention. The need for mechanical ventilation may be short- or long-term depending on the specific disorder, and will usually require the placement of an artificial airway for protection against aspiration. An endotracheal tube is generally preferred for ventilation of less than 2 weeks' duration, while a tracheostomy is the airway of choice for longer-term ventilation.

Noninvasive ventilatory techniques such as continuous positive airway pressure (CPAP) and noninvasive positive pressure ventilation (NPPV) are indicated in situations in which the potential for aspiration is low and ventilation is short-term, such as nocturnal ventilation for a patient with postpolio syndrome. Mobilization of secretions is accomplished with a combination of aerosol therapy, chest physiotherapy, effective coughing, and suctioning for patients unable to effectively cough on their own. Techniques and equipment such as high frequency chest compression (HFCC) using a device such as the THAIR-py vest, intrapulmonary percussive ventilation (IPV) equipment (Percussionaire, Sand Point, Idaho), or "artificial cough machines" using a mechanical insufflation-exsufflation (MI-E)

device (J. H. Emerson Co., Cambridge, Mass) may all be useful in improving secretion removal.

In patients who can maintain adequate ventilation but cannot take a deep breath, hyperinflation therapy utilizing intermittent positive-pressure breathing (IPPB) is indicated to treat and prevent further atelectasis as well as to provide adequate volume for coughing. In patients who are recovering from muscular weakness, changing them from IPPB to incentive spirometry should be considered when the VC routinely exceeds 15 mL/kg. Patients who are not permanently paralyzed and are recovering from their disease should have a regular program of breathing retraining and exercise conditioning to assist them in regaining the muscular energy necessary for spontaneous ventilation and effective coughing.

Patients requiring mechanical ventilation due to neuromuscular disease often have normal or near-normal lung function and ventilatory drive. Ventilatory muscle weakness predisposes these patients to the development of atelectasis and pneumonia. Because of this, aggressive bronchial hygiene and use of techniques to maintain adequate lung inflation are often required. Large tidal volumes (12 to 15 mL/kg), moderate to high inspiratory flow rates ($\geq$60 L/min), and the judicious use of PEEP (5 to 10 cm H_2O) may be indicated in these patients.[34] Total ventilatory support may be required using synchronized intermittent mandatory ventilation (SIMV) or assist-control ventilation, depending on the patient's ability to spontaneously breathe. Chest physiotherapy, aerosolized bronchodilator use, adequate humidification, and careful attention to the patient's airway should be included in the patient's respiratory care plan. Ventilator weaning and discontinuance should be considered based on assessment of the patient's disease state or condition, measurement of appropriate indexes used to predict success, and optimization of the patient's overall condition.

CRITICAL CONTENT

RESPIRATORY CARE OF THE PATIENT WITH NEUROMUSCULAR DISEASE

- Frequent assessment of ventilatory function
- Airway maintenance and care
- Bronchial hygiene procedures
- Hyperinflation techniques
- Oxygen therapy
- Assisted ventilation, short- and long-term ventilation, and invasive and noninvasive PPV
- Pulmonary rehabilitation and patient and caregiver education

SITE- AND AGE-SPECIFIC CONSIDERATIONS AND COSTS AND ETHICAL ISSUES

Most neuromuscular disorders are to a greater or lesser degree chronic in nature, therefore site-specific care encompasses a spectrum from acute care, through both inpatient and outpatient rehabilitation, and finally to home care. With regard to age-specific considerations, some neuromuscular disorders are both age- and gender-specific,

Duchenne's muscular dystrophy being an example, while other disorders such as GBS have only minor gender or age predilections. Also, advancing age is associated with increased susceptibility to diseases and disorders of all kinds.

The economic impact of neuromuscular disorders is significant. Because the majority of these patients require both acute and chronic care, including both rehabilitation and home care, the direct cost (ie, cost related to care) is enormous. As an example, the estimated annual cost of treating *Campylobacter*-associated GBS is estimated to be as high as $1.8 billion in 1995 dollars.[19] The indirect costs related to lost productivity are also large. In another example, one cross-sectional multicenter study looked at the total direct costs over 1 year for all cases of SCI. These costs included emergency medical services, hospitalizations, attendant care, equipment, supplies, medications, environmental modifications, physician and outpatient services, nursing homes, household assistance, vocational rehabilitation, and other miscellaneous items. These costs, in 1995 dollars, amount to an estimated $7.736 billion.[35]

We live in an era when advances in life-sustaining technology have dramatically enhanced the ability to prolong life, even in the face of terminal illness. This fact, coupled with the devastating effects most neuromuscular disorders have on patients and their families, means ethical considerations are of prime importance. Issues such as informed consent, quality of life, artificial life support measures, palliative care, advanced directives, and end-of-life decisions become a source of concern and debate for the patient, the family, and the caregivers. The reader should refer to Chapter 5 for a complete description of these aspects of health care across the continuum of care.

HEALTH PROMOTION AND QUALITY-OF-LIFE ISSUES

Because of the chronic and debilitating nature of most neuromuscular disorders, many of these patients require extensive daily care, so educating the patient and caregivers is of utmost importance. As a respiratory therapist you will be providing care to patients with neuromuscular disorders in a variety of settings, and in many of these situations you will have the opportunity to provide patients and their caregivers with needed education at the same time you are providing respiratory care. Even though the patient may be receiving care in an acute care hospital, their education on provision of self-care should begin as soon as possible.

The quality of a patient's life is influenced to some degree by the amount of their dependence on others. Providing the patient with the ability to be self-sufficient (to the degree their disability permits) is a step toward returning some of their sense of self-worth. This is an important aspect of improving the quality of life for many of these patients.

INTRODUCTION TO CASE STUDIES

Now you proceed with the most exciting part of this chapter, that of working through two hypothetical cases. Your instructors will assign you to work on specific critical thinking exercises and group critical thinking exercises, depending on the available time, types of patients you are likely to encounter in your clinical rotations, and resources available. Please check with your instructor to verify which case(s) and exercises you should complete, individually or working in groups. Your instructor may also direct you to develop learning issues as part of your problem-based learning (PBL) process or assign specific, predetermined learning issues that have been developed for this chapter. Please check with your program faculty before proceeding with the following cases.

CASE STUDY 1

NICHOLAS NUMB

Initial History

Mr. Numb, a 33-year-old Caucasian male who works as a personal fitness trainer, was in his usual state of good health until yesterday morning. When he awoke he noticed numbness and tingling in his feet, which was accompanied by difficulty getting out of bed. Throughout the course of the day, he felt tired and drained, with walking becoming increasingly difficult. This morning, along with difficulty walking, he had trouble eating his breakfast without choking, which prompted him to seek medical attention. He presented in his primary care physician's office with complaints of fatigue, muscle aches, difficulty walking and swallowing, and shortness of breath with minor physical exertion. He denies any recent illness or prior pulmonary disease and

states that the only time he sought medical care within the past year is for a routine flu shot 4 days prior to this incident.

 Critical Thinking Exercise 1

PRIORITIZING PATIENT CARE

Explain how you would prioritize your assessment of this patient based on his presenting symptomatology.

Physical Examination (Performed in His Physician's Office)

Appearance: A well nourished 33-year-old Caucasian male, height 6 feet 1 inch, weight 175 lb, in no obvious respiratory distress, conscious, alert, and oriented to time, place, and person.

CASE STUDY 1 *(continued)*

Vital signs

HR	112/min
RR	22/min
BP	155/105
SpO$_2$	N/A
Temp.	36.8°C

HEENT	Normal in appearance, pupils equal, round, and reactive to light and accommodation (PERRLA), no ptosis with repeated eye blinking, cranial nerves intact, scalenes and sternocleidomastoids intact but weak, with difficulty swallowing.
Chest	
Inspection	Normal thoracic configuration.
Auscultation	Clear and equal breath sounds but diminished bilaterally.
CV	Normal S$_1$ and S$_2$ heart sounds with no gallops or murmurs.
Extremities	Significant weakness in the lower extremities with absent deep tendon reflexes, some minor weakness in the upper extremities with diminished deep tendon reflexes.

Critical Thinking Exercise 2

MAKING INFERENCES BY CLUSTERING DATA

a. What inference can you make about the potential for this patient to develop pneumonia, and why?

b. Practice clustering the data that lead you to this inference by identifying all the data that led you to make the above inference.

One hour later: Following his physician's physical examination, Nick is admitted to the hospital and placed in the medical intensive care unit for observation.

Critical Thinking Exercise 3

ANTICIPATING FINDINGS

a. What additional data would you obtain for your assessment of this patient in the intensive care unit?

b. Why would you look for and collect specific findings?

c. What specific findings do you anticipate and how would they guide your management of this patient?

CLINICAL DATA IMMEDIATELY AFTER ADMISSION TO THE ICU

Vital signs

HR	118/min
RR	26/min
BP	150/110
SpO$_2$	N/A
Temp.	37.1°C

Chest	
Auscultation	Bilaterally clear and equal but diminished in the bases.

CASE STUDY 1 *(continued)*

CBC

WBC	11,000/mm^3
Hgb	13.8 g/dL
Hct	40%
RBC	4.4 million/mm^3
Neutrophils	66%
Lymphocytes	18%
Monocytes	8%
Eosinophils	4%
Basophils	1%
Bands	3%
Electrolytes	normal

PFT data

MIP	−30 cm H$_2$O
VC	2.13 L

ABG room air

pH	7.42
Pco$_2$	35
Po$_2$	88
HCO$_3^-$	22.5
BE	−1
Sao$_2$	96.6%

Radiology

AP chest	Eight rib inspiration, no infiltrates, masses, or other abnormalities.

Critical Thinking Exercise 4

PROBLEM SOLVING USING CLINICAL DATA

What does the above clinical data suggest about this patient's diagnosis? Explain the rationale for your interpretation.

Critical Thinking Exercise 5

ANTICIPATING PROBLEMS AND SOLUTIONS

a. How will you determine how this patient's condition is progressing?
b. What problems would you anticipate?
c. What recommendations would you make based on each specific finding?

CLINICAL DATA 6 HOURS AFTER ADMISSION TO THE ICU

Vital signs

HR	132/min
RR	36/min
BP	148/95
Spo$_2$	N/A
Temp.	38.1°C

Chest

Auscultation	Diminished bilaterally but clear.

ABG room air

pH	7.45
Pco$_2$	32
Po$_2$	86
HCO$_3^-$	22.3
BE	−0
Sao$_2$	96.6%

PFTs

MIP	−20 cm H$_2$O
VC	1.10 L

CASE STUDY 1 (continued)

Radiology

AP chest	Poor inspiratory effort with bibasilar atelectasis.
Spinal tap	Increased protein levels in the cerebrospinal fluid, otherwise normal.

Case summary 36 hours after ICU admittance: The diagnosis of Guillain-Barré syndrome was made based on the history, laboratory findings, and bedside spirometry. An order for daily plasmapheresis was written. On the basis of the vital signs, MIP, and VC, the patient was electively intubated with a #8.5 oral endotracheal tube and placed on mechanical ventilation. A chest x-ray confirmed proper tube placement. The initial settings were SIMV mode, set respiratory rate 10 and a total respiratory rate of 18, tidal volume 1000 mL, inspiratory flow rate of 60 L/min, FIO_2 0.35 with no PEEP. An ABG was obtained after 30 minutes of mechanical ventilation, with the following results:

ABG 35% SIMV 10

pH	7.43
PCO_2	36
PO_2	114
HCO_3^-	23.0
BE	−1
SaO_2	99%

Clinical summary over 10 days: Over the next 10 days, the patient was maintained on mechanical ventilation on the same settings. On day 7, spirometry performed with Mr. Numb off the ventilator yielded these data: VC 1.83 L, MIP −24 cm H_2O, and spontaneous Vt varying between 150 and 300 mL. Vital signs were stable,

the patient felt stronger, paresthesia in his legs was diminished, deep tendon reflexes were returning and his chest x-ray demonstrated clearing of the atelectasis. Scant amounts of colorless secretions were suctioned from the airway. ABG results while on the ventilator were:

ABG 30% SIMV 10

pH	7.39
PCO_2	39
PO_2	95
HCO_3^-	24.0
BE	−0
SaO_2	98%

Case conclusion through day 20: Throughout the next week, the patient continued to show steady improvement in muscle strength and ventilatory parameters. Weaning was initiated, and on day 19 spirometry results revealed a VC 2.64 L, MIP -38 cm H_2O, and spontaneous Vt averaging 400 mL. ABG results done on an SIMV rate of 4 were:

ABG 30% SIMV 4

pH	7.41
PCO_2	41
PO_2	98
HCO_3^-	24.0
BE	0
SaO_2	98%

The patient was extubated that afternoon without incident. Over the course of the next 2 days his breath sounds remained clear with a weak but improving cough, normal vital signs, and improving ventilatory parameters. On day 21 he was transferred to a medical floor and was discharged 4 days later without further incident.

CASE STUDY 1 *(continued)*

Group CT Exercise

PRO/CON DEBATE

One group of students should present the argument that Mr. Numb needs to be trached after his third day of mechanical ventilation. Provide data, evidence, and reasons to support this recommendation. Be sure to explain why this decision is the best one at the time and what could happen if there are any further delays.

A second group should use the same case and develop the argument that Mr. Numb should **not** be trached at this point in his hospitalization. Again, provide data, evidence, and reasons to support this recommendation. Be sure to explain why this decision is the correct one at this time.

The entire class should discuss which side was more effective and who won the debate. Did the team who won the debate support the most valid medical position, or was their argument just presented more effectively?

CASE STUDY 2

WENDY WEEK

Initial History

Ms. Week, a 28-year-old Caucasian female who works as a registered nurse, was in her usual state of excellent health until yesterday afternoon. Shortly after arriving at work for her evening shift, she noticed diplopia while reading a patient's chart. As the evening progressed, she began to experience dysphonia, and was unusually fatigued while performing routine nursing duties. While on her dinner break, she found that she could not adequately chew her food, and this was accompanied by dysphagia. Upon hearing the symptoms, her nurse manager sent her to the emergency department (ED) for evaluation and treatment. She denies any recent illness or past medical problems.

Critical Thinking Exercise 1

PRIORITIZING PATIENT CARE

Explain how you would prioritize your assessment of this patient based on her presenting symptoms?

Physical Examination (Performed in the ED)

Appearance: A well-nourished 28-year-old Caucasian female, height 5 feet 7 inches, weight 125 lb, anxious, in no obvious respiratory distress, conscious, alert, and oriented to time, place, and person.

Vital signs

HR	72/min
RR	26/min
BP	132/74
SpO_2	N/A
Temp.	37.1°C

HEENT	Normal in appearance, pupils equal, round, and reactive to light, but sluggish to accommodate (PERRLA), significant ptosis with repeated eye blinking, has difficulty maintaining her gaze in an upward direction while keeping her eyes open, cranial nerves intact, scalenes and sternocleidomastoids intact but weak, with difficulty swallowing and speaking clearly when asked to count loudly from 1 to 100.

CASE STUDY 2 *(continued)*

Chest

Inspection	Normal thoracic configuration.
Auscultation	Clear and equal breath sounds but diminished bilaterally.
CV	Normal S_1 and S_2 heart sounds with no gallops or murmurs.
Extremities	Generalized upper and lower extremity weakness with normal deep tendon reflexes. She was unable to hold her arms abducted in the horizontal position for more than 15 seconds.

Critical Thinking Exercise 2

MAKING INFERENCES BY CLUSTERING DATA

a. What inference can you make about the potential for this patient to develop pulmonary problems, and why?

b. Practice clustering data by identifying all the data that lead you to make the above inference.

Critical Thinking Exercise 3

ANTICIPATING FINDINGS

a. What additional data would you obtain for your assessment of Ms. Week?

b. Why collect these particular data?

c. What specific findings do you anticipate and how would they guide your management of Ms. Week?

Clinical data immediately after admission to the medical floor: Based on the ED exam, Ms. Week is admitted to the medical floor of the hospital. Additional data collected at this time are as follows:

Vital signs

HR	94/min
RR	28/min
BP	128/82
SpO_2	N/A
Temp.	37.1°C

Chest

Auscultation	Bilaterally clear and equal but diminished in the bases.

CBC

WBC	6000/mm³
Hgb	13.2 g/dL
Hct	38%
RBC	4.5 million/mm³
Neutrophils	66%
Lymphocytes	18%
Monocytes	8%
Eosinophils	4%
Basophils	1%
Bands	3%
Electrolytes	normal

PFT data

MIP	–32 cm H_2O
VC	2.46 L

ABG room air

pH	7.39
Pco_2	42
Po_2	86
HCO_3^-	23.5
BE	0
Sao_2	97%

Radiology

AP chest	Eight rib inspiration, no infiltrates, masses, or other abnormalities.

CASE STUDY 2 *(continued)*

Tensilon (Anticholinesterase) Test

Edrophonium chloride (Tensilon) 2 mg given intravenously over a 15-second period. No response was noted after 30 seconds and an additional 8 mg was administered. Within 15 seconds there was a notable improvement in her ability to blink her eyes, her ocular range of motion, and her hand grip strength. These improvements only lasted for about 5 to 10 minutes.

Serologic testing: Testing reveals a positive antibody binding test for AChR antibodies.

Critical Thinking Exercise 4

PROBLEM SOLVING USING CLINICAL DATA

a. What do the clinical data suggest about this patient's diagnosis? Explain the rationale for your interpretation.

b. Based on the information you have, what if any additional data might assist you in the diagnosis? Explain your rationale.

The patient is transferred to the medical intensive care unit (MICU) for evaluation and monitoring following review of her initial clinical data.

Two to six hours after admission to the MICU: A diagnosis of myasthenia gravis is made on the basis of the patient's symptoms and the results of laboratory testing. Ms. Week is started on pyridostigmine bromide, and alternate-day prednisone.

Critical Thinking Exercise 5

ANTICIPATING PROBLEMS AND SOLUTIONS

a. How will you monitor this patient's condition to determine if further intervention is required?

b. What pulmonary problems would you anticipate?

Six hours after admission to the MICU, the patient begins to experience progressive weakness despite increasing amounts of pyridostigmine. She begins to experience bradycardia, diaphoresis, and excessive lacrimation, accompanied by gastrointestinal symptoms, including abdominal cramps, nausea, vomiting, and diarrhea.

Vital signs

HR	128/min
RR	34/min
BP	142/92
SpO_2	N/A
Temp.	37.4°C

Chest

Auscultation	Diminished bilaterally but clear.

ABG room air

pH	7.45
PCO_2	35
PO_2	76
HCO_3^-	22.5
BE	–0
SaO_2	95.6%

PFTs

MIP	–30 cm H_2O
VC	2.10 L

Radiology

AP chest	Poor inspiratory effort, with minimal bibasilar atelectasis.

CASE STUDY 2 *(continued)*

Case summary, days 1 to 5: A cholinergic crisis was suspected, so the pyridostigmine was temporarily withdrawn and the patient's muscarinic symptoms subsided over the next 4 hours. Serial monitoring of her VC and MIP every 4 hours demonstrated that the patient's spontaneous ventilatory ability remained adequate to maintain normal blood gas values. Over the next 2 days, with pharmacotherapy the patient steadily regained strength. On day 3, bedside spirometry revealed VC 2.89 L, MIP -40 cm H_2O, and spontaneous V_T varying between 350 and 450 mL. Vital signs were stable, and her chest x-ray demonstrated clearing of the atelectasis. The patient was transferred to a general medical floor, and after another 2 days was discharged without incident.

 Group Critical Thinking Exercise 1

DECISION MAKING: DEVELOPING A LONG-TERM CARE PLAN

Use the information from Ms. Week's case to develop a long-term care plan for her to manage her MG. Describe your care plan for discharge

from the hospital and for long-term care, if required. Describe what outcome measures you will utilize to assess the effectiveness of Ms. Week's disease management. Discuss the prognosis and quality of life expected for Ms. Week.

 Group Critical Thinking Exercise 2

COMMUNICATION, NEGOTIATION, AND ETHICS

Suppose Ms. Week's condition continued to deteriorate, and the medical decision was that intubation and mechanical ventilation were required. However, Ms. Week states she should "just be allowed to die." Have a group of students research the various arguments for why Ms. Week should allow the intubation to take place. Each member of the group should practice the role of a health practitioner who is discussing this situation with her. Have the two or three most convincing students role play this role in front of the entire class and have the class judge who did the best job of communicating with Ms. Week. The entire class may discuss what made the winning argument so convincing.

 KEY POINTS

- Neuromuscular disease comprises a group of disorders in which the primary pathophysiological manifestation is, ultimately, failure of the ventilatory pump to adequately move air into the lungs.

- Because neuromuscular diseases inhibit inspiration, they are by definition, restrictive diseases.

- The primary clinical manifestation of ventilatory pump failure is hypoventilation, resulting in hypercapnia, hypoxemia, and acidosis. Long term clinical manifestations vary with the dis-

order but can include secretion accumulation, atelectasis, and lower airway infection.

- Neuromuscular disorders can be categorized into four basic groups according to the component of the ventilatory pump which is affected: 1) disorders of the muscles, 2) disorders of the neuromuscular junction, 3) disorders of the peripheral motor nerves, and 4) disorders of the central nervous system (including the cerebrum or brain, and the spinal cord).

- Control of breathing is provided by the medullary center in the brain stem.

- Medullary output is modified by two groups of chemoreceptors, the central chemoreceptors and peripheral chemoreceptors, including the carotid and aortic body chemoreceptors as well as the input from the pontine apneustic and pneumotaxic centers.

- Three types of vagally mediated sensory receptors are found in the lungs that provide input to the medullary center, the irritant receptors, the bronchopulmonary stretch receptors, and the C-fiber receptors.

- Output from the respiratory control center in the brain descends to the anterior horn cells of the spinal column.

- The muscles of ventilation include the diaphragm, the external and internal intercostas, the muscles of the anterior abdominal wall, and the accessory muscles of ventilation.

- The primary muscle of inspiration is the diaphragm, accounting for the majority of work done during quiet breathing. It is innervated bilaterally by the phrenic nerves, which have their origin in cervical nerves C3, C4, and C5.

- A disorder of the muscle not related to a change in the innervation of the muscle is termed a myopathy.

- Dystrophy refers to the destruction and regeneration of muscle fibers, and the eventual replacement of the muscle fibers by fibrous and fatty connective tissue.

- The two most frequently encountered muscular dystrophies (MDs) are *Duchenne's and Becker's dystrophies.*

- Usually beginning early in life, both MDs are characterized by painless weakness, most prominently in the pelvic girdle and thighs, less prominently in the shoulders, and least often in the distal extremities.

- *Polymyositis-dermatomyositis* is a rare disease of the muscles, falling into the broad category of idiopathic inflammatory myopathies.

- Disorders of the neuromuscular junction are caused by three basic pathophysiological mechanisms: 1) impaired postsynaptic membrane receptor mechanisms, 2) a deficiency in neurotransmitter synthesis and/or release, and 3) depolarizing or nondepolarizing blockade of acetylcholine binding sites by drugs and poisons.

- Myasthenia gravis (MG) is an acquired antigen-specific autoimmune disease characterized by weakness and fatigability that is exacerbated with repetitive effort.

- MG is caused by circulating antibodies that damage the acetylcholine receptors (AChRs) within the muscle fiber plasma membrane, causing both a qualitative and quantitative deficiency in their function.

- Diagnosis of MG is made on the basis of clinical history, the presence of circulating AchR antibodies, electromyographic findings and the results of anticholionersterase testing.

- Primary treatment of the patient with MG includes anticholinesterases, corticosteroids, azathioprine, plasmapheresis, and thymectomy.

- Treatment of pulmonary MG symptoms includes assisted ventilation, hyperinflation techniques, and bronchial hygiene procedures as indicated.

- Lambert-Eaton myasthenic syndrome (LEMS) is an acquired autoimmune disorder in which circulating autoantibodies cause a deficiency in voltage-sensitive calcium channels on the axon terminal plasma membranes.

- A characteristic of LEMS is that with repeated stimulation, muscular output briefly grows stronger rather than weaker, as in MG.

- LEMS is strongly associated with small cell carcinoma of the lung.

- Treatment of pulmonary symptoms in LEMS, if present, include bronchial hygiene procedures, hyperinflation techniques, and assisted ventilation as indicated.

- Botulism is a neuroparalytic disorder caused by a neurotoxin produced by the anaerobic, gram positive, spore forming, bacterium, *Clostridium botulinum.*

- Botulism symptoms usually begin in 12 to 24 hours with gastrointestinal manifestations including nausea, vomiting, and abdominal pain. Cranial nerve musculature is affected first, causing diplopia, dysarthria, dysphagia, and dysphonia.

- Botulism treatment includes administration of antitoxin, elimation of residual toxin from the gastrointestinal tract, mechanical ventilatory support as indicated, and general supportive measures.

- Tetanus is a neurologic syndrome caused by a neurotoxin produced by the anaerobic, gram positive, spore forming, bacterium, *Clostridium tetani.*

- Diagnosis of tetanus is made largely on the basis of the clinical picture.

- Treatment includes stabilization, wound debridement, antibiotic therapy, human tetanus immune globulin, muscle relaxants, and supportive care, including maintenance of a protected, patent airway, and mechanical ventilation if acute respiratory failure ensues.

- Prevention of tetanus through immunization is the key to control of the disease.

- Diseases of the peripheral motor nerves affect one or more of the three basic components of a peripheral motor neuron, 1) the neuron cell body, 2) the axon, and 3) the Schwann cell or its product, the myelin sheath.

- *Guillain-Barré Syndrome* (GBS) is a disorder characterized by acute, ascending symmetrical flaccid paralysis of voluntary musculature, including those supplied by the cranial nerves and those controlling ventilation, with associated loss of deep tendon reflexes and increased cerebrospinal fluid (CSF) protein.

- Diagnosis of GBS is usually made on the basis of history, clinical progression, and abnormally high CSF protein concentration.

- Management of GBS should include admission to the ICU with careful and frequent monitoring of vital signs, SpO_2, and bedside spirometry, including vital capacity (VC) and maximum inspiratory pressure (MIP).

- Because GBS patients are prone to airway compromise, early intervention to protect the airway should be considered, even in the absence of obvious ventilatory impairment. VC ≤10–15 mL/kg and MIP ≤20–30 cm H_2O mandate intubation with mechanical ventilatory support.

- Treatment of GBS is largely supportive and, along with mechanical ventilation, should include vigilant airway care, fluid and nutritional support, prophylactic anticoagulant therapy to prevent venous thrombosis and resultant pulmonary embolism, rotating bed care to prevent decubitus ulcers, and physical therapy to keep joints mobile and prevent muscle contractures.

- *Poliomyelitis* or *acute anterior poliomyelitis* is an acute illness that selectively invades and kills motor neurons of the brain stem and spinal cord, resulting in asymmetric flaccid paralysis.

- Poliomyelitis is rarely seen in the United States, and thus can be difficult to diagnose.

- Postpolio syndrome, occurring months to years later, is a phenomenon of slow progressive weakness and fatigue usually adding to the weakness in already affected muscles.

- *Amyotrophic lateral sclerosis (ALS)* is a fatal degenerative disorder of the anterior horn cells and corticospinal tract of the spinal column characterized by slow, progressive paralysis of voluntary musculature.

- The onset of ALS is insidious, with weakness occurring in the limbs, trunk, including the muscles of ventilation, and pharynx, and may be symmetric or asymmetric with upper or lower motor neuron involvement predominating.

- ALS treatment is supportive and includes mechanical ventilation as indicated.

- The extent of neurologic deficit secondary to spinal cord injury (SCI) depends on the extent and location of the injury to the cord. Transection of the spinal cord above the level of C3 results in the loss of all ventilatory muscle function, requiring permanent long-term mechanical ventilation, while injury to the cord between C3 and C5 preserves some diaphragmatic function.

- Effective coughing is a major problem for spinal cord patients. These patients are therefore susceptible to accumulated secretions, atelectasis, and lower airway infection.

- Hospital care for SCI includes aggressive bronchial hygiene, rotating bed therapy to reduce decubitus ulcer formation, maintenance of fluid-electrolyte and nutritional status, and measures to prevent venous thrombosis.

- Long term mechanical ventilatory support may be required for SCI, depending on the location and extent of cord injury.

- A variety of drugs have the ability to directly suppress the medullary respiratory center resulting in hypoventilation, including narcotics, hypnotics, and sedatives.

- Indications for intubation of the drug overdose patient include depressed ventilation, as indicated by ABG findings of acute respiratory failure, hemodynamic instability as demonstrated by cardiac dysrhythmias and hypotension, and poor mentation as measured by a standardized reference such as the Glasgow Coma Scale.

- Complications include concomitant cardiopulmonary disease, aspiration secondary to the presence of the drug overdose and the development of acute lung injury (ALI) secondary to the drug, e.g., heroin.

- These problems are treated with some combination of supplemental oxygen therapy, bronchial hygiene procedures, hyperinflation techniques, assisted ventilation, long-term ventilation, and pulmonary rehabilitation.

- VC, MIP, and maximum expiratory pressure (MEP) are useful measures of ventilatory muscle strength.

- A MEP of ≥ 40 cm H_2O is necessary for an effective cough to clear pulmonary secretions.

- VC ≤ 10 mL/kg and MIP < -20 to -30 cm H_2O are associated with impending ventilatory failure and need for ventilatory support. A rapid shallow breathing index (f/V_T) of > 105 is associated with difficulty in maintaining effective spontaneous ventilation.

- Often, the decision to intubate and mechanically ventilate the patient is made when MIP declines to ≤ -30 cm H_2O and VC falls to $\leq 10-15$ mL/kg or ≤ 1.0 L, independent of blood gas findings.

- Management of the patient with a neuromuscular disorder should be focused on the complications by ensuring adequate ventilation, maintaining and protecting the airway, mobilizing secretions, and treating and preventing further atelectasis.

- Patients requiring mechanical ventilation due to neuromuscular disease often have normal or near normal lung function and ventilatory drive. However, ventilatory muscle weakness predisposes these patients to the development of atelectasis and pneumonia.

- Because the majority of neuromuscular disease patients require both acute and chronic care, including both rehabilitation and home care, the cost is enormous.

- Because of the devastating nature of some neuromuscular disorders, issues such as informed consent, quality of life, artificial life support measures, palliative care, advanced directives, and end of life decisions become a source of concern and debate for the patient, the family, and the caregivers.

- Because of the chronic and debilitating nature of most neuromuscular disorders, many of these patients require extensive daily care, thus educating the patient and the caregivers is of utmost importance.

REFERENCES

1. Coleridge HM, Coleridge JC. Pulmonary reflexes: Neural mechanisms of pulmonary defense. *Annu Rev Physiol.* 1994;56:69–91.

2. Murray JF, Nadel JA. *Textbook of Respiratory Medicine.* 2nd ed. Philadelphia: Saunders; 1994.

3. Bennett JC, Plum F. *Cecil Textbook of Medicine.* 20th ed. Philadelphia: Saunders; 1996.

4. Van den Bergh PY, Tome EM, Fardeau M. Etiology and pathogenesis of the muscular dystrophies. *Acta Neurologica Belgica.* 1995;95:123–141.

5. McDonald CM, Abresch RT, Carter GT, et al. Profiles of neuromuscular diseases. Duchenne muscular dystrophy. *Am J Phys Med Rehabil.* 1995;74 (Suppl 5):S70–S92.

6. Weidensaul D, Imam T, Holyst MM, et al. Polymyositis, pulmonary fibrosis and hepatitis C. *Arthritis Rheum.* 1995;38:437–439.

7. Marie I, Hatron PY, Hachulla E, et al. Pulmonary involvement in polymyositis and dermatomyositis. *J Rheumatol.* 1998;25:1336–1343.

8. Mastaglia FL, Phuillips BA, Zilko P. Treatment of inflammatory myopathies. *Muscle Nerve.* 1997;20: 651–664.

9. Dalakas MC. Controlled studies with high-dose intravenous immunoglobulin in the treatment of dermatomyositis, inclusion body myositis, and polymyositis. *Neurology.* 1998;51(6 Suppl 5): S37–S45.

10. Infante AJ, Infante PD, Jackson CE, et al. Evidence against chronic antigen-specific T lymphocyte activation in myasthenia gravis. *J Neurosci Res.* 1996; 45:492–499.

11. Truffault F, Cohen-Kaminsky S, Khalil I, et al. Altered intrathymic T-cell repertoire in human myasthenia gravis. *Ann Neurol.* 1997;41:731–741.

12. Marx A, Wilisch A, Schultz A, et al. Pathogenesis of myasthenia gravis. *Virchows Archiv.* 1997; 430:355–364.

13. O'Neill JH, Murray NM, Newsom-Davis J. The Lambert-Eaton myasthenic syndrome. A review of 50 cases. *Brain.* 1988;111:577–596.

14. Shapiro RL, Hatheway C, Swerdlow DL. Botulism in the United States: a clinical and epidemiologic review. *Ann Intern Med.* 1998;129:221–228.

15. Steffen R, Mellin J, Woodall JP, et al. Preparation for emergency relief after biological warfare. *J Infect.* 1997;34:127–132.

16. Ernst ME, Klepser ME, Fouts M, et al. Tetanus: Pathophysiology and management. *Ann Pharmacother.* 1997;31:1507–1513.

17. Bardenheier B, Prevots DR, Khetsuriani N, et al. Tetanus surveillance-United States, 1995-1997. *Morbid Mortal.* 1998;47:1–13.

18. Gergen PJ, McQuillan GM, Kiely M, et al. Comments in *N Engl J Med.* 1995;332:761–766.

19. Hughes RA, Rees JH. Clinical and epidemiologic features of Guillain-Barré syndrome. *J Infect Dis.* 1997;176(Suppl 2):S92–S98.

20. Buzby JC, Allos BM, Roberts T. The economic burden of Campylobacter-associated Guillain-Barré syndrome. *J Infect Dis.* 1997;176(Suppl 2):S192–S197.

21. Meythaler JM, DeVivo MJ, Braswell WC. Rehabilitation outcomes of patients who have developed Guillain-Barré syndrome. *Am J Phys Med Rehabil.* 1997;76:411–419.

22. Meythaler JM. Rehabilitation of Guillain-Barré syndrome. *Arch Phys Med Rehabil.* 1997;78: 872–879.

23. Prevots DR, Sutter RW. Assessment of Guillain-Barré syndrome mortality and morbidity in the United States: implications for acute flaccid paralysis surveillance. *J Infect Dis.* 1997;175(Suppl 1): S151–S155.

24. Weibel RE, Benor DE. Reporting vaccine-associated paralytic poliomyelitis: concordance between the CDC and the National Vaccine Injury Compensation Program. *Am J Pub Health.* 1996;86: 734–737.

25. Hull HF, Birmingham ME, Melgaard B, et al. Progress toward global polio eradication. *J Infect Dis.* 1997;175(Suppl 1):S4–S9.

26. Ernstoff B, Wetterqvist H, Kvist H, et al. Endurance training effect on individuals with postpoliomyelitis. *Arch Phys Med Rehabil.* 1996;77:843–848.

27. Jackson CE, Bryan WW. Amyotrophic lateral sclerosis. *Semin Neurol.* 1998;18:27–39.

28. Nelson LM. Epidemiology of ALS. *Clin Neurosci.* 1995–1996;3:327–331.

29. Morrison BM, Morrison JH, Gordon JW. Superoxide dismutase and neurofilament transgenic mod-

els of amyotrophic lateral sclerosis. *J Exp Zool.* 1998;282:32–47.

30. Liu D. The role of free radicals in amyotrophic lateral sclerosis. *J Molec Neurosci.* 1996;7:159–167.

31. Shaw PJ, Ince PG. Glutamate, excitotoxicity and amyotrophic lateral sclerosis. *J Neurol.* 1997;244 (Suppl 2):S3–S14.

32. Davanipour Z, Sobel E, Bowman JD, et al. Amyotrophic lateral sclerosis and occupational exposure to electromagnetic fields. *Bioelectromagnetics.* 1997;18:28–35.

33. Vinceti M, Guidetti D, Pinotti M, et al. Amyotrophic lateral sclerosis after long-term exposure to drinking water with high selenium content. *Epidemiology.* 1996;7:529–532.

34. Slutsky AS. Mechanical ventilation. American College of Chest Physicians Consensus Conference. *Chest.* 1993;104:1833–1859.

35. DeVivo MJ. Causes and costs of spinal cord injury in the United States. *Spinal Cord.* 1997;35:809.

22

ACUTE RESPIRATORY DISTRESS SYNDROME (ARDS)

John Wright, Orna Molayeme, Paul Bellamy, and Melvin A. Welch Jr.

In giving advice, seek to help,
not to please your friend
SOLON, ANCIENT GREECE
600 BC

LEARNING OBJECTIVES

1. Describe facts, descriptions, and definitions related to acute respiratory failure and ARDS.
2. Discuss the etiology, pathophysiology, and clinical features of ARDS.
3. Discuss the management of mechanical ventilation of patients with ARDS.
4. Apply specific formulas and theory to assist in clinical decision making in the management of a patient with ARDS.
5. Apply the critical thinking skills of prioritizing, making inferences, anticipating, negotiating, communicating, decision making, and reflecting by completing exercises in case examples of ARDS.
6. Apply strategies to promote critical thinking in the respiratory care management of patients with ARDS through completion of chapter exercises and group discussion.
7. Use clinical case examples in the chapter to perform an initial patient assessment, using the clinical data presented.
8. Interpret clinical data from the case examples, including history, physical examination, lab data, radiographic data, and hemodynamic data to make recommendations for respiratory care management.

9. Develop care plans for the patients in the case examples, including recommendations for therapy, with consideration of the cost, ethical, and quality-of-life issues.
10. Communicate facts, evidence, and arguments to support evaluations and recommendations proposed in the care plan for the patient with ARDS.
11. Practice the skill of negotiating in an attempt to gain acceptance of your proposed care plan for the patient with ARDS.
12. Evaluate treatment and outcomes of interventions in order to propose changes in the care plan.
13. Describe the role of the respiratory therapist in the diagnosis, treatment, and management of ARDS.

KEY WORDS

Acute Respiratory
  Distress Syndrome
  (ARDS)
Acute Respiratory
  Failure (ARF)
Auto-PEEP
Barotrauma

Delta P
Extracorporeal
  Membrane Oxygenation
  (ECMO)
Hemodynamics
High-Frequency
  Ventilation (HFV)

Inverse Ratio Ventilation
Morbidity
Mortality
Nitric Oxide
Pressure Control
  Ventilation (PCV)
Protective Lung Strategy

Pulmonary Vascular
  Resistance (PVR)
Sepsis
Systemic Vascular
  Resistance (SVR)
Tachypnea
Volutrauma

INTRODUCTION

Acute respiratory distress syndrome (ARDS), initially described in 1967,[1] is a severe form of acute respiratory failure that has become firmly established in the medical terminology. ARDS is one of the most common diagnoses in the critical care setting, with an estimate of more than 150,000 cases occurring annually in the United States.[2] The mortality rate for ARDS appears to have declined over the last two decades from 60% to a current level of 40%.[3] Although a specific treatment has not been developed, tremendous progress has been made in understanding the pathophysiology and clinical outcomes. Even without the identification of specific new treatments, the overall mortality of ARDS has steadily improved in recent years.

Acute respiratory failure (ARF) develops when the work of breathing (WOB) is too high or gas exchange is severely impeded. Acute pulmonary edema is a form of ARF that represents a spectrum of lung injury resulting in abnormal fluid accumulation in the lung alveoli and parenchyma. The fluid accumulation is caused by acute illnesses associated with increased pulmonary venous pressure (ie, hydrostatic pulmonary edema) or acute lung injury (ALI), in which the normal barriers to fluid movements are damaged (ie, nonhydrostatic pulmonary edema).

ARDS refers to those patients with ALI who have severe gas exchange problems.[4] Severe gas exchange problems generally present themselves as ventilatory failure, hypoxic failure, or both. Ventilatory failure results in elevated $Paco_2$ levels while hypoxic failure is defined by a lower-than-normal Pao_2 level (Table 22-1).

To some extent, the pulmonary condition itself tends to indicate what type of acute respiratory failure may develop. Classical causes of acute respiratory failure (ie, atelectasis, pneumonia, and bronchospasm) are usually not associated with an alteration in the underlying pulmonary architecture. Physiologic hallmarks for these conditions include hypoxemia, reduced functional residual capacity (FRC), and a normal pulmonary vascular resistance (PVR). Fortunately, most patients with acute respiratory failure fall into the classical group and have a good prognosis. There is, however, a large population of patients who fall into the other category (ie, ARDS) of ARF.

Patients with ARDS have some similarity in physiological hallmarks such as hypoxemia and

---

TABLE 22-1   SEVERE GAS EXCHANGE PROBLEMS

VENTILATORY FAILURE	HYPOXIC FAILURE
$Paco_2$ >50 mm Hg Acute form: acidotic pH Chronic form: renal compensation	Pao_2 <60 mm Hg with an Fio_2 >0.50 **Caused by:** Ventilation/perfusion mismatch (eg, secretions, bronchospasm). Shunting (eg, edema, pneumonia, atelectasis, mucus plugs). Diffusion impairment Low Fio_2 (eg, altitude, closed-space fire). Hypercapnia on room air (eg, drug overdose). Combinations of the above.

reduced FRC. However, patients in this group usually have an elevated PVR. In contrast to the classical group, the basal pulmonary architecture is significantly destroyed in ARDS and the prognosis is less favorable.

CRITICAL CONTENT

ARDS VS. CLASSIC ARF

ARDS	Classic ARF
More severe gas exchange problems	Less severe gas exchange problems
Basal pulmonary architecture destroyed	Pulmonary architecture intact
Increased PVR	Normal PVR
Prognosis less favorable	Prognosis more favorable

ETIOLOGY

ARDS is a severe form of acute respiratory failure due to a large variety of massive, often unrelated, insults to the lung (Table 22-2). All these diverse problems are grouped together because they share a common feature: a systemic inflammatory reaction that may result in injury to the capillary endothelium and damage to pulmonary surfactant, resulting in significant changes in pulmonary mechanics and function. In spite of this common feature, a universally accepted definition of the syndrome does not exist.

The condition may be a consequence of direct pulmonary damage such as aspiration or trauma, or the indirect result of a systemic process, such as sepsis. In very general terms, ARDS refers to the acute onset of noncardiogenic pulmonary edema that is due to increased permeability of the capillary endothelium and subsequently the alveolar epithelium. In more specific terms, the term ARDS encompasses the clinical and pathophysiologic changes that take place when there is damage to the microvascular endothelium or the alveolar epithelium commonly seen in ALI. Secondary responses include an increased permeability, interstitial edema,

TABLE 22-2   RISK FACTORS FOR ALI/ARDS[5]

Primary
Pneumonia (viral, bacterial, fungal)
Aspiration of gastric contents
Pulmonary contusion
Irritant gas inhalation (eg, phosgene, cocaine, smoke, high concentrations of oxygen)
Near-drowning

Secondary
Sepsis
Prolonged systemic hypotension/shock
Pancreatitis
Drugs (salicylates, thiazides)
Sickle cell crisis
Burn injuries (chemical- or heat-induced)
Multiple trauma
Gynecologic (abruptio placentae, amniotic embolism, eclampsia)
Fulminant hepatic failure
Multiple drug transfusions

and alveolar flooding. Subsequently, gas exchange deteriorates and metabolic abnormalities occur.

PATHOPHYSIOLOGY AND RELATED THEORY

Damage to the Capillary Endothelium

Any one of the risk factors listed in Table 22-2 can initiate a systemic inflammatory process that is associated with widespread microvascular endothelial injury. When such injury occurs in the pulmonary capillaries, protein-rich fluid leaks into the pulmonary interstitium. The lymphatic system typically drains excess fluid and protein from the interstitium. Back-up drainage systems become functional if the lymphatic system is overwhelmed. However, the pulmonary capillary leakage can exceed the capacities of all drainage systems, eventually leading to alveolar flooding.

The injury process involves the release of various agents that act directly on the capillary endothelium or may affect it through immunologic mediators. For example, when gram-negative bacteremia occurs, the bacterial endotoxin does not cause endothelial damage directly; it causes neutrophils and macrophages to adhere to endothelial surfaces and release a variety of inflammatory mediators that can cause further injury. Vasoactive substances may cause pulmonary vasoconstriction, exacerbating the microvascular injury.

Among the mediators, the key players are prostaglandins, endotoxins, and interleukins. The mediators spread and intensify the situation. For example, bacterial endotoxin moves through the bloodstream, often initiating a cascade of biochemical reactions that can lead to septic shock, organ failure, and death.

The initial mediators cause the abnormal release of cytokines, small proteins that usually help the body kill bacteria. However, cytokines may cause abnormalities when they are released in large quantities. A variety of cytokines and other molecular mediators are involved in the pathogenesis of ARDS and sepsis.

Destruction of the Alveolar Epithelium

The alveolar epithelial barrier, which is relatively impermeable, can become damaged by the inflammation, further facilitating the influx of fluid, neutrophils (PMNs), and inflammatory by-products. During this process, PMN-activating cytokines such as interleukin 8 can also infiltrate the lungs. The inflammatory fluids entering alveolar and interstitial spaces can decrease lung compliance and alveoli can eventually become flooded or consolidated. Surfactant is usually impaired by the presence of inflammatory agents and protein, causing atelectasis and compromising gas exchange. The atelectasis leads to a further decrease in compliance.

Because of the injury to the pulmonary capillary endothelium, the normal vascular response to alveolar hypoxemia does not occur, contributing to excessive blood flow to nonaerated alveoli (ie, alveoli with atelectasis or consolidation). As this occurs, ventilation/perfusion mismatching and intra-

pulmonary shunting become severe. The overall result of these processes is refractory hypoxemia, stiff lungs, and respiratory distress. In addition, in some areas there is microvascular obstruction by fibrotic thrombi, aggregates of platelets, or PMNs. This results in increased deadspace if the related alveoli are spared.

For years it was believed that ARDS affected the lung in an even, diffuse manner, in part because the plain chest x-rays looked diffusely abnormal. However, recent studies[6,7] have shown that ARDS affects the lung in a patchy manner. As a result of this uneven distribution of disease process, there will be uneven distribution of inspiratory gas, resulting in ventilation/perfusion mismatching. There is also the potential of mechanical ventilation pressures to produce damage when applied to an unevenly diseased lung.

Right-to-left shunting is caused by perfusion through areas of alveolar edema and atelectasis. This progressive shunting, combined with ventilation-perfusion mismatching, causes an increased A-aO_2 gradient, which, as it progresses to the severe stages, even interferes with CO_2 elimination. As the severity of the disease increases, a higher F_{IO_2} level is required to maintain an acceptable Pa_{O_2}. Ventilation-perfusion mismatching and right-to-left shunting sometimes lead to profound arterial hypoxemia even in the face of appropriate therapy.

Areas with high V/Q result in an increased physiological deadspace. Deadspace can increase to over twice the normal level in ARDS. Increased deadspace interferes with the efficiency of CO_2 elimination and accounts for the increased arterial-end tidal CO_2 gradient seen in ARDS.

Since gravity has such a profound effect on hydrostatic pressures and the distribution of fluid in the lung, the disease process primarily affects the lower, often described as "gravity dependent," regions of the lung. The upper independent region of the lung is usually less affected.

The ARDS-affected lung can be differentiated and described according to three general regions or zones. The "healthy" (ie, upper nondependent) zone typically has adequate gas exchange but tends to become overdistended. The other two zones are less compliant, and therefore direct a relatively larger portion of the tidal volume to the healthy zone, resulting in overdistention. The "recruitable" middle zone can participate in gas exchange once a critical opening pressure is achieved, which opens the otherwise atelectatic alveoli. The third zone (ie, lower dependent) can be described as the non-aerated consolidated region of the lung, which is generally believed to be "nonrecruitable," no matter what maneuvers are applied. For the supine patient these lung zones may actually represent the anterior, midthoracic, and posterior chest. Therefore edema mostly occurs in the posterior region in the supine patient.

The concept of the three zones can help the respiratory therapist realize that only a small portion of the lung is involved in gas exchange. The

CRITICAL CONTENT

KEY FACTS ABOUT ARDS

- ARDS is a consequence of pulmonary damage either by direct means, such as by aspiration or trauma, or indirectly, as the result of a systemic process such as sepsis or pancreatitis.
- ARDS refers to the acute onset of noncardiogenic pulmonary edema due to a systemic inflammatory process that is associated with injury to the pulmonary capillaries and the release of immunologic mediators.
- Alveolar flooding leads to atelectasis and consolidation, which leads to low FRC, refractory hypoxemia, and low lung compliance.
- The disease process is patchy and uneven, not uniform as previously believed, and affected lungs can be divided into three zones: an upper nondependent zone that remains normal, a midlung zone that may be thought of as "recruitable," and a lower dependent zone that is consolidated ("nonrecruitable").

residual open portion of the lung must support the gas exchange required for the entire body. For example, the healthy zone may correlate in size to the lung of a 20-kg child, yet it is providing gas exchange for a 75-kg adult.

Exudative Phase

The exudative phase occurs during the first 3 days of ARDS. During this phase, there is damage to the pulmonary capillary endothelium, destruction of the alveolar epithelium, and an influx of inflammatory agents as described above. Hyaline membranes develop in the absence of alveolar epithelium, and type I pneumocytes are destroyed. The initial insult is marked by respiratory alkalosis and hypoxemia. The ARDS condition may be limited to the exudative phase or it may progress to the fibroproliferative phase.

Fibroproliferative Phase

Three to seven days after the onset of ARDS, a process of lung repair commences. During this period, there is a proliferation of type 2 alveolar cells, collagen formation in the interstitium, and a migration of fibroblasts into the intraalveolar exudate. This is often considered the silent stage; circulation is apparently stable and the patient appears to be doing well. However, pulmonary compliance is decreasing as fibrosis develops and the P_{AO_2}–P_{aO_2} gradient is increasing. The degree of pulmonary disability is determined by the degree of fibrosis.

Chronic Phase

A chronic (fibrotic) phase develops over the next 10 to 14 days if the inflammatory process continues. This phase includes emphysematous changes, areas of fibrosis, pulmonary vascular obliteration, and lung destruction.[5] The extent to which the pulmonary architecture is remodeled can vary greatly. Extensive fibrosis and obliteration of the pulmonary vasculature prevent the architecture from returning to normal and leave the patient who progresses to this stage with a severe respiratory disability.

POTENTIAL PHASES OF ARDS*

- Exudative phase—first 3 days: Damage to pulmonary capillary endothelium, destruction of the alveolar epithelium, and an influx of inflammatory agents
- Fibroproliferative phase—days 3 to 7: Lung repair, fibrosis develops, increasing P_{AO_2}–P_{aO_2} gradient
- Chronic phase—days 7 to 21: Emphysematous changes, areas of fibrosis, pulmonary vascular obliteration, and lung destruction; extent of damage can vary greatly

*Note: A patient's progression may stop at any point; not all ARDS cases progress to all phases described above.

Multiple Organ Dysfunction Syndrome (MODS)

Multiple organ dysfunction syndrome (MODS) refers to acute organ injuries associated with widespread systemic illness. ARDS is closely related to MODS since it often leads to or is a result of the failure of another organ. As one organ system fails, toxins and/or inflammatory factors are released systemically, placing other systems at risk for organ failure. Hence, an acute lung injury may instigate an inflammatory response, which subsequently causes additional lung injury (ie, ARDS) as well as systemic organ injury. On the other hand, a nonpulmonary condition such as pancreatitis can release inflammatory factors that lead to ARDS. Other factors that may predispose a patient to ARDS and/or MODS include high severity of the primary illness and comorbid disease. In systemic illnesses such as sepsis, ARDS is often the first sign of organ failure after circulatory dysfunction. Other organ dysfunction and failure usually come later (eg, kidney and/or liver).

CLINICAL FEATURES

Because the onset of ARDS may be sudden or insidious, any patient presenting with a predispos-

ing condition (see Table 22-2) should be viewed with a high degree of suspicion. Early clinical features include dyspnea, tachypnea, and anxiety, as well as pulmonary edema, refractory hypoxemia (ie, P_{aO_2} <60 mm Hg on F_{IO_2} ≥0.35), and a chest radiograph showing diffuse bilateral infiltrates, especially in the lower dependent lung zones. The clinical features of both hydrostatic and nonhydrostatic pulmonary edema are similar, making it difficult to differentiate between these two forms of respiratory failure. Both forms of pulmonary edema include symptoms of dyspnea, tachypnea, and anxiety. Lung compliance and lung volumes are decreased with either form.

A review of the history and physical examination can assist in the differential diagnosis. If the patient has any of the risk factors for ARDS listed in Table 22-2, a diagnosis of ARDS is more likely. Similarly, the presence of risk factors for hydrostatic pulmonary edema (eg, congestive heart failure) increase the probability that the respiratory failure is not due to ARDS (see Chapter 18 for more on hydrostatic [ie, cardiogenic] pulmonary edema).

Although chest radiographs for both forms of pulmonary edema appear similar, ARDS is more often associated with air bronchograms, a normal heart size, sparing of the costophrenic angles, and peripheral alveolar infiltrates. A more definitive differential diagnosis is often dependent upon the insertion of a pulmonary artery catheter to obtain hemodynamic measurements.

Pulmonary artery (PAP) and pulmonary artery wedge pressure (PAWP) values can differentiate cardiogenic pulmonary edema from ARDS. In cardiogenic pulmonary edema, the PAWP is increased, cardiac output (CO) is decreased, and pulmonary hypertension (if present) is secondary to pulmonary venous congestion. Thus, although there may be pulmonary hypertension, a significant pulmonary artery diastolic pressure (PAD) to wedge pressure (PAWP) gradient is nonexistent. Since there is no significant pressure drop across the lungs, there is no significant elevation of the pulmonary vascular resistance (PVR).

Conversely, in ARDS, the PAWP is usually normal, and CO is normal or increased. Pulmonary hypertension is often present in the mild to moderate range, while the pulmonary artery diastolic pressure (PAD) to wedge pressure (PAWP) gradient is usually elevated to more than 5 mm Hg, thus reflecting an elevation of the PVR.

Having said this, it is important to point out that patients receiving mechanical ventilation, especially those on positive end-expiratory pressure (PEEP), can present with misleading clinical features. Pressures obtained by the pulmonary artery catheter can misrepresent hemodynamic status because alveolar pressures may exceed capillary hydrostatic pressure in certain areas of the lung.[9] Capillary narrowing or collapse can occur, disrupting the continuous column of blood from the catheter tip to the left heart, if the pulmonary artery catheter is positioned in a vessel in which alveolar pressure is greater than capillary hydrostatic pressure. This invalidates the accuracy of the PAWP measurement. Fortunately, the catheter is balloon-tipped and flow-directed so it almost always goes to well-perfused areas.

CRITICAL CONTENT

CLINICAL PRESENTATION OF ARDS VS. CARDIO-GENIC PULMONARY EDEMA

Similarities shared between ARDS and cardiogenic pulmonary edema: Early features of dyspnea, tachypnea, refractory hypoxemia, diffuse bilateral infiltrates

Differences between ARDS and cardiogenic pulmonary edema: In ARDS, the PAWP is usually **normal** and the PVR is often **increased,** but in cardiogenic pulmonary edema, the PAWP is **increased** and the PVR is **normal**

Typical Laboratory Findings

Once the presence of gas exchange abnormalities, alveolar edema, and metabolic abnormalities have been established, ARDS is more easily identified by the parameters listed in Table 22-3.[4] Typical arterial blood gases (ABGs) will reflect the right-to-left shunting and ventilation/perfusion mismatch-

TABLE 22-3   CLINICAL FEATURES OF ARDS

1. A worsening hypoxemia as indicated by $PaO_2/FIO_2 \leq 200$, regardless of PEEP, or $PaO_2/PAO_2 < 0.2$ (or $PaO_2 < 50$ mm Hg on $FIO_2 > 0.60$)
2. Static compliance <40 mL/cm H_2O
3. Bilateral pulmonary infiltrates on chest x-ray
4. PCWP ≤ 18 mm Hg
5. No clinical evidence of elevated left atrial pressure (ie, CHF)

ing previously described. The patient's FRC will decrease because many lung units have atelectasis or are filled with fluid. Therefore the severity of the syndrome can be assessed in part by the degree of hypoxemia and tachypnea. In addition to the relationship between PaO_2 and FIO_2 previously described, the PaO_2/FIO_2 ratio can assist in the diagnosis of ARDS. A PaO_2/FIO_2 ratio <200 is a commonly accepted criterion for ARDS.

Ventilation/perfusion mismatching associated with the syndrome will result in increased dead-space ventilation. Normal physiological deadspace can be roughly estimated as 1 mL per pound of ideal body weight. For example, a 150-lb patient would have a physiological deadspace of 150 mL. The deadspace/tidal volume ratio (ie, the ratio of ineffective to effective ventilation) is normally 0.3. In ARDS this ratio (commonly referred to as V_{DS}/V_T) increases to 0.6 to 0.9.

To compensate for the increased deadspace ventilation, and for a variety of other complex reasons, a patient with ARDS will become tachypneic, often with decreasing tidal volumes. This combination of decreasing tidal volume and increasing respiratory rate may itself lead to an increased V_{DS}/V_T ratio. As the condition worsens, the respiratory rate often rises to an even higher level with a further decrease in tidal volume. This situation eventually leads to a vicious cycle of progressively less efficient ventilation, which often ultimately leads to hypercapneic respiratory failure. Clinically, this decreasing efficiency of ventilation in later stages of ARDS presents as a combination of increased minute volume, without the anticipated degree of hyperventilation (lowering of the Pa_{CO_2}). It is important to note that areas of vascular injury without alveolar injury also contribute to the increase in deadspace seen with ARDS.

At the cellular level, an inadequate oxygen supply will initiate production of excessive amounts of lactate. When cellular oxygen decreases to a critical level, normal aerobic metabolism shifts to anaerobic metabolism, in which lactate is produced. Therefore lactate serves as an indicator of the imbalance between tissue oxygen demand and supply. An elevated lactate level can be caused by hypoperfusion of tissues, significantly impaired arterial oxygen content, or both. Thus an elevated lactate level should alert the clinician to the probability of inadequate oxygenation at the cellular level.

The extent to which a patient will exhibit any or all of these findings depends on the severity of the patient's condition. Therefore early identification of the syndrome alerts the respiratory therapist to potential impending pathophysiological conditions and should invoke early intervention. The presence of an illness responsible for ALI (eg, aspiration, multisystem trauma, sepsis) combined with respiratory failure should trigger further, more detailed assessment, with ARDS in mind as a potential diagnosis.

The therapist will need to consider the physical examination data, the history of present illness (HPI), past medical history, and the aforementioned laboratory findings to differentiate ARDS from other causes of pulmonary hypertension and acute respiratory failure.

CRITICAL CONTENT

TYPICAL LAB FINDINGS WITH ARDS

- Refractory hypoxemia, Pa_{O_2}/Fi_{O_2} <200
- If patient is hypoxic, increased serum lactate present
- Reduced FRC
- Hyperventilation (early); hypoventilation (late)
- V_{DS}/V_T increases up to 0.6 to 0.9

TREATMENT AND MANAGEMENT

Because of the substantial morbidity and mortality of ARDS, recent research efforts have focused on developing new treatments and preventing the destructive pathophysiological process. New approaches include improved supportive therapy (eg, nutrition, gastrointestinal bleeding prophylaxis, venous thrombosis prevention), new mechanical ventilation modes and strategies, and new pharmacologic approaches focused on interrupting the underlying disease process. The reduced mortality seen recently undoubtedly comes from improvements in overall care delivered in ICUs by better-trained respiratory therapists, physicians, and nurses.

The medical treatment of ARDS concentrates on three major areas: 1) reversing the underlying disorder, 2) blocking the specific mechanism of injury to the alveolar-capillary membrane, and 3) providing supportive care while minimizing the pathological consequences of ALI. The first two areas of concentration attempt to prevent the development of ARDS, while the third area investigates methods to decrease morbidity and mortality once it occurs. The care plan for reversing underlying disorders can vary considerably, depending on the specific precipitating cause, and therefore will not be addressed in this chapter. However, medical treatment for the second and third major areas are described in this chapter.

Blocking the Specific Mechanism of Injury to the Alveolar-Capillary Membrane

All aspects of specific treatment are highly controversial, primarily due to the inconclusive results. It is difficult to design human studies in which the lung injury is well-defined, end points are clearly established, and other factors are highly controlled. Thus investigations have not provided a clear-cut answer to blocking the specific mechanism of injury to the alveolar-capillary membrane. However, general guidelines include 1) stabilizing neutrophils that are capable of being activated by and producing most of the potential inflammatory and toxic products associated with ALI, and 2) inactivating the toxic products. Neutrophil stabilization is addressed by neutralizing those mediators responsible for their activation, including complement, cytokines, and endotoxin. Toxic products that need inactivation include degradative proteases, oxygen-derived free radicals, arachidonic acid metabolites, and platelet activating factor.

Pharmacological Therapy

See Table 22-4 for a list of factors that can result in alveolar-capillary injury and pharmacological interventions that can possibly minimize or prevent such injury.

Supportive Care: Minimizing the Pathological Consequences of ALI

Treatment for ARDS is largely supportive. There are three major areas of supportive measures: 1) recognizing and preventing complications, 2) minimizing edema formation, and 3) maintaining tissue oxygenation while reducing exacerbating factors.

Recognizing and Preventing Complications. A primary goal of supportive care is to recognize and prevent complications. A list of potential complications for various organ systems is shown in Table 22-5. Since the lung has already been injured, an additional pulmonary complication would be defined as a secondary lung injury. Complications of this type can be categorized as nosocomial (ie, acquired

TABLE 22-4   COMMON PROBLEMS WITH ARDS AND INTERVENTIONS TO CONSIDER

FACTORS THAT CAN RESULT IN ALVEOLAR-CAPILLARY INJURY	PHARMACOLOGICAL INTERVENTION(S) TO CONSIDER

Mediators that activate polymorphonuclear leukocytes (PMNs):	General against all PMN mediators
	    Corticosteroids
	    General antiinflammatory agents
	    Prostaglandin E_1

Specific PMN mediators
    Complement
    Proinflammatory cytokines
 	
    Endotoxin
	Specific Interventions
	    Corticosteroids
	    Antiinflammatory cytokines
	    Anti-tumor necrosis factor monoclonal antibody
	    Tumor necrosis factor soluble receptor
	    Monoclonal antibodies (eg, HA-1A, E5)

Toxic products released from PMNs
    Degradative proteases
 	
    Oxygen free radicals
 	
    Arachidonic acid metabolite
    (eg, thromboxane)
 	
    Platelet activating factor (PAF)
	
	    Alpha-1 antitrypsin
	    Exogenous surfactant
	    Nitric oxide
	    Corticosteroids
	    Oxygen free radical scavengers
	    Ketoconazole
	    Prostacyclin
	    Prostaglandin E_1
	    Corticosteroids
	    Urokinase

T A B L E 2 2 - 5 **ARDS: COMPLICATIONS OF MEDICAL TREATMENT**

Pulmonary	Hematologic
Oxygen toxicity	Disseminated
Pulmonary fibrosis	intravascular
Barotrauma	coagulation (DIC)
Pulmonary emboli	Anemia
	Thrombocytopenia
Cardiac	
Low cardiac output	**Renal**
Arrhythmia	Renal failure
Hypotension	Fluid retention
Infection	**Gastrointestinal**
Sepsis	Hemorrhage
Nosocomial	Pneumoperitoneum
pneumonia	Ileus
	Gastric distention

Other
Psychiatric
Endocrine
Hepatic
Neurologic

in a hospital) or iatrogenic (ie, an adverse condition induced by treatment). Common complications to recognize and avoid include aspiration, barotrauma/volutrauma (defined later in this chapter), nosocomial infection, and oxygen toxicity. Methods for avoiding (or at least minimizing) common complications will be discussed later in this chapter.

Minimizing Edema Formation. The loss of alveolar-capillary membrane integrity allows the formation of edema in great quantities, even at low hydrostatic pressures. Therefore microvascular hydrostatic pressure, indicated by the pulmonary artery wedge pressure (PAWP), is maintained as low as possible to minimize fluid flux. Diuretics do not necessarily decrease lung water significantly. Attempts to use diuretics to decrease lung water can result in inadequate systemic circulation to the tissues. Since cardiac output plays a key role in

oxygen delivery (Do_2), administration of fluids may be indicated to preserve cardiac performance, even in the presence of wet lungs. The goal is to maintain the lowest possible PAWP that is consistent with adequate cardiac output.

The type of pulmonary edema associated with ARDS can result in the buildup of great quantities of fluid even at low driving pressures. As mentioned previously, this low-pressure-gradient edema is due to increased permeability of the alveolar-capillary membrane. To minimize fluid flux, microvascular hydrostatic pressure (ie, PAWP) is maintained at the lowest possible level. Hemodynamic monitoring becomes essential as fluid therapy is administered to maintain an adequate cardiac output in the presence of wet lungs. Diuretics can be given in an attempt to decrease alveolar fluid buildup. However, inadequate tissue perfusion (ie, at the microvascular level) is a potentially significant side effect of such diuresis. Minimizing pulmonary edema formation must therefore be carefully balanced with fluid therapy for adequate cardiac output/oxygen delivery/tissue perfusion. Patients who are hypovolemic often do not tolerate PEEP (ie, they suffer decreased cardiac output) as well as those who are euvolemic.

Several options of fluid therapy are available. However, there has been an ongoing debate whether to use colloids or crystalloids on patients with adequate hematocrit (>30%). Proponents of colloid solutions (eg, albumin) argue that they are more effective for intravascular volume expansion. These proponents also argue that gas exchange worsens when crystalloid solutions are used because much of the solution ends up in the alveoli and pulmonary interstitium. Colloidal osmotic pressure can also decrease as a result of infusions of large volumes of crystalloids.

Those favoring crystalloid therapy believe that osmotic pressure differences driving fluid into the vascular space cannot be generated, since the barriers restricting the movement of colloid from the vascular space into the lungs are not functioning normally when the lung is injured. Proponents of crystalloid therapy warn that colloid solutions may actually compound the formation of edema.

Packed red blood cells are often used when patients have a low hematocrit or a low PAWP. There is a twofold advantage to administering packed red blood cells in this scenario: packed RBCs increase the oxygen carrying capacity of the blood and they also expand intravascular volume with a product that remains in the vascular space. Administration of systemic vasodilator agents can lower systemic afterload, thus improving CO while maintaining low pulmonary vascular pressures. Inotropic agents can then be used to support blood pressure. Caution should be taken when vasodilators are used, especially in the later stages of ARDS when they can interfere with the advantages of hypoxic vasoconstriction (ie, maintaining V/Q matching by decreasing perfusion to alveoli that are not ventilated). See Table 22-6 for a list of methods to minimize edema formation.

CRITICAL CONTENT

MINIMIZING EDEMA FORMATION

- Loss of alveolar-capillary membrane integrity allows for easy formation of edema
- Goal is to maintain the lowest possible PAWP consistent with adequate CO
- Hemodynamic monitoring is essential as fluid therapy is administered in order to maintain adequate CO in the presence of wet lungs
- Ongoing debate over whether to use colloids or crystalloids
- Diuretics used for minimizing pulmonary edema must be carefully balanced with fluid therapy to maintain adequate cardiac output/oxygen delivery/tissue perfusion

Maintaining Tissue Oxygenation. With the potential threat of MODS, and tissue hypoxia in general, it is essential that adequate oxygen delivery (Do_2) be maintained in patients with ARDS. Adequate oxygen delivery can be addressed by minimizing oxygen demand and/or increasing Do_2. Strategies for minimizing oxygen demand focus on

TABLE 22-6   METHODS FOR MINIMIZING EDEMA FORMATION

- Administer fluids *but* maintain lowest possible PAWP that is consistent with an adequate cardiac output
- Respiratory therapy interventions (see Table 22-7)
- Colloids, crystalloids, packed red blood cells, vasodilators, inotropes (see pharmacological therapy section)

reducing the metabolic rate. Examples of these strategies include pain control, anxiety control, and regulation of body temperature (ie, fever control).

Since Do_2 is the product of CO and Cao_2, anything that increases either of these variables will increase Do_2. Therefore Do_2 can be increased by elevating the CO, increasing the level of hemoglobin, or increasing the amount of oxygen in the blood. CO can be elevated by supporting the cardiovascular system by means of inotropic agents and/or fluids. Cardiovascular support should avoid hypotension [ie, keep systolic BP >90 and mean arterial pressure (MAP) >60] and maintain adequate urine output.

Hemoglobin can be increased by administration of packed red blood cells and/or prevention of blood loss. The general consensus is to keep the hemoglobin level ≥10 or the hematocrit ≥30%.

CRITICAL CONTENT

MAINTAINING ADEQUATE TISSUE OXYGENATION

- Tissue oxygenation is dependent on a balance between oxygen supply and demand
- **Minimize demand** (minimize metabolic rate): Strategies include pain, anxiety, and fever control
- **Optimize supply** (optimize Do_2): Strategies include optimizing CO (inotropics/fluids) and optimizing Cao_2 (Hb, Pao_2)

Conventional as well as new, nontraditional respiratory therapy strategies for increasing the level of oxygen will be discussed in detail later in the chapter.

Supplemental Oxygen.　In the early stages of ARDS, the patient is likely to require supplemental oxygen due to the effects that pulmonary edema has on gas exchange. However, a correlation between ARDS and need for supplemental oxygen may not be obvious in the earliest stage of the syndrome. The patient most likely will appear mildly hypoxemic, will require minimal oxygen therapy (eg, nasal cannula), and the development of ARDS may not be easily foreseen.

The patient's respiratory rate and oxygen requirements will increase as the level of respiratory distress increases. Oxygen should be titrated according to the patient's clinical status. Oxygen titration in this setting usually leads to the use of high-flow systems.

Increasing the FIO_2 is the simplest method of achieving adequate oxygenation. If, however, the primary cause of hypoxemia is shunting within the lung, supplemental oxygen alone will not correct the hypoxemia. The goal is to obtain adequate oxygenation with the lowest possible FIO_2 to avoid the toxic effects of high levels of oxygen.

Oxygen toxicity can lead to lung injury if high levels of supplemental oxygen (ie, $FIO_2 > 0.60$) are administered for more than 24 hours. Oxygen toxicity can worsen lung fibrosis and the ARDS condition. In addition, the time required for lung injury to occur decreases as the FIO_2 is increased above 0.60. Therefore respiratory therapy interventions that can decrease the FIO_2 should be considered as soon as the risk of oxygen toxicity becomes high. On the other hand, one should never let concern for oxygen toxicity lead one to tolerate inadequate oxygen delivery or tissue oxygenation.

In the early stages of ARDS, supplemental oxygen may be the only form of respiratory therapy required. However, the pathophysiological effects of fully developed ARDS result in stiff, noncompliant lungs, leading to an increased WOB, progressive refractory hypoxemia, and possibly respiratory failure. The patient should therefore be monitored for tachypnea, dyspnea, progressive hypoxemia (eg, with pulse oximetry), and other indicators of impending respiratory failure. See Table 22-7 for a list of respiratory therapy interventions used for ARDS.

Conventional Mechanical Ventilation.　If the patient's clinical condition deteriorates further and respiratory failure develops, then intubation and invasive mechanical ventilation is indicated. In ARDS, the WOB may consume 25% to 50% of the body's total oxygen consumption ($\dot{V}O_2$) (normal range is 2% to 5%). Mechanical ventilation can reduce the WOB, allowing redirection of oxygenated blood from respiratory muscles to vital organs. An additional result of this increased WOB in these critically ill patients is increased carbon dioxide production due to an elevated metabolic rate from the additional muscle expenditure of energy. As a result, patients with ARDS often require an increased minute ventilation just to maintain normocapnia.

The relatively larger tidal volumes provided by mechanical ventilation can increase oxygenation by improving the V/Q matching (ie, by ventilating areas of the lung that were not adequately ventilated during spontaneous respirations). The more efficient movement of gas can assist with the removal of CO_2 as well, improving ABG results. Conventional mechanical ventilation (Table 22-8) has traditionally been adjusted to deliver large tidal volumes (ie, 10 to 15 mL/kg) to prevent hypoxemia and the development of atelectasis. Conventional mechanical ventilation settings were chosen to achieve normal ABGs by providing tidal volumes and respiratory rates well tolerated by the structurally normal lung.

In the conventional volume assist-control mode, the patient receives the set VT each time the ventilator is triggered. Therefore the total respiratory rate dictates the minute ventilation whenever the set respiratory rate is below the total respiratory rate. For example, if the patient's respiratory drive causes him or her to breathe at a total respiratory rate of 24, any respiratory rate setting from 1 to 24 will yield the same minute ventilation. The primary

TABLE 22-7 RESPIRATORY THERAPY INTERVENTIONS FOR ARDS

INADEQUATE OXYGENATION/VENTILATION	RESPIRATORY THERAPY INTERVENTION
Oxygen delivery	Supplemental O_2 (nonintubated patients)
	Optimization of ventilator pressure settings (protective lung strategy)
	Prone positioning
	Nitric oxide
	Surfactant
	Partial liquid ventilation
	Extracorporeal membrane oxygenation (ECMO)
	Possibly one or more of the other interventions listed below
Impending respiratory failure	NPPV
	Conventional mechanical ventilation
	Supplemental O_2 (nonintubated patients)
	Optimization of ventilator pressure settings (protective lung strategy)
	Possibly one or more of the other interventions listed above
V/Q mismatch	Supplemental O_2 (nonintubated patients)
	Optimization of ventilator pressure settings (protective lung strategy)
	Prone positioning
	Surfactant
	NPPV
	Conventional mechanical ventilation
	Possibly any of the other interventions listed above
Oxygen consumption	Possibly one of more of the interventions listed above
Increased work of breathing	Supplemental O_2 (nonintubated patients)
	Optimization of ventilator pressure settings (protective lung strategy)
	NPPV
	Conventional mechanical ventilation
	Possibly one or more of the other interventions listed above
Pulmonary hypertension	Nitric oxide
Vascular leakage	Minimize tidal volume and minute ventilation
	Optimization of ventilator pressure settings (protective lung strategy)
	Permissive hypercapnia
Barotrauma/volutrauma	Optimization of ventilator pressure settings (protective lung strategy)
	Permissive hypercapnia (protective lung strategy)

TABLE 22-8   TRADITIONAL CONVENTIONAL VENTILATOR SETTINGS

- An FIO_2 that provides a PaO_2 >60 mm Hg
- Tidal volumes of 10 to 15 mL/kg
- Volume ventilation in the assist-control (a/c) mode
- Respiratory rate of 12 to 20 bpm
- A PEEP level that assists in improving oxygenation when FIO_2 alone is not generating a PaO_2 >60 mm Hg

function of the set respiratory rate in this situation is to serve as a backup rate in case the patient becomes fatigued or stops initiating breaths for any reason (ie, sedation, paralysis).

As with supplemental oxygen systems, increasing the FIO_2 is the simplest method for improving oxygen delivery during mechanical ventilation. The goal is to obtain adequate oxygen delivery with the lowest possible FIO_2 in order to avoid the detrimental effects of oxygen toxicity.

Positive end-expiratory pressure (PEEP) can be used to further improve oxygenation by increasing the FRC. The FRC is increased as collapsed or unstable alveoli are recruited by the end-expiratory pressure. When collapsed alveoli are opened up and ventilated, shunting is reduced, resulting in improved oxygenation. This process does not actually reduce edema, but shifts it out of the alveolar space to the interstitium, allowing for better gas exchange. If hypoxemia requires the FIO_2 to be increased toward the toxic range (ie, an FIO_2 >0.60), PEEP should be considered.

Optimizing the Pressure-Volume Relationship.
When Ashbaugh and colleagues initially described ARDS in 1967,[1] large tidal volumes and high levels of PEEP (ie, the conventional approach) were recommended to recruit collapsed alveoli. It has been known for many years, however, that mechanical ventilation itself can damage the lung.[11] High inspiratory pressures and large tidal volumes can lead to overinflation of healthy alveoli, which over time can result in barotrauma.[12] Conversely, if the

PEEP is set too low, lung injury can occur because alveoli are allowed to collapse and reopen during each respiratory cycle,[13] creating excessive shear forces.[14]

The complications associated with conventional mechanical ventilation (eg, volutrauma and O_2 toxicity) can potentially be minimized by utilizing various nonconventional mechanical ventilation strategies. Recent studies[15,16] describe the heterogenous pulmonary pathology seen in ARDS and have demonstrated that alveolar overdistention is responsible for much of the iatrogenic damage during mechanical ventilation, not elevated airway pressures. Hence the term "volutrauma" is probably more appropriate to describe this damage than the long-used term, "barotrauma."

During conventional ventilation, the well-aerated healthy (ie, upper, independent) lung zone probably receives most of the tidal volume, often resulting in alveolar overdistention. Tidal volumes closer to the physiologic norm (ie, 5 to 7 mL/kg) are more appropriate for patients with ARDS.[17] By delivering smaller tidal volumes, volutrauma is less likely to occur.

Pressure control ventilation (PCV) offers several potential advantages over volume ventilation with regard to treatment of ARDS (Table 22-9). A longer inspiratory time and a decelerating flow pattern allow for better gas distribution. In addition,

TABLE 22-9   ADVANTAGES OF PRESSURE CONTROL VENTILATION OVER VOLUME VENTILATION[22]

- PIP is limited
- Inspiratory time is adjustable
- A longer inspiratory time often provides better gas distribution and exchange
- A decelerating flow pattern allows for rapid flow at the onset of inspiration when the delivered gas is traveling through the larger airways and a tapering flow as the delivered gas approaches increasingly smaller airways at the end of inspiration

PCV is ideal for optimizing the pressure-volume relationship because changes in volume can be observed as the therapist adjusts airway pressures.

The pressure-volume relationship can be optimized by using a protective lung strategy. Ventilation is optimized with a protective lung strategy by attempting to obtain complete alveolar recruitment. The technique consists of two basic interventions: 1) open the lung through alveolar recruitment and 2) stabilize the lung by keeping it open.

Pressure control ventilation is ideal for applying a protective lung strategy because airway pressures and inspiratory time can be regulated. In addition, the rapid initial inspiratory flow rate enables the ventilator to achieve the desired pressure level quickly, minimizing the time during which the alveoli are exposed to lower pressure levels that might make them collapse. This rapid initial inspiratory flow also appears useful at meeting high inspiratory flow demands generated by the patient, thus increasing the probability of patient synchronization and comfort.

A protective lung strategy is based on setting the PEEP at or slightly above the lungs' lower inflection point (LIP) to prevent alveolar collapse and to minimize injury from repeated opening and closing (Fig. 22-1).[10] The delta P (ie, the inspiratory pressure level involved in delivering a tidal volume) is then adjusted to a level at or below the lungs' upper inflection point (UIP) to minimize overdistention of lung units.

To determine the LIP and UIP, a static pressure-volume curve is required. To obtain a static condition, no flow of air can be present, therefore sedation may be required to create such a situation. The LIP can be obtained by slowly increasing the PEEP from 0 cm H_2O until a disproportionate increase in volume occurs (hence only pressure ventilation should be used). The sudden rise in volume correlates with the PEEP reaching a critical minimum pressure, resulting in extensive alveolar recruitment. By setting the PEEP at or slightly above this point, massive alveolar collapse will be minimized, significantly enhancing oxygenation and ventilation.

In a similar fashion the UIP is obtained by slowly decreasing the peak inspiratory pressure (PIP) from approximately 30 or 40 cm H_2O until a sudden, yet significant, decrease in volume occurs. The UIP represents the point above which additional pressure does not significantly further open the lung. Above the UIP, overdistention is very likely to occur. By adjusting the PIP to a level just below the UIP, the respiratory therapist is maximizing the tidal volume while simultaneously avoiding overdistention.

Although the static pressure-volume loop can be drawn on paper by plotting the volumes associated with various pressure levels, a real time

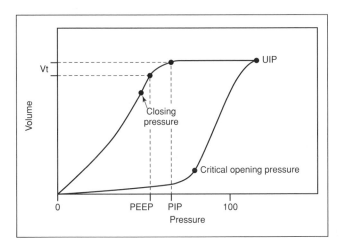

FIGURE 22-1 An inspiratory static pressure-volume curve indicates two inflection points: the critical opening pressure (also referred to as the lower inflection point or LIP) and the upper inflection point (UIP). The LIP represents the critical opening pressure of a great number of alveoli and the UIP reflects near-maximal lung volumes, a point beyond which further increases in pressure yield only minimal increases in volume (ie, beyond this point overdistention occurs). Traditional tidal volumes of 10 to 15 mL/kg tend to exceed the UIP, leading to overdistention. To minimize chances of volutrauma, tidal volumes should be set below the UIP but above the closing pressure, the point where a small decrease in pressure leads to a sudden and significant drop in volume. During ARDS, PEEP applied at levels above the LIP may minimize lung injury due to shear forces by preventing end-expiratory alveolar collapse.[10]

pressure-volume graphical display is preferred. Ventilation can be optimized much faster by observing real time pressure and volume waveforms as adjustments are made. Keep in mind that a truly static pressure-volume curve can only be obtained when flow is zero. Verify zero flow by means of the flow waveform or a digital flow measurement.

CRITICAL CONTENT

OPTIMIZING THE LUNG PRESSURE-VOLUME RELATIONSHIP: PROTECTIVE LUNG STRATEGY

While the patient is on pressure control ventilation: Set the PEEP at or slightly above the lungs' lower inflection point (LIP) to prevent alveolar collapse and minimize injury from repeated opening and closing. Set the peak pressure at or below the lungs' upper inflection point (UIP) to minimize overdistention of lung units.

Various Forms of Pressure Ventilation. There are various forms of pressure ventilation available to choose from. Each of them has at one time or another been advocated for use on patients with ARDS. The most recognized form is pressure control ventilation (PCV). This pressure-limited, time-cycled mode is available on most modern microprocessor ventilators. It can be used much like traditional volume assist-control ventilation, the primary difference being the need to monitor for fluctuations in tidal volume as the patient's condition changes over time. The potential advantages of PCV over traditional volume-based ventilation in ARDS have been previously discussed. What follows is a brief introduction to some variations in use of pressure-based modes of ventilation that have at various times been advocated for use on patients with ARDS.

High-Frequency Ventilation (HFV). Another form of pressure ventilation is high-frequency ventilation (HFV). This form of pressure ventilation involves a significant decrease in delta P and hence

tidal volume (eg, ≤3 to 5 mL/kg), and a simultaneous increase in the set respiratory rate (eg, 90 to 300 breaths per minute [bpm]). Usually, with high respiratory rates gas movement via diffusion occurs higher in the respiratory tract, minimizing deadspace and allowing gas exchange to occur at smaller tidal volumes. As in traditional pressure ventilation, most alveolar recruitment is achieved by setting the PEEP at or slightly above the LIP. Overdistention in HFV is less likely since peak airway pressures are significantly lower (ie, well below the UIP).

High-frequency positive pressure ventilation (HFPPV) and high-frequency jet ventilation (HFJV) are two variations of high-frequency ventilation used on adult patients. HFPPV utilizes respiratory rates of 60 to 100 bpm with tidal volumes of 3 to 5 mL/kg. This form of high-frequency ventilation can be administered through a conventional ventilator. HFJV is usually delivered by means of a special ventilator in conjunction with a conventional ventilator. Respiratory rates of 100 to 150 bpm and tidal volumes of 1 to 4 mL/kg are often used during HFJV.

High-frequency oscillation (HFO) is predominantly used on neonatal patients. This system varies significantly from HFPPV and HFJV. High-frequency oscillation is delivered at a rate of 100 to 3000 cycles per minute. Tidal volumes are lower than normal physiologic deadspace volume. Some HFOs employ active exhalation, whereby a volume of gas is actually "sucked out" of the patient during the expiratory phase. Detailed discussion of these highly specialized forms of mechanical ventilation is beyond the scope or intent of this chapter. The reader is referred to the medical literature for more specific details.

Inverse Ratio Ventilation (IRV). If adequate oxygenation is not achieved with conventional PCV, inverse ratio ventilation (IRV) is sometimes initiated (PC-IRV). In an attempt to improve oxygenation, the inspiratory time is extended, exceeding the time allocated for expiratory time. For example, the inspiratory:expiratory ratio (I:E) in conventional ventilation is greater than 1:2, while an I:E ratio in

IRV might be 2:1 or 3:1. The result is air trapping at the end of expiration. The pressure generated by this effect is called auto-PEEP and has a PEEP-like effect on FRC and oxygenation. Since the inverse I:E ratio is not natural and is quite uncomfortable, patients usually require heavy sedation with or without paralysis. Anecdotally, PC-IRV may be helpful in maintaining gas exchange when other more conventional approaches fail; however, it must be used with considerable caution.

This approach to ventilation should only be attempted by very experienced clinicians, who can rapidly recognize and respond to the potential side effects. Decreased cardiac output due to air trapping (auto-PEEP effect) and volutrauma are potential serious complications. These complications are most likely to occur as the disease process begins to reverse and the lungs become more compliant. Therefore PC-IRV should not be used without an experienced care team. It is also recommended that a pulmonary artery catheter be utilized in these situations to monitor cardiac output and oxygen delivery during these potentially risky procedures.

Airway Pressure Release Ventilation (APRV). APRV is similar to IRV in the sense that ventilation can occur at lower peak airway pressures. The I:E ratio is often inverse as in IRV. However, during APRV the patient breathes spontaneously from the circuit while the ventilator fluctuates between two separate CPAP levels. Tidal volume is augmented by the higher CPAP level. Pressure is then periodically dropped to the lower CPAP level, facilitating the elimination of CO_2 and reducing mean airway pressure.

The amount of time spent at each CPAP level is adjustable. Like IRV, expiratory time (ie, time spent at the lower CPAP level) is usually kept short to minimize the loss of FRC. Since patients can breathe spontaneously, they may tolerate APRV better than IRV. Oxygenation may be the result of auto-PEEP (ie, end-expiratory pressure caused by breath stacking).

CRITICAL CONTENT

Pressure ventilation can take various forms:
- PCV—The standard, basic form of pressure ventilation
- HFV—Numerous subtypes exist (HFPPV, HFJV, HFO)
- PC-IRV—PCV with inverse I:E ratios (use with caution!)
- APRV—Allows spontaneous ventilation with fluctuating baseline pressures; interesting concept, but there is little published support for its use

Optimizing Oxygenation of the Ventilator Patient. It is important to note that in the advanced stages of ARDS, ABGs and pulse oximetry cannot be effectively used to assess tissue oxygenation because they do not account for the complex hemodynamic conditions that often exist at this stage of disease. Therefore, for a respiratory therapist to advocate attempts to optimize tissue oxygenation, he or she must understand and utilize the following equations:

Oxygen delivery

Do_2 = cardiac output × arterial O_2 content × 10

= cardiac output × [(1.34 × Hb × Sao_2) + (0.003 × Pao_2)] × 10

Normal Do_2 = 640 to 1400 mL/min

Oxygen consumption (oxygen uptake)

$\dot{V}o_2$ = cardiac output × arterial-venous difference in O_2 content × 10

= cardiac output × {[1.34 × Hb × (Sao_2 − $S\bar{v}o_2$)] + (0.003 × Pao_2)} × 10

Normal $\dot{V}o_2$ = 180 to 280 mL/min

The metabolic requirements of the tissue determines $\dot{V}_{O_2}$, unless D_{O_2} falls below this level, at which time $\dot{V}_{O_2}$ is directly dependent upon D_{O_2}[18] (Fig. 22-2). Figure 22-2 shows the relationship between D_{O_2} and $\dot{V}_{O_2}$. The slope on the graph represents the situation in which an increase in $\dot{V}_{O_2}$ is directly related to an increase in D_{O_2}. Through use of various techniques (eg, transfusion, inotropic agents, increasing the F_{IO_2} and/or PEEP) the D_{O_2} should be increased until it reaches the plateau level, when the relationship changes. In the plateau region of the graph, significant increases in D_{O_2} are matched with, at best, trivial incremental increases in $\dot{V}_{O_2}$. Tissue oxygenation, therefore, is optimized at the top of the slope just as the graph plateaus. There is in effect nothing more to be gained by further increases in D_{O_2} once the plateau is reached. $\dot{V}_{O_2}$ and D_{O_2} can be maximized by 1) volume expansion, 2) transfusion, 3) inotropic drugs, or 4) various manipulations of the mechanical ventilator (discussed previously).

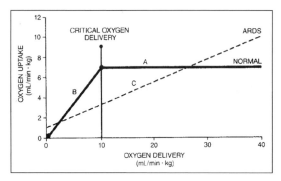

FIGURE 22-2 Graph of D_{O_2} versus $\dot{V}_{O_2}$. Under normal conditions, oxygen uptake (ie, consumption) is optimized at the plateau level (A).[18] Increases in oxygen delivery are not required (and usually do not occur) after the point of critical oxygen delivery. Prior to achieving the point of critical oxygen delivery (B), oxygen uptake is directly dependent upon increases in oxygen delivery. During ARDS (C), higher levels of oxygen delivery are required to accommodate higher-than-normal levels of oxygen uptake. A plateau and the point of critical oxygen delivery may not exist or may exist at very high levels of oxygen delivery and uptake. The elevated requirement for oxygen delivery is due to impaired oxygen extraction, which implies that tissue hypoxia is present. Tissue hypoxia may predispose the patient to MODS.

If a pulmonary artery catheter is not available, optimization of oxygenation becomes more difficult. In such a situation, hemodynamic compromise should be prevented by ensuring that blood pressure is adequate (ie, systolic blood pressure >90 mm Hg and mean blood pressure is >60 mm Hg), urine output is adequate, and lactic acidosis does not develop. However, these noninvasive measures are not always reliable indicators of the adequacy of CO.

Ideal monitoring would involve an accurate tissue oxygenation measurement. Until such technology is developed, tissue oxygenation should be optimized by the previously described method. However, even once tissue oxygen assessment is available, new questions arise (eg, which tissue[s] should be measured) because CO may be heterogeneously distributed.

Additional Treatment and Management Strategies

Research and clinical experience have produced additional strategies for the treatment and management of ARDS. New strategies include the administration of a nontraditional medical gas such as nitric oxide and prone positioning of the patient. The following strategies provide additional options for your clinical approach to treating the patient with ARDS.

Nitric Oxide. There are two reasons for using nitric oxide (NO) in ARDS: 1) as a selective vasodilator, inhaled NO can dilate the pulmonary circulation but not the systemic circulation (this is due to its very rapid inactivation by hemoglobin) and 2) inhaled NO should selectively dilate **only** the areas of the pulmonary vasculature that are in contact with ventilated alveoli (avoiding an increase in blood flow through capillaries perfusing shunted alveoli). The overall effect should be a reduction in pulmonary artery pressure and an increase in arterial oxygenation.

A decrease in pulmonary arterial pressure is noted in patients with reactive pulmonary vessels within seconds of the inhalation of NO. As such, inhaled NO seems to be a very good test of vaso-responsiveness in patients with primary pulmonary hypertension. Pulmonary vasodilation ceases within minutes of its discontinuation.

Inspired concentrations of 5 to 80 parts per million (ppm) have decreased pulmonary artery pressure in adults.[19] However, Bigatello and colleagues[20] showed that a lower mean pulmonary artery pressure and a higher Pao_2 occurred when 2 to 20 ppm was inhaled. The inspired concentration of NO is measured by either a chemiluminescence or an electrochemical analyzer. Rossaint and co-workers[21] also showed that systemic oxygenation improves with the administration of NO.

A positive response is usually defined as an increase in Pao_2/Fio_2 of >20%. However, patients may be variably responsive to NO inhalation at different times during their clinical course. The lack of success at any one time does not preclude a beneficial response several days later. In addition, the hemodynamic and respiratory effects of NO may occur at different dose ranges. The concentration of inspired NO is adjusted to cause the desired effect and then slowly reduced as the patient's condition improves. Rapid withdrawal of inhaled NO can result in hypoxemia and hemodynamic insufficiency. Therefore gradual discontinuation (weaning) is advised.

Side effects associated with NO include the formation of nitrogen dioxide (NO_2) and methemoglobin. The rate of conversion of NO to NO_2 is directly proportional to the square of the NO concentration, the residence time of NO in oxygen, and the Fio_2. Therefore, there is an incentive to lower the dose and duration of NO and lower the Fio_2. NO_2 is highly toxic to the respiratory epithelium, and pulmonary edema usually follows several hours later. NO combines with hemoglobin to form methemoglobin. A level of <3% is usually accepted in the clinical setting.

Certain safety measures should be taken to minimize unnecessary complications. Scavenging exhaled gas, monitoring NO and NO_2 levels, and obtaining a daily methemoglobin measurement should be performed. A scavenger system can be implemented to prevent exposure of caretakers to

TABLE 22-10   VARIABLES AFFECTING THE EFFICACY OF NITRIC OXIDE IN THE TREATMENT OF ARDS[22]

- Timing: early vs. late
- Primary vs. secondary forms of lung injuries
- Dose
- Responders vs. nonresponders

the gas by incorporating a suction system or absorption system into the expiratory side of the circuit.

Before working with NO, the clinician should be familiar with the hazards of using this gas. Also, when using NO to treat ARDS, certain variables can affect the success of the treatment (Table 22-10).

Prospective randomized trials have had variable results. Patients with high pulmonary vascular resistance seem to benefit the most from NO. Recent studies have shown that NO is associated with significant improvement in oxygenation and hemodynamics, but not with survival or number of days of intubation. In fact, the beneficial effect of NO inhalation may only last for 48 hours.[22]

Inhaled NO remains a treatment for ARDS with uncertain promise. However, due to the many uncertainties usually associated with an experimental drug, NO should be used with guarded caution. In the absence of clear benefit in randomized controlled trials, the use of NO remains experimental.

CRITICAL CONTENT

INHALED NITRIC OXIDE

- Inspired concentrations of 5 to 80 ppm of NO selectively vasodilates the pulmonary vasculature, which improves V/Q and therefore oxygenation, and reduces pulmonary hypertension.
- Concentration should be adjusted to cause the desired effect, then slowly reduced as the patient's condition improves.

- Gradual weaning is advised to avoid adverse hypoxemic and hemodynamic responses.
- Side effects of NO include formation of NO_2 and methemoglobin.
- Benefits of NO are unclear in randomized controlled trials, and its use remains experimental.

Permissive Hypercapnia.   Another approach to minimize or avoid the complications of volutrauma and oxygen toxicity is through the practice of permissive hypercapnia. In general, permissive hypercapnia is a clinical strategy that allows the $Paco_2$ to increase above normal values, provided the pH is within a specified range. The intent is to provide adequate oxygenation and minimize the risk of volutrauma by accepting a level of hypoventilation that is felt to be safely tolerated by the human body.

Permissive hypercapnia is often initiated when the PIP is >40 cm H_2O. In such a situation, the PIP is lowered to <40 cm H_2O (by lowering tidal volume if in a volume mode) and the $Paco_2$ is allowed to climb. Increases in $Paco_2$ to levels as high as 65 to 80 mm Hg are sometimes achieved. The degree of hypoventilation is considered acceptable as long

CRITICAL CONTENT

PERMISSIVE HYPERCAPNIA

- Permissive hypercapnia is a clinical strategy that allows the $Paco_2$ to increase above normal values provided the pH is within an acceptable range (eg, >7.25).
- The acidosis is often corrected over time by renal compensation or through administration of sodium bicarbonate.
- Sedation and paralysis are often required.
- It is contraindicated in patients with hemodynamic instability or increased ICP.

as the pH is >7.25. The acidosis is often corrected in several days by either renal compensation[23] or administration of sodium bicarbonate. Sedation and paralysis are often required. Permissive hypercapnia is contraindicated in patients who have hemodynamic instability or increased intracranial pressure (ICP).

Surfactant.   Surfactant is the endogenous substance that decreases alveolar surface tension and prevents atelectasis. Surfactant function has long been known to be defective in ARDS. Evidence that surfactant therapy improves the outcome in ARDS is not very convincing. For example, nebulized surfactant has been shown to be ineffective. However, in an animal model, a combination of surfactant and nitric oxide was more effective in treating ARDS than either treatment alone.[24] The results of larger clinical trials will be needed to clarify the role of surfactant therapy in treating ARDS.

Partial Liquid Ventilation.   Partial liquid ventilation involves the use of a traditional mechanical ventilator as well as instillation of perfluorocarbon (PFC) liquid into the lungs. The PFC is instilled to the point of filling up the lungs to their functional residual capacity. This is determined by seeing the liquid at the level of the airway just at the end of exhalation. A standard ventilator can be attached to the airway to provide some tidal ventilation. The evaporation of the PFC must be matched with periodic additional instillation of the liquid into the lungs. Full liquid ventilation requires a special ventilator system and is beyond the scope of our brief review in this chapter.

In animal models, partial liquid ventilation with small volumes of PFC improved gas exchange and increased survival time in experimental ARDS.[25,26] The improvements observed in gas exchange have been attributed to a higher V/Q ratio due to recruitment of atelectatic alveoli, displacement of alveolar exudate by the PFC mixture, and redistribution of the blood flow to the regions with increased ventilation.

In patients with ARDS, partial liquid ventilation appears to be a promising alternative therapy.

Recommendations regarding the use of partial liquid ventilation for the treatment of ARDS are pending the results of ongoing, multicenter clinical trials.

Extracorporeal Membrane Oxygenation (ECMO). ECMO is an alternative form of treatment that does not necessarily involve mechanical ventilation. ECMO utilizes a system that is similar to the cardiopulmonary bypass equipment used for open heart surgeries. A large portion of the patient's cardiac output circulates through an artificial lung where CO_2 is removed and oxygen added. Since ventilation and oxygenation are occurring in the artificial lung, mechanical ventilation is decreased to minimize its associated complications such as barotrauma. A recent study showed successful treatment of ARDS with high survival rates.[27] As with the other alternative forms of therapy for ARDS being briefly reviewed here, more research is needed to confirm the proper role of ECMO in the treatment of ARDS.

Prone Positioning. It has been proposed that patients with ARDS can benefit from being repositioned, due to the heterogeneous distribution of lung injury. By positioning the patient in the prone position, the well-ventilated healthy (ie, upper, nondependent) lung zone becomes dependent. Some patients have improvement in ventilation/perfusion matching while others do not. All patients with ARDS who have been repositioned need specialized nursing care. The labor involved can become cost-prohibitive because the benefits of repositioning are often transient, requiring routine repositioning. Recommendations regarding the use of prone positioning for the treatment of ARDS are pending the results of clinical trials.

APPLYING CONCEPTS TO COMMON PROBLEMS

In general, the most common problems with ARDS include reversing the underlying disorder, blocking the mechanism of alveolar capillary injury, and minimizing the pathological consequences of ALI through supportive measures. More specifically, common problems associated with or observed during supportive measures include inadequatee tissue oxygenation, increased WOB, ventilation-perfusion mismatch, pulmonary hypertension, alveolar-capillary membrane injury, pulmonary edema, and impending respiratory failure. Refer to Tables 22-4, 22-6, and 22-7 for the list of interventions to consider.

In addition to the above common problems, there are three specific ones that will be briefly discussed below: vascular leakage, barotrauma/volutrauma, and ventilator-associated pneumonia.

Vascular Leakage. There are two categories of pulmonary arterioles: alveolar blood vessels and extraalveolar blood vessels. The alveolar blood vessels surround and come into contact with the alveolar walls. The pressure exerted on these vessels is equal to the pressure exerted on the alveoli.

Extraalveolar vessels are influenced by pressures like the pleural pressure that leads to alveolar expansion. While the alveolar vessels are compressed by the expansion of the alveoli during positive pressure ventilation (PPV), the extraalveolar vessels expand with the lung. PPV causes the pressure inside the extraalveolar vessels to exceed the pressure outside the vessels as the lungs expand and contract. This causes vascular leakage into the pulmonary spaces. As a result, fluid accumulates in the pulmonary extracellular spaces, which is a major complication of ARDS that is enhanced by PPV.

The amount of vascular leakage is directly related to the size of the tidal volume from PPV.[28] The leakage occurs whether the volume is delivered by high or low peak pressures.[29] Based on these findings, the clinician should keep tidal volumes and minute ventilation to a minimum. This provides theoretical support for approaches to mechanical ventilation such as permissive hypercapnia and pressure ventilation with low tidal volumes as described previously.

Barotrauma/Volutrauma. Barotrauma/volutrauma is a common problem when treating ARDS. Because the ARDS-affected lung has a heterogeneous quality (see pathophysiology section), the independent (upper) regions of the lung tend to be more compliant than lower, more involved areas, and therefore predispose these more compliant areas to be overdistended and subject to barotrauma/volutrauma. Refer to Table 22-7 for recommended interventions.

Ventilator-Associated Pneumonia (VAP). Chastre and colleagues[30] showed that microbiologically provable VAP occurs far more often in patients with ARDS than in other ventilated patients. Because ARDS patients are treated with antibiotics early in the course of their syndrome, the onset of a VAP is frequently delayed after the first week of mechanical ventilation, and it is usually caused by methicillin-resistant *Staphylococcus aureus* (MRSA) and other multidrug-resistant organisms. Refer to Table 22-7 for recommended interventions.

CONSIDERATION OF COSTS AND ETHICAL ISSUES

Cost considerations for the management of ARDS are virtually impossible to ascertain for the same reason that the mortality statistics differ significantly: the heterogeneity of the disease and the lack of a consistent definition of ARDS. Although 150,000 cases of ARDS were reported last year in the United States alone, an estimate of foreign cases is not obtainable.[31]

There continues to be difficulty in establishing a precise definition of ARDS, because this syndrome occurs in a heterogeneous group of patients. Differences within the patient population may account for variations in outcomes. For example, the etiologies of ARDS and the definition itself may not be the same at a community hospital and a university medical center.[32]

Insurance companies, Medicare, and Medicaid pay for most of the care provided to patients with ARDS. Both expensive (eg, pharmacological agents) as well as inexpensive solutions have had limited success in treating ARDS. Until a standardized approach is developed, a reasonable system for measuring and controlling the costs of

ARDS is unlikely to be possible.[33] Respiratory therapists can help control the costs of care by being aware of the various alternative forms of treatment, sharing knowledge with other clinicians, and avoiding the use of inappropriate and unnecessary clinical strategies.

An ethical issue commonly associated with ARDS is terminal weaning. Due to the high mortality rate, life support equipment is often intentionally withdrawn when a situation becomes hopeless. The type of care (ie, aggressive vs. palliative) provided should correlate with the likelihood of death versus the desire for life-sustaining treatment (Fig. 22-3).

The respiratory therapist should be fully aware of terminal weaning plans and should interact with the family accordingly. Most terminal weaning protocols alternate between sedating the patient and incrementally withdrawing support from the mechanical ventilator. For example, the set respiratory rate is decreased from 12 to 8 bpm. At a designated time or if the patient becomes distressed,

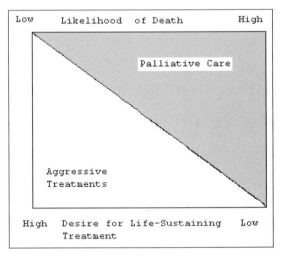

FIGURE 22-3 The balance between aggressive treatments and palliative care depends upon the likelihood of death and the desire for life-sustaining treatments. If the likelihood of death is low, the desire for life-sustaining treatments is usually high. If the likelihood of death increases, the need for palliative care increases and the need for aggressive treatments decreases. The balance, of course, changes with the status of the patient.

sedation is administered. The respiratory rate is again decreased and followed by a higher level of sedation. As this process continues, the patient's respiratory drive is diminished, along with any discomfort or agitation. Once the family has agreed to the terminal weaning process, the aforementioned technique should transpire over a relatively short period of time.

Respiratory therapists may have difficulty dealing with terminal weaning from an emotional standpoint or due to religious beliefs. The respiratory therapy supervisor should consider such factors when the work assignment is made.

The treatment of ARDS presents other ethical dilemmas and cost issues. For example, potentially effective interventions such as monoclonal antibodies and partial liquid ventilation are available; however, they are presently experimental and require that a consent be administered. In addition, they are very expensive and labor intensive. Therefore some of the ethical questions raised by these facts are: Do we provide this therapy for all patients with ARDS? and How does an institution decide who will receive these advanced forms of treatment? The standard cost question is: Who will pay for these expensive interventions? From a scientific and financial standpoint, the medical community should ask itself whether it is worth investing in a potentially advantageous new intervention. In other words, will clinical advancements eventually offset the financial investment in terms of both improvement of patient care and cost effectiveness?

A good example of a relatively new but very expensive therapy for which we are searching for appropriate guidelines for use is inhaled nitric oxide. At the time of this writing, nitric oxide has been approved for use in neonates (≥ 34 weeks gestational age) with hypoxic respiratory failure. The current cost is approximately $3000 per day. Respiratory therapists should know that administering NO can generate a significant cost to the hospital. Although nitric oxide is usually nonreimbursable and expensive to the hospital, should it be used if it provides some benefit to the patient? Like many other questions raised in today's health care

environment, this question is multifaceted and difficult to answer.

In terms of both human lives and medical resource utilization, the cumulative cost of ARDS and MODS remains unacceptably high. The results of ongoing investigations may provide insights into the pathogenesis and treatment of ARDS and assist in addressing cost issues.

CRITICAL CONTENT

COSTS AND ETHICAL ISSUES IN ARDS

- The total cost for treating ARDS is unknown due to the heterogeneity of the disease and the lack of a finite definition of the syndrome.
- Until a standardized approach to treatment is developed, a workable system for measuring and controlling the costs of ARDS is unlikely to be possible.
- The respiratory therapist should be fully aware of terminal weaning plans.
- The ethical issues include questions about who should receive various expensive new forms of experimental therapy.

PROGNOSTIC FACTORS AND OUTCOMES

Respiratory failure accounts for 20% of the deaths from ARDS, while a combination of sepsis and multiple organ dysfunction syndrome (MODS) causes the remaining 80%. ARDS mortality increases with organ failure; isolated respiratory failure has a 40% mortality rate while the failure of two organs yields a 54% rate, three organs 72%, four organs 84%, and five organs 100%.[34,35]

The difference between survivors and nonsurvivors is as follows: survivors had a higher oxygen delivery and a higher oxygen consumption, while nonsurvivors had lower values in these clinical indices, as well as more organ failure and acidosis. Other prognostic indicators are listed in Table 22-11.

TABLE 22-11   FACTORS CONTRIBUTING
TO ARDS MORTALITY[34]

- <10% bands on peripheral smear
- Persistent acidemia
- HCO_3^- <20
- BUN >65
- Steroids have no beneficial effect

The prognosis for survival in ARDS depends primarily on three variables: the associated clinical disorder, the development of infection, and the development of nonpulmonary organ failure. According to Bell and colleagues[36] infection increased the rate of multiple organ system failure from 47% to 93%. With regards to bacteremic patients, survivors had identifiable sources while nonsurvivors often had occult pneumonia.

Many ARDS patients recover with hardly a trace of their life-threatening disease. However, some develop adult bronchopulmonary dysplasia. About one third of recovered ARDS patients present with signs of bronchial hyperactivity, while others have restrictive defects. Willms and co-workers[32] found that 29% of the nonsurvivors died from respiratory failure alone. In a large prospective series of ARDS patients, Suchyta and associates[37] found that 45% of nonsurvivors died of "pure" respiratory failure. These studies suggest that there is an urgent need for more effective forms of respiratory support. Table 22-12 lists some of the more common post-ARDS outcomes. In 80% of the survivors, chest radiographs return to normal. However, persistent infiltrates and hyperinflation have been noted. Central airway obstruction is a likely cause of late-onset dyspnea in ARDS survivors. This is a potentially fatal but often surgically correctable problem.

The most common abnormality found in ARDS survivors is a reduced carbon monoxide diffusion capacity (Dco). Elliott and co-workers[38] showed that prior cigarette smoking is not responsible for the abnormal Dco.

Normal or slightly reduced Pa_{O_2} values have been found in most ARDS survivors.[39] Hypoxemia at rest is noted in approximately 15% of survivors and is brought on by associated exercise in 36% after the first year of recovery.[40] Supplemental oxygen is usually not required at rest. It may be required during physical activity for patients who have a Dco less than 30% of predicted. Severe hypoxemia with moderate exertion is uncommon 6 months after ARDS.[41] Forced vital capacity (FVC), total lung capacity (TLC), forced expiratory volume in 1 second (FEV_1), and forced expiratory flow in midexpiration ($FEF_{25\%-75\%}$) increase from about 50% to 90% of the predicted value within 6 to 9 months. The range of pulmonary function recovery is broad. Some patients return to normal pulmonary function soon after ARDS. Most patients show only a mild restrictive pattern, in which FVC and FEV_1 are reduced proportionately. A minority of patients show severe restrictive impairment.[42]

Patients less than 20 years old and patients over 50 years old seem to be more prone to persistent restrictive impairment after ARDS.[43] The effects of therapeutic interventions on the developing lung and the inability of the aged lung to regenerate could be the underlying factors predisposing these younger and older patients to complications during the recovery period.

TABLE 22-12   POST-ARDS OUTCOMES[42,45,46]

- Most ARDS survivors recover without disability, although some degree of impairment is common.
- Recovery occurs quickly during the first 3 to 6 months and more slowly in subsequent months.
- Within 1 year after the onset of ARDS, pulmonary function recovery reaches a plateau. At that time, any abnormality that is present is likely to be permanent.
- The long-term pulmonary function outcome of survivors does not seem to be influenced by the initial cause of ARDS.

Residual pulmonary impairment correlated with low thoracic compliance, high pulmonary artery pressures, high PEEP levels, and longer duration of mechanical ventilation.[43] The presence of a pneumothorax affects survival (66% in nonsurvivors vs. 46% in survivors) and appears to be related to the structural changes occurring with time. The incidence of pneumothorax (48.8% of the entire population) was significantly higher in late ARDS (87%) vs. intermediate ARDS (46%) and early ARDS (30%).

Patient outcomes and intensity of care are the products of the interaction of the patient and the caregiver and the caregiver's response (Fig. 22-3).[33] The clinical caregiver's response varies from hospital to hospital, from unit to unit, from physician to physician, and by the same physician over time. Respiratory therapists are no different. The clinical response is influenced by training (eg, respiratory therapist vs. nurse), clinical setting (eg, community hospital vs. tertiary care center), pharmacopeia (eg, US vs. Germany), available equipment or expertise (eg, nuclear magnetic resonance scanner, newest generation of ventilator), financial and community

CRITICAL CONTENT

SURVIVAL IN ARDS

- The prognosis for survival in ARDS depends primarily on three variables: the associated clinical disorder, the development of infection, and the development of nonpulmonary organ failure.
- Survivors have a higher DO_2 and a higher $\dot{V}O_2$, while nonsurvivors had lower values in these clinical indices, as well as more organ failure and acidosis.
- The most common abnormality found in survivors is a reduced DCO.
- Residual lung impairment (mild restrictive disorder) is seen in most survivors.
- Normal or slightly reduced PaO_2 values have been found in most survivors.

imperatives, experience level, and recent exposure to clinical reports and lectures. Recent experiences may dramatically alter the decisions made by the clinician from one day to the next.

In deciding on a strategy for rehabilitative care, prognostic factors and predicted outcomes must be considered. One should use a strategy that seeks to improve outcomes by minimizing or preventing iatrogenic lung injury. This approach should be taken early in the course of ARDS. Optimal treatment and management of both acute and rehabilitative care may be clarified as further studies are conducted.

SUMMARY

Since its initial description in 1967, ARDS has become one of the most common diagnoses in the critical care setting. ARDS has been, and remains, one of the biggest treatment challenges for the health care professional. As such it presents numerous opportunities for respiratory therapists to optimize the use of critical thinking skills.

Improvement in outcomes is most likely multifactorial, and is attributable to advances in supportive care, earlier detection, more effective treatment of comorbid diseases (eg, nosocomial infections), and the broad application of innovative mechanical ventilation techniques. However, the cumulative cost of ARDS and MODS, both in terms of human lives and medical resource utilization, remains unacceptably high. The medical community awaits the results of ongoing investigations that may provide insights into the pathogenesis and treatment of ARDS.

INTRODUCTION TO CASE STUDIES

Now you proceed with the most exciting part of this chapter, that of working through two hypothetical cases. Your instructors will assign you to work on specific critical thinking exercises and group critical thinking exercises, depending on the available time, types of patients you are likely to encounter in your clinical rotations, and resources available. Please check with your instructor to verify which case(s) and exercises you should complete, individually or in groups. Your instructor may also direct you to develop learning

issues as part of your problem-based learning (PBL) process or assign specific, predetermined learning issues that have been developed for this chapter. Please check with your program faculty before proceeding with the following cases.

CASE STUDY 1

MS. AMY ARD

Day 1: Initial History

Ms. Amy Ard is a 30-year-old woman who was feeling fine until the day before admission, when she began having a fever, emesis, and malaise. Throughout the night Ms. Ard's symptoms continued and caused her to go to the local emergency room (ER) at 5 AM. Prompted by physician interview questions, Amy states that she does not have any shortness of breath, orthopnea, coughing, sputum production, hemoptysis, wheezing, or chest pain.

Physical Examination

General	Patient is alert, oriented ×3, and anxious. Upon admission her weight was 60 kg. She presents with dry mouth and axillae.
Chest	Breath sounds indicated crackles at the right base.
Labs	WBC of 18,000/mm³, Hb. 8.7 g/dL, an anion gap is present, serum ketones are large, and blood sugar is high.

Vital signs

HR	110/min
RR	19/min
BP	125/85
SpO$_2$	93% NC 4 L/min
Temp.	40°C

Critical Thinking Exercise 1

MAKING INFERENCES BY CLUSTERING DATA

a. What inference can you make about the potential for this patient to develop pneumonia?

b. Identify and group (cluster) the data that lead you to this inference.

Based on the preliminary data, the admitting diagnosis of diabetic ketoacidosis (DKA) is made. In addition, pneumonia is suspected and therefore "rule out pneumonia" is also listed in the progress notes under diagnosis. Antibiotics, insulin, and fluids are administered. Blood, urine, and sputum cultures are ordered.

Day 2, 0630 hours: Ms. Ard becomes hypotensive (ie, blood pressure decreases to 70/palpable). Fluids and vasopressors are administered. The patient vomits and aspirates. Ms. Ard develops moderate respiratory distress (ie, respiratory rate of 28 bpm), using accessory muscles. SpO$_2$ is 90%. Breath sounds reveal fine, bilateral, inspiratory crackles. The patient is awake and alert. Additional lab results reveal that a pneumococcal bacteremia is present along with acute renal failure.

Critical Thinking Exercise 2

PRIORITIZING PATIENT CARE

What specific objective data would you use to determine if this patient has a higher priority than your other patients?

CASE STUDY 1 *(continued)*

The 4 L/min nasal cannula is replaced by a high-flow system (ie, 50% cool aerosol mask). SpO_2 is 93%. Ms. Ard's respiratory rate is 30 bpm. She looks anxious and fatigued.

Critical Thinking Exercise 3

ANTICIPATING PROBLEMS AND SOLUTIONS

a. Given the latest data, what problems do you anticipate?

b. What is your proposed solution(s) to these anticipated problem(s)?

Day 2, 1230 hours: Ms. Ard's respiratory rate increases to 34 bpm while the SpO_2 decreases to 88%. The patient is intubated and then admitted to the medical intensive care unit (MICU). Ms. Ard is placed on mechanical ventilation with the following settings: Volume ventilation, assist/control mode, FIO_2 = 1.0, ventilator respiratory rate = 16 bpm, VT = 800 mL, PIP = 48 cm H_2O, PEEP = 5 cm H_2O. A pulmonary artery catheter is inserted. An ABG reveals:

ABG volume A/C 100%

pH	7.21
PCO_2	36
PO_2	49
HCO_3^-	14
BE	–13
SaO_2	82%

Critical Thinking Exercise 4

PROBLEM SOLVING USING CLINICAL DATA

a. What is the primary problem(s) regarding ventilation and oxygenation?

b. What solution(s) do you recommend?

Day 2, 1300 hours: The PEEP level is increased to 10 cm H_2O. SpO_2 is 91%.

Day 2, 2100 hours: The SpO_2 has decreased to 87%. The PEEP is increased to 15 cm H_2O, resulting in a SpO_2 of 93%.

Day 3, 0800 hours: The PEEP is increased to 17 cm H_2O. SpO_2 is 99%. Chest auscultation reveals bilateral inspiratory crackles. This saturation value is confirmed by an ABG (see below). The PIP is now 68 mm Hg. Urine output is normal and blood pressure is 130/70.

ABG volume A/C 100%

pH	7.30
PCO_2	50
PO_2	141
HCO_3^-	25
BE	–2
SaO_2	100%

Critical Thinking Exercise 5

REFLECTING AND DECISION MAKING

a. Reflect on the thought process that was used to correct inadequate oxygenation during mechanical ventilation. Explain what assumptions were made about the patient's lungs and disease process that caused the ventilator adjustments to be made.

b. Describe two typical ventilator adjustments that you could make to correct inadequate oxygenation.

A chest radiograph was taken (see Fig. 22-4).

(continued)

CASE STUDY 1 *(continued)*

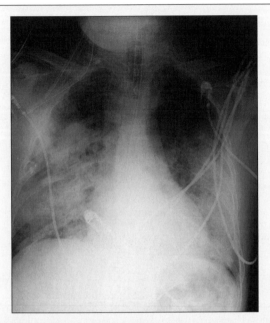

FIGURE 22-4 The chest radiograph shows diffuse air-space filling with air bronchograms in the left lung consistent with pneumonia, cardiogenic pulmonary edema, or ARDS.

 Critical Thinking Exercise 6

ANTICIPATING PROBLEMS AND SOLUTIONS

a. Should an elevated PIP generate a concern or is the "plateau" pressure more of a concern? Explain.

b. What ventilator management strategy could maintain oxygenation yet decrease the PIP?

Day 3, 0930 hours: The nurse obtains the following hemodynamic measurements: PAWP (wedge pressure) 24 mm Hg, cardiac output 3.0 L/min. Diuresis is ordered for the elevated PAWP.

Day 3, 1000 Hours: The attending physician expresses a concern for the PEEP level and is worried about absorption atelectasis and barotrauma. He writes orders for sedation with morphine and paralysis with vecuronium. He also writes an

order to decrease the PEEP level to 15 cm H_2O. You implement the change in PEEP. As a result, the PIP is now 58 cm H_2O.

 Critical Thinking Exercise 7

PROBLEM SOLVING USING CLINICAL DATA

When the PEEP was reduced by 2 cm H_2O (from 17 to 15 cm H_2O), what does the drop in PIP from 68 to 58 cm H_2O tell you about the patient's lung condition? (What problem was being caused by the PEEP of 17 that has now been lessened by decreasing the PEEP to 15?)

Day 3, 1100 hours: Concerned about the effect that a decrease in the PEEP level might have on oxygenation, you request another ABG. The results are as follows:

ABG Volume A/C 100%

pH	7.36
P_{CO_2}	48
P_{O_2}	118
HCO_3^-	23
BE	−1
Sa_{O_2}	100%

You notice that the Sp_{O_2} is 99%.

 Critical Thinking Exercise 8

COMMUNICATION AND DECISION MAKING

a. Why is it important to relay this information to the physician as opposed to simply accepting the saturation as a positive clinical sign?

b. What complications of mechanical ventilation are you trying to avoid?

c. What adjustments would you suggest to the physician?

CASE STUDY 1 *(continued)*

The physician thanks you for contacting him and writes an order to decrease the F_{IO_2} to 90% and then decrease the PEEP to 13 cm H_2O if oxygen saturation remains >93%. On 90% oxygen and a PEEP of 13 cm H_2O, the ABGs are listed below. A chest radiograph is taken (see Fig. 22-5).

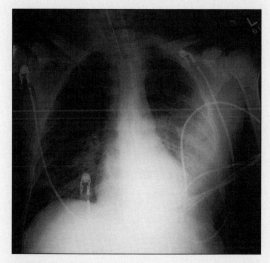

FIGURE 22-5 Ms. Ard's second chest radiograph.

ABG volume A/C 100%

pH	7.39
P_{CO_2}	45
P_{O_2}	142
HCO_3^-	27
BE	+1.5
Sa_{O_2}	100%

Day 3, 1530 hours: You suggest implementing a protective lung strategy (ie, decreasing tidal volume to 6 mL/kg and prolonging the inspiratory time) to the physician. You describe the benefits of treating the ARDS lung as a "small" lung instead of a "stiff" lung. The physician does not agree with your suggestion. He is concerned about the unstable status of the PIP and wants a guaranteed tidal volume. The physician recommends that in-line albuterol treatments be initiated.

 Group Critical Thinking Exercise 1

PRO/CON DEBATE: BRONCHODILATORS FOR ARDS PATIENTS

Two groups should be assigned to present the arguments for and against the use of beta$_2$ agonists in patients with ARDS. One group should present the pro and another the con positions for this practice. After the debate the entire class should discuss: Which side presented their case more effectively? What was it that made their arguments more effective?

 Critical Thinking Exercise 9

NEGOTIATING

a. What do you say to the physician to persuade him or her to use pressure assist/control ventilation or a protective lung strategy?

b. What response do you anticipate? Explain why you expect this response.

You present the information described in Tables 22-13 and 22-14 in an attempt to persuade the physician to try pressure assist/control. The physician has not had experience with pressure assist/control and asks you to provide supportive literature. You present the articles listed in Table 22-15. He reviews the articles, remains somewhat skeptical, but decides to accept "in principle" your suggestion.

 Critical Thinking Exercise 10

DECISION MAKING

Now you have the decision making ability *and* increased responsibility for the outcome. Do you try pressure assist/control and a protective lung strategy or do you stay with the known outcome of volume ventilation?

(continued)

CASE STUDY 1 *(continued)*

TABLE 22-13 PRESSURE ASSIST/CONTROL OVERVIEW

- Peak inspiratory pressure can be controlled (ie, limited so as not to exceed a predetermined value).
- The peak inspiratory pressure level can be maintained for a specified duration as determined by the inspiratory time.
- Since the inspiratory time is adjustable, the I:E ratio is variable.
- Pressure assist/control is flow responsive, enabling it to instantaneously adapt to changes in compliance, resistance, and patient effort.
- The decelerating flow pattern provides even gas distribution by generating slower, more laminar flow toward the end of inspiration as positive pressure interfaces with progressively smaller airways.
- A relatively longer inspiratory time enhances gas distribution.

You decide to convert to pressure assist/control. The mode is changed to pressure assist/control (pressure control). Upon your recommendations, the physician writes an order for the following ventilator settings: FIO_2 0.90, RR 24 bpm, PEEP 13 cm H_2O, PIP (PEEP plus delta P) 38 cm H_2O, inspiratory time = 1.0 seconds. On these settings, the tidal volume is 550 mL and the SpO_2 is 99%.

Day 3, 1600 Hours: The physician is pleased that you were able to oxygenate the patient at a lower PIP. He wants to lower the FIO_2 and the PEEP

TABLE 22-14 PRESSURE ASSIST/CONTROL: CONSEQUENCES OF MORE EVEN GAS DISTRIBUTION

- Reduction in V/Q mismatch
- Improved gas exchange
- Improved compliance
- Lower airway pressures

TABLE 22-15 SUPPORTIVE LITERATURE

- Abraham and Yoshihara[47] compared volume assist/control (volume control) with pressure assist/control (pressure control). They found that pressure assist/control increased PaO_2, DO_2, and VO_2.
- Rappaport et al[48] did a prospective, randomized study and found no difference in mortality between pressure control and volume control; pressure control was associated with a faster improvement in compliance; and pressure control decreased duration of mechanical ventilation.

while maintaining adequate oxygenation. After several manipulations of the ventilator settings, the SpO_2 increases to 100%. The new ventilator settings are: FIO_2 = 0.75, RR 24, PEEP 8 cm H_2O, PIP (PEEP plus delta P) 33 cm H_2O, inspiratory time 1.5 seconds. Cardiac output is now 3.8 L/min. PaO_2 is 124 mm Hg and SaO_2 is 99%. *Congratulations!* You successfully decreased the FIO_2 and the PEEP and still maintained a SpO_2 at 100%.

At this point, the nurse measures the patient's blood pressure. The value is 100/55. The physician and nurse are concerned about the significant decrease in blood pressure and attribute it to the most recent changes in ventilator settings and the pressure assist/control mode itself. They bring their concerns to your attention.

 Critical Thinking Exercise 11

CLINICAL PROBLEM SOLVING USING GRAPHIC DATA

a. Examine Fig. 22-6. This graphic tracing was obtained from Ms. Ard at this time. Analyze this graphic to determine what is occurring as a result of her current ventilator settings.

b. Based on your findings, what would you recommend be done?

CASE STUDY 1 *(continued)*

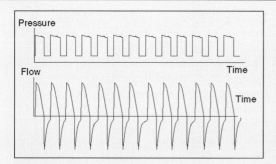

FIGURE 22-6 Pressure and flow/time graphic for Ms. Ard.

Critical Thinking Exercise 12

CLINICAL PROBLEM SOLVING

a. Reflect on the ventilator setting changes on day 2 from 1300 to 0800 hours.
b. What clinical parameters were overlooked?
c. Based on your initial assessment and findings, was the patient being managed appropriately on the previous shift?

You recall the variables associated with oxygenation (review Table 22-16). Upon reviewing this information, you realize that you have been so busy adjusting the ventilator settings according to ABGs and the pulse oximeter, that you neglected to consider the bigger picture of oxyge-

TABLE 22-16 OXYGEN-DERIVED VARIABLES

GENERAL VARIABLE	SPECIFIC CLINICAL MARKER
Tissue input	Pao_2, Sao_2, Cao_2, Do_2
Tissue utilization	$\dot{V}o_2$, O_2 extraction ratio[a]
Tissue output	$P\bar{v}o_2$, $S\bar{v}o_2$, lactate level

[a]O_2 Extraction ratio = $\dot{V}o_2/Do_2$; normal O_2 extraction = 250/1000 = 25%; maximum = 75%

nation while adjusting PEEP. In addition, although the set PEEP is 8 cm H_2O, an auto-PEEP of 3 cm H_2O is detected. Therefore the total PEEP (ie, set PEEP plus auto-PEEP) is 11 cm H_2O.

Critical Thinking Exercise 13

TREND ANALYSIS/REFLECTION ON THE DECISION MAKING PROCESS

a. Assess the patient's oxygenation status by reviewing all the data in Table 22-17. What is your conclusion regarding oxygenation and the PEEP settings given this information?
b. Reflect on how the clinical decisions were being made regarding PEEP adjustments and this patient's oxygenation. Was focusing on arterial oxygenation parameters alone sufficient to reflect the overall picture?

TABLE 22-17 Pao$_2$ VERSUS Do$_2$

PEEP (cm H_2O)	Pao$_2$ (mm HG)	Sao$_2$ (%)	CO (L/min)	O$_2$ DELIVERY (mL/min)	BLOOD PRESSURE (mm Hg)
17	141	100	3.0	501	130/70
15	118	100	3.1	528	118/66
13	142	100	3.5	591	130/65
11	124	99	3.8	632	100/55

(continued)

CASE STUDY 1 *(continued)*

After seeing the trend summary, the physician requests the calculation of oxygen delivery every shift and after every change in ventilator settings and after every change in hemodynamic status. In an attempt to further optimize the patient's ventilator settings, you obtain an order to titrate the PEEP level to further improve oxygen delivery.

Day 4: You decrease the total PEEP level to 9 cm H_2O. An ABG and an update on the hemodynamic parameters reveals:

ABG pressure A/C 75%

pH	7.30
Pco_2	60
Po_2	115
HCO_3^-	29
BE	+1
Sao_2	100%

Total PEEP (cm H_2O)	9
Pao_2 (mm Hg)	115
Sao_2 (%)	100
CO (L/min)	4.6
O_2 delivery (mL/min)	774
Blood pressure (mm Hg)	100/50

The patient easily tolerates a decrease to 60% oxygen. You decrease the total PEEP level to 7 cm H_2O. The pulse oximeter display indicates that the SpO_2 is 97%. The most recent ABG and selected hemodynamic parameters are as follows:

ABG pressure A/C 60%

pH	7.35
Pco_2	45
Po_2	92
HCO_3^-	25
BE	−2
Sao_2	97%

Total PEEP (cm H_2O)	7
Pao_2 (mm Hg)	92
Sao_2 (%)	97
CO (L/min)	6.1
O_2 delivery (mL/min)	1011
Blood pressure (mm Hg)	110/50

A more comprehensive review of the trend in oxygen delivery can now be documented (see Table 22-18). As can be seen, oxygen delivery is a useful parameter to follow when making adjustments of PEEP.

TABLE 22-18 Pao_2 VERSUS Do_2

PEEP (cm H_2O)	Pao_2 (mm Hg)	Sao_2 (%)	CO (L/min)	O_2 DELIVERY (mL/min)	BLOOD PRESSURE (mm Hg)
17	141	100	3.0	501	130/70
15	118	100	3.1	528	118/66
13	142	100	3.5	591	130/65
11	124	99	3.8	632	100/55
9	115	100	4.6	774	100/50
7	92	97	6.1	1011	110/50

CASE STUDY 1 (*continued*)

Critical Thinking Exercise 14

TREND ANALYSIS/EXPLORING INCONSISTENCIES

a. Review the data in Table 22-18. Which of the data do not seem consistent with your initial expectations, given the increasing oxygen delivery that is occurring with decreases in PEEP?
b. Explain how it is possible for these data to be accurate, in spite of the initial appearance of not being what you would have expected.

The fact that many clinicians rely on pulse oximeters and ABGs instead of oxygen delivery calculations reinforces the following quote by 19th-century English writer Samuel Butler: "Life is the art of drawing sufficient conclusions from insufficient premises."

Days 5 through 12: The paralytic agent and sedation are discontinued. The aforementioned method of maximizing oxygen delivery was repeat-

edly used until the patient required 40% oxygen. The pulmonary artery catheter was removed and the patient began weaning from the ventilator.

Day 19: Patient goes home on insulin and is scheduled for periodic dialysis.

Group Critical Thinking Exercise 2

PRO/CON DEBATE: VOLUME VS. PRESSURE VENTILATION

One group of students is assigned to present the argument that Ms. Ard should have remained on volume ventilation while titrating PEEP to optimize oxygen delivery. After the group discussion, this group's designated leader will list the advantages of this ventilator management strategy. A second group of students is assigned to develop an argument supporting the conversion to pressure control ventilation. Again, the designated leader will list the advantages after the discussion. The entire class then discusses which strategy they feel is most effective and why. Was the best strategy selected because of clinical facts or because of a more effective presentation?

CASE STUDY 2

MS. NANCY NITRIC

Postop Day 1

Use the definitions listed in Table 22-19 and the hemodynamic norms listed in Table 22-20 during the following case study.

You are assigned to a patient named Ms. Nancy Nitric, who has been on mechanical ventilation following her lung transplant surgery. The following ventilator settings have not changed since her arrival in the ICU from the OR: Volume ventilation: assist/control mode, FIO_2 0.9, mandatory rate 14 bpm, VT 550 mL. PEEP was not initiated because the surgeons were concerned about

the effect of positive pressure on the anastomoses. Additional data: PIP 42 cm H_2O, MAP 14 cm H_2O, urine output is normal. A pulmonary artery catheter is inserted. The PCWP = 13 mm Hg, MPAP is 39 mm Hg, PVR 424 dyne/second/cm⁵. Hemoglobin is 14 gm/dL, methemoglobin 0.9%, CO 4.9 L/min, DO_2 823 mL/min, SaO_2 90%.

The patient has been receiving continuous intravenous infusions of vasoactive drugs as well as a low dose of dopamine. The patient has been sedated with the intravenous morphine and diazepam.

(continued)

CASE STUDY 2 *(continued)*

TABLE 22-19 DEFINITIONS OF SYSTEM FAILURE

- Renal failure is defined as a serum creatinine concentration ≥3 mg/dL.
- Liver failure is defined as a serum bilirubin concentration ≥4 mg/dL.
- Coagulopathy is defined as:
    A platelet count ≤90,000/mm^3 and prothrombin time ≥1.5 times the control
    OR
    Partial thromboplastin time ≥1.5 times the control
    OR
    Hematocrit ≤20%

TABLE 22-20 HEMODYNAMIC NORMS

Pulmonary artery pressure (PAP)
Normal PAP = 15 to 30 mm Hg (systolic)
               5 to 12 mm Hg (diastolic)

Mean pulmonary artery pressure (MPAP)
MPAP = [(2 × pulmonary diastolic)
     + pulmonary systolic]/3
Normal MPAP = 11 to 18 mm Hg

Pulmonary capillary wedge pressure (PCWP)
Normal PCWP = 5 to 15 mm Hg

Pulmonary vascular resistance (PVR)
PVR = [(MPAP − PCWP)/CO] × 79.9
Normal PVR = 150 to 250
    dyne/second/cm^5

Oxygen delivery (DO$_2$)
DO_2 = cardiac output × O$_2$ content × 10
DO_2 = cardiac output × [(1.34 × Hb
    × SaO$_2$) + (0.003 × PaO$_2$)] × 10
Normal DO_2 = 640 to 1400 mL/min

Oxygen consumption (V̇O$_2$)
$\dot{V}O_2$ = cardiac output × arterial-venous
    difference in O$_2$ content
$\dot{V}O_2$ = cardiac output × [1.34 × Hb
    × (SaO$_2$ −S$\bar{v}$O$_2$)] + (0.003 × PaO$_2$) × 10
Normal $\dot{V}O_2$ = 180 to 280 mL/min

Critical Thinking Exercise 1

PRIORITIZING PATIENT CARE

a. Explain how you would prioritize this patient based on the clinical data.
b. What specific objective data would you use to determine if this patient has a higher priority than your other patients?
c. If Ms. Nitric is the first patient you see on your shift, how would you know if she is your highest clinical priority?

Critical Thinking Exercise 2

MAKING INFERENCES BY CLUSTERING DATA

a. What inference can you make about Ms. Nitric's pulmonary condition?
b. Which of the patient's hemodynamic measurements did you use to make an inference regarding the patient's pulmonary condition?

Critical Thinking Exercise 3

DECISION MAKING

An ICU intensivist has assumed responsibility for medical management of Ms. Nitric. This physician is considering changing the patient to pressure control ventilation at this time and she asks for your opinion regarding ventilator management.

a. Would you support switching to PC ventilation at this time? Support your recommendation by giving reasons why or why not.

After discussion, the physician orders the following parameters: FIO$_2$ 0.9, ventilator RR 14 bpm, PEEP = 0 cm H$_2$O. Inspiratory pressure

CASE STUDY 2 *(continued)*

level 28 cm H_2O, inspiratory time 1.0 seconds. Observed data: MAP 9 cm H_2O, SpO_2 89%, Hb 14 gm/dL. Cardiac output is 5.1 L/min, urine output is 50 mL over the past 6 hours. Serum creatinine concentration is 6 mg/dL.

The physician is pleased with the decrease in airway pressures, but is not satisfied with the oxygen saturation. Hence, she writes an order to apply PEEP at 5 cm H_2O.

Critical Thinking Exercise 4

ANTICIPATING PROBLEMS

What problems do you anticipate may develop with the application of PEEP? (Explain how and why you anticipate the problems that will develop in this patient.)

You inform the physician of the surgeon's concern about PEEP and its effect on the surgical repair site. The doctor insists on applying PEEP. Again, you express your reservations with regard to applying PEEP and recommend nitric oxide, explaining how it can also assist in decreasing pulmonary artery pressure. The physician accepts your arguments and asks for your recommendation regarding the dose and specific orders. You suggest an initial dose of 5 ppm. After initiating the NO, the following data are obtained: MPAP 36 mm Hg, SaO_2 93%, PVR 360 dyne/second/cm^5, DO_2 890 mL/min, methemoglobin 1.1%, cardiac output 5.1 L/min.

Critical Thinking Exercise 5

PROBLEM SOLVING: EVALUATION

a. Has the patient's oxygenation improved with the use of NO and PEEP? Explain.
b. Did the nitric oxide have an effect on the PVR? Explain your answer.

Postop day 2: The physician is pleased with the clinical improvements. She orders the nitric oxide dose to be increased to 20 ppm in increments of 2 ppm. The following data were obtained at a dose of 20 ppm: MPAP 34 mm Hg, PCWP 14 mm Hg, cardiac output 4.8 L/min, tidal volume increased 10%.

ABG pressure A/C 75%

pH	7.38
PCO_2	44
PO_2	90
HCO_3^-	26
BE	+0.5
SaO_2	96%

You ascertain that the increase in tidal volume is due to an improvement in lung compliance. Pink, frothy secretions are observed during suctioning.

Critical Thinking Exercise 6

DECISION MAKING/NEGOTIATING

a. The physician wants to increase the NO level to 25 ppm. Analyze the data and determine if you would support this recommendation.
b. What would your recommendation be at this time?
c. How would you negotiate with the physician to have your recommendation implemented?

Postop day 3: The physician writes an order to measure methemoglobin values daily. Attempts are made to decrease the nitric oxide dose, but each attempt to completely discontinue the NO causes the patient to rapidly develop hypoxemia and hemodynamic instability.

(continued)

CASE STUDY 2 (continued)

Critical Thinking Exercise 7

PROBLEM SOLVING

Given the difficulty described above, how would you proceed to solve this problem?

The nitric oxide level was decreased to 15 ppm. The patient's pulmonary artery pressure (mean) and oxygen saturation levels remained stable. The NO level was successfully decreased by 10 ppm over the next 2 hours, resulting in a level of 5 ppm. Attempts to wean the nitric oxide level below 5 ppm were associated with significant hypoxemia and hemodynamic instability. Such negative effects were quickly ameliorated by returning to the previous level (ie, 5 ppm) of NO. Over the next several days, attempts to completely wean the nitric oxide were successful. Nitric oxide therapy was continued for a total of 8 days.

Critical Thinking Exercise 8

PROBLEM SOLVING:
EVALUATION AND ANALYSIS

a. Is nitric oxide effectively treating the problem of pulmonary hypertension?

b. Discuss your analysis of the overall effectiveness of the decision to use NO in this patient situation. Overall, was it beneficial or not? Support your evaluation with specific reasons.

Ms. Nitric's clinical course deteriorated due to multiple organ failure. She expired on the 11th day after surgery.

Group Critical Thinking Exercise 1

DECISION MAKING CONSIDERING COSTS AND ETHICS

The hospital budget only allows for a limited number of nitric oxide systems. The CEO wants input from the respiratory therapy department on criteria for patient selection. Divide the class into two groups. Group A will discuss criteria for determining which patients receive nitric oxide (pro NO). Group B will discuss outcomes (con NO). Each group should use evidence-based clinical research to support its arguments. The debate is then presented in front of the class. Discuss the strengths and weaknesses of the arguments presented. Discuss cost and ethical issues.

KEY POINTS

- The similarities of clinical presentation of acute respiratory distress syndrome (ARDS) when compared to cardiogenic pulmonary edema are early features of dyspnea, tachypnea, refractory hypoxemia, and diffuse bilateral infiltrates.

- ARDS differences when compared to cardiogenic pulmonary edema are:

    in ARDS, pulmonary artery wedge pressure (PAWP) usually *normal*, and pulmonary vascular resistance (PVR) often *increased*,

    in cardiogenic pulmonary edema, PAWP *increased*, with PVR *normal*

- ARDS refers to the acute onset of noncardiogenic pulmonary edema that is due to increased permeability of the capillary endothelium and subsequently the alveolar epithelium

- Surfactant is usually impaired by the presence of inflammatory agents and protein, causing atelectasis and compromising gas exchange.

- The overall result of the processes involved in ARDS are refractory hypoxemia, stiff lungs, and respiratory distress.

- ARDs affects the lung in an uneven, patchy manner, resulting in an uneven distribution of the disease process and an uneven distribution of inspiratory gas, resulting in ventilation/perfusion mismatching.

- ARDS is closely related to multiple organ dysfunction syndrome (MODS) since, as one organ system fails, toxins and/or inflammatory factors are released systemically, placing other symptoms at risk for organ failure.

- The medical treatment of ARDS concentrates on three major areas: 1) reversing the underlying disorder; 2) blocking the specific mechanism of injury to the alveolar-capillary membrane, and 3) providing supportive care while minimizing the pathological consequences of acute lung injury.

- Human studies regarding blocking the specific mechanism of injury to the alveolar-capillary membrane remain inconclusive.

- Treatment for ARDS is largely supportive. There are three major areas of supportive measures: 1) recognizing and preventing complications, 2) minimizing edema formation, and 3) maintaining tissue oxygenation while reducing exacerbating factors.

- Recognizing and preventing complications is very important in that it prevents an additional pulmonary complication (ie, either nosocomial or iatrogenic).

- Regarding treatment for minimizing edema formation:
  - loss of A-c membrane integrity allows for easy formation of edema
  - goal to maintain the lowest possible PAWP consistent with adequate CO
  - hemodynamic monitoring essential, as fluid therapy is administered to maintain adequate cardiac output in the presence of wet lungs
  - ongoing debate whether to use colloids or crystalloids
  - diuretics used for minimizing pulmonary edema formation must be carefully balanced with fluid therapy to maintain adequate cardiac output and oxygen delivery to the tissues

- Treatment to maintain adequate tissue oxygenation is dependent upon balance between oxygen **supply** and **demand**. Goals include:
  - **minimizing demand** (minimizing metabolic rate) by such strategies as pain, anxiety, and fever control
  - **optimizing supply** (optimizing Do_2) by such strategies as optimizing CO (inotropics/fluids) and optimizing CaO_2 (Hb, Pao_2)

- The complications associated with conventional mechanical ventilation (eg, volutrauma and O_2 toxicity) can potentially be minimized by utilizing various nonconventional mechanical ventilation strategies.

- When a patient is on pressure control ventilation and you are attempting to optimize the lung pressure-volume relationship by utilizing a "protective lung strategy," you should set the PEEP at or slightly above the lungs' lower inflection point (LIP) (to prevent alveolar collapse and minimize injury from repeated opening and closing), and set the PIP at or below the lungs' upper inflection point (UIP) to minimize lung overdistention.

- Pressure ventilation can take on various forms:
  - PCV—the standard, basic form of pressure ventilation
  - HFV—numerous subtypes exist (HFPPV, HFJV, HVO)
  - PC-IRV—PCV with inverse I:E ratios (Use with caution!)
  - APRV—allows spontaneous ventilation with fluctuating baseline pressures; interesting concept, but little evidence published to support its use

- Inhaled nitric oxide (NO) concentrations of 5 to 80 ppm selectively vasodilate the pulmonary vasculature which improves V/Q and therefore oxygenation as well as reduces pulmonary hypertension.

- NO concentration is adjusted to the desired effect, then, slowly reduced as the patient's condition improves with gradual weaning advised to avoid adverse hypoxemic and hemdynamic responses.

- Side effects with NO include formation of NO_2 and methemoglobin.

- Respiratory therapists can help control the cost of care by being aware of the various alternative forms of treatment, sharing knowledge with other clinicians, and avoiding the use of inappropriate and unnecessary clinical strategies.

- Ethical issues include who receives various (expensive) forms of therapy for which outcome data are lacking (experimental therapy)

- The prognosis for survival in ARDS depends primarily on three variables: the associated clinical disorder, the development of infection, and the development of nonpulmonary organ failure.

SUGGESTED RESOURCES: WEB SITES

http://www.aarc.org
This web site for the American Association for Respiratory Care provides easy access to several other web sites by selecting "RC Links." From "RC Links":
a. A Medline search can be started by selecting "Resources" and then "Grateful Med."
b. National Institutes of Health clinical trials can be reviewed by selecting "Government"
c. The *Journal of the American Medical Association*, the *New England Journal of Medicine*, and other professional journals can be obtained by selecting "Publications."
d. "Virtual Hospital" can be accessed by selecting the category labeled as such.

http://www.pathguy.com/lectures/resp.htm
This web site provides a view from the microscope. Photos of tissues affected by ARDS and other respiratory diseases are available.

http://www.lungusa.org/diseases/ards_factsheet.html
Sponsored by the American Lung Association, this web site provides important information about ARDS and other respiratory diseases.

http://www.geocities.com
Easy to understand medical and research information on ARDS is provided and updated frequently. This site includes FAQs (frequently asked questions), articles, current issues and discussions, support for ARDS patients and families, education, and other information resources.

http://www.ahealthyme.com
A basic overview of ARDS and other conditions is provided by this site.

REFERENCES

1. Ashbaugh DG, Bigelow DB, Petty TL, et al. Adult respiratory distress in adults. *Lancet.* 1967;2:319–323.

2. Murray GF. Mechanisms of acute respiratory failure. *Am Rev Respir Dis.* 1977;115:1071–1078.

3. Milberg JA, Davis DR, Steinberg KP, et al. Improved survival of patients with adult respiratory distress syndrome (ARDS): 1983-1993. *JAMA.* 1995;273:306–309.

4. Bernard GR, et al: The American-European consensus conference on ARDS: Definitions, mechanisms, relevant outcomes, and clinical trial coordination. *Am J Respir Crit Care Med.* 1994;149:818–824.

5. Tomashefski JF. Pulmonary pathology of adult respiratory distress syndrome. *Clin Chest Med.* 1990;11:593–619.

6. Gattinoni L, Presenti A, Torresin A. Adult respiratory distress syndrome profiles by computed tomography. *J Thorac Imaging.* 1986;1:25–30.

7. Maunder RJ, Shuman WP, McHugh JW, et al. Preservation of normal lung regions in the adult respiratory distress syndrome. *JAMA.* 1986;255:2463–2465.

8. West JB. State of the art: Ventilation-perfusion relationships. *Am Rev Respir Dis.* 1977;116:919–943.

9. Rajacich N, Burchard KW, Hasan FM. Central venous pressure and pulmonary capillary wedge pressure as estimates of left atrial pressure: Effects of PEEP and catheter tip malposition. *Crit Care Med.* 1989;17:7–11.

10. Amato MBS, Barbas CSV, Medeiros DM, et al. Beneficial effects of the "open lung approach" with low distending pressures in acute respiratory distress syndrome. *Am J Respir Crit Care Med.* 1995;152:1835–1846.

11. Verbrugge SJC, Bohm SH, Gommers D, et al. Surfactant impairment after mechanical ventilation with large alveolar surface area changes and effects of positive end-expiratory pressure. *Br J Anesth.* 1998;80:360–364.

12. Dreyfuss D, Saumon G. Role of tidal volume, FRC, and end-inspiratory volume in the development of pulmonary edema following mechanical ventilation. *Am Rev Respir Dis.* 1993;148:1194–1203.

13. Amato MBP, Barbas CSV, Pastore L, et al. Minimizing barotrauma in ARDS: protective effects of PEEP and the hazards of driving and plateau pressures. *Am J Respir Crit Care Med.* 1996;153:375 (abst).

14. Taskar V, John J, Evander E, et al. Surfactant dysfunction makes the lungs vulnerable to repetitive collapse and re-expansion. *Am J Physiol.* 1997;155:313–320.

15. Hickling KG, Henderson SJ, Jackson R. Low mortality associated with low volume, pressure limited ventilation with permissive hypercapnia in severe respiratory distress syndrome. *Intensive Care Med.* 1990;16:372–377.

16. Marini JJ. New approaches to the ventilatory management of the adult respiratory distress syndrome. *J Crit Care.* 1992;87:256–257.

17. Roupie E, et al. Titration of tidal volume and induced hypercapnia in acute respiratory distress syndrome. *Am J Respir Crit Care Med.* 1995;152:121–128.

18. Cain SM. Supply dependency of oxygen uptake in ARDS: myth or reality? *Am J Med Sci.* 1984;288:119–124.

19. Pepke-Zaba J, Higenbottam TW, Dinh-Xuan AT, et al. Inhaled nitric oxide as a cause of selective pulmonary vasodilation in pulmonary hypertension. *Lancet.* 1991;338:1173–1174.

20. Bigatello LM, Hurforn WE, Kacmarek RM, et al. Prolonged inhalation of low concentrations of nitric oxide in patients with severe adult respiratory distress syndrome: effects on pulmonary hemodynamics and oxygenation. *Anesthesiology.* 1994;80:761.

21. Rossaint R, Falke KF, Lopez F, et al. Inhaled nitric oxide for the adult respiratory distress syndrome. *N Engl J Med.* 1993;328:399–405.

22. Manktelow C, Bigatello L, Hess D, et al. Physiological determinants of the response to inhaled nitric oxide in patients with the acute respiratory distress syndrome. *Anesthesiology.* 1997;87:297.

23. Lessard MR. New concepts in mechanical ventilation for ARDS. *Can J Anesth.* 1996;43:R50.

24. Zhu GF, Sun B, Niu SF, et al. Combined surfactant therapy and inhaled nitric oxide in rabbits with oleic acid-induced acute respiratory distress syndrome. *Am J Respir Crit Care Med.* 1998;158:437.

25. Kaisers U, Max M, Walter J, et al. Partial liquid ventilation with small volumes of FC 3280 increases survival time in experimental ARDS. *Eur Respir J.* 1997;10:1955.

26. Overbeck MC, Pranikoff T, Yadao CM, et al. Efficacy of perfluorocarbon partial liquid ventilation in a large animal model of acute respiratory failure. *Crit Care Med.* 1996;24:7.

27. Lewandowski K, Rossaint R, Pappert D, et al. High survival rate in 122 ARDS patients managed according to a clinical algorithm including extracorporeal membrane oxygenation. *Intensive Care Med.* 1997;23:819.

28. Corbridge T, et al. Adverse effects of large tidal volumes and low PEEP in canine acid aspiration. *Am Rev Respir Dis.* 1990;142:311.

29. Parker J, et al. Lung edema caused by high peak inspiratory pressure in dogs: role of increased microvascular filtration pressure and permeability. *Am Rev Respir Dis.* 1990;142:321–328.

30. Chastre J, Trouillet JL, Vuagnat A, et al. Nosocomial pneumonia in patients with adult respiratory distress syndrome. *Am J Respir Crit Care Med.* 1998;157(4 Part 1):1165.

31. Bernard GR, Artigas A, Brigham KL, et al. Report of the American-European Consensus Conference on ARDS: definitions, mechanisms, relevant outcomes and clinical trial coordination. *Intensive Care Med.* 1994;20:225–232.

32. Willms D, Nield M, Gocka I. Adult respiratory distress syndrome: Outcome in a community hospital. *Am J Crit Care.* 1994;3:337–341.

33. Morris AH. Cost-benefit considerations in managing oxygenation failure. *Respir Care.* 1993;38:829.

34. Montgomery AB, Stager MA, Carrico CJ, et al. Causes of mortality of patients with the adult respiratory distress syndrome. *Am Rev Respir Dis.* 1985;132:485–489.

35. Sloane PJ, et al. A multicenter registry of patients with acute respiratory distress syndrome: Physiology and outcome. *Am Rev Respir Dis.* 1992;146:419–426.

36. Bell RC, Coalson JJ, Smith JD, et al. Multiple organ system failure and infection in the adult respiratory distress syndrome. *Ann Intern Med.* 1983;99: 293–298.

37. Suchyta MR, Clemmer TP, Elliott CG, et al. The adult respiratory distress syndrome: a report of survival and modifying factors. *Chest.* 1992;101: 1074–1079.

38. Elliott CG, Rasmussen BY, Crapo RO, et al. Prediction of pulmonary function abnormalities after adult respiratory distress syndrome. *Am Rev Respir Dis.* 1987;135:634–638.

39. Schwartz DB, Bone RC, Balk RA, et al. Hepatic dysfunction in the adult respiratory distress syndrome. *Chest.* 1989;95:871–875.

40. Fanconi S, Kraemer R, Weber J, et al. Long-term sequelae in children surviving adult respiratory distress syndrome. *J Pediatr.* 1985;106:218–222.

41. Buchser E, Leuenberger PH, Chiolero R, et al. Reduced pulmonary capillary blood volume as a long-term sequela of adult respiratory distress syndrome. *Chest.* 1985;87:608–611.

42. Peters JI, Bell RC, Prihoda TJ, et al. Clinical determinants of abnormalities in pulmonary function in survivors of the adult respiratory distress syndrome. *Am Rev Respir Dis.* 1989;139:1163–1168.

43. Ghio AJ, Elliott CG, Crapo RO, et al. Impairment after respiratory distress syndrome. *Am Rev Respir Dis.* 1989;139:1158–1162.

44. Gattinoni L, Bombino M, Pelosi P, et al. Lung structure and function in different stages of severe adult respiratory distress syndrome. *JAMA.* 1994;271: 1772.

45. Lakshminarayan S, Stanford RE, Petty TL. Prognosis after recovery from adult respiratory distress syndrome. *Am Rev Respir Dis.* 1976;133:7–16.

46. Elliott CG, Morris AH, Cengiz M. Pulmonary function and exercise gas exchange in survivors of adult respiratory distress syndrome. *Am Rev Respir Dis.* 1981;123:492–495.

47. Abraham E, Yoshihara G. Cardiorespiratory effects of pressure controlled ventilation in severe respiratory failure. *Chest.* 1990;98:1445–1449.

48. Rappaport S, Shpiner R, Yoshihara G, et al. Randomized, prospective trial of pressure-limited versus volume-controlled ventilation in severe respiratory failure. *Crit Care Med.* 1994;22:22–32.

23

RESPIRATORY DISTRESS SYNDROME OF THE NEONATE

J. M. Cairo and Tara Orfanello Jones

*Information is not knowledge
and knowledge is not wisdom.*
—FRANK ZAPPA

LEARNING OBJECTIVES

1. Describe the most common factors that contribute to the incidence of respiratory distress syndrome (RDS) of the newborn.
2. Discuss the pathophysiology and clinical manifestations of RDS.
3. Provide information on various conditions that can complicate the diagnosis of RDS.
4. Describe various strategies that can be used to minimize the incidence of RDS.
5. Apply critical thinking skills of prioritizing, anticipating, and decision making in the management of neonates with RDS.
6. Interpret clinical data from case examples to make appropriate therapeutic interventions, including selection and implementation of mechanical ventilation.
7. Describe various strategies that can be used in the diagnosis and treatment of a neonate with RDS that is complicated by the presence of primary pulmonary hypertension.
8. Evaluate treatment outcomes following therapeutic intervention, such as the successful implementation of mechanical ventilation.

KEY WORDS

Apgar Scoring
Continuous Positive Airway Pressure (CPAP)
High Frequency Ventilation (HFV)
Hyaline Membrane Disease
Neutral Thermal Environment
Nutritional Support
Prematurity
Respiratory Distress Syndrome (RDS) of the Neonate
Surfactant Deficiency

INTRODUCTION

Respiratory distress syndrome (RDS) of the neonate (also known as infant respiratory distress syndrome or hyaline membrane disease) is the most common cause of morbidity and mortality in newborn infants.[1] Despite improvements in perinatal care, RDS remains a major public health concern, affecting approximately 25,000 infants each year in the United States. Indeed, it is estimated that RDS complicates 1% of all births worldwide and is responsible for nearly 30% of all neonatal deaths.

Although neonatal RDS was first described in 1903, its etiology was not determined until the latter half of the 20th century. Groundbreaking studies by Avery and colleagues[2] in the late 1950s demonstrated that the underlying problem in RDS is a deficiency of surfactant production in the terminal airspaces due to immaturity of the pulmonary system. Subsequent studies by other investigators have confirmed this hypothesis and shown that the incidence of RDS is inversely related to gestational age.[3] Moreover, these epidemiological data have demonstrated that 60% of all infants born before 30 weeks gestation are afflicted with RDS. The incidence decreases to 30% for infants born between 30 and 34 weeks gestation, and is relatively rare in infants who reach a gestational age of 39 weeks.

A number of other perinatal factors besides prematurity can increase the incidence of RDS, including low birthweight, abnormal placental conditions, umbilical cord compression and prolapse, and prenatal maternal complications, such as diabetes, hyper- and hypotension, shock, anemia, and hemorrhage. Respiratory distress syndrome occurs more often in males than females. It also occurs at a higher rate in the second-born and subsequent births in cases of multiple gestation. The incidence of RDS is significantly higher in premature infants born by abdominal surgery

CRITICAL CONTENT

The most common factors known to contribute to the incidence of RDS are:

- Prematurity (<32 weeks gestation)
- Low birthweight
- Abnormal placental conditions
- Prenatal maternal complications, such as diabetes mellitus, hyper- and hypotension, shock, anemia, and hemorrhage
- Caesarian delivery

(elective caesarian section) when compared to infants delivered vaginally following a normal course of labor.[4]

PATHOGENESIS OF RESPIRATORY DISTRESS SYNDROME OF THE NEONATE

As already described, the underlying problem in respiratory distress syndrome of the neonate is a deficiency of pulmonary surfactant in the terminal airspaces. Pulmonary surfactant is initially produced in small amounts by the fetus beginning about the 22nd week of gestation. A major surge in surfactant production occurs between the 32nd and 34th weeks of gestation. (See critical content box for more detailed information about surfactant.) Infants born before 32 weeks of gestation therefore typically demonstrate inadequate surfactant production. This lack of surfactant causes an increase in alveolar surface tension, which leads to alveolar collapse on expiration. The infant attempts to compensate for the increased surface tension and maintain alveolar patency by generating higher-than-normal intrathoracic pressure gradients. Unfortunately the neonatal chest wall is fairly compliant (ie, soft and pliable) and it is therefore easily pulled inward as the infant makes greater inspiratory efforts, thus resulting in the common clinical finding of chest wall "retractions." With continued effort, the infant begins to experience respiratory muscle fatigue, which leads to a reduced alveolar expansion, progressive atelectasis, and decreased pulmonary compliance.

These alterations in respiratory mechanics (increased chest wall compliance combined with decreased lung compliance) are manifested as a reduction in functional residual capacity (FRC). When coupled with the presence of an immature alveolar-capillary network, alveolar collapse (shunt) and ventilation-perfusion imbalances occur, ultimately leading to progressive hypoxemia, hypercarbia, and respiratory acidosis. If the hypoxemia persists, the infant becomes hypoxic and must resort to anaerobic metabolism to meet the increased metabolic needs, thus leading to a metabolic acidosis.

The structural changes that occur in the lungs of neonates with RDS are remarkably consistent. Initially, bronchial membrane edema and hemorrhage occur, giving the lungs a dark red, liver-like appearance. As the disease progresses, damage to the capillary endothelial cells caused by hypoxia and acidosis causes an increase in pulmonary capillary permeability. This increased capillary permeability along with the aforementioned increased alveolar surface tension promotes the leakage of protein-rich fluid into the alveoli and the formation of characteristic hyaline membranes. (It is worth noting that these hyaline membranes are similar in appearance to those seen in patients with acute respiratory distress syndrome.) Although the development of hyaline membranes has always been of interest, one should not lose sight of the fact that the primary pathophysiologic changes that are responsible for the abnormal gas exchange are

CRITICAL CONTENT

PULMONARY SURFACTANT

Pulmonary surfactant is composed of a mixture of lipids and proteins that are secreted by alveolar type II cells. It consists of approximately 90% phospholipids and 10% proteins. The phospholipid portion consists primarily of dipalmitoyl phosphatidylcholine (DPPC) with smaller amounts of unsaturated phosphatidylcholine, phosphatidylinositol, phosphatidylethanolamine, and neutral lipids. The protein components are glycoproteins that are designated as surfactant-associated protein A (SP-A), B (SP-B), C (SP-C), and D (SP-D). These surfactant-associated proteins serve multiple roles, such as promoting phospholipid reabsorption, enhancing immune response, and enhancing fluid clearance. Pulmonary surfactant reduces alveolar surface tension through the absorption of lipids to form a phospholipid monolayer at the air-liquid interface in alveoli.[6,7]

the diffuse pulmonary edema and atelectasis and their effects on FRC and work of breathing as described earlier. The disease process is generally self-limiting because after about 72 hours, pulmonary macrophages appear and phagocytose the hyaline membranes. Complete resolution of the disease typically occurs within 5 to 7 days, provided that further pulmonary damage has not occurred during treatment.[5]

PRENATAL DIAGNOSIS

Prenatal diagnosis of RDS is not feasible; however, several laboratory tests have been developed to predict the risk of developing RDS.[5,8] The most commonly performed test involves determination of the lecithin/sphingomyelin (L/S) ratio of amniotic fluid obtained via amniocentesis. It is generally accepted that an L/S ratio ≥2:1 indicates that a sufficient amount of surfactant is present to minimize the risk of RDS. Ratios less than 2:1 suggest the possibility of RDS and that delivery should be delayed as long as possible to allow greater fetal lung maturation to occur. Several other tests that most clinicians feel are not as reliable as those used to quantify the L/S ratio can be used to assess fetal lung maturation. These include the Clement's bubble test (shake test) and various spectrophotometric analysis techniques designed to determine the presence of adequate amounts of surfactant in amniotic fluid.

CLINICAL MANIFESTATIONS

Infants born with RDS typically demonstrate the signs of labored breathing and respiratory distress at birth or within the first hours following delivery. Many of these infants will present with abnormal Apgar scores. *Apgar scoring* is a technique for performing a rapid physical assessment of a neonate. Premature infants born before 32 weeks gestation or who are depressed due to asphyxia present with poor Apgar scores both at 1 minute and at 5 minutes after delivery. (See critical content box for a description of Apgar scoring.) Neonates born before 28 weeks gestation will also show characteristic signs of immaturity, including low birthweight, reduced muscle tone, thin, translucent skin, fine downy hair, smooth soles, small nipples, and immature genitalia. More mature and stronger infants (those born after 32 weeks gestation) may demonstrate higher Apgar scores at birth and have a more delayed and slowly progressive course of RDS.

CRITICAL CONTENT

APGAR SCORING

Assessment is typically performed at set time intervals after delivery. Five physical signs are assessed, including heart rate, respiratory rate, muscle tone, reflex irritability, and skin color (ie, the presence of cyanosis or pallor). Each physical sign is rated as 0, 1, or 2 points, depending on the severity of the finding. For example, severe depression warrants a score 0 whereas mild to moderate depression is rated as 1. A score of 2 is reserved for normal findings. The Apgar score is normally assessed at 1 minute and again at 5 minutes of age. If the 5-minute score is less than 7, additional scores are usually assessed every 5 minutes for up to 20 minutes. The term "Apgar scoring" is named for Virginia Apgar, the physician who first proposed this type of assessment.[9]

The Apgar score is an objective method of quantifying the newborn's condition. It is therefore useful for conveying information about the overall status and response to resuscitation. However, resuscitation must be initiated before the score is assigned. Therefore, the Apgar score is not used to determine the need for resuscitation, what resuscitation steps are necessary, or when to use them. Three of the five Apgar parameters (respiration, heart rate, and color) are used to direct resuscitation efforts. The precise sequence of resuscitation steps is thoroughly described in the neonatal resuscitation textbook published by the American Academy of Pediatrics.[10]

The classic signs of respiratory distress include tachypnea (respiratory rate >60 breaths per minute), cyanosis on room air, nasal flaring, substernal and intercostal retractions, abdominal distension, and expiratory grunting. Paradoxical (ie, see-saw) respirations in which the chest wall moves inward and the abdomen moves outward on inspiration and vice versa on expiration are commonly seen, and indicate an increase in the work of breathing. This breathing pattern can also suggest the presence of respiratory muscle fatigue and imminent respiratory failure.

Chest radiographs of infants with RDS are characterized by a diffuse reticulogranular (ground-glass) pattern and hypoexpansion. Neonates delivered closer to term may have a less specific hazy infiltrate. As we will discuss subsequently, radiographs from infants with RDS are similar to those obtained from infants with group B streptococcal infection.

Measurements of respiratory mechanics demonstrate a characteristic restrictive pattern. Total lung capacity (TLC), inspiratory capacity (IC), vital capacity (VC), functional residual capacity (FRC), and residual volume (RV) are decreased.[11] Although the infant's chest wall compliance is high, static lung compliance is significantly reduced due to the presence of diffuse atelectasis and edema.

Arterial blood gas analysis demonstrates all of the signs of ventilatory failure: acidosis, hypercapnia, and hypoxemia. During the early stages of RDS, the acidosis is the result of acute ventilatory failure and the associated increase in $Paco_2$. As the disease progresses, the pH tends to remain decreased due to the presence of a metabolic acidosis associated with lactic acid accumulation that results from hypoxemia and anaerobic metabolism. The hypercapnia of RDS may occur with hypoventilation associated with respiratory muscle fatigue, or from V/Q mismatch. The hypoxemia is primarily from the alveolar edema and atelectasis (intrapulmonary shunting) described earlier. The presence of intracardiac shunts, such as a patent ductus arteriosus (PDA), or persistent pulmonary hypertension of the newborn (PPHN) can also contribute to venous admixture and the resultant hypoxemia.

Hemodynamic problems are also common in these patients. Alveolar hypoxia leads to pulmonary arteriolar constriction and elevation in pulmonary vascular pressures. This is often further aggravated by the development of acidosis, which causes further pulmonary hypertension. If the systemic vascular pressures remain low, and the pulmonary hypertension is significant, a right-to-left ("cyanotic") shunt may occur through fetal pathways (ie, foramen ovale and ductus arteriosus), creating a condition referred to as PPHN. In these situations, the neonate's condition improves with therapy (eg, fluid administration, oxygen therapy), and as systemic vascular pressures increase, the shunt typically reverses and becomes left-to-right. In this latter case, the increased blood flow to the right heart and into the pulmonary circulation ultimately leads to pulmonary congestion, increased pulmonary capillary leakage into the alveoli, and pulmonary edema. The development of a left-to-right PDA shunt often confounds the diagnosis, as it typically occurs as the infant's RDS is beginning to improve with therapy, thus slowing, or sometimes stopping altogether, improvement of the infant's condition.

CRITICAL CONTENT

**TYPICAL CLINICAL PRESENTATION
OF AN INFANT WITH RDS**

- Respiratory distress at or shortly after birth
- Tachypnea
- Room air cyanosis
- Nasal flaring
- Subcostal and intercostal retractions
- "See-saw" respiration (paradoxical abdominal and chest movement)
- Expiratory grunting
- Chest radiographs show a reticular, groundglass appearance with hypoexpansion of the lungs

DIFFERENTIAL DIAGNOSIS OF RDS

The differential diagnosis of RDS should include assessment for the presence of systemic illnesses with pulmonary manifestations, such as viral or bacterial pneumonia, sepsis, congenital heart disease, and aspiration syndrome (clear fluid, blood, or meconium). A less serious form of respiratory distress in the newborn, which is called transient tachypnea of the newborn (TTN), should also be considered in the differential diagnosis of RDS.

Neonatal Pneumonia

A number of viruses and bacteria can cause pneumonia in neonates. Viral agents include herpes virus, cytomegalovirus, rubella, varicella zoster, and respiratory syncytial virus. Bacteria that are most often associated with this type of pneumonia include group B streptococci, *Escherichia coli, Listeria monocytogenes, Klebsiella pneumoniae,* and *Treponema pallidum.* Beta-hemolytic streptococcal infection is by far the most serious type of pneumonia that can affect neonates.

Group B streptococcal infections should be suspected in cases in which maternal fever and ammonitis are present, or when premature rupture of the membranes (PROM) occurs more than 12 hours prior to delivery. (Beta-hemolytic streptococci are normal inhabitants of maternal cervical and vaginal tissue.) Symptoms associated with group B streptococcal pneumonia may appear within several hours after birth or may not appear for several days. Generalized sepsis may appear simultaneously with the signs of pneumonia, but pneumonia is considered the primary event. Preterm infants typically demonstrate gross alveolar involvement, whereas term or near-term infants may show a diffuse or localized involvement.[5]

Physical signs of pneumonia include generalized listlessness, irritability, and poor feeding. Although hematology studies involving white blood cell counts are not always reliable in diagnosing infection, neutropenia usually indicates sepsis or the presence of a severe infection. Leukocytosis with the number of mature leukocytes representing only about 20% of the total leukocyte count (ie, shift to the left) may also indicate the presence of group B streptococcal pneumonia.[11]

Persistent Pulmonary Hypertension of the Newborn (PPHN)

Persistent pulmonary hypertension of the newborn (previously known as persistent fetal circulation, or PFC) develops in the presence of a right-to-left (cyanotic) shunt through a patent ductus arteriosus and foramen ovale. As previously described, PPHN occurs when fetal shunts fail to close at birth due to hypoxia and acidosis, and systemic hypotension combined with significant pulmonary hypertension occur. PPHN is often preceded by intrauterine asphyxia, and it is commonly associated with other conditions that lead to hypoxia and hypoventilation, such as the presence of severe RDS, meconium aspiration, and pneumonia. With the requirement of development of pulmonary hypertension as a key precipitating factor, PPHN is much more common in larger, less premature infants whose pulmonary vasculature is capable of developing a sustained vasoconstrictive response to the hypoxia and acidosis.

Apgar scores for these neonates are typically lower at 1 and 5 minutes. Tachypnea, mild to moderate respiratory distress, and hypoxemia are typically noted with and without cyanosis. Chest radiographic findings are usually normal except that pulmonary vascular markings may be diminished. Although breath sounds are normal, auscultation of the heart reveals the presence of a holosystolic murmur.[5]

Diagnosis of PPHN has typically been accomplished using the hyperoxia test, pre- and postductal arterial blood gas sampling, and the hyperoxia-hyperventilation test. The hyperoxia test involves administration of 100% oxygen via an oxyhood. Infants who maintain a Pao_2 >100 mm Hg are thought to have disease of the lung parenchyma, while infants with a Pao_2 <50 mm Hg are thought to have evidence of a right-to-left

shunt. A Pao_2 between 50 and 100 mm Hg suggests the presence of a parenchymal disease or a cardiovascular defect. Noninvasive measurements of pre- and postductal Pao_2 can be obtained using transcutaneous monitoring. In these studies, a difference in Pao_2 >15 mm Hg indicates the presence of significant shunting of blood through the ductus arteriosus. In the hyperoxia-hyperventilation test the infant is hyperventilated with a manual resuscitator with 100% oxygen. The level of hyperventilation is determined by ventilating the infant to a $Paco_2$ of 20 to 25 mm Hg (a range that will yield the greatest level of pulmonary vasodilation). In those infants with PPHN, the Pao_2 will typically rise to 100 mm Hg or higher. If the Pao_2 fails to rise to this level with hyperventilation, it suggests the possibility that a congenital cardiac defect (eg, atrial or ventricular septal defect, tetralogy of Fallot, transposition of the great vessels) may be present. Identification of congenital cardiac defects, as well as confirmation of the presence of a PDA, can be accomplished with echocardiography studies or other invasive cardiac catheterization studies.

CRITICAL CONTENT

COMMON TESTS USED TO DIAGNOSE PPHN

- Hyperoxia test
- Pre- and postductal blood gas sampling
- Hyperoxia-hyperventilation test
- Doppler (color) echocardiography

Patent Ductus Arteriosus and Heart Failure (Acyanotic, Left-to-Right Shunt)

Patent ductus arteriosus is a common finding in premature infants weighing less than 1500 grams. PDA may occur in isolation or may accompany other types of pathology, including RDS and other types of congenital cardiac defects, such as ventricular septal defects and transposition of the great vessels. Isolated PDA is often seen in patients with congenital rubella. PDA is also often seen in infants born at high altitude. PDA is very often seen associated with RDS, although its manifestations are often not apparent until the RDS begins to resolve.

PDA should be suspected in those infants who demonstrate a continuous or machine-like murmur on auscultation of the heart, bounding pulses, low diastolic pressures (<26 mm Hg), a wide pulse pressure, and an active precordium.[12] Congestive heart failure (CHF), pulmonary infections, and failure to thrive are also commonly noted in these infants.[5] Definitive diagnosis of PDA can be accomplished with echocardiography, particularly with color Doppler echocardiography. These studies can demonstrate the direction in which blood is shunting through the ductus arteriosus (ie, either right-to-left or left-to-right), along with evidence of left atrial and ventricular enlargement and flattening of the interventricular septum.

Acyanotic PDA shunting should also be suspected in an infant who was beginning to recover from RDS as evidenced by reductions in oxygen concentrations and levels of ventilatory support as might be anticipated in uncomplicated RDS, but who then relatively suddenly stops improving, or acutely worsens in their clinical condition. This often occurs on days 4 to 7, when the hypoxemia and acidosis of the RDS has been effectively treated and the patient's pulmonary vascular pressures begin to fall. The falling pulmonary artery pressure allows systemic (aortic) pressure to create flow from the aorta to the pulmonary artery, hence the development of excessive pulmonary blood flow. This increased pulmonary blood flow results in pulmonary edema and decreasing compliance (recognized by the unexpected clinical deterioration). This leads to the eventual development of CHF if the condition persists for a long enough period of time. The scenario above often occurs in the very premature infant. In these infants the ductus arteriosus often fails to close at birth, but the magnitude of blood flow through the ductus does not become great enough to detect until the recovery phase of the RDS causes the fall in pulmonary vascular pressures.

Meconium Aspiration Syndrome (MAS)

Aspiration syndromes, particularly meconium aspiration syndrome (MAS), can lead to an acquired surfactant deficiency, even in near-term or postterm infants. In fact, MAS can only develop in infants who are delivered at or near term. It is generally believed that the infant must be of at least 36 weeks gestation to have sufficient meconium to present an aspiration danger. The typical scenario in which MAS occurs is that of a large term or postterm infant who is asphyxiated before or during the delivery process.

The presence of meconium-stained amniotic fluid or yellow staining of nails and umbilical cord should alert the clinician to the possibility of MAS. The definitive diagnosis of MAS, however, requires the direct visualization of meconium below the vocal cords. The presence of respiratory distress, including tachypnea, nasal flaring, grunting, and cyanosis are common findings in these infants. Coarse bronchial breath sounds and prolonged expirations are also heard. Hypoxemia, hypercarbia, and metabolic acidosis usually develop during the first 24 hours after birth in moderately affected neonates.

CRITICAL CONTENT

MECONIUM ASPIRATION

Meconium is a viscous green liquid that is composed of undigested amniotic fluid, squamous epithelial cells, and vernix, that is normally found in the fetal bowel.[5] When the fetus experiences hypoxia in utero, blood flow is redistributed away from the fetal lungs, spleen, kidneys, and intestines, to the heart and brain to preserve the integrity of these vital organs. This reduction in blood flow to the intestines results in vasoconstriction of the intestinal vasculature, increased peristalsis, and sphincter relaxation, along with passage of the meconium into the amniotic fluid. The asphyxiated fetus demonstrates deep, gasping respiratory movements, and aspiration of meconium and amniotic fluid occurs.

Chest radiographs of infants with meconium aspiration syndrome demonstrate alveolar hyperinflation with depressed diaphragms. Areas of decreased aeration are typically interspersed with areas of hyperlucency, resulting in a pattern of irregular densities throughout the lung fields. Nonspecific consolidation of various lung lobes is also present. Pleural fluid accumulation and air leaks, particularly pneumomediastinum and pneumothorax, are also commonly seen.[5]

Transient Tachypnea of the Newborn (TTN)

Transient tachypnea of the newborn is a milder form of respiratory distress in neonates. As its name implies, it is characterized by higher-than-normal respiratory rates (>100 breaths/min). It is also characterized by cyanosis, mild hypoxemia, and a mixed acidosis that develops several hours after a normal delivery (ie, Apgar scores at 1 and 5 minutes are typically normal). Chest radiographs demonstrate pulmonary congestion with patchy infiltrates. It is believed that this mild, short duration of respiratory distress is related to delayed fetal lung fluid absorption by the neonate's lymphatic system following birth.

TTN occurs most often in near-term and term infants who experience intrauterine asphyxia. Evidence of maternal bleeding, diabetes, and prolapsed umbilical cord, as well as maternal analgesia and anesthesia are often implicated in the etiology of

CRITICAL CONTENT

COMMON CONDITIONS THAT SHOULD BE CONSIDERED IN THE DIFFERENTIAL DIAGNOSIS OF RDS

- Neonatal pneumonia (particularly group B streptococcal infections)
- Persistent pulmonary hypertension of the newborn
- Patent ductus arteriosus (acyanotic left-to-right shunting)

TTN. It is generally self-limiting and tends to resolve by 48 hours after birth when the infant is treated with low concentration oxygen therapy.

MANAGEMENT OF RDS

Prevention Strategies

The preferred approach to managing an infant with RDS is to minimize or avoid the development of the problem. Probably the most effective means of minimizing high-risk situations is to provide effective prenatal care of the mother and fetus. In cases where RDS appears likely, there have been a number of preventive approaches proposed during the past 25 years, including administration of maternal glucocorticoids (which is thought to accelerate the natural biochemical development of surfactants), minimizing the damage to existing surfactant by avoiding birth asphyxiation to the greatest extent possible, and the now-common approach of preventing or minimizing the severity through prophylactic direct administration of surfactants to the neonate's lungs, either at or shortly after birth.

Management Strategies

Management strategies for infants with RDS should focus on providing support for adequate respiratory and cardiovascular function. Specifically, respiratory care procedures should be directed toward treating and subsequently preventing atelectasis, hypoxemia, and hypercarbia.[13,14] Oxygen therapy, initiation of ventilatory support, maintenance of a neutral thermal environment, administration of exogenous surfactants, antibiotics and appropriate fluid and electrolyte therapy, and providing adequate nutritional support form the foundation for successful care of these infants.

Surfactant Therapy. Perhaps no single therapy has had as great an impact on the morbidity and mortality of the premature infant than the use of exogenous surfactant replacement therapy. Beginning in 1990, when the FDA approved the first commercially available surfactants, there have been numerous published reports of the effectiveness of this type of therapy.[14] Not only has surfactant therapy demonstrated improved outcomes with RDS infants, but also it appears to be a factor involved in the lowering of the gestational age of viability. Many extremely premature, extremely low birth-weight infants are now surviving that would likely not have done so just a few years ago.

Many factors appear to influence the effectiveness of surfactant therapy.[15] There are various types of surfactants, methods of administration, infant-specific factors (not all RDS infants respond the same), and dosing schemes, as well as different times when the surfactant is first introduced. These all appear to be potentially important variables. For instance, controversy continues over when (in the course of the disease) surfactant should be administered. Very early administration (ie, immediately after delivery of a high-risk infant) is referred to as using a "prophylactic" approach. Waiting until clear clinical signs of RDS develop before beginning surfactant therapy is referred to as using the "rescue" approach. Both sides of this controversy have their advocates and reports of success. This complicated topic is beyond the scope of this chapter, and the reader is encouraged to further research this subject as you develop your understanding of management approaches to treatment of the RDS infant.

Oxygen Therapy.

Maintenance of adequate oxygenation with the lowest possible FIO_2 should be based on frequent monitoring of arterial blood gases through both noninvasive and invasive techniques. It is generally agreed that the infant's PaO_2 should be maintained in the range of 50 to 70 mm Hg with a $PaCO_2$ <60 mm Hg and a pH between 7.25 and 7.50.[16] Oxygen therapy with adequate humidity can be administered via an oxygen hood or through a nasal cannula. These methods of delivery have been shown to be quite effective for spontaneously breathing neonates.

Continuous Positive Airway Pressure (CPAP).

Failure to achieve an appropriate oxygen tension by oxygen therapy alone should prompt the therapist to suggest more aggressive strategies, such as the application of continuous distending pressure to the infant's airways with continuous positive airway pressure. CPAP administered through nasal prongs has been shown to be a quite effective means of treating hypoxemia by increasing the FRC and thus preventing atelectasis.[5] Nasal CPAP is indicated if the infant's PaO_2 is ≤50 mm Hg while receiving an FIO_2 >0.60. CPAP support usually begins between 4 and 6 cm H_2O. CPAP levels may be increased in 2-cm H_2O increments until an acceptable PaO_2 is achieved. Judicious adjustments in the level of CPAP are essential because excessive levels will result in reductions in cardiac output and hypercapnia.

Due to the higher incidence of failure of CPAP alone in lower birthweight infants, CPAP is often bypassed, and the infant will go directly from oxygen therapy to some form of mechanical assistance. This is a decision best made by an experienced clinician, who is able to assess the entire clinical picture and thus provide an individualized approach to care.

Mechanical Ventilation.

The decision to initiate intermittent positive pressure ventilation should be considered for infants who demonstrate ventilatory failure (ie, $PaCO_2$ >60 mm Hg and a pH <7.25) or severe apneic episodes. However, endotracheal intubation and mechanical ventilatory support are usually initiated at delivery for very premature infants and those neonates that have experienced significant perinatal asphyxia, even if the initial ABGs do not meet the above mentioned criteria. The incidence of failure of less aggressive measures is so high that experienced clinicians do not usually wait for deterioration to reach the point of extremely poor blood gas results. Ventilatory support for near-term and term infants is sometimes delayed until there are clear signs of respiratory distress, such as central cyanosis, grunting, nasal flaring, and substernal and intercostal retractions.

The goal of mechanical ventilatory support for infants with RDS should be to use the lowest possible mean airway pressures and FIO_2 to ensure adequate alveolar ventilation and tissue oxygenation. Achieving this goal will reduce the risks of oxygen toxicity, barotrauma, and other serious complications associated with positive pressure ventilation. Although there are a variety of ventilatory strategies that can be used for these infants, it is generally accepted that the use of a time-cycled, pressure-limited ventilator is preferred. This type of ventilatory support can provide a wide range of inspiratory to expiratory ratios (I:E) and inspiratory times along with positive end-expiratory pressure (PEEP). Short inspiratory times (eg, .25 to .40 second) resulting in smaller I:E ratios (eg, I:E ratios ≤1:1) are typically used initially, but may not be adequate to ensure sufficient time for oxygenation. Inspiratory holds may be used to allow for better distribution of ventilation on inspiration and thus more time for gas exchange. Inverse I:E ratios (ie, inspiratory times exceeding expiratory times) may also be beneficial but should be administered with caution because of the potential for cardiovascular compromise.

FIO_2 should be adjusted to ensure that the neonate's Pao_2 is maintained in a range of 50 to 70 mm Hg. PEEP levels of 4 to 6 cm H_2O are usually sufficient to prevent airway collapse on expiration and maintain adequate oxygenation. Higher levels of PEEP should be used judiciously to avoid the risk of barotrauma and hemodynamic compromise that is associated with elevated mean airway pressures.

High-frequency ventilation (HFV) delivered through either a high-frequency jet ventilator or a high-frequency oscillator may be effective for the infant who cannot be adequately ventilated and oxygenated with conventional ventilatory strategies. The main advantage of using this approach over conventional ventilators is related to the fact that high-frequency ventilation can be accomplished at significantly lower mean airway pressures than with conventional ventilatory modes. Those patients likely to develop severe RDS should probably be considered for early intervention with HFV, rather than waiting for conventional strategies to fail.

Maintenance of Neutral Thermal Environment (NTE). Maintenance of a neutral thermal environment for infants with RDS represents a considerable challenge for neonatal practitioners.

Although temperature assessment by measurements of rectal and axillary temperature can be used to assess core temperature, both of these techniques may be poor indicators of thermal balance in a cold environment. Furthermore, both techniques can only be performed intermittently and require unnecessary stimulation of the infant. Keep in mind that just because the infant's core temperature is normal, it does not necessarily follow that the infant is in an NTE. The key requirement for NTE is that the infant must be maintaining a normal core temperature while expending minimal metabolic energy (measured by oxygen consumption). If the infant is maintaining a normal core temperature, but has increased his or her metabolism to generate the heat to do so, the infant is not in an NTE, but is within what is referred to as their thermoregulatory range. This is the range of environmental temperatures over which the infant is able to maintain a normal core temperature through alteration of their metabolic rate.

Skin sensors that are placed on the face, abdomen, or thorax can provide a reasonable alternative for measuring environmental temperature and mediating the infant's response.[5] Servo-controlled radiant warmers that utilize skin sensors are used routinely to ensure that the infant's environmental temperature is maintained so that the skin temperature is 36°C to 36.5°C. Maintenance of skin temperature in this range results in maintaining the infant in a NTE.

The radiant warmer temperature range that must be maintained to keep an infant in their NTE depends on whether the infant is naked or clothed and on his or her gestational age and body weight. Temperatures of 23°C to 32°C can be used for infants who are clothed, while a temperature range of 32°C to 35°C is typically required for naked infants. The temperature range required to maintain NTE is lower for larger, term infants and becomes higher for lower birthweight (LBW), premature infants. The smaller the body mass, the higher the ratio of skin surface area to body mass. This, combined with minimal insulating subcutaneous fat in LBW infants causes excessive loss of body heat, thus the need to keep the surrounding temperature at a higher range to maintain normal core temperature with minimal energy expenditure (ie, maintain a NTE).

It is important to recognize that a cold infant will typically respond poorly to therapeutic interventions. In addition, if the infant is not in an NTE, he or she is expending metabolic energy to maintain their core temperature. This consumes additional oxygen and increases carbon dioxide production, thus requiring increased ventilation and consumption of vital nutrient stores, factors which limit or prevent growth. In a worst-case scenario, the infant may resort to a catabolic state (ie, may consume their own tissue proteins for the fuel necessary to maintain their metabolic rate).

General Supportive Care.   The immune response of neonates, particularly the response of premature infants, is immature and unable to protect the newborn against many pathogenic organisms. Consequently, these infants are susceptible to a variety of infections, most notably bacterial pneumonia. As discussed earlier, bacterial pneumonia must be considered in the differential diagnosis of RDS. As a result, antibiotic therapy should be administered when pneumonia is suspected. Definitive diagnosis of systemic infections can be accomplished through blood cultures and sensitivity studies and should ultimately be used to guide the choice of antibiotic.

Management of fluid and electrolyte and nutritional balance are essential for the successful treatment of neonates with RDS. It is important to understand that total body water and the distribution of fluids within the extracellular and intracellular spaces vary with gestational age and change after birth. For example, the intracellular fluid increases from about 20% of the total body weight at 32 weeks gestation to 33% of the body weight at term and to about 40% of the body weight at 3 months following birth. Conversely, the extracellular fluid decreases from nearly 80% of the body weight at 32 weeks gestation to 45% of the body weight at term. Eventually, the extracellular fluid will make up only about 25% of the total body weight at 3 months of age.[5] The timing of these changes can vary considerably in infants with

TABLE 23-1   NUTRITIONAL REQUIREMENTS FOR NEWBORNS[14]

Water	140–150 mL/kg/day
Calories	100–120 kcal/kg/day
Protein	7%–16% of calories
Fat	35%–55% of calories
Carbohydrates	35%–65% of calories

RDS. Recognition of fluid and electrolyte imbalances should be based upon history and physical findings and the results of clinical laboratory studies.

Fluid and electrolyte disturbances are most often associated with excessive insensible water loss through the skin and respiratory system, the presence of congenital cardiac defects, particularly those leading to congestive heart failure, and gastrointestinal problems such as necrotizing enterocolitis. Regardless of the etiology, fluid and electrolyte administration should be directed toward correcting acidosis, hypoglycemia, hypovolemia, and hypotension.[5]

Nutritional Management.   Nutritional support is an important concern in the care of neonates with RDS. The approach that is used to meet the nutritional requirements for these infants can vary considerably depending on the severity of their disease, whether the infant is receiving ventilatory support through an endotracheal tube, the gestational age of the infant, and if the infant has an effective sucking reflex and can tolerate oral feedings. Intravenous therapy, along with nasogastric, orogastric, and gastrostomy tubes can be used to feed both premature and term infants who are critically ill and cannot tolerate oral feedings. Infants who can tolerate oral feedings can receive the appropriate nutrients through conventional techniques (eg, bottle feeding) (Table 23–1).

CONSIDERATION OF COSTS AND ETHICAL ISSUES

Although the cost of care for newborns with RDS appears to have been reduced somewhat after the introduction of exogenous surfactant therapy,[17] these costs are still considerable. A recent investigation into the economics of treatment of RDS concluded that depending on birthweight, the expected cost of initial hospitalization for RDS care ranged from $124,022 per survivor from smaller infants (birthweight 500 to 1000 g) to $29,606 for larger infants (birthweight >1500 g).[18] The difficulty with assessing these data is that this only includes the initial hospitalization, not the cost of ongoing care that many of these survivors will ultimately require.

An additional major factor that complicates any assessment of the financial impact of RDS is that some of these RDS survivors go on to have various degrees of chronic lung disease, and/or

lifelong neurological complications. Even though there has been a decreased mortality associated with improved care, surfactant use, and other advances, there has been no reduction seen in the incidence of chronic lung diseases.[15]

Many infants who would have likely died previously are now surviving. This is certainly viewed by many as progress in the care of these infants. However, factored into this is the reality that while some of these infants go on to live normal lives, others have major medical and/or neurological handicaps. The ethical issues raised by this are potentially overwhelming and unfortunately beyond the scope of this chapter. The reader is encouraged to investigate these topics as time and interest allow.

CASE STUDY 1

BABY BOY GRUNTER

Initial Case Scenario

You are called to a high-risk delivery of a 17-year-old gravida 1, para 0 female who presents with PROM and abdominal contractions. The baby's estimated gestational age is 27 weeks as determined by the mother's last menstrual period. The mother reports that she is not taking any medications and denies substance abuse; however, traces of heroin were found in her blood at the time of delivery.

Data Obtained During Initial Maternal History and Physical Examination

Vital signs

HR	120/min
RR	16/min
BP	125/80
SpO$_2$	N/A
Temp.	99.1°F

General Appearance: The mother appears malnourished and very anxious. Lung sounds are clear on auscultation and she does not demonstrate any signs of respiratory distress.

Critical Thinking Exercise 1

ANTICIPATING POTENTIAL PROBLEMS AND SOLUTIONS

Maternal substance abuse can adversely affect the fetus. Several factors should be considered when you are preparing for the delivery of these high-risk neonates.

a. How will the presence of narcotics in the mother's blood potentially affect the neonate?

b. What should you anticipate about the baby's condition and how would you treat it?

c. What types of respiratory equipment should be available in the delivery room for a high-risk delivery?

d. Classify Baby Grunter as "Term" or "Pre-Term" and "AGA," "SGA," or "LGA" and explain how this will help you anticipate the problems he or she will be at high risk for.

Following an 8-hour period of intense labor, a 720-gram male is delivered by vaginal breech

CASE STUDY 1 *(continued)*

extraction. Upon delivery, the baby presents with cyanosis and no spontaneous respirations or heart rate. His Apgar score at 1 minute is 3.

Critical Thinking Exercise 2

PRIORITIZING PATIENT CARE

a. What are the immediate priorities [ie, what action(s) should immediately be taken]? Give the reason(s) for each recommendation.
b. Would the 1-minute Apgar be needed to dictate what action should be taken? Explain why or why not.

Group Critical Thinking Exercise 1

PRENATAL CARE

Providing adequate prenatal care, particularly to indigent mothers, is a major public health concern.

a. What are the components of a well-designed prenatal care plan?
b. Identify some of the social, ethical, and political concerns that can interfere with the provision of adequate prenatal care.

Upon completion of this group project, the results of the group's research can be presented to the full class for their reaction and input.

After several minutes and the initiation of the actions you recommended, his heart rate increases from 65 bpm to 123 bpm and the neonate begins to breathe spontaneously. However, his respirations are labored and paradoxical. After a moderate amount of clear fluid is suctioned through the endotracheal tube, his pulse oximeter saturation increases from 55% to 86%. His 5-minute Apgar score is 4. Umbilical artery

and venous catheters are inserted and the neonate is transferred to the NICU. Upon admission to the NICU arterial blood gases are obtained and a chest radiograph is ordered. Blood cultures are drawn and sent to the laboratory for analysis. The results of ABG analysis while he is being manually ventilated with 100% oxygen are:

ABG #1

pH	7.14
P_{CO_2}	71
P_{O_2}	48
HCO_3^-	23.5 mEq/L
BE	−10
Sa_{O_2}	64%

Additional Physical Exam and Lab Findings

General	There is no evidence of meconium in the placental fluid.
HEENT	Soft and flat fontanels and an intact palate.
Chest	Auscultation of the chest reveals bilateral coarse breath sounds.
CV	Cardiac auscultation reveals a regular rate and rhythm and no evidence of murmurs. Arterial blood pressure determined with a blood pressure cuff placed over the left arm is 81/65 mm Hg.
Abdomen	Physical exam of the neonate demonstrates a nontender, nondistended abdomen.
Radiograph	The initial chest radiograph reveals mild haziness in both lung bases.

(continued)

CASE STUDY 1 *(continued)*

Critical Thinking Exercise 3

**MAKING INFERENCES
BY CLUSTERING
DATA/DECISION MAKING**

Accurate interpretation of clinical and historical findings as well as laboratory tests forms the basis for selecting the working diagnosis and initial treatment plan.

a. Based on the data presented, what diagnosis would you suggest?

b. Identify the data that lead you to your initial inference regarding the diagnosis. (Explain how each piece of data led you to your inference.)

c. Briefly describe those conditions that should be ruled out in a differential diagnosis of this newborn and how will this be accomplished.

d. At this point what are the therapeutic interventions that are needed? Briefly give your reasons for each recommendation you make.

Shortly after NICU admission, mechanical ventilation is initiated using a time-cycled, pressure-limited ventilator.

Mechanical Ventilatory Support

Initial ventilator settings

RR	34
I-Time	0.34 sec
PIP	24 cm H_2O
PEEP	4 cm H_2O
FIO_2	0.80

Twenty minutes after initiation of mechanical ventilatory support, arterial blood gas analysis and blood chemistries are obtained. The results of the ABGs are:

ABG #2 vent: 80%

pH	7.32
Pco_2	50
Po_2	45
HCO_3^-	25 mEq/L
BE	−1.5
Sao_2	84%

Lab data

Na^+	138 mEq/L
K^+	4.1 mEq/L
Cl^-	100 mEq/L

Critical Thinking Exercise 4

**CLINICAL "PROBLEM SOLVING":
IDENTIFYING THE THERAPEUTIC
OPTIONS AND DECISION MAKING**

Given the continuing difficulty with maintaining adequate oxygenation of Baby Grunter, the physician asks you what the options are to improve oxygenation in this patient.

a. Identify at least three therapeutic options that might lead to improved oxygenation in this patient. Briefly explain the theoretical basis for how each option may result in improved oxygenation.

b. Which option would you recommend at this time? Support your decision by stating the reasons you think it is the best option at this time.

Group Critical Thinking Exercise 2

**NEGOTIATION
WITH THE PHYSICIAN**

Assign students in a group to select an option they identified in Critical Thinking Exercise 4b and present their arguments for their option to another student who will role-play the physician (or the instructor may role-play the physician). This can be presented before the entire class. Which students made effective arguments? The class can discuss the various approaches to negotiation with a physician when a therapist has a clinical recommendation. What are the characteristics of an effective argument?

CASE STUDY 1 *(continued)*

Age 12 hours: After consultation with the attending neonatologist, it is decided that the neonate will receive four doses of exogenous surfactant.

 Critical Thinking Exercise 5

ANTICIPATING RESPONSES TO THERAPY

a. Identify the desirable therapeutic responses to surfactant therapy, including what you would monitor to recognize when they are occurring.

b. What complications do you anticipate might occur and what would you monitor to recognize if they are developing?

 Group Critical Thinking Exercise 3

PRO/CON DEBATE: RESCUE VERSUS PROPHYLACTIC USE OF SURFACTANT THERAPY

There is considerable debate as to the most effective use of surfactant replacement therapy. Discuss the pros and cons of administering surfactant before there is evidence of severe respiratory distress. One group should present the pros to prophylactic (ie, early) use, while the other presents the con position, making the case for rescue use only. This debate can be presented in front of the entire class, followed by participation of the remaining students if desired.

After the first dose of surfactant, the PIP was decreased to 22 cm H_2O. The PIP remained stable at 20 cm H_2O following the administration of the three subsequent doses. Subsequent chest radiographs revealed continued atelectasis and bilateral ground-glass appearance, and blood gases demonstrated a persistent acidosis with hypoxemia on an FIO_2 of 0.80. Approximately 45 minutes after receiving the last dose of exogenous surfactant, Baby Grunter becomes agitated and

demonstrates signs of increased respiratory distress. Pulse oximetry readings show a rapid decline in oxygen saturation (SpO_2 of 75%), his heart rate increases to 170/min, and his mean arterial pressure rises to 95 mm Hg. Breath sounds are significantly decreased on the right side of the chest, and severe retractions are noted. A stat chest radiograph was ordered.

 Critical Thinking Exercise 6

CLINICAL PROBLEM SOLVING/DECISION MAKING

a. Given the relatively acute clinical deterioration, what is the most likely differential diagnosis at this time?

b. What is the appropriate response to this most recent crisis?

c. What was most likely the etiology of this problem?

Age 36 hours: After Baby Grunter received the appropriate treatment for the acute deterioration he stabilized, but showed no signs of significant clinical improvement. After further consultation with the neonatologist, it was decided that conventional mechanical ventilation would be discontinued and a high-frequency ventilation strategy using a high-frequency oscillator would be attempted.

Initial HFOV settings

Frequency	15 Hz
Amplitude	26 cm H_2O
Mean Airway Pressure	11 cm H_2O
FIO_2	0.55

Rib expansion as noted on the most recent chest radiograph was 10.5 at an MAP of 14 (immediately prior to placement on HFO). Arterial blood

(continued)

CASE STUDY 1 (*continued*)

gases drawn after 30 minutes of HFOV demonstrate the following results:

ABG #3 HFO 55%

pH	7.35
Pco$_2$	45
Po$_2$	60
HCO$_3^-$	25 mEq/L
BE	−1
Sao$_2$	90%

Group Critical Thinking Exercise 4

REFLECTION ON DECISION MAKING: HFV VERSUS CONVENTIONAL VENTILATION

Initially the decision in this case was to start with conventional ventilation.

a. Was this obviously a bad decision at the time? Discuss why it was, or why it was not. Support your position with reasons.

b. Examine and reflect on the decision to go to HFV. What do you think the reasons were behind this decision being made *at this point in time* in the patient's management?

During the subsequent 12 hours, the F$_{IO_2}$ is reduced to 0.45. The baby remains stable for the next 36 hours and a decision is made to wean him from the HFOV.

Critical Thinking Exercise 7

PROBLEM SOLVING: WEANING FROM MECHANICAL VENTILATOR SUPPORT

Describe the appropriate parameters and steps for weaning an infant from a high-frequency oscillator.

Age 96 hours: After successfully weaning from the HFOV, the infant is placed on SIMV at minimal settings.

SIMV settings

RR	10/min
I-Time	0.33 sec
PIP	12 cm H$_2$O
PEEP	5 cm H$_2$O
F$_{IO_2}$	0.28

Arterial blood gases drawn after 30 minutes of SIMV demonstrate the following results:

ABG #4 SIMV 28%

pH	7.35
Pco$_2$	42
Po$_2$	75
HCO$_3^-$	23 mEq/L
BE	−2.5
Sao$_2$	96%

The infant remains stable on these settings for the next 8 hours and the decision is made to discontinue the SIMV and place him on CPAP with 4 cm H$_2$O and an F$_{IO_2}$ of 0.24. The infant's condition, including vital signs, ABGs, and pulse oximetry remain stable for the next 24 hours while being maintained on these minimal ventilator settings. Baby Grunter is extubated the next morning and placed in an incubator on room air.

Critical Thinking Exercise 8

ANTICIPATING PROBLEMS AND SOLUTIONS: EXTUBATION

a. What types of equipment should you have at the bedside when extubating Baby Grunter?

b. What are the potential problems that can develop upon extubation? How will you recognize if these problems develop?

c. What is the appropriate treatment for the infant after extubation?

CASE STUDY 2

BABY BLUE

Initial Evaluation

You are asked to evaluate an infant with cyanosis and tachypnea. Upon reviewing the infant's history, you learn that the baby is a 39-week gestation, 5500-gram, 1-week-old female born to a mother with uncontrolled diabetes (IDDM). Shortly after birth, the infant was diagnosed with respiratory distress syndrome and treated with surfactant replacement and mechanical ventilation. Initial chest radiographs revealed the characteristic bilateral ground-glass appearance, which resolved over about 2 days on mechanical ventilation. Subsequent laboratory tests and chest radiographs showed resolution of the RDS on day 4 of therapy, and the infant was extubated and placed on nasal CPAP of 5 cm H_2O for 2 days. She was then weaned from the nasal CPAP and placed on a nasal cannula at a flow of 0.5 L/min. Approximately 12 hours after the initiation of the oxygen via the nasal cannula, the infant demonstrated signs of cyanosis and tachypnea.

Critical Thinking Exercise 1

ANTICIPATING/INITIAL ASSESSMENT

Using the clinical history provided:

a. Classify Baby Blue as "Term" or "Pre-Term" and "AGA," "SGA," or "LGA" and explain how this will help you anticipate the problems she will be at high risk for. List various conditions that should be considered in the differential diagnosis of this infant based on this analysis and her resultant classification.

b. Describe the tests that can be performed in the differential diagnosis of the origin of this patient's cyanosis.

Current vital signs and physical examination and lab data:

Chest	Clear bilateral breath sounds.
CV	Holosystolic murmur.
Radiograph	Decreased pulmonary vascular markings.

Vital signs

HR	135/min
RR	74/min
BP	90/50
SpO_2	74%
Temp.	N/A

You place the infant under an oxyhood with 100% oxygen and obtain an ABG:

ABG #1 100% oxyhood

pH	7.21
Pco_2	57
Po_2	44
HCO_3^-	22.5 mEq/L
BE	−8
Sao_2	63%

The physician asks you to perform a pre- and postductal arterial blood gas measurement. Blood samples are obtained from the right radial artery and from the umbilical artery.

Pre- and postductal blood Po_2

Right radial Pao_2	105 mm Hg
Umbilical artery Pao_2	50 mm Hg

(continued)

CASE STUDY 2 *(continued)*

Critical Thinking Exercise 2

CLINICAL ASSESSMENT AND PROBLEM SOLVING

a. What can you infer from the pre- and post-ductal blood gas result?

b. Demonstrate with a schematic diagram how this differential in P_{O_2} can occur.

c. How can these data be used to develop a sound diagnostic strategy to determine the etiology of this infant's problem?

You are asked by the attending neonatal cardiologist to perform a hyperventilation-hyperoxia test. The results of this test are below:

Hyperoxia-hyperventilation test results

pHa	7.57
Pa_{CO_2}	22 mm Hg
Pa_{O_2}	85 mm Hg

Critical Thinking Exercise 3

INTERPRETING DATA FROM SPECIALIZED TESTS

The hyperoxia-hyperventilation test is performed specifically to identify the presence of PPHN.

a. Why is it important to maintain a low Pa_{CO_2} during this procedure? Explain the physiological basis of this test and how it can be used in the diagnosis of PPHN.

b. How can this test be performed in a safe and effective manner?

c. Describe newer methods of gathering the same information. Is there a lower risk involved for the patient with these newer methods?

After consulting with the neonatologist, the decision is made to administer inhaled nitric oxide. The infant is intubated and nitric oxide (NO) therapy is administered at 20 ppm via a time-cycled, pressure-limited mechanical ventilator. After 24 hours of NO therapy the infant's Pa_{O_2} increases to 75 mm Hg on an F_{IO_2} of 0.30. Within 48 hours, the infant's Pa_{O_2} increases to 95 mm Hg and remains stable as the NO is weaned to 5 ppm. Over the next 6 hours the NO is weaned to zero, and is subsequently discontinued. The baby is released to the step-down unit for observation. She continues to be stable and is discharged 8 days later.

Critical Thinking Exercise 4

NITRIC OXIDE THERAPY: COSTS AND ETHICAL CONCERNS

NO therapy is relatively new. Like all new therapies it takes some time to determine where and when the therapy is cost effective. Because of the considerable costs involved, NO therapy has stirred considerable debate among clinicians.

a. Describe the indications for instituting nitric oxide therapy. What are the potential hazards of this type of therapy? Describe the precautions that must be taken to prevent adverse side effects during this type of therapy.

b. Is NO therapy reasonable in this specific situation? Cite specific reasons why you feel it is or is not appropriate in this situation.

c. Why is such therapy so controversial? How do ethics become involved in the consideration of this type of therapy?

KEY POINTS

- Respiratory distress syndrome (RDS) of the neonate (also known as infant respiratory distress syndrome or hyaline membrane disease) is the most common cause of mortality and morbidity in newborn infants.

- Despite improvements in perinatal care, RDS remains a major public health concern, affecting approximately 25,000 infants each year in the United States, and it is responsible for nearly 30% of all neonatal deaths.

- The incidence of RDS is inversely related to gestational age and is relatively rare in infants who reach a gestational age of 39 weeks.

- The underlying problem in respiratory distress syndrome of the neonate is a deficiency in the amount of pulmonary surfactant initially produced by the fetus in the terminal airspaces.

- The lack of surfactant causes an increase in alveolar surface tension, which leads to alveolar collapse on expiration.

- A number of perinatal factors besides prematurity can increase the incidence of RDS, including low birth weight, prenatal maternal conditions, and multiple gestations.

- Prenatal diagnosis of RDS is not feasible; however, several laboratory tests have been developed to predict the risk of developing RDS, most notably the L/S ratio.

- The classic signs of respiratory distress include tachypnea (respiratory rate >60 breaths per minute), cyanosis on room air, nasal flaring, substernal and intercostal retractions, abdominal distension, and expiratory grunting.

- The differential diagnosis of RDS should include assessment for the presence of systemic illnesses with pulmonary manifestations, such as viral or bacterial pneumonia, sepsis, congenital heart disease, and aspiration syndrome (clear fluid, blood, or meconium).

- A less serious form of respiratory distress in the newborn, which is called transient tachypnea of the newborn (TTN), should also be considered in the differential diagnosis of RDS.

- PPHN develops in the presence of a right-to-left (cyanotic) shunt through a PDA and FO, and is commonly associated with severe RDS or other causes of significant hypoxemia and hypoventilation, eg, intrauterine asphyxia, MAS, or pneumonia.

- PDA is very often associated with RDS, although its manifestations are often not apparent until the RDS begins to resolve.

- Postdelivery management of infants with RDS should focus on providing adequate respiratory and cardiovascular support directed at treating and preventing atelectasis, hypoxemia, and hypercarbia.

- No single therapy has probably had as big an impact on the morbidity and mortality of premature infants as the use of exogenous surfactant replacement.

- The effectiveness of surfactant replacement therapy is influenced by the type of surfactant used, methods of administration, and timing of when the therapy is initiated.

- The goal of mechanical ventilatory support should be to use the lowest mean airway pressures and F_{IO_2} to ensure adequate alveolar ventilation and tissue oxygenation.

- Maintenance of a neutral thermal environment, adequate nutritional support, and fluid and electrolyte balance are essential to providing optimum care for infants with RDS.

REFERENCES

1. Avery GB. *Neonatology: Pathophysiology and Management of the Newborn.* 3rd ed. Philadelphia: Lippincott; 1987.

2. Avery ME, Mead J. Surface properties in relation to atelectasis and hyaline membrane disease. *Am J Dis Child.* 1959;97:513–523.

3. Hulsey TC, Alexander GR, Robillary PY, et al: Hyaline membrane disease. The role of ethnicity and maternal risk factors. *Am J Obstet Gynecol.* 1993;168:572–576.

4. Dinwiddie RM. *Diagnosis and Management of Paediatric Respiratory Disease.* 2nd ed. New York: Churchill-Livingstone; 1997.

5. Aloan CA, Hill TV. *Respiratory Care of the Newborn and Child.* 2nd ed. Philadelphia: Lippincott; 1997.

6. Robbins C, Green R, Lasker M, et al. The lung of the premature infant: Pathophysiology of disease and newer therapies. *Mount Sinai J Med.* 1994; 61:416–423.

7. Poulain FR, Clements JA. Pulmonary surfactant therapy. *West J Med.* 1995;162:43–50.

8. Koff PB, et al. *Neonatal and Pediatric Respiratory Care.* 2nd ed. St Louis: Mosby; 1993.

9. Apgar V. A proposal for a new method of evaluation of the newborn infant. *Curr Res Anesth Analg.* 1953;32:260.

10. Kattwinkel J, et al. *Neonatal Resuscitation Textbook.* 4th ed. Elk Grove Village, IL: American Academy of Pediatrics; 2000:1–11.

11. Niermeyer S. Respiratory distress syndrome. In: *Pediatric Decision Making.* 3rd ed. St. Louis: Mosby; 1991.

12. Askins DF. *Acute Respiratory Care of the Neonate.* 2nd ed. Petaluma, Calif: NICU Ink Publishers; 1997.

13. Whitsett JA, Pryhuber GS, Rice WR, et al. Acute respiratory disorders. In: Avery GB, Fletcher MA, MacDonald MG, eds. *Neonatology: Pathophysiology and Management of the Newborn.* 4th ed. Philadelphia: Lippincott; 1994.

14. Jobe AH. Pulmonary surfactant therapy. *N Engl J Med.* 1993;328:861–868.

15. Hoekstra RE. Surfactants in the treatment and prevention of RDS. *Neonatal Resp Dis* (Tufts Univ School of Med) 1999;1–12

16. Whitaker K. *Comprehensive Perinatal and Neonatal Respiratory Care.* 2nd ed. Albany: Delmar; 1997.

17. Schwartz RM, Luby AM, et al. Effect of surfactant on morbidity, mortality, and resource use in newborn infants weighing 500 to 1500 g. *N Engl J Med.* 1994;330:1476–1480.

18. Neil N, Sullivan SD, Lessler DS. The economics of treatment for infants with respiratory distress syndrome. *Med Dec Making.* 1998;18:44–51.

INDEX

Note: Page numbers followed by *f* and *t* refer to figures and tables, respectively.